SOCIAL AN[D]
BEHAVIOURAL SC[IENCES]
FOR NURSES

SOCIAL AND BEHAVIOURAL SCIENCES FOR NURSES

PSYCHOLOGY, SOCIOLOGY AND COMMUNICATION FOR PROJECT 2000

Dr. N.H. Groenman | Dr. O.D'A. Slevin
M.A. Buckenham | J. van Dalen
N.P.J. Wetzels | R.J.J. Zewald

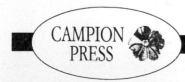
CAMPION PRESS

— *Campion Integrated Studies Series* —

British Library Cataloguing-in-Publication Data

302/GRO

Groenman, N. H.
Social and behavioural sciences for nurses,
I. Title II. Slevin, O. D'A. III. Buckenham, M. A.
300

ISBN 1-873732-03-1

Cover design:	Artisan Graphics, Edinburgh
Basic layout:	Studio Blanche, Noordwijk
Drawings:	Wim Hoogstraten, Leiden
	Ton Wollenberg, Utrecht
Cartoons:	Ivo Winnubst, Almere
Photographs:	University Hospital (AV-dienst), Maastricht / ANP, Amsterdam
	I. van Gelder, Wassenaar / Gemini Hospital, Den Helder
	Harper & Row, New York / Hollandse Hoogte, Amsterdam
	Queen Wilhelmina Fund, Amsterdam / D. Langeveld, Lisse / Leer, Amsterdam
	Van Loghum Slaterus, Deventer / L. Merks, Zaltbommel / NIPG, Leiden
	Harry Pelgrim, Heerewaarden / W. van der Putten, Oegstgeest
	Spaarnestad, Haarlem / Youth for Christ, Driebergen / A. Vermeulen, Den Helder
	B. de Wit, Oegstgeest

Acknowledgements: We are grateful to Blackwell Scientific Publications for permission to reproduce the tables on page 124, and to Hodder & Stoughton for permission to reproduce the extract on page 192.

Printed by Groen bv, Leiden, The Netherlands
Bound by Jansenbinders, Leiden, The Netherlands

First published 1992   ISBN   1-873732-03-1

© 1991 SMD EDUCATIONAL PUBLISHERS | LEIDEN | THE NETHERLANDS
Series co-ordination: J.R.M. Arets and J.P. Vaessen

© 1992 CAMPION PRESS LIMITED
384 Lanark Road
Edinburgh   EH13 0LX

Preface

Social and Behavioural Sciences for Nurses is a psychology, social sciences and social skills textbook for health care students. It is one of the texts in the Campion Integrated Studies series in which patients and clients are regarded as independent individuals with an active input into their own treatment; their subjective needs are the starting point for care.

In common with the other titles in the series, Social and Behavioural Sciences for Nurses is presented in modular format with clearly defined learning outcomes for each chapter and assignments throughout the book to encourage independent study. The theoretical aspects of the subject areas are demonstrated and made relevant by numerous practical case studies, and questions for self-testing are included at the end of each module.

In the United Kingdom, as elsewhere in Europe, nursing is undergoing major changes to enable it to meet the demands for health care as we approach the 21st century. The new Project 2000 qualifying nurse education in the United Kingdom is directed towards preparing the student for a new role of 'knowledgeable doer'. That is, a practitioner who is: orientated toward health promotion and health education as well as care of the ill and disabled; capable of meeting the needs of patients or clients in ever-changing circumstances, in hospital or community settings; educated rather than trained, with practice founded on a sound knowledge base and a capacity to approach nursing problems in a critical and reflective manner. The new nursing will be informed by a broad range of scientific, philosophical and humanities-based disciplines.

This book addresses the social and behavioural sciences which will contribute to a deeper understanding of the process of nursing. It will be particularly useful for Project 2000 students during their common foundation studies where consideration is given to adult (including the elderly), children's, mental health and mental handicap nursing. The text addresses development across the life span and includes chapters on mental health, learning difficulties and somatic-medical psychology. Sociological perspectives are covered comprehensively with chapters devoted to health and illness and to the interpersonal skills relevant to nursing. With its detailed coverage of psychological and social sciences the book can be used as a course reader for the full three-year course leading to registration as a nurse.

The book will also make a contribution to post-qualifying education and development, as the nurse proceeds to proficiency in primary practice and subsequently to more advanced practitioner roles. Those involved in other caring professions such as physiotherapy, occupational therapy, speech therapy and social work will also find the book of great value. The authors consider that many medical and (university) nursing students will also benefit from the book's contents.

Psychologists and social scientists are far from unanimous in answering the question, 'What is the best scientific approach?', when considering individual or social behaviour. Atkinson et al. (1987) state, 'There is no "right" or "wrong" approach to the study of psychology. Most psychologists take an eclectic viewpoint, using a synthesis of several approaches to explain psychological phenomena.' The authors are aware of this problem. They view psychology and sociology as empirical sciences and have consciously avoided 'preaching' a particular orientation as the only true approach. Against this background, they have attempted to do proper justice to those modern psychological and sociological developments which have had significant application to the integrated approach in patient and client care.

Module 1 comprises a review of the psychological field. The social role of the psychologist is examined, as is behavioural methodology in general. This general survey is followed by a more detailed discussion of five important psychological approaches: neurobiological, behavioural, cognitive, psychoanalytic and humanistic.

Module 2 addresses the discipline of developmental psychology. It is not assumed in this module that human development comes to a halt when 'adulthood' is reached. Consequently, a good deal of attention is paid to the development of the adult and to that of the older person. Physical, socio-emotional and cognitive development, together with their interrelationships, are discussed systematically for each perceived stage of the individual's life.

Module 3 approaches human behaviour in its social context, drawing on the contributions from the disciplines of sociology and social psychology. The individual is presented as a social being, functioning through the social relationships and social links of which he is part. This module also includes a chapter on illness as a social phenomenon. Questions like: 'When are you ill?' and 'Who decides whether or not you are ill?' are discussed here. A final chapter in this module addresses the issues of family, community and the elderly in society.

Module 4 looks at psychology related to health. Illness is presented as both a stressor and a reaction to stress. An explanatory model is provided in order to give a better understanding of the many different individual reactions to ill-

ness. The consequences of these upon nursing care are also presented, highlighting the links with the material studied in Module 5. The psychological aspects of so-called functional complaints like stress headaches and lower back pain are examined as are the psychology of psychiatry and the area of learning difficulty. A chapter which looks at psychological treatment and counselling is also included. Examples are used to illustrate how patients contending with emotional problems can be supported through their illness.

Module 5 relates to the theory and practice of social skills in the professional nursing situation. The authors define social skills as a special type of 'nursing procedure'. These are skills which, like other nursing techniques are mastered through the acquisition, rehearsal and practical application of knowledge. Various conversational modes are discussed. The use of social skills in therapeutic interventions and the nature and importance of the nurse-patient relationship are addressed.

Cooperation within a group context and the chairing of meetings are examined theoretically, alternating with exercises which can be carried out individually or in groups. Nurses – particularly senior ones – have to negotiate with other health service staff during policy meetings. How should nurses prepare for and act du-ring negotiations of this nature? The module is rounded off with a discussion of the negotiating process and the management of conflict.

For convenience the authors refer to the nurse throughout in the female gender. Patients are referred to in the male gender unless this is obviously inappropriate. In the module on developmental psychology, children are both male and female. No bias towards either sex is intended.

We wish to thank the following for allowing their photographs to be used in this book:
- staff and patients at Leighton Hospital, Mid Cheshire Hospitals Trust;
- staff and students of the Cheshire College of Health Care Studies;

- management and staff of Macclesfield District Psychology Service, Macclesfield Health Authority;
- Women's Voluntary Service, Leighton Hospital.

The authors welcome any critical comments on their work.

Spring 1992   Dr. N.H. Groenman
                     Dr. O.D'A. Slevin
                     M.A. Buckenham
                     J. van Dalen
                     N.P.J. Wetzels
                     R.J.J. Zewald

Contents

Module 1

PSYCHOLOGY: A GENERAL INTRODUCTION

Introduction to Module 1

Since the 1960s interest in human behaviour has grown enormously in the industrialized countries. In broad social terms, the importance of the so-called social sciences has been recognized, as a result of which, more and more psychologists, sociologists, welfare and social workers have been employed in the health and welfare sectors.

This module will focus explicitly upon the role of the psychologist. The first chapter will examine the different aspects of psychology in general, and the different types of psychologist will also be discussed:
– occupational psychologist;
– child psychologist;
– educational psychologist;
– experimental psychologist;
– clinical psychologist.

It is primarily the clinical psychologist whom nursing staff will encounter on a regular basis during their day-to-day work. This is due not least to the fact that medical psychology (which we will look at in Module 4) is a specific field of clinical psychology.

It is no longer acceptable that patients in health care institutions should be treated without due attention being paid to the impact of being ill upon human behaviour and communication. This explains the key role played by the psychologist, whose work relates to the origins and development of human behaviour. The welfare aspects of care have also increased in importance as far as nursing care is concerned, which is why some knowledge of psychology is a vital part of modern nursing.

Psychology offers a number of different ways of explaining reality, which means that behaviour can be explained in more than one way. When talking about psychology, therefore, we refer to 'schools', 'theories' or 'systems'.

In Chapter 2 of this module, we will look at five schools, namely:
– neurobiological;
– behavioural;
– cognitive;
– psychoanalytical;
– humanistic (phenomenological).

The leading representatives of each approach are discussed in this module, together with their theories. A brief description of the impact of the treatment upon the patient is also provided. It is not, however, the aim of this book to come down in favour of any one of the schools of psychology which are described here.

1

Psychology

1. Introduction

Psychology has much to offer nurses and other health care professionals in their understanding of, and dealings with people. Within the sphere of the nurse's role will be encountered psychologists whose importance in the treatment of patients rests on their greater understanding of this area of knowledge.

In the first section of this chapter, the different roles which psychologists can play will be examined in more detail.

It is not only the psychologist, of course, who is involved in the study of human behaviour. Other disciplines also make a contribution, including psychiatry, sociology and education.

The second section describes the different types of psychologist, with particular attention paid to the clinical psychologist.

The final section concentrates upon the different aspects of psychology as a science.

Learning outcomes

After studying this chapter the student should be able to:
– define and explain what is meant by psychology;
– describe the place and significance of psychology with respect to psychiatry and sociology;
– define the working area of at least three types of psychologist, including the clinical psychologist;
– define and explain what is meant by medical psychology;
– define the following:
  • the concept of science;
  • four characteristics of a theory;
  • the scientific method.

2. Psychology; a brief survey of the field

Study activity
1. Try to define as accurately as possible what psychologists do.

Psychologists are concerned with many different questions, both personal and social. They seek to answer questions like:
– How does one bring up a child to be a stable and happy personality?
– How can mental illness be avoided?

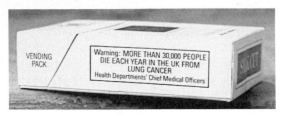

Figure 1.1.1

- In what way does stress influence the incidence of physical complaints?

These are general questions, but psychologists are also called upon to advise on more specific matters. Examples include:
- What is the best method for helping this patient conquer his nicotine addiction?
- How should the different instruments on the dashboard of a car be set out in order to ensure that the likelihood of errors of judgement, particularly at crucial moments, is as small as possible?
- How do you make an effective television advert?
- How do you formulate a study programme for a child with learning difficulties?
- What is the best way to prepare a patient for an operation?

Looking at this list of examples – which is far from exhaustive – you will realize that it is no simple task to define what psychology is. In general terms, psychologists are concerned with what people think, feel and want, and with how to deal with them. There are also psychologists, however, who are interested in the behaviour of apes, or of pigeons and rats.

Psychology translates literally as 'the science of the soul', although it is no longer defined in those terms. Modern psychologists would say that they record and interpret 'expressions of people's behaviour', thus defining psychology as 'the science of human behaviour'. We then have to state what we mean by expressions of human behaviour. Behaviour comprises all of the activities which can be observed and recorded, such as walking, talking, problem-solving, nursing someone and suffering pain. Everything we know about one another is picked up from our perception of each other's behaviour. Psychology seeks to identify behavioural laws on the basis of our behaviour, the different ways in which we express ourselves, and how we communicate something of ourselves to others.

In order to discover laws of behaviour, it is necessary to build up an understanding of the factors which cause and influence behaviour. Behaviour is influenced by strictly physical factors: someone with a broken leg cannot run, someone who is seriously ill does not (usually) feel alert and happy.
Environmental factors also influence our behaviour: you behave differently at a Christmas party on a hospital ward compared with a similar party at home.
A long-term environmental factor is the manner of a person's upbringing. It makes a world of difference if you were taken seriously and valued during your childhood and teenage years, or if you were treated as worthless and as a burden.
Hereditary factors also play a role. We know that there are strong arguments for assuming that intelligence, for instance, is partially determined by hereditary factors.
You might, by now, have gained the impression that only external factors go towards determining behaviour: in fact, nothing could be further from the truth. We are, of course, able to reason for ourselves – we consult our own feelings and we then decide what line of behaviour to pursue.

As indicated earlier, psychology used to be defined as the study of the soul (or of the mind). 'Soul' or 'mind' are ways of referring to thoughts and the processes of the human will. People viewed the soul and/or mind as the cause of behaviour. We have already seen that this view is incorrect: social circumstances and the past development of the individual also have an enormous impact upon behaviour.

The mind can only be 'directly' studied in one way, through the self-observation method (or, to use a fancier term, introspection): that is to say, by allowing the person to investigate for himself what is going on inside him. This can yield useful information.

Study activity

2. Give at least three examples of introspection on the basis of your own experiences.

In scientific terms introspection is an unreliable method because it is not possible to check the answers given by the individual questioned. Even when the person answers in good faith, he cannot state accurately in what order his thoughts are strung together. The aim of science is to make universally applicable statements which can be proved or refuted. Consequently, there is an important tendency in the field of psychology which argues that the introspective method may not be used. Supporters of this view state that in place of self-observation (introspection) the psychologist should only use the observation method. This method is based upon the expression of feelings, thoughts and decisions. An example of such expression is as follows: the patient cries and says he is sad. The fact that the patient is crying and saying he is sad can be observed by more than one person. Therefore, it is possible to check observations.

Incidentally, more and more psychologists are objecting to the 'science of (human) behaviour' tag. The protesters acknowledge that self-observation is an inferior scientific method to that of observation, but many feel that it is going too far to conclude that feelings, thoughts, etc. – in short, the mental processes – cannot be studied. Psychologists are not just interested in behaviour for its own sake, but also for what it reveals about the subject's feelings, thoughts and hence their mental processes. Therefore, the most common definition of psychology is: 'the science of (human) behaviour and the mental processes'.

You will have noticed that we keep placing the word 'human' in brackets before the word 'behaviour'. Psychologists who are only interested in behavioural processes can also study the behaviour of animals.

At the beginning of this chapter we said that the (clinical) psychologist might be asked for an answer to the question, 'What is the best way of helping a patient (Mr. Smith) to give up smoking?' The answer will rarely be one hundred percent correct, because it is based upon knowledge of a 'general' nature. The (clinical) psychologist knows how an anti-smoking therapy programme ought generally to be implemented in the case of a patient like Mr. Smith. That is not to say that the psychologist can control Mr. Smith as if he were a puppet on a string, but neither is there any reason to expect that Mr. Smith will react differently to the same therapy programme which has already been used with other patients.

People sometimes think that a psychologist has X-ray eyes – that he has the power to look straight through other people and to see precisely what motivates them. That is not true, of course. Instead, the psychologist has learned to study people's behaviour and to use his knowledge to draw certain conclusions from this.

The psychologist does not control the patient like a puppet on a string

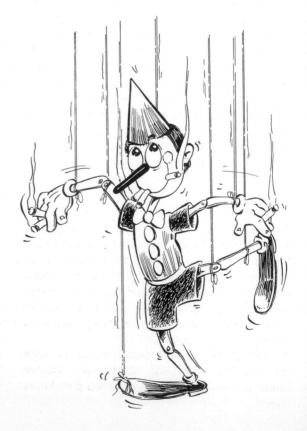

There are other disciplines apart from psychology which relate to human behaviour. The most obvious example is *psychiatry*. Psychiatry and psychology are sometimes confused. A psychiatrist is a doctor – a specialist physician. He has studied medicine. Consequently, the psychiatrist knows the biological basis of human behaviour. In addition, during his period of specialization, he will also have picked up a good deal of psychological know-how. This knowledge is concerned in particular with aspects of abnormal human behaviour.

Psychology is an autonomous academic discipline, comprising a thorough study of the origin and subsequent development of human behaviour. Psychologists also engage systematically in the study of human behaviour as manifested under extreme circumstances– during a (serious) illness, for example. The clinical psychologist and the psychiatrist have a large area in common, formed by their knowledge of abnormal behaviour and by psychotherapy. Psychotherapy is an area common to both, in that it relates to treatment methods for various forms of behavioural disorder which are purely psychological in character. Abnormal behaviour is another common area, even though this might be viewed from differing standpoints: from the point of view of medical psychopathology (psychiatry) on the one hand, and as a behaviour disorder (clinical psychology) on the other. There is a danger that psychiatry is becoming too concerned with the psychological aspects of abnormal behaviour and not sufficiently so with its biological determinants.

A second example is *sociology*. Sociologists are concerned with the study of groups of people and with the relationships which exist between these groups. An example of a question which a sociologist might be asked is: 'How, in general terms, do doctors give instructions to nursing staff?' Sociologists also study social processes. An example of this is: 'Why do many nurses not belong to a trade union?'
Psychologists are concerned primarily with the individual person: 'Why does Doctor Baker always make snide comments to Sister Hart?'

Study activity
3. Illustrate the position occupied by psychology compared to psychiatry and sociology using practical examples.

3. What is a psychologist?

The title 'Psychologist' is safeguarded in many countries. In Great Britain it is the title 'Chartered Psychologist' which is protected. Not just anyone can call themselves a chartered psychologist. Only someone who has successfully fulfilled the criteria of the British Psychological Society can use this title. Within the field of psychology itself there are a number of schools, and psychologists work in extremely diverse fields.
Types of psychologist include: occupational psychologist, child psychologist, educational psychologist, experimental psychologist and clinical psychologist. The working area of the clinical psychologist has already been mentioned in the previous section.

An *occupational psychologist* works in a company or any other organization which manufactures goods or provides services. His job within a company includes personnel selection, ergonomic research (adjusting the working situation to the people who work within it), answering questions regarding the welfare of employees, and so on. The occupational psychologist studies the many aspects which can be identified in the relationship between the employee and his company, and seeks to harmonize these to as great an extent as possible.

A *child psychologist* is concerned with the development of the individual from child to adult; this relates predominantly to the study of intelligence, language and personality. In schools, for instance, he will work with children with learning and educational problems. His concern may mainly be with children who have learning difficulties or who have emotional problems. The work comprises both treatment and guidance on the one hand, and prevention on the other.

Educational psychologists are interested in the

way teaching methods influence the learning process. They are also involved in research into such things as the influence of personality and socio-economic factors upon learning. Educational psychologists are also concerned with the best way of testing knowledge, and they help develop school progress tests. They also contribute to the development of educational goals. Their work is concerned not only with individual pupils, but also with the planning of the general educational process.

The *experimental psychologist* is occupied primarily with research. In most cases this is fundamental research carried out in the laboratory (figure 1.1.2). Such research may concern the motor system, observation, the functioning of the brain, etc.

The *clinical psychologist* is the type of psychologist whom nursing staff will encounter in their professional work. He is concerned with individuals who are in need of assistance. To put it more precisely: the clinical psychologist is interested in behaviour which is viewed by the individual himself or by those around him as undesirable.

Examples of behaviour which are experienced as undesirable by the actual patient may be expressed as follows:
- 'I feel so sad.'
- 'I always feel hunted.'
- 'I'm so frightened on the street.'
- 'My wife wants to divorce me.'
- 'My son hits me.'
- 'Things aren't working out any more on the sex front.'

The clinical psychologist seeks ways of changing the problem behaviour. Alternatively, he can also try to alter the way in which this behaviour is experienced. In cases of this nature it is generally a question of acceptance problems. An example of this is homosexuality. A few years ago, it was felt necessary to 'cure' homosexuality, whereas now the objective is to help

Figure 1.1.2
The 'fine motor system' is studied in the psychological laboratory

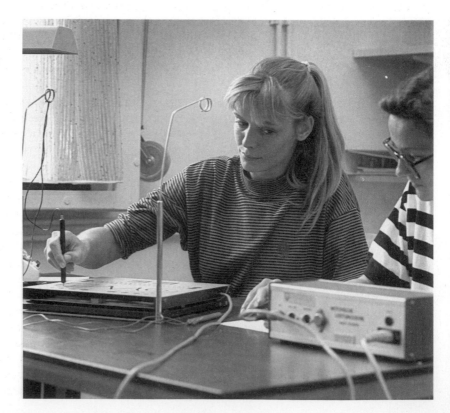

the individual to come to terms with it. Although the clinical psychologist is generally concerned with an individual with problems, it is often necessary to use the person's relationships (in the family, with his or her partner) in solving those problems.

Many clinical psychologists also work psycho-therapeutically, treating people's behavioural or emotional problems. The clinical psychologist is viewed as a specialist in a precise psychological field. In most countries, an Institute of Psychologists keeps a Register of Clinical Psychologists. In order to be included in this register, the psychologist has to work under supervision for four years after passing his master's examination in psychology. Several years of further training are then required before he can work as a psychologist. There are various forms of psychotherapy, which have grown out of the different schools of psychology. The oldest form is psychoanalysis, while a more recent version is behavioural therapy. Clinical psychology has interfaces with many forms of health care. Some clinical psychologists have set up independently, but most are attached to institutions like hospitals, psychiatric clinics and convalescent homes. Most hospitals have a clinical psychology department.

Study activity
4. Describe the difference between the psychological welfare aspects of nursing care and the treatment provided by the clinical psychologist.

A recent development in the field of clinical psychology is the heightened attention which has been paid to occupational psychology. Questions such as unemployment, disability, early retirement and preparation for retirement are demanding ever more attention. The occupational psychologist has, for instance, been teaching individual employees to cope better with stress in the workplace. The clinical psychologist can organize courses which are geared towards the prevention of back complaints: the company's profit can be increased by a clear reduction in the amount of working time lost through illness.

A specific component of clinical psychology is *medical psychology*. Medical psychology consists of the application of clinical psychology in the somatic-medical, psychiatric and learning difficulties situations. Medical psychologists in the somatic area are concerned with the emotional problems associated with physical suffering. An example of this is the grief felt by a patient with an incurable illness. They are also occupied with physical conditions which relate to psychological conflicts and stress. Examples of this are conditions like gastro-intestinal complaints or post-coronary syndrome. So-called functional complaints also belong to the working field of the medical psychologist. Functional complaints relate to physical experiences on the part of the patient for which the doctor cannot provide an explanation. Examples include various forms of headache and lower back pain. The medical psychologist is also interested in the manner in which the doctor and the nurse talk to the patient. The nature of the relationship between doctor and patient is important, as this has been shown to influence the incidence, persistence, cure and prevention of physical conditions.

This book will pay particular attention to the work of clinical psychologists who are active in the medical situation. We will, therefore, be returning to the examples referred to above.

Finally, a comment on the relationship between psychology and everyday knowledge. We all build up knowledge of our fellow humans, so why is psychology necessary – after all, don't we all live together as people? Psychology may be presented as an objective form of everyday human knowledge which has been expressed in words and can hence be transferred. Everyday knowledge is usually implicit: 'It's hard to put into words, it's just the way I feel.' Answers like this are not enough for the psychologist. The interpretation of general human knowledge is also highly subject to the mood the questioner happens to be in at the time, his prejudices and errors in his thinking. The psychologist has special know-how and techniques for ensuring that the patient does not fall victim to such arbitrary circumstances. As an experienced scientist, he seeks to arrive at objective knowledge and to cancel out the influence of subjectivity to as great an extent as possible.

4. Psychology as a science

a. Science

A dictionary definition of science might be given as: 'A systematically ordered body of knowledge'. If we wish to qualify a particular field of study as 'science', that knowledge has to meet a number of criteria. These are: truth, objectivity, intersubjectivity and rationality.

As far as *truth* is concerned, scientific knowledge is not something which can be viewed as absolutely true under all circumstances. Knowledge is the interpretation of the interconnection between established facts. When new facts arise, we are sometimes obliged to alter our interpretation of the connection between facts which were already known.

In seeking the truth, the scientist tries to be as *objective* as possible. That is to say, he will attempt to keep the influence of his own subjective observation to as limited a degree as possible. In so doing, he acknowledges that strict objectivity is not possible. A person, that is the scientist making a subjective judgement, is always needed in order to observe the actual occurrences.

Strictly speaking, therefore, objectivity means striving to achieve maximum *intersubjectivity*. That is to say that in gathering knowledge, the scientist will use methods whose reliability has been acknowledged by (as far as possible) other scientists. Agreement is then seen to exist between different people, with their own subjective interpretations, regarding a particulare method.

The rules by which a scientist ought to abide in collecting facts and interpreting the connections between those facts are strictly *rational*. They arise through logical reasoning. The simple collection of facts does not complete the scientific researcher's task. He also has to indicate *why* these facts occur. In other words, he has to explain the established facts. 'Explain' means that he describes the relationship between the

actual occurrences. The accuracy of the description is demonstrated if, on the basis of the provided explanation, the reoccurrence of the facts can be predicted. Perhaps it will now be apparent why the truth of scientific theories can *never* be absolute. Theories are replaced in the course of time by different, better theories.

b. Characteristics of a theory

Science is not just a collection of unconnected statements about factual reality. Scientific practitioners seek to achieve a systematic approach in their knowledge. They systematically order their statements regarding the connections between actual occurrences, with the result being known as a 'theory'. Therefore, a theory is a rationally derived proposition regarding the connections between actual occurrences. The methods used in formulating a theory have been mutually agreed by scientists. The accuracy of a theoretical statement is tested by means of prediction.

A theory is subject to a number of requirements:
- *Logical consistency*. This means that the theory must not contain any propositions which contradict one another.
- *Testability*. A theory must give rise to propositions which can be supported or refuted by means of empirical data. To put it more briefly, the theory must allow actual occurrences to be predicted.
- *Simplicity* (Parsimony). If several theories exist in a particular field, preference will be given to the most simple. The 'simplicity' of a theory means that as few concepts as possible are required in order to explain the phenomena. These concepts should themselves also be as uncomplicated as possible.
- *Compatibility*. If several theories are available, preference will be given to the one which is most compatible with other theories.

c. The scientific method

The empirical cycle was described by the Dutch scientist de Groot (1961) and scientific research can proceed in accordance with this cycle. 'Empirical' is: taking experience as the source of knowledge. 'Experience' is: observing facts. 'Knowledge' is: interpreting the connections between those facts. As we have already stated, knowledge is an interpretation of the interconnections between established facts.

The empirical cycle described by de Groot consists of five stages:

- *Observation*: the collection and grouping of facts.
- *Induction*: the postulation of connections between the facts. These postulated connections are known as hypotheses.
- *Deduction*: the derivation of particular consequences from these hypotheses. These take the form of predictions which can be tested.
- *Testing the hypotheses*. This is subject to a number of requirements. Testing must occur in such a way that the same results can, in principle, be obtained by different researchers. This can be achieved by standardizing the research situation.
- *Evaluation of the results of the test*. Was the prediction correct? The extent to which the prediction comes true has a further impact upon the theory.

d. Empirical cycle and the nursing process

De Groot's empirical cycle for scientific research is very similar to the different stages of the nursing process. The nursing process is a problem-oriented approach based on a problem-solving technique (Open University, 1984). Whilst the nursing process is conceived as having four steps, namely assessment, planning, implementation and evaluation (Marriner, 1975), the empirical cycle and the nursing process can be represented as follows:

Empirical cycle	Nursing process
1. Observation	1. Assessment (Observation)
2. Induction: hypothesis	2. Planning; to include:
3. Deduction: realization	3. formulation of nursing goals
4. Testing	4. Implementation
5. Evaluation	5. Evaluation

Observation is the first stage in both cycles. This is followed by the formulation of hypotheses, or planning. Planning also takes in the third stage of the empirical cycle, namely the realization of the hypotheses through the establishment of nursing goals. This is followed by implementation (the testing of the hypotheses), with the extra step in the nursing process of generalization/stabilization. Both cycles then finish with the evaluation of the process as a whole.

e. Scientific research and psychology

The objective of psychology as a science is to acquire knowledge of actual behaviour patterns, that is, of behaviour. Behaviour acts as an indicator of mental processes. A number of research methods exist within the field of psychology. We will look at several of these.

Basic experimental research takes place in the laboratory, under strictly controlled conditions. Laboratory conditions are most suited for determining the influence of a single factor, or variable as it is termed, upon whatever is being studied. This type of research, and the manner in which it is carried out, is very similar to the kind of research done in the physics laboratory, for instance. Research into the senses (proprioception, sight, hearing, taste, feeling and smell)

Nursing research 'in the field'

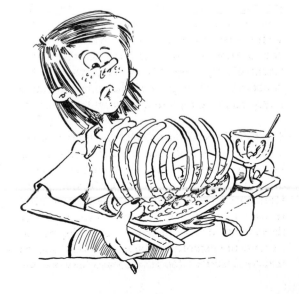

generally occurs under conditions of this type. A perfume manufacturer might, for instance, ask whether the addition of a particular substance will make a perfume more attractive.

Research also occurs 'in the field'. This refers to the careful observation of animals or humans in their natural environment. This method of research has been used in the following study. The natural environment was a hospital ward with six beds. The researcher was studying the extent to which disturbances during the serving of the daily hot meal had an influence upon the 'eating behaviour' of the patients on the ward. Disturbances were taken to include the appearance on the ward of a doctor, nurse, dietician, etc., while the patients were eating their main meal. The researcher noted the portions which were brought into the ward and then weighed the amount of leftover food. She also noted the number of times the ward was entered during the meal-time by a third party. In the case of patients who were not feeling well, such disturbances had a marked effect – the patient stopped eating the meal. In general terms, however, she was able to conclude that actual food intake was barely affected by disturbances, although there were individual differences between patients. (Deutekom, Philipsen and Ten Hoor, 1991).

A commonly applied method of psychological research is the use of questionnaires. This method allows particular details of larger groups of people to be collected. This method is used in order to study the political preferences of the general public, during elections, for instance. Market research into such things as the use of a particular brand of margarine is another example of this kind of study. It is more difficult than many people think to draw up the type of questionnaire required for such studies. One problem is that the questions must not be suggestive; therefore, a question like 'Sunrise cooking oil splashes a lot less when frying than Goldtex, doesn't it?' would not be acceptable. When applying the questionnaire method, trained interviewers use a pretested questionnaire. The questions have to be answered by a representative group of people comprising individuals from the population group to be studied.

The best-known research instrument of the psychologist is the psychological test. Tests can be used to collect important data in a relatively simple way, regarding for example interests, attitudes and achievements. There are intelligence tests, personality tests, career choice tests, school progress tests, and so on. The characteristic of a test is that two scores are always compared, that of the person being studied and that of (part of) a population group. The latter is generally an average score. An intelligence quotient, for instance, is always a comparison between the individual score and the average score of the rest of the population. This principle of comparison also applies to research into personality traits. If you want to determine how neurotic someone is by using a test for neurotic behaviour, you compare that individual's score with the average score of the population.

The carrying out of research can give rise to ethical problems. The question is to what extent you are justified in using people as test subjects for purposes of research. Participation in research should occur on a voluntary basis and with the informed consent of the individual. If the nature of the research makes it impossible to inform the subject fully about what is going to happen, this should be done as soon as possible afterwards. The privacy of the participating individual must not be violated. Psychologists' organizations have formulated strict rules in this regard.

Hospitals usually have a Medical Ethics Committee. The ethical character of every piece of research undertaken in the hospital has to be examined and approved in advance by this committee. Under no circumstances may patients be used as test subjects in a study without their knowing it and without having given their permission.

Some psychologists use test animals in order to study processes which are deemed to be fundamental to numerous animal species and humans. This type of research is also subject to rules, in order to prevent animals being used unnecessarily for experimental purposes, and to ensure that the test animals are properly treated.

5. Summary

Psychology is a science with a wide range of methods and techniques.
The scientific method, as defined by De Groot, is very similar to the individual stages of the nursing process.

The different types of psychologists were identified and the following were examined in particular in this chapter:
– the clinical psychologist;
– the medical psychologist.

This attention is justified, because the clinical psychologist forms part of the multi-disciplinary health care team.
Clearly, medical psychology is a vital area for the working practice of the nurse.

2

Movements in psychology

1. Introduction

As yet, psychology as a science has not come up with a single all-embracing theory. In other words, we do not yet have one single theory which can explain and predict psychological reality in its entirety.

There have been five main movements in the development of psychology as a science:
– neurobiological;
– behavioural;
– cognitive;
– psychoanalytical;
– humanistic (phenomenological).

Each psychological movement or school, trend or approach, has its own point of view from which it addresses the study of reality. Each psychological movement also has its own research methods and methodology of treatment.

The five schools of psychology referred to above will be discussed in this chapter. The key representatives of each approach will be introduced, and their theories will be explained. Finally, the impact of each approach upon patient treatment will be briefly examined.

Learning outcomes

After studying this chapter, the student should be able to:
– provide a general description and comparison of five psychological movements;
– describe and explain the following aspects of the five psychological movements:
  • the most important research methods;
  • the key representatives;
  • the treatment approach.

2. Movements in psychology; a global orientation

Behaviour can be explained in a variety of ways, and the different explanations can often all be correct simultaneously.

For example: you see someone in a restaurant sitting comfortably and relaxed smoking a cigarette after his meal. How would you explain this behaviour? Several explanations are possible:

– The nicotine level in the person's 'internal environment' has dropped during the meal. Consequently, he feels compelled to raise his nicotine level once again.
– The end of the meal acts as a stimulus for which the response is smoking. This is a stimulus-response relationship, in other words, a learned habit.
– The entire group in the restaurant lights up cigarettes. He does not wish to break the pattern (or: he doesn't wish to feel left out) and so he lights up too.

There are a number of (often highly divergent) approaches in psychology, also referred to as explanatory systems or theories. Each of these approaches uses its own set of concepts and its own form of therapy. There is no such thing as *the* theory of psychology.

Atkinson et al. (1987) put it thus: 'Put another way, all of these approaches have something important to say about human nature, and few psychologists would insist that only one of them contained the whole truth'.

It cannot be stated that any one of the approaches is correct, and that the others are wrong. Each approach has its advantages and drawbacks. The following approaches are usually distinguished: the neurobiological, the behavioural, the cognitive, the psychoanalytical and the humanistic approach. In its own way, each approach ultimately leads to the same goal: a better understanding of people's behaviour. Which approach is favoured at a given time depends upon a number of purely practical and pragmatic factors. The most important of these is the type of problem for which help is sought. A phobia (a serious anxiety syndrome), for instance, can be dealt with more rapidly and easily using the behavioural approach than by using the humanistic. Other factors, however, certainly play a part as well, including the university where the psychologist in question studied, his personal preference and expertise, and also the preference of the team to which the psychologist belongs. If he works within a team (a treatment team on a psychiatric ward for instance) which is used to psychoanalytical explanations, he will tend to go along with that approach.

Every study topic within the field of psychology can be approached from a number of different viewpoints.

Smoking has been cited as an example.

A second example is the study of *aggression*. Psychologists from the five movements listed above accentuate different aspects of aggression. Consequently, if the aggression is seen as a problem, each will opt for a different form of treatment.

A physiological psychologist taking the neurobiological approach will be interested in the mechanisms in the brain which are responsible for the incidence of aggression. He will argue that these brain mechanisms should be influenced, through the administration of a medication, for instance. This approach is found in biological psychology.

A psychologist who follows the behavioural approach will study the learning experiences which have resulted in a person behaving aggressively. He will state that the person in question has learned that aggression seemingly pays. His therapy will be aimed at depriving aggression of its rewarding character. A good example of this is a child's temper tantrum.

A cognitive psychologist will try to discover how people interpret particular occurrences which make them angry. Such a psychologist will investigate why it is that this person thinks that every time someone bumps into him, it was done deliberately and with malicious intent.

The psychologist taking the psychoanalytical approach will try to find out what earlier experiences have influenced control of aggression. He will ask how this person was treated during his early childhood years, by whom, and what stood in his way to such an extent that he now goes into an uncontrollable rage at the least provocation.

The humanistic psychologist, finally, will focus upon those aspects of society which promote aggression by blocking the individual's needs. This psychologist asks what is wrong with the current situation which makes the person in question feel so boxed-in. The answer could lie in a bad marriage, problems at work, or similar factors.

Each approach will lead to a different way of tackling the problem of aggression. The neuropsychologist seeks a cure which will inhibit aggression.

The behavioural psychologist tries to change the person's direct, everyday environment.

The cognitive psychologist tries to teach the person to interpret the situation differently.

The psychoanalytical psychologist tries to determine which childhood experiences are influencing the person in his aggression problem.

The humanistic psychologist emphasizes the creation of a situation from which the person can develop, ceasing to be aggressive in the process.

These approaches do not rule one another out. Each can make a valuable contribution to the understanding of human behaviour, and the treatment of disruptions in that behaviour.

Study activity

1. On the basis of this general orientation, try to indicate which psychological movement has the greatest appeal for you.

3. The neurobiological approach

The case of Diane

Diane is now forty-five years old, and has suffered in the past year from bouts of depression which have been growing in intensity.

According to Diane, it began gradually. In the beginning she felt tired and listless. As the months passed her listlessness and dissatisfaction with her situation grew. She didn't feel like doing anything. She became indifferent to more and more things – even her friends.

She feels literally nothing for her husband who left her two years ago to live abroad with a young woman. She has no children, nor any will to live. The compulsion to die is in the centre of her mind. She feels that death would get her out of the swamp into which she is sinking ever deeper.

The neurobiological approach is based on the assumption that processes in the brain and nervous system have an important impact upon human behaviour. Behaviour, from blinking to much more complex forms of behaviour like

Figure 1.2.1
Drive on or stop?

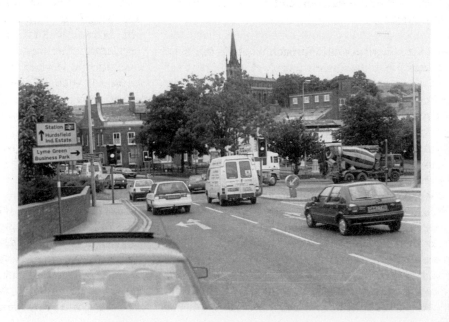

driving a car or solving a mathematical sum, depends upon physical processes, more specifically those in the brain and in the central nervous system. For example: you are driving a car and you have to stop for an amber light which is about to change to red (figure 1.2.1). First of all, you have to receive the amber light image on the retina of your eye. Your eye then sends a signal to your brain, where the signal is processed. The memory recognizes the amber light as a signal that you have to stop. A number of processes now occur in your brain's cortical areas: can I stop, given the speed at which I'm travelling, can I make it through, and are there any police about? A signal is then sent by the brain to the muscles of your leg and foot. We assume that the signal in question means 'stop'. The brain has to know where your foot is, and then tell it where to move to, namely the brake-pedal. At the same time, your eyes monitor whether the car is actually stopping, and any necessary corrections are made, once again via processes in your brain. Stopping for a red light appears to be an automatic reflex, but in order for this to occur, a number of different messages have to be sent to and from the brain. If something goes wrong with these messages (in the eye, in the connections with the brain, in the memory, in the cortical areas where decisions appear to be made, in the connection to the foot or in the foot itself) that behaviour can no longer be implemented.

Psychologists who approach the study of human behaviour from the neurobiological point of view are called neuropsychologists. These psychologists are involved in research into the functioning of the nervous system, and more specifically the central part, namely the brain. In general terms, the research method used in neuropsychology is based on the following principle. A particular human function, speech for instance, is controlled by a particular part of the brain. If part of the brain is damaged or destroyed, no new brain cells are created. Consequently, the destruction of part of the brain means that a particular human function is lost. This explanation appears to coincide with reality in the case of patients with speech problems following a brain haemorrhage. The neurobiological approach would have made even more progress than it already has if that were the end of the story. It appears, however, that adjoining parts of the brain can take over the lost function, (plasticity) although sometimes only partially. The brain can, as it were, compensate for the loss. This ability to compensate is much greater in children than in adults.

Working on the principle that there is a close relationship between a specific location in the brain and a form of behaviour, a variety of methods have been developed for testing this relationship. We will list a number of these.

Studying the evolution of the brain
This is done by comparing the human brain with that of animal species which are close to humans in evolutionary terms (apes, for instance) or by comparing the development of the brain in an animal and a human embryo. This kind of research provides information regarding the function of different areas of the brain, and how this function develops over time, that is, during evolution and during the life of a human.

Studying illness or brain damage
Certain illnesses, a tumour for instance, can attack particular areas of the brain. Injuries such as a gunshot wound or a head wound resulting from a car accident can also damage the brain. By studying the behaviour of the patient (i.e. symptoms of the illness process), it is possible to discover the function for which the damaged area of the brain is customarily responsible. If a person who has suffered damage to a particular part of his brain is transformed from an easy-going individual into someone easily provoked to anger, the damaged area is likely to be involved with regulating aggression.

Studying brain degeneration
If a particular area of the brain has been destroyed, the nerves linked to that area will wither away. It is possible to study the development of such nerves using a microscope. This provides information regarding the connections between different parts of the brain.

Study by stimulation
The stimulation of a particular area of the brain using weak electrical currents has an effect upon behaviour. Patients are sometimes asked during a brain operation to report what experiences they have during the stimulation of different areas of the brain. Sometimes they feel something in their body, or suddenly recall a particular memory. Studies of this kind carried out on animals like rats and apes include the permanent implantation of electrodes into the brain so that part of the brain can be stimulated repeatedly.

Studying the electrical activity of nerves
When nerve cells are active, electrical activity is generated. This activity can be measured. Electro-encephalography (EEG), in which electrodes are stuck to the head, can be used to record brain activity. When a test subject engages in a particular activity, such as reading a book, it can be seen which parts of the brain are active at that moment. The EEG rhythm of someone who is active and concentrating is entirely different to that of someone at rest.

The results of research carried out from the neurobiological angle are also important for illness processes resulting from the lack of a particular substance in the brain. Generally speaking, therefore, treatment based on this approach will consist of an attempt to deal with this physical situation, through the administration of medication for instance, or by operating. An example is Parkinson's Disease; this condition appears to be caused primarily by a lack of dopamine in the brain. Certain forms of depressive behaviour can be convincingly explained by the inadequate functioning of physiochemical processes in the brain. The treatment of such conditions, either through medication or surgically, is not the job of the psychologist but of medical doctors. Psychologists who work using the neurobiological approach are found primarily in research laboratories, but also to an increasing extent in the clinic. Neuropsychologists in the clinic are occupied for the most part with diagnostics, that is, with questions like: what influence will a particular brain injury have upon this patient in terms of his intelligence, language, attention and concentration, memory, action and personality? The neuropsychologist can answer these questions using a variety of test methods.

Clinically-employed neuropsychologists can, however, also be occupied with different therapy programmes in convalescent institutions, for instance, where they oversee the recovery of patients with brain injuries. An example of such a therapy programme is the so-called 'cognitive retraining programme'. Programmes of this nature are designed literally to relearn how to think in an ordered manner. This programme of therapy will be prescribed for certain patients whose thought processes have been disrupted by a brain injury. They have to learn once again how to solve an everyday problem, such as keeping an appointment or working the washing machine.

Study activity
  2. **a.** Carefully study the case of Diane at the beginning of this section.
  b. Describe how this psychological movement would explain, diagnose and treat Diane's depression.

4. The behavioural approach

Practitioners of this approach are primarily occupied with behaviour. Behaviour can be seen, heard, felt or detected by the researcher. Examples are eating, walking, talking, going pale, sweating, panting, saying 'ouch'.

A second characteristic of practitioners of this approach is that they believe that internal processes play a secondary role in the generation and continuation of behaviour. The behavioural approach attaches greater importance to influences from the surrounding environment.

Here is an example:
Sally (3 years old) whinges: she demands a sweet in a whiny voice. Why doesn't she simply ask for a sweet? Because she won't get one if she asks, but she will if she whines about it. A reaction from Sally's environment (being given a sweet) determines whether she whinges or asks.

Behaviour is felt to be influenced in the first place by factors which precede that behaviour.

For example:
Someone hits you, so you hit back or run away.

Secondly, behaviour is said to be influenced by factors which follow it.

For example:
Why do you pick up a ringing telephone? Because you will receive a message which might be important to you. Here too, then, it is a factor outside the individual in question which determines his behaviour (picking up the telephone).

The second feature is closely related to a third: almost all forms of behaviour are learned. Sally's whining and the picking up of a telephone are both forms of learned behaviour. No distinction is made here between appropriate and inappropriate behaviour, between normal and abnormal behaviour and between stable and neurotic behaviour. Inappropriate behaviour, neurotic behaviour and abnormal behaviour are all learned.

For example:
You have a colleague who does not pay attention during discussions at work. The fact that someone else is speaking does not prevent him from interrupting and expressing his own opinion in a loud and unashamed manner.

Why is this? Because he has learned that his inappropriate behaviour means that his opinion is heard. Undesirable behaviour can also occur because the required form of behaviour for a particular situation has never been learned.

For example:
A woman is afraid in company, she does not dare go to parties, and so stays at home: she has a phobia about social contact.

Why? She has not learned how to make contact, or how to 'chat'; she simply does not know how to do it.

A fourth characteristic of the behavioural approach to psychology is the heavy emphasis which is placed upon scientific research. Behaviour has to be measured (how often did the colleague interrupt during working discussions; for how long did Sally whine?).
Behaviour has to be related to the factors which precede and follow it:
– How did the group react to their colleague's rude behaviour?
– How did Sally's mother react to her whining?

It must be possible to predict changes in behaviour.

For example:
Give Sally a sweet when she is playing quietly, and do not react, including becoming angry, when she whinges. The prediction will then be that the desired behaviour – playing quietly – increases in frequency and that the undesired behaviour – whining – decreases in frequency.

Picking up the telephone:
learned behaviour

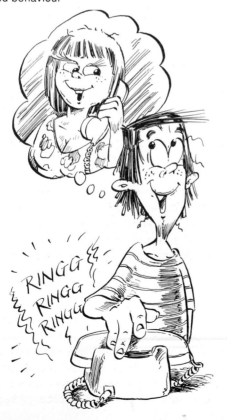

RINGG
RINGG
RINGG

Take note: the whining will decrease after first increasing sharply for a short period during negation. This is a typical characteristic of *extinction*. We will say more about extinction in due course.

As scientifically-trained behaviour experts, every psychologist will, of course, be convinced of the importance of research. Nevertheless, it is the behaviourally-oriented psychologist who places the greatest emphasis upon this aspect of the discipline, although the difference in emphasis is relative rather than absolute.

If such emphasis is placed upon observable behaviour, what about what goes on inside the person? One of the pioneers of this field, the American J.B. Watson (1913) stated that psychology ought to be concerned solely with observable behaviour. Psychology should not occupy itself with conscious processes, that is, with what we experience. Only one person can have any knowledge of conscious processes. If someone is afraid, he alone feels that fear. It can, however, be deduced from his behaviour that he is afraid. Watson believed that psychology cannot be concerned with personal experiences, not because they do not exist, but because they cannot be directly observed and recorded. The inner world can only be explored by an intermediate path. This path comprises the messages which the person being studied communicates about his interior. The researcher uses the self-observation method (introspection) in cases of this nature. Watson mistrusted the results of research based on introspection. In practice, however, things are never quite so black and white. What a person experiences is expressed in his behaviour. A person who is frightened says 'I'm afraid', he sweats, his heartbeat increases in frequency and he avoids whatever it is he is afraid of. These are all examples of behaviour from which it can be deduced that he is afraid.

Nowadays there are few psychologists who regard themselves as strict followers of Watson. The modern psychologist however, is still heavily influenced by his way of thinking: emphasis is placed upon behaviour with reference to emotions, thought processes, and so forth.

The greatest weight is placed on the observation and cataloguing of behaviour and, not the least important by any means, upon predicting behaviour.

A critical comment: it is not the case that all behaviour is learned. Nor is it so that all behaviour continues due to learning processes. This may be shown using three examples:
– A person who has suffered serious brain damage in an accident shows signs of cognitive breakdown. These signs of breakdown, including failure to recognize members of his family and the inability to pronounce certain words, are examples of behaviour which have not resulted from a learning process. They are the result of a radical physical trauma. A person who breaks his leg cannot walk as before. This inability to walk is not the result of a learning process. The invalid will only be able to learn to walk again when one condition has been satisfied, namely that his leg has healed.
– A great deal of what is said about growth and maturation in Module 2, 'Developmental Psychology' relates to processes which are preconditions for learning. That means that a certain form of maturation and growth first has to be completed before a particular learning process can occur (figure 1.2.2). An example is riding a bike. This motor action cannot be learned until the body has reached a certain size. The neurological system also has to be developed to such an extent that it can control the muscles. The same applies to the balance system.
– There are more and more indications from the field of ethology (the area of biology concerned with the behaviour of animals) that both humans and animals display forms of behaviour which derive from heredity. These forms of behaviour do not exist as a consequence of a learning process, but because they are established genetically. Examples include making yourself look physically bigger (standing up straight, shoulders back) when resolutely stating your opinion, and making yourself look small (huddling up, lowering the head) when accepting a justified rebuke.

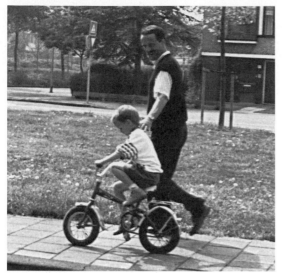

Figure 1.2.2
Learning to ride a bike:
growth and maturation play a role

The behavioural orientation plays a major role in modern psychology, and has proved highly successful. The results of the scientific research carried out in this manner lend themselves particularly well to therapeutic application in the medical field. Functional complaints, for instance, can be readily explained using this form of psychology. We will deal with this in much greater detail in due course.

We turn now to the question of how we learn behaviour.
In the first instance we learn by association: because two events occur at the same time, we learn that they are related. Secondly, we learn that because we as people like to experience pleasure and avoid pain, we are more likely to do things if they are followed by nice experiences. We avoid doing things which are followed by an unpleasant experience, like pain.

Two terms are very important within the behavioural approach: 'stimulus' and 'response'. A stimulus can be both external or internal. External stimuli are changes in the environment of an organism (a human, animal or plant) which result in a particular reaction. Internal stimuli come from within the organism itself. Examples in the case of humans are pain sensations or feeling one's own heartbeat. Response literally

means answer – the reaction of the organism to the stimulus.

Four scientists played a key role in the founding and development of the behavioural approach: Pavlov, Watson (to whom we have already referred), Skinner and Bandura.

The first, Ivan Petrovitch Pavlov (1849–1936) was a Russian physiologist who began his career as an expert in nutrition. As part of his work, he developed a procedure for studying behaviour and discovered an important principle of learning. Pavlov studied salivation in dogs by placing meat powder on their tongues. He discovered by chance that the dogs began to salivate as soon as they saw the assistant who brought their food, or even when they simply heard his footsteps. A stimulus (the assistant) which did not initially elicit this response, now caused salivation. This was because the man in question brought the dogs the meat powder. Even without meat powder, his presence was henceforth enough to cause the dogs to salivate. Pavlov investigated the phenomenon further by causing a bell to be rung just before the dogs were given meat powder. After this had been done several times, the dogs began to salivate as soon as they heard the bell. This process was later to be given the name 'classical conditioning'. Classical conditioning is illustrated in diagram 1.2.1.

The most important element in classical conditioning is the stimulus. A previously *neutral stimulus* can elicit a response by association with (i.e. coinciding with) a stimulus which automatically elicits that response. If the assistant had not brought food, the dog would never have salivated upon seeing or hearing him. Nor will a normal dog salivate when it hears a bell ringing. It was only because the bell had rung on a number of occasions when the dog was fed that its ringing led to salivation.
The neutral stimulus (in this case the bell) is called a *conditioned stimulus*, because it can only elicit the response after the process of classical conditioning. This stimulus which automatically elicits the response (in this case the meat powder) is called an *unconditioned stimulus*.

Diagram 1.2.1
Classical conditioning

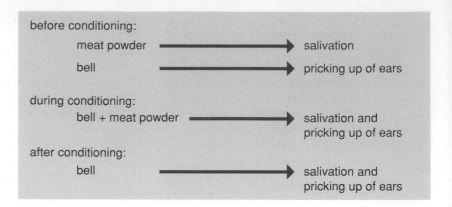

before conditioning:
    meat powder ⟶ salivation
    bell ⟶ pricking up of ears

during conditioning:
    bell + meat powder ⟶ salivation and pricking up of ears

after conditioning:
    bell ⟶ salivation and pricking up of ears

Will Pavlov's dog continue to salivate every time it hears a bell ringing? That depends. If it always receives food after the bell has rung, then it will continue to respond in this way. If, however, the bell rings a number of times and the dog does not receive any food, it will eventually cease to react by salivating. Therefore, if the conditioned stimulus is provided on a number of occasions without the unconditioned stimulus, the response will cease to be elicited after a time. This phenomenon is known as *extinction*. Extinction is not quite the same as unlearning, but the response fades and gradually reduces. This occurs naturally.

Conditioning occurs automatically and so does extinction. After all, the dog cannot decide for itself whether or not to salivate.

It is not only the conditioned stimulus (the bell) which can elicit the response. Stimuli which resemble the conditioned stimulus can also draw the same response. A different bell will, therefore, also lead to salivation. This principle is known as *generalization*. It can explain why people sometimes respond to new situations which are similar to known situations. The opposite of generalization is *discrimination*: distinguishing between stimuli, and hence reacting to one stimulus and not to another. If one stimulus is followed by the unconditioned stimulus and the other is not, the response will be elicited by one but not by the other. Imagine then that Pavlov had used two bells, a bell with a high tone and one with a low tone, and that the dog had been given meat powder only after the high bell was sounded and not after the ringing of the low bell. In this case, the dog would only salivate when it

heard the high bell ringing, and not when it heard the low bell. In other words, it would have learned to distinguish between the two bells.

Pavlov discovered an important phenomenon through experiments of this sort, namely that a conflict can lead to a neurosis. (According to the thinking of the behavioural school, a neurosis is a form of learned and at the same time inappropriate and/or undesirable behaviour. An example of a neurosis is a phobia, such as an extreme and irrational fear of lifts). Pavlov taught dogs to salivate upon seeing a circle and not upon seeing an ellipse. He then changed the form of the ellipse so that it appeared more and more like a circle. At the point where it became impossible to distinguish the circle from the ellipse any more, the dog began to move in a restless fashion, bite at its restraints and to bark loudly whenever it was brought near to the research room. It displayed behaviour comparable with that of humans when they are extremely anxious or neurotic.

The principles of classical conditioning have been applied primarily to the occurrence of phobias. Previously innocuous stimuli (the street, for instance) can cause anxiety due to association with another stimulus, such as a serious accident. The person in question becomes anxious whenever he is in the street, and will thus avoid going out. Another example of classical conditioning is the child who having received an injection from a person in a white coat, becomes anxious about anyone wearing similar clothes. The white coat was previously a neutral stimulus, but its coincidence with the injection has now turned it into a stimulus which elicits anxiety.

B.F. Skinner (1904–1990) is the most influential behaviourist. Skinner studied English literature and wanted to become a writer. Having read the work of Pavlov, he began to study psychology, after which he concentrated primarily upon animal research with rats and pigeons. He was particularly interested in the manipulation and control of behaviour. Skinner discovered, for instance, how to get a pigeon to peck at a button. When it did so, it was rewarded with food.

The basis of Skinner's *operant conditioning* (also referred to as instrumental conditioning) was the control of behaviour by changing rewards and punishments in the environment. The key element in the operant approach is the response. A response can vary between a simple reflex such as salivation, to complex behaviour like the solution of a problem. A response is an observable piece of behaviour which can be linked with events in the environment. The essence of operant conditioning is that a response increases in frequency when it is followed by a positive consequence, something pleasant, or in technical terms a *reinforcer*. Such a consequence might be expressed as C+. Skinner defined something as a reinforcing consequence if it served to increase the frequency of the response preceding it. There are many forms of reinforcer: material reinforcers such as money or a present; activity reinforcers, like watching TV or playing a game; social reinforcers like attention, a pat on the back or a compliment. What is a reinforcer for one person need not be so for another.
Not everyone is equally susceptible to a compli-
ment, and not everyone finds it pleasant to watch TV.
Diagram 1.2.2 illustrates operant conditioning

What do all these symbols mean? We will take as an example the picking up of a ringing telephone. We know that the following series of actions is *not* innate (i.e. an inborn, unlearned response): 1. hearing the telephone ring, 2. picking up the receiver, 3. hearing a message. This is a learned action. The S (stimulus) in the diagram represents hearing the telephone ring. If you do not know what that means, you can react in a number of ways: with R1 (response 1), for instance (= looking around in surprise), but also with R3 (= kicking the telephone away) or with R2 (= picking up the receiver). Picking up the receiver is the only action to be followed by a reinforcing consequence (C+), namely the message which is communicated. In time, therefore, the ringing of the phone will be followed solely by the picking up of the receiver.

There are a number of clear differences between operant and classical conditioning. The most important is as follows:
In classical conditioning, the individual is passive and the response is elicited automatically (the dog cannot do anything about it, nor does it need to: hearing the bell leads automatically to salivation). In the case of operant conditioning, the individual is active: the individual selects a particular behavioural response, and a reinforcer follows from the environment. The pigeon pecks the button and is rewarded with

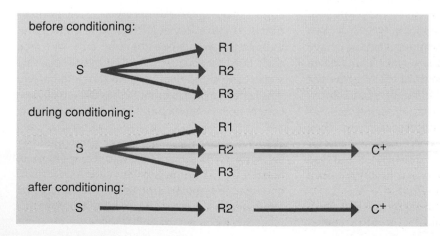

Diagram 1.2.2
Operant conditioning

food; the human picks up the phone because of the message which follows. It is because a subject-initiated action occurs that the term *instrumental conditioning* is also used. A key characteristic of operant conditioning is the fact that the response can be refused.

Behaviour is not only channelled in a particular direction when it is followed by a positive consequence, but also if it enables the individual to avoid a negative consequence. Therefore, the 'avoidance of something negative' is also a reinforcer (memory aid: remember the following rule from mathematics: negative times negative equals positive). An example of a *negative reinforcer* is as follows: if a child does his homework he does not have to help do the washing up. Doing his homework is thus rewarded by not having to wash up.

Extinction can also occur in operant conditioning. This happens when a particular piece of behaviour is no longer followed by a reinforcer. In order to ensure than certain behaviour no longer occurs, one has to remove its positive consequences. No reinforcer may be allowed to follow undesirable behaviour. We have already given the example of Sally whining for her sweet. The whining (this is the undesired behaviour to be unlearned) is no longer followed by a sweet. Unfortunately, a characteristic of extinction is that, at the beginning of this 'unlearning process', the undesired behaviour becomes more marked – in some cases to an extreme degree. Therefore, for the first day or even days, Sally whines even more. If the parents cave in at this point, they will be worse off than when they started. If they give in to Sally's even stronger whinging and whining, they will have taught her that she has got to make a big fuss in order to get a sweet. Instead of teaching her not to whine, they will have taught her to throw tantrums. If they hold out, though – and especially if, while ignoring her tantrums, they give her a sweet during desirable behaviour (playing quietly) – after a few days the crying and screaming for sweets will disappear from Sally's repertoire of behaviour.
Extinction is not the same as *punishment*. Punishment is the infliction of a negative conse-

quence following undesirable behaviour. The consequences of punishment are not so clear. Furthermore, punishment often has negative side-effects such as aggression or fear. The linkage of a negative consequence to an undesirable form of behaviour has repercussions which are difficult to predict. You know what you are trying to have 'unlearned' in this way, but not what you are going to get in its place. A happy child who bites his nails can be turned into a fearful, crushed child who does not bite his nails. Punishment and a negative reinforcer are widely confused. Punishment hinges upon the *inflicting* of a negative consequence. A negative reinforcer is where something negative ceases to be inflicted. If the effect of an action is the cessation of punishment, then that is negative reinforcement.

Operant conditioning can also be used to teach new behaviour. New behaviour is understood to mean the following.
In the case of animals, it refers to behaviour which would never be displayed in the natural environment, for instance, a pigeon causing a little lift to rise by pulling on a string, in order to gain access to the food located in the lift.
The learning of new behaviour occurs according to the principle of *shaping*. First of all, any behaviour is rewarded – behaviour which approximates to the new behaviour to be learned – and this is a step in the right direction. The response then has to move more and more in the desired direction in order to lead to reinforcement. An example is when a child is learning to speak. In the beginning, the parents reward the child for any babble he produces. Great attention is paid to every noise the child utters. After a time, the parents pay attention only when the child makes a noise which resembles an existing word. The child then has to pronounce real words before hearing that he has done well, and finally he has to come out with a full sentence.

We have already touched on the behaviourally-oriented psychologist's views of inappropriate behaviour. Inappropriate behaviour is a form of undesirable but learned behaviour. The person has just failed to learn a particular response (this is a certain form of behaviour) or else has learned an undesirable form of behaviour in its place. In order to change the undesirable form of behaviour, you have to determine precisely what is serving to reinforce it. You then miss out this reinforcer on each occasion that the undesirable behaviour occurs. From the treatment point of view, it is not advisable to deprive the person of the reinforcer in question. It should, however, be administered after the person has displayed other, desirable behaviour. In this way, you subject the undesirable behaviour to extinction (i.e. it disappears) and a desirable form of behaviour increases in frequency. After a short period of increase on the part of the undesirable behaviour (a characteristic of extinction) it will decrease in frequency. Because the reinforcement is now linked with the desirable form of behaviour, this will increase in frequency.

An example:
There is a very troublesome patient on the ward. He is aggressive, pushy and continually demands attention where none is really required. This is undesirable behaviour. Desirable behaviour would be that he remains quietly in his room and only rings when necessary. The way to change this behaviour is not to pay him any attention when he is aggressive and pushy. He should be given attention, the nurse should go to him, do something pleasant with him, when he has been quiet in his room for a while. What might be expected in such a situation is that, after a short period during which the patient becomes totally impossible, he will then calm down.

A number of observations.
Firstly: you only embark upon a course of action of this nature if corrective comments have had absolutely no effect.
Secondly: this patient still has to get his 'share' of attention, which is not an easy matter. It is much easier to react to a bell than to no bell.
Thirdly: imagine that part of the 'totally impossible behaviour' comprises a protest to hospital management about 'scandalous neglect from the nursing staff'. As you will appreciate, behavioural therapy has to be properly organized – do not try it off your own bat.

Another critical comment should be made at this point. We acted at the beginning of this section as if a person's 'internal' world could not be studied in a reliable manner. That is not correct. It can indeed be done. As early as 1932, Edward Tolman published the results of an ingeniously conceived experiment. He demonstrated that rats, without ever having been in a particular maze, could learn its plan with great precision. When moving through the maze towards a piece of food, the rats did not make any mistakes. The rats were transported around the maze a number of times in a kind of 'chair-lift' arrangement. All they could do was look around – they could neither walk nor sniff. They were transported by a variety of routes to a place where a piece of food was located. It appeared that simply by looking, the rats had learned the plan of the maze. No matter where they were introduced into the maze, they never made a mistake in the route to be taken. Tolman concluded two things.

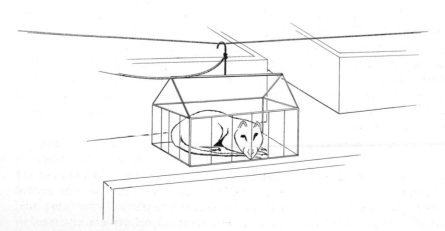

Figure 1.2.3
The rat is transported around the maze in its 'lift' and thus learns the precise plan of the maze

Firstly: another behaviour determinant must be assumed between the stimulus (the maze) and the response (running in the maze because of the reinforcer: the piece of food) (figure 1.2.3). This other behaviour determinant is 'knowledge of the plan of the maze'. And secondly: this 'knowledge' factor could be readily studied. In psychologists' jargon the knowledge factor is called the 'cognitive factor'. Bandura (1977) incorporated the cognitive factor in his theory of 'social learning'.

Albert Bandura (1977) was the pioneer of *social learning theory*. He adhered to the operant approach towards the shaping and maintenance of behaviour. The operant view creates the impression that behaviour is determined solely by the environment. In the example cited earlier, the environment is the telephone message which elicits the proper response to the ringing telephone. Bandura felt that there is a continuous interaction between behaviour and the environment. The environment shapes the behaviour of the person, but, he argues, the 'behaving' person also acts upon the environment, thereby changing it. It is difficult for Skinner (1972) to explain individual differences between people. He states: 'They have a different learning history'. Taken to its extreme, the implication of this view would be that if you bring up two children in an identical manner, you would end up with two identical adults. Bandura has much less difficulty in explaining the individual differences between people. Individual behaviour arises from the interaction between environment and individual.

Bandura is of the opinion that it is useful to add another factor between stimulus and response. We referred to this factor above as the 'cognitive factor'. Perhaps a more apt and descriptive term is the 'organism factor', with 'O' as its symbol. This O-factor consists of all those characteristics of a person which make him an individual. It is the factor which determines the individual's reaction to the environment.

Apart from the repeated influence of behaviour and environment, the social learning theory has a second important characteristic, namely the view that many pieces of behaviour are acquired without direct reinforcement. We also learn certain behaviour patterns because we have seen other people using them, we watch, we imitate. This type of learning is called *vicarious-learning*. People learn by observing the behaviour of others, and by witnessing the consequences of that behaviour. The other person acts, as it were, as a model. According to the social learning theory, reinforcement is not necessary for learning, although it does facilitate it. When someone sees another person doing something, that behaviour is registered in his repertoire of behaviour. For example: there is a crisis on the ward. A patient suddenly has a cardiac arrest. A student is the first to notice, and, more or less in a panic, alerts the person in charge. The student sees that this person reacts in a calm, business-like and highly efficient manner, carrying out a series of necessary actions. The 'model-learning' effect of this will be that the student will tend, in the event of something similar occurring, to act in the same calm and efficient manner.

It would appear in this example that reinforcement has diminished in importance. That is not so, as in this case it is reinforcement which determines the implementation of the behaviour. In the example, the head of the ward carried out a number of actions in an adequate manner, and the correct implementation of these actions was determined by their immediate reinforcement. The student sees that the resuscitation equipment is used, and so he will do the same on similar occasions in the future. The correct technical use of the equipment is learned by direct reinforcement and not so much by model-learning.

Because we see a great many different examples of behaviour around us, you might say that we have numerous patterns for model-learning. The kind of behaviour we display in a specific situation will depend upon the reinforcement we expect as a result.

In other words, reinforcement determines the implementation of behaviour. Reinforcement can take on a variety of forms. In the first place, there is reinforcement of the kind we saw in classical and operant conditioning. This occurs directly in the form of a material reward (children: sweets; adults: money), the approval or disapproval of others, or the cessation of an annoying situation.

The social learning theory adds two forms to these. In the first case, reinforcement is provided by the person's seeing someone else being rewarded for particular behaviour. An example might be where a colleague rewards a sick child. You notice that a colleague carries out a painful nursing process on a sick child without the child crying, screaming and tensing up as he does when you carry out a similar action. You notice that your colleague first distracts the child by telling him a story and causing him to relax. The action is carried out during the telling of the story. The next time you do it the same way.

A second form of reinforcement added by the social learning theory is where the person reinforces himself by approving of his own behaviour. Other people can criticize your behaviour, even on a repeated basis, and yet you don't change your behaviour. Why not? Because you think that your behaviour is correct. You reinforce yourself.

To sum up: behaviour depends upon the situation in which one finds oneself (the student on the ward), the significance which the person attaches to a particular situation (crisis situation), reinforcement for similar behaviour in the past (immediately alert person in charge), the observation of others in such a situation (calmly fetching resuscitation equipment). The appreciation which the person in charge displays towards your behaviour, and your own opinion on the matter will then determine whether you continue to behave in the same way.

Study activity
3. **a.** Carefully study the case of Diane on page 30.
   b. Describe how this psychological movement would explain, diagnose and treat Diane's depression.

5. The cognitive approach

People think and reason. The suggestion implicit in Section 4 is that the human mind is simply a kind of serving hatch, or perhaps a telephone switchboard where stimuli are received and responses sent out. We all know from our own experience that this is not the case. The fact that you can read and understand this text is, in itself, an indication that Watson's views are not strictly true. The word 'happy' is simply a quantity of ink shaped in a special way (figure 1.2.4). The reader attaches the significance of a pleasurable emotion to this quantity of ink. The 'telephone switchboard' is not passive, it is active. A much better conclusion would be to state that we are not like telephone switchboards at all. Other examples could be given: our perception system attaches the significance of 'a nocturne by Chopin' and 'beautiful!' to 'a large number of audible stimuli'.

Figure 1.2.4
Only ink, but meaning too

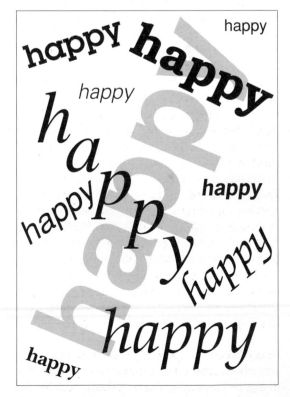

Cognition is a term which refers to mental processes like thinking, reasoning, perceiving, remembering. Thanks to cognition, we can solve problems, form an idea of a planned holiday, remember things from the past.

The *cognitive approach* derives from a reaction against the behavioural approach. Cognitive psychologists work on the principle that there is something else between environment and behaviour, namely what the person thinks, believes or expects. We came to the conclusion in the previous section that the behavioural approach does not deny the presence of cognitive processes. However, those who adhere to the behavioural approach assume that these processes cannot be studied in an objective manner. The cognitively-oriented psychologist would respond to this as follows, 'If we do not have methods for studying these cognitive processes, then we should develop research methods which will allow us to do this in an objective manner. To act as if they don't exist is to throw the baby out with the bathwater.' The cognitively-oriented psychologist will argue that it is precisely thinking, perception, and so on in which the psychologist is interested – motor activity (i.e. behaviour) is only interesting because it relates to these cognitive activities.

The cognitive psychologist allocates a central role to cognitive processes in determining behaviour. Disrupted cognitive processes lead to disrupted behaviour. For example: a person who feels, 'I'm worthless' (a cognition) will behave in a timid and socially withdrawn manner. By changing his cognitions, the disruption in his behaviour can also be changed. Therefore, if we succeed in convincing the person in question that he can achieve a lot (a cognition), he will feel happier in company with others, and will no longer act in such a timid manner.

A distinction may be made here between the content and the structure of thought. The thought content is *what someone is thinking* at a particular moment; you can ask the person about this. The thought structure is the *way in which someone thinks*; it is the manner by which someone arrives at the content of the thought, the

patterns which can be detected in thought. It is very important to distinguish between these two (content and structure). For example: two people wake up in the morning and notice that they have a pain in the back (a perception: a thought content). One thinks: 'I must have sat in a draught yesterday – I must keep my back warm today.' The other thinks: 'I put too much strain on my back yesterday. If I'm not careful I'll end up like my Dad with his two hernia operations, and eventually in a wheelchair. I'd better stay in bed for a couple of days.' Two different cognitive processes have the result that the significance attached to the experience of pain is totally different.

Two instances of these cognitive processes are as follows:

- *Expectations*: these are thoughts directed towards future events, such as the expectation that you will or will not be able to do something ('Learn French? There's no point, I could never learn that language'), or the expectation that you will pass or fail an exam ('Driving test tomorrow – I won't bother reading the Highway Code again, I know it well enough already').

- *Providing meaning*. People continually provide a meaning for what happens to them or to their environment. We continually interpret the events around us and evaluate our own input into them. Here is another example. The driving test has gone badly, particularly as far as the questions were concerned. One person might say: 'I really am daft, spending the night before the test out on the town!' While another person might say: 'The questions were far too difficult, and everyone fails the first time anyway.' These interpretations lead to different feelings and hence to different behaviour.

Important representatives of the cognitive approach are Wolfgang Köhler, Edward Tolman and Jean Piaget.

Wolfgang Köhler was a German psychologist who emigrated to the United States just before World War Two. He carried out a series of experiments using chimpanzees (Köhler, 1925) (figure 1.2.5). He was able to demonstrate on the

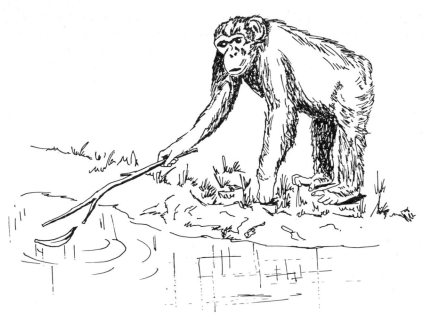

Figure 1.2.5
The ape pulled the
banana towards itself
using the stick

basis of these that learning does not simply consist of a series of stimulus-response associations (the telephone switchboard idea), but that cognitive factors are also important. A famous test designed by Köhler is as follows.

The chimpanzee sits in a cage. Just in front of the cage is a stick. A little further away is a banana. The chimpanzee first tries to reach the banana by holding its arm through the bars of the cage, but it cannot reach. It can, however, reach the stick. It takes it, but at first does nothing with it. The ape studies the situation for some time, and then suddenly takes the stick and uses it to pull the banana towards itself.

A few days after this experiment, Köhler put the same ape in a slightly different situation, a different cage, a different, longer stick and the banana was positioned further away. Without any further reflection, the chimp took the stick and pulled the banana towards itself.

A few days later again, Köhler put the ape in a room in which a bunch of bananas was suspended from the ceiling. The room also contained a number of sturdy boxes. The ape tried to reach the bananas from a standing position, but found itself to be too short. After a little bit of trying, but still relatively quickly, the ape stacked the boxes on top of each other beneath the bananas, climbed on top of them and took the entire bunch.

In these experiments, the chimpanzee solved problems using three cognitive factors.

The first is 'insight' (characteristic: suddenly acting in a goal-oriented manner), the second is called 'availability' (characteristic: once learned, always learned) and the third is called 'transfer' (characteristic: what has been learned in one situation can be used again in another similar situation).

We do, of course, recognize in this many of our own experiences with learning – the sudden perception of the solution, the 'Aha-experience'. Insight is a general phenomenon in human learning, in the solving of a problem or a puzzle, for instance. Everyone has had the experience of having searched for a solution to a problem when that solution suddenly pops into their head: the 'Aha-experience'.

A number of factors are important with respect to learning through insight:
– *Insight* depends upon the orderly arrangement of the components of the problem. If the elements of the situation which are important to the solution of the problem are arranged in such a way that their relationship is clear, insight will arrive at an earlier stage. It is easier for Köhler's chimpanzee to solve the problem when the stick is located near the banana than when the stick is located on the

other side of the cage. As far as humans are concerned, this arrangement of the different elements of the situation does not occur in reality but mentally. We are not very good at finding solutions if we have too few clues; nor are we successful when offered a disordered quantity of information. We are then obliged first to sift the information to determine what is relevant and what is irrelevant. Therefore, a well-ordered workplace and a tidy desk help us to spend an evening studying effectively.

– If a solution has been found through insight, it can be repeated immediately. The route which we followed in finding the solution remains directly *available*. If we have suddenly found a solution by puzzling through the problem ourselves, we see the correct solution relatively quickly in comparable problem situations. The situation is entirely different, however, if use was made of conditioning principles during the learning process. In that case, the repeated execution of the desired behaviour on a second occasion will only be slightly faster than on the first. The organism learns the desired behaviour very slowly.

– A solution which is found through insight can be applied to new situations: it can be *transferred*. It is a cognitive solution, the subject has a particular goal in sight, and has found a means of achieving it. This means, this method, can also be used for other goals. Consequently, we are capable of abstracting solutions from the concrete situation in which the solution was found. The ape learned how to use the stick (concrete) but also how to use an implement (abstract) in a problem situation.

A second representative of the cognitive school is Edward Tolman. Tolman believed that a great deal of conditioning, such as that described for the behavioural approach, does, in fact, consist of the learning of a meaning. The sequence bell-saliva-meat (see Section 4) is interpreted in the following way by Tolman: the test animal has learned that 'the sound of a bell' means 'meat is coming', and salivation begins. The animal has learned that one thing follows the other. This is called 'sign learning'. As far as Pavlov and Watson were concerned, the sequence bell-saliva-meat is one without further value. Tolman, however, argues that the test animal displays certain behaviour because it expects that something will follow. What is learned is not the execution of a response, but the formation of an expectation: the expectation that something (meat, for example) will follow. An expectation is a 'cognitive image' of the situation. According to Tolman's reasoning, it would be understandable if one response were to be replaced without any problem by another response leading to the same expected result. In the previous section we gave the example of the rat which learned the layout of a maze from a moving cage, that is, without it walking through the maze itself. 'Sitting in a cage' could easily be substituted in this case by 'walking the route'. The behaviour is controlled by the expectation that the reinforcement was present at a known location in the maze. Another well-know example relates to the rat which swims to its goal after it had learned to walk to it. If the maze is filled with water, the rat will swim along the correct route without error. Therefore, the rat has not learned the response (walking through the maze) but has learned a particular plan of the maze. It has, as it were, a map of the maze in its head (a cognitive map). The learning of meaning, of expectation, is learning with understanding – it is not conditioning.

A third important representative of the cognitive approach is the Swiss psychologist Jean Piaget. Piaget studied the development of cognitive structures. Following years of intensive observation of children, he formulated a theory of cognitive development. This theory is generally accepted. Piaget's theory is based upon four stages of cognitive development: (Piaget, 1952).

Sensorimotor stage (0–2 years)
There is a close relationship between motor activity and perception. Grasping, holding, dropping and trying again are a means of practicing motor actions, but also of getting to know the objects held. The child learns that there is a relationship between his actions and the consequences of these. Some actions and the associated

consequences are great fun for the child, such as 'throwing teddy on the floor over and over again', followed by 'getting teddy back again', because father keeps picking him up. The child also learns that an object does not change if you look at it from a different angle, or if you look at it over something else. This phenomenon is called *object permanence*. This is demonstrated by the fact that a baby of a few months age will start looking around for an object which has been hidden. A baby of 5 months does not know if a ball still exists when it is hidden under a cloth; he will not look for it. When he is 8 months old, he will lift up the cloth to look for the ball underneath it. Every parent makes grateful use of this stage when playing 'peekaboo'; the parent holds a doll behind the newspaper and the child looks surprised because he does not know where the doll has gone. The parent then suddenly pushes the doll above the paper and calls 'peekaboo'. The child is delighted: the doll was gone, but now it is back again!

Preoperational stage (2–7 years)

The second stage distinguished by Piaget is called the preoperational stage. The child learns in this stage how to deal with symbols, including words. Words refer to things but are not those actual things – they symbolize them. The word 'mother' refers to mother, but is not mother herself. The child runs through the room with a stick between his legs and says 'I'm riding a horse.' The stick represents the horse, it is not the horse itself. Therefore, children aged between 3 and 4 years speak and think in symbols, but they do not yet use those symbols correctly, hence the term preoperational. A good example of incorrect use of symbols during this stage is the so-called conservation problem. *Conservation* has the following meaning: the quantity of something does not change when its shape changes, and the weight of something does not alter when it is put together in a different manner. The volume of a liquid, for instance, does not change when it is placed in a different shape glass. A brain-teaser for children of this age is the question: 'What is heavier, a pound of feathers or a pound of lead?' One of Piaget's best-known experiments concerned the conservation of volume.

There are two glasses on a table: one short, wide glass, and one tall, narrow glass. The short glass contains a certain amount of water. The water from the short glass is poured into the tall glass while the child watches.

The child is asked whether there is the same amount of water in the tall glass as there was in the short glass. A four year-old will answer that there is more water in the tall glass, because the water level is higher. A seven year-old, who has grasped the concept of conservation, will answer that there is the same amount of water. No water has been lost and the water level is higher, but the glass is narrower (see figure 2.5.5).

Operational stages (7–11 years, and 11–15+ years)

Piaget then identified the operational stages. These are the stages during which children 'operate' with or handle different symbols correctly. Piaget distinguishes between the concrete operational and the formal operational stages. The concrete operational stage is said to be characteristic for children aged between about 7 and 11 years, while the formal operational stage is for children aged between about 11 and 15 years and older.

The *concrete operational stage* is characterized by correct use of abstract terms in relation to concrete matters. For example: the child knows without difficulty the (sometimes complicated) route home from a friend's house. When he comes to a corner, he knows whether to turn left or right, but if you ask him to describe the route or to sketch it, he will be unable to do so. He cannot abstract from the concrete situation, but if you place him at a random point along the route, he will be perfectly able to go home directly.

Children also learn during this stage to order objects in groups and series. These objects have to be present in concrete form: 'Do you see that basket of fruit? Count how many pears are in it', or: 'Take the red and yellow marbles out of this bag', or: 'Put these blocks in a row, starting with the smallest and ending with the biggest.'

When they reach the *formal operational stage* (11–15 years), children are able to draw a map of their route. They will do this in a systematic manner, beginning either at their own or their friend's house. Perhaps they will even begin in the middle of the route and work out the drawing to either side, but they will not connect the first turn to the right with the fourth turn to the left. A characteristic of the formal operational stage is that the problem is solved in a systematic manner. The system used might, of course, be inconvenient or even wrong (i.e. not leading to the concrete solution). However, the characteristic feature is the use of a system, a plan. In short: children learn during this stage how to think in an abstract manner, thus allowing the child to solve a problem by 'mentally' developing and testing a solution.

Here is an example:
A child is given three tubes of colourless liquid. The combination of two or three of these will result in a red colour. The child's task is to find out which combination of liquids will provide the red colour. A young child will try to get the red colour by mixing the liquids at random. An older child, by contrast, will consider the problem first, and will then systematically explore all the options. Hence, first mix liquid 1 with liquid 2, then 1 with 3, then 2 with 3 and finally, 1 with 2 and 3. In this way, he is sure to find the solution to the problem.

Piaget's theory of cognitive (intellectual) development is generally accepted. The sequence of sensorimotor, preoperational, concrete operational and formal operational is not disputed. The ages indicated by Piaget have, however, come in for some criticism. There is a tendency to lower Piaget's age thresholds somewhat. There has also been criticism of the concept of 'stages'. This term suggests that upon reaching his seventh birthday, a child will suddenly know that a pound of lead is obviously the same weight as a pound of feathers, while a day earlier, he would have sworn that the pound of lead was obviously a lot heavier. Cognititve development does in fact proceed very gradually. The stating of ages is an attempt to indicate the likely times for these stages to be present and not definitive statements of fact and is not a major obstacle to the use of the concept.

The cognitive approach is geared primarily towards the manner in which people solve problems. The next stage is – how can you teach problem-solving to people who are not yet very good at it? You might characterize your own school career as a carefully planned attempt to master problem-solving methods, and to teach you how to solve systematically the problems which you will encounter in your work.

It is also apparent that in clinical practice patients are taught systematically how to solve particular problems. From self-injection for diabetics, to, 'How do I remember my appointments?' for a brain-damaged trauma patient in a convalescent home. In the latter case, the patient is taught to develop a strategy for dealing with his problems of forgetfulness. An example of such a strategy is: 'If I don't know what time it is, I have to look at my watch.' Or a second example, in which the strategy comprises two steps: 1. Write down the appointment in your diary, stating the correct day and the correct time; 2. Look at your watch to see what time it is, look in your diary to see if you've got an appointment.' 'Cognitive retrainers' work with the patient to discover the problem and the goal in a given situation. The patient then has to determine which steps will lead to that goal, carry out those steps one by one, and check that they are getting nearer their goal. If that is not the case, they have to adjust their intermediate steps.

Study activity
4. a. Carefully study the case of Diane at the beginning of Section 3.
   b. Describe how this psychological movement would explain, diagnose and treat Diane's depression.

6. The psychoanalytical approach

The founder of the *psychoanalytical approach* was Sigmund Freud (1856–1939) (figure 1.2.6). Freud, and the school which he founded, have had an enormous influence upon the development of psychology in its totality. This is even more the case with regard to clinical and medical psychology (see Stafford-Clark, 1965).

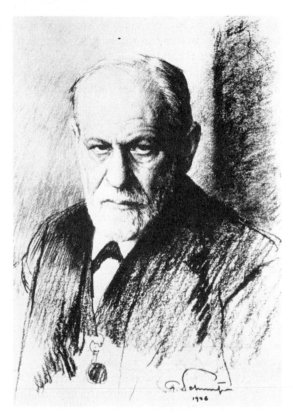

Figure 1.2.6
Sigmund Freud (1856–1939)

Freud was a Viennese doctor who specialised in neurology. He was often confronted in his practice with patients suffering from so-called 'hysterical' symptoms. This was the term given in the late 19th century to paralysis and complaints of exhaustion for which no scientific explanation was apparent. These inexplicable symptoms captured Freud's imagination. In 1886 he spent a year studying under the famous French psychiatrist Jean Charcot, who had successfully treated patients of this kind using hypnosis. Upon returning to Vienna, Freud tried out various kinds of therapeutic techniques on his own patients. He was working at this time in close conjunction with Joseph Breuer, a Viennese general practitioner. Breuer taught Freud the importance of 'catharsis'.

Catharsis is an intense feeling of liberation caused by the free expression of emotions, and the reliving of an intense emotional experience. The relief which is often felt after weeping is also a form of catharsis. The idea that you should not bottle up unpleasant feelings but should express them is commonplace nowadays. This idea is based on catharsis. In order to achieve catharsis, Freud developed the method of free association. This entails that the patient lies on the couch and talks about all the thoughts which come into his head, however unimportant or threatening they might appear. By analysing and interpreting these free associations, Freud succeeded in making his patients aware of their deeper, unconscious feelings and emotions.

Freud worked on the principle that it is emotion above all which motivates human behaviour. These emotions are for the most part unconscious in character. We are not aware of them, or else only vaguely, and yet they determine our behaviour. Freud studied the connections between the conscious and unconscious impulses. The visible and perceptible results of these connections are our thoughts and feelings, and for others, our visible behaviour. The result of the trial of strength between these impulses determines the specific character or personality of the individual. Apart from studying the personality as manifested at present, Freud also investigated the manner in which the personality was shaped during the individual's life. In addition to his ideas on personality, Freud also wrote on developmental psychology, which has also had a great impact upon the field as a whole. Freud's interest in the individual personality of the patient and its development can be summed up as follows: the emphasis in Freud's work lies upon the recognition of individual differences.

An image of the human mind (in Freud's work the interaction between conscious and unconscious impulses) which is regularly used by psychoanalysis is that of an iceberg. The part above water stands for our conscious experiences, that is, what we feel, think and can describe as such. A much greater part of the iceberg is located under water. It is invisible, unreachable, but still has a tremendous impact: just think of the sad end of the Titanic. The part under water represents the unconscious. The unconscious consists of wishes, impulses and all sorts of memory which we cannot, at least not at will, bring into our conscious experience. In order to properly understand Freud's theory, it is essential that we recognise the ability of such unconscious things to influence our thoughts, feelings and behaviour.

Freud attempted to study these unconscious elements using a variety of methods. His teacher, Charcot, used hypnosis, but Freud was unable to achieve good therapeutic results using this method. His best experiences were with 'free association', with the patient recounting his experiences without reserve. The story might be illogical, incoherent and its content might relate to entirely unacceptable matters. Nevertheless, Freud then tried to discover its underlying coherence, that is, the unconscious impulses which it revealed. He then communicated this interpretation gradually and carefully to the patient. The patient recognized the accuracy of the interpretation through an intense feeling of liberation – catharsis. If the therapist revealed his interpretation too quickly, the patient might react with rage, dismay and anxiety.

According to Freud, the individual personality is made up of three important systems: the 'id', the 'ego' and the 'superego'.

The *id* is the first part, the original form of the personality. It is already present in a baby. The ego and the superego develop from the id over the course of a number of years. The id comprises fundamental biological impulses, such as the need to eat and to drink, to avoid pain, to express aggression, and to gain sexual pleasure. The id is, therefore, closely associated with biological processes, and functions according to the principle of gratification. This is an old-fashioned term, and basically means: the id seeks to avoid pain and to obtain pleasure, without any concern for the continued existence of the individual. The id is demanding, impulsive, irrational and selfish in its search for pleasurable sensations.

It is sometimes said that, according to Freud, the id motivates the individual purely and simply to carry out sexual acts. That is not the case. The id motivates the individual to seek nice, pleasant experiences and to avoid the unpleasant. Sexual experiences are pleasant for the emotionally stable person, but there are pleasurable experiences other than sex. These pleasure seeking forces are sometimes referred to as *libido*. The gratification principle of the id lies at the heart of those other pleasurable experiences too. In the adult, the id is in the submerged part of the iceberg, i.e. it is in the unconscious part of the mind.

The baby learns pretty quickly that it is not always possible to get your own way immediately. Even as a baby you often have to postpone the satisfaction of your needs from time to time. You can't wee in your nappy any more, you have to do it in the potty. Learning to take account of reality gives rise to the ego. The *ego* has the role of keeping an eye on reality. The function of the ego is to express the wishes of the id in a manner which corresponds with reality (and with the requirements imposed by the superego, as we will see in a moment). The ego works in accordance with the reality principle: the satisfaction of needs is postponed until the most appropriate time. Being the part of the mind in touch with reality, it is in its totality in the exposed part of the iceberg, i.e. the conscious part of the mind. The ego, you might say, mediates between the needs of the id and the requirements of the superego.

The *superego* arises as we begin to view the standards and values of our parents or our social environment as our own. The child no longer washes his hands before eating because father says he has to, but because 'it's the done thing' or because 'a voice' inside him says that it is necessary. His conscience is speaking. If the child does not follow his conscience, he will feel guilty.

Freud is of the opinion that, at an unconscious level, the child is actually very afraid of losing his parents' affection. At a conscious level this anxiety is experienced in the form of guilt. The superego develops in response to the rewards and punishments of the parents: it is the internal representation of the standards and values of the society as taught by parents and other educators. It comprises the conscience and ideals and is responsible for controlling behaviour in accordance with social rules. The superego checks whether a particular action is right or wrong. It rewards appropriate, good behaviour with the experience of satisfaction, and it punishes inappropriate, bad behaviour with a sense of guilt. By acting as the conscience, i.e. preventing undesirable impulses from entering the conscious mind (the ego) from the unconscious mind (the id), it by definition occupies the barrier between id and ego and sees into both the unconscious and conscious mind.

This can occur on a very primitive level, in which case the person will think in a very uncompromising manner, and will be a real perfectionist. The superego imposes very high demands upon behaviour, but it can also be more understanding and flexible. People who are lucky enough to have a superego which functions in this manner are able to put their values and standards (i.e. their principles) into perspective and to adapt them to the situation.

Therefore: the id seeks pleasurable and good feelings, irrespective of whether these can be achieved, the superego is concerned with behaviour which is entirely appropriate to social values and standards, and the ego mediates in the resultant conflict. The result of this mediation is our behaviour, our experiences, our thinking. The conflict between the id and superego with the ego as mediator is, therefore, the motivation of our behaviour.

Because society condemns the free expression of aggression and sexuality, these desires cannot always be met at any desired moment. The more limitations which a child experiences, the greater the likelihood of conflict. People who wish to express a desire, but expect to be punished for it, become anxious. Just because an unacceptable wish is not carried out does not mean that it simply goes away. The ego has two ways of carrying out forbidden wishes of this nature in a manner acceptable to the superego. The first way is to select a 'disguised' means of expression. Participation in, or even spectating at aggressive sports can be an expression of such an impulse. Viewed from the point of view of Freud's theory, the increasing aggressiveness displayed on the football field is seen in a remarkable light. And what should we make of squabbling politicians or lawyers who earn their money by arguing in public (in a highly refined manner, of course – the superego has to be satisfied!) (figure 1.2.7)? The growing popularity of soft porn, whether or not on television, also takes on a special significance from this Freudian point of view.

A second way open to the ego is to use what are known as 'defence mechanisms'. This term refers to an unconscious process which protects

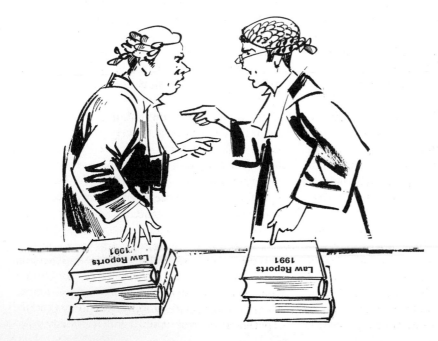

Figure 1.2.7
Arguing in public in a refined manner

the personality from the experience of anxiety, by twisting reality a little; a defence mechanism adjusts the experience of reality. The reality for a woman might be that she discovers a lump in her breast. This experience can be so frightening that she simply 'denies' that there is a lump. 'It's just a hard spot, nothing more,' she will say aloud to herself. This does nothing to change the lump, but the way in which it is experienced is altered.

We all make use of defence mechanisms from time to time. We are, in fact, unable not to use them. We use them when we find ourselves in a frightening situation which we cannot readily control. If we cannot effectively change the fear-inducing aspects of a situation, we alter our experience of that situation. Many defence mechanisms have been described – here are a few of them:

– Repression

Freud referred to the most common defence mechanism as 'repression'. This is a defence against an internal threat. Repression serves to push thoughts out of the conscious mind. An example is 'forgetting' a traumatic childhood experience, such as incest. Memory loss can also be a form of repression. Freud argued that there are certain desires from our childhood which all of us repress. All boys repress their feelings of sexual attraction to their mothers. The same applies to their sense of rivalry and enmity towards their fathers. Freud called this the Oedipus complex (see page 52).

– Displacement

Displacement is a means of transferring emotional feelings which have originated from one situation, to another (normally unrelated) situation. The classic example is of the husband who is angry but rather afraid of his wife, so he kicks the cat. He 'displaces' his anger from one object to another.
Displacement also happens in health care situations: the nurse, angry about an unfair comment made by the ward sister, takes it out on the patient: the patient, hurt because his wife did not turn up at visiting time, behaves unpleasantly towards the nurse.

– Denial

If reality becomes too threatening, giving rise to too much anxiety, a person can deny that it exists. The parents of a terminally ill child can refuse to accept that there is something wrong with their child, even though they have been kept fully informed of the diagnosis and prognosis. Another example is that of a wife, whose husband has died, continuing to lay the table for her dead husband or 'hearing' his footsteps. We have already given the example of the woman with a lump in her breast.

– Rationalization

Rationalization means 'providing a logical and socially desirable reason for something you do'. Rationalization can help, for instance, to overcome disappointment when a goal is not achieved, like: 'I don't need a driving licence anyway, public transport is excellent these days, and all those exhaust fumes are bad for the environment.' If that was really how you felt, then why did you spend all that money on driving lessons, and go through all the aggravation of failing the test so many times? It is also a way of providing an acceptable motive for your behaviour. It is often a good excuse.

– Reaction formation

It is sometimes possible to conceal a desire by strongly expressing the opposite. For example: a mother of an unwanted child feels guilty about her negative feelings. In order to quiet her guilty conscience she spoils the child and is overanxious about all aspects of his upbringing. He is not allowed to play with other children ('they're so rough, they'll hurt you'). He has to wear a thick coat, even when it is warm out ('you catch cold so easily, you're such a sensitive type'). The mother thinks she is caring for her child properly, but viewed closely her behaviour can have a harmful effect on the development of the child's personality.

– Projection

Everyone has undesirable characteristics which they would rather not admit to. Projection shields the person from recognizing these characteristics by attributing them in an exaggerated manner to other people. If you convince yourself that everyone cheats in exams, you will find it easier to take in a crib-sheet. Or: 'I'm not a pain in the neck, the ward sister is.' You can then happily make life difficult for her, it is what she deserves, after all.

– *Intellectualization*
Intellectualization is an attempt to distance oneself from an emotionally threatening situation, by dealing with it in abstract intellectual terms. This kind of defence often occurs with people employed in the health sector. A nurse who is continually confronted with serious human suffering cannot, for reasons of sheer self-protection, become emotionally involved with each patient. A certain degree of distance is necessary in order to be able to function properly. In this way, a sore becomes an ulcer, cancer becomes a tumour and the cutting off of a breast becomes mastectomy.

– *Identification*
If we feel intensely threatened, one way of surviving is to 'become like the threat'. You start to think and feel like the person threatening you. You become convinced of the reasonableness of his actions, and thus adopt them. The horrors inflicted in concentration camps by camp elders (themselves prisoners, but appointed head of a barracks) upon fellow inmates are understandable from the point of view of this defence mechanism. A similar reaction often occurs during a kidnap where the victim is often remarkably mild afterwards about those who threatened him with death. We also recognize the phenomenon, albeit in a much milder form, in our own situation. The young houseman, entirely convinced during his student days of the need to treat patients humanely, is overwhelmed by a multitude of (threatening) responsibilities and is quick to drop this conviction.

– *Regression*
Regression means that an individual falls back upon an earlier form of satisfaction characteristic of an earlier stage in his development. Regression occurs in stressful settings where the patient, unable to cope with his present situation, constantly demands comfort and attention, a reversion to the behaviour of his childhood. Regression as

a defence mechanism is also commonly found in elderly patients.

The psychoanalytical approach is based upon a theory of the personality, but also a theory of the development of human emotions. We have already discussed this. Freud is of the opinion that the first five years of a person's life are extremely important for the development of the human personality. During these first five years we go through a number of stages. The way in which these stages are completed is important to the manner in which the personality goes on to function during adulthood. Freud called these the 'psychosexual stages'. During each of these stages, the child has a different bodily zone where he experiences pleasurable feelings.

As we have mentioned before, there continues to be widespread misunderstanding of Freud's view, and so we will state it once again in more explicit terms. Freud continually used the word 'sexuality', particularly in his description of the development of the child. He did not use 'sexuality' in the sense of adult sexuality as we understand it. He used the term in a more transferrable manner, in the sense of seeking to achieve a pleasurable sensation by building up tension and then releasing it.

Psychosexual development from childhood to adulthood, as described by Freud, occurs in five stages:
– *The oral stage* (0–1 year).
During this stage, the mouth is the primary erogenous zone. Babies experience pleasure by sucking and later by biting. Traces of this are to be found in adult behaviour in the shape of smoking, eating, chewing gum and kissing.

– *The anal stage* (2–3 years)
During this stage, the anus is the primary erogenous zone. The retention and then expulsion of faeces first causes the build up and then the release of tension, thus causing a sensation of pleasure. Meanness is said to be an expression of anal characteristics in adults.

– *The genital stage* (4–5 years)
The sexual organs become the erogenous zone

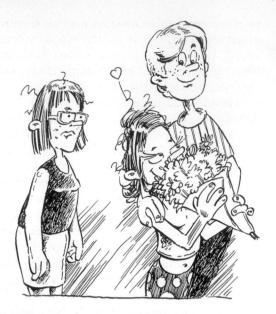

The three of us: how about Oedipus?

during this period. Children discover their sexual organs in a playful manner, and get to know the associated pleasant feeling. They discover the biological difference between the sexes. A characteristic process of repression occurs during this stage. Boys begin to see their fathers as a rival for the love of their mothers, and react with anxiety, as their fathers are so much stronger. This can be physically damaging or as Freud expressed it in symbolic terms, it can emasculate him. The fear of physical harm is called penis anxiety or castration fear. This leads to what Freud called the Oedipus complex, after the Greek tragedy by Sophocles in which Oedipus unwittingly killed his father and married his mother. This whole collection of feelings may be characterized in the following way: in his imagination every young boy experiences his father as a rival for the love of the mother. This Oedipal problem is manageable because the boy identifies with the father, and through him shares in the love of his mother. The process of identification also brings about the further development of the superego.

Freud is less forthcoming about Oedipal development in girls. Boys are afraid of physical harm, while girls realize they have already been damaged. The enmity associated with this ex-

perience is called penis envy. The girl blames her mother for this lack. Mother allowed her to be born without a penis, or else mother carried out the threat of physical harm. She chooses the father as the object of her affection. Freudians sometimes refer to the equivalent of the Oedipus complex in girls as the Electra complex after a character in another play by Sophocles who was in love with her father and has her mother killed. The Oedipus complex is also managed by girls through identification. By identifying with her mother, she shares in the love of her father. Once again, the process of identification brings about the further development of the superego. During this stage the child learns how to develop relationships with other people.

Study activity
5. Give two situations in which the adult is confronted by his or her own Oedipus complex.

– *The latency period* (6–13 years)
This stage features a reduction in attention to the body. It is a stage during which attention is focused more upon cognitive development, and does, of course, coincide more or less with the primary school period. The child then reaches puberty, the beginning of the next stage.

– *Puberty* (14+ years)
It is during this stage that adult sexuality develops.

These five stages of development do not always proceed without problems. If a problem occurs, fixation in a particular stage can result. Fixation means that if someone experiences too little (or too much!) pleasure during a particular stage, he remains in that stage. Therefore, that person spends the rest of his life seeking the same sort of gratification as is customary during the stage in which he is fixated. For instance the seeking of satisfaction in eating, drinking or smoking could be explained as that person being fixated in the oral stage. A characteristic of anal fixation is pronounced neatness, orderliness, saving and resistance to pressure exercised from outside.

Within this theory personality developement is linked to physical development and stops at puberty. This idea is not universally accepted.

Erik Erikson worked in the Freudian tradition. He adapted the psychoanalytical theory of development in the following way. Erikson (1950) did not refer to psychosexual stages but to *psychosocial* stages. As far as Erikson was concerned, development does not stop at puberty. He believed that essential things also happen during adulthood. Erikson argued that the individual is confronted during each stage by a social problem characteristic of that stage. The manner in which he learns to deal with this social problem determines the style in which his further development will progress.

The child in his first year of life (during the oral phase, according to Freud) is confronted with the problem: 'Can I trust my fellow humans, or is thorough mistrust the only justifiable approach?' Children who 'opt' for a thorough mistrust on the basis of a bad experience with their parents or the people looking after them, will always be mistrustful of their fellows. A child should develop trust in other people during this stage, as this is necessary for a properly balanced personality. During the second year of life (the anal stage, according to Freud), the fundamental problem lies in the question: 'Am I someone in my own right, or am I dependent upon others?' The child learns to control himself and develops a sense of being able 'to take life on'.

Aged 3 to 5 years (roughly corresponding with Freud's genital stage), the child wrestles with the question: 'Can I take initiatives for myself, or should I feel guilty about wanting to do this?' The child learns through this process how to undertake activities for himself, and how to determine the goal and direction of his behaviour.

From the sixth year to puberty (approximately the latency period) the child struggles with the contradictory experiences of 'industry' versus 'feelings of failure'. If the child manages to solve this conflict effectively, he develops a sense of being competent in a variety of skills, including intellectual, social and physical abilities. Although the child is fully aware that when he moves to his new school (upon transfer from primary to secondary school) he will leave some friends and have to make new ones, he is not afraid of the confrontation with all those other children, because he knows he can cope.

During adolescence, the individual battles with feelings of confusion regarding his identity: 'Who am I?', 'Am I what I do?', 'What do I want?', 'Well, if that's how it's got to be...' This stage is rounded off favourably if the adolescent feels himself to be a stable and unique personality. He knows what he is worth, and that is more than a little. This personality is able to cope with uncertainty and doubt, and can even use these as sources of inspiration. Finding one's own identity is the major problem of the adolescent. On the basis of this understanding of his own identity, decisions are taken which are of enormous importance to the further course of his life in the areas of education, career and sexual orientation, for instance.

The young adult is faced with the problem which Erikson identified using the terms 'intimacy' and 'isolation'. How do you form close, meaningful relationships while not 'losing' yourself in them. How can you remain yourself, while closely attaching yourself to someone or something else? This relates in particular to the selection or otherwise of a lifetime partner, or with the conscious choice of a particular job.

This can be illustrated using a few questions.

Are you still the same John Smith, now that they think of you as that tall student on ward 4?

Are you someone else now that you're married and you've changed your name to Mrs. Johnson instead of Anne Smith?

To what extent will you, as a young woman, tolerate your social status being largely determined by your husband's profession?

The following exchange illustrates this idea:

'Have you heard, Sandra's new boyfriend is a joiner on a building-site?' 'Really? Well, I would have thought that she could have done a lot better than that. Her father's a lawyer isn't he? Perhaps she'll come to her senses and it won't last long.'

Erikson distinguishes two further stages, namely middle adulthood and the ageing years.

The characteristic problem of middle adulthood is to find a balance between the satisfaction of 'I'm now doing the work I always wanted to' and 'I don't seem to have time to do anything else but work.' Also: 'Everything's going great with the family' and 'I'm just a cook and cleaner around here.' This problem is dealt with favourably if the person in question feels jointly responsible for his or her family and society, but also knows how to keep a healthy distance. Erikson described the ageing years as being characterized by 'despair' versus 'integrity'. On the one hand: 'Was that it? Is that what I worked so hard for?', and on the other a feeling of satisfaction: 'I am content. Things are fine.'

Erikson's contribution is important for two main reasons. Firstly he recognized that human development does not stop at puberty. He correctly points out that human development continues through adulthood, middle age and the ageing years. Secondly, the importance of the social context in which a person lives is emphasized. Human beings are not simply creatures who develop in accordance with biological rules; social factors also play a significant role.

The psychoanalytical approach has a number of implications for the treatment of patients. According to Freud, all mental problems relate to an attempt to satisfy impulses from an earlier stage of development. A conflict arises between a particular desire (id) and the recognition that to express that desire could be risky (ego). This leads to the development of a symptom such as fear. The symptom is only the expression of a deeper cause. There is no point, according to psychoanalysis, in treating the symptom (i.e. the observable behaviour), because the symptom will then express itself in a different manner. The true cause (the unconscious conflict) has not, after all, been removed. The method for changing behaviour is through free association, which means that the patient tells the therapist everything which occurs to him.

Many pertinent objections have been raised against the psychoanalytical approach. Freud's theory is based upon his experience over the course of fifty years in treating neurotic patients. In other words, it is founded on case studies. Modern psychology does not accept case studies as final reference material in demonstrating the value of a theory. Freud also studied patients, that is to say, emotionally disturbed individuals. Any conclusions drawn from research of this nature need not relate to healthy, emotionally normal individuals. The themes which Freud considered important were those which prevailed in turn-of-the-century Europe. The themes of the current age could be entirely different. A closely related aspect is the fact that Freud's theories are hopelessly discriminatory. It is pointed out that Freud had little understanding of women: after all, didn't he say that they were just castrated men? In short, there is much to criticize in Freud and his approach to the human personality. This does not, however, diminish the fact that he had a great influence upon the creation of modern clinical psychology. For that reason alone, we have to take him seriously.

Study activity
  6. **a.** Carefully study the case of Diane at the beginning of Section 3.
  b. Describe how this psychological movement would explain, diagnose and treat Diane's depression.

7. The humanistic (phenomenological) approach

The adherents of the so-called humanistic approach feel that it is the subjective experiences of the individual which are, in fact, the most important. This approach is less concerned with the impulses which have led to the current situation of the individual as described in the theories of Freud. Nor do they stress overt, observable behaviour in the manner of the behaviourally-oriented psychologist. According to psychologists of the humanistic orientation, what is really important is the personal view of the world and interpretation of events (the individual's *phenomenology*), his life in the here and now.
In order to understand what someone thinks about his present life, the psychologist has to get to know that person's opinions, his outlook on

life, and his values, standards and experiences. The psychologist must, in a manner of speaking, get into the other person's skin and look at the world through his eyes.

The emphasis which humanistic psychology places upon personal experiences has led to a lively exchange of views with supporters of the so-called cognitive school. Cognitive psychologists are interested in the structures and processes of thought. The humanists, by contrast, place heavy emphasis upon personal experience or feeling. Both groups are convinced that there is a powerful interaction between thinking and feeling. Both theories are a reaction against the strict behaviourism of Pavlov and Skinner.

The term 'humanistic' can be misleading. It does not signify a belief system, but is used instead to emphasize the fact that the field concentrates upon the characteristic properties of human beings. According to the humanists, these characteristics are the individual's ability to determine the course of his own life, and free will.

The humanistic school of psychology has had a significant impact upon psychology as a whole. Its influence has increased sharply during the last twenty years. Incidentally, its influence has extended beyond psychology. Like the Freudian approach, it has influenced social thinking in general. Society as a whole has been permeated with the positive values of a number of concepts from humanistic psychology. Terms and slogans like: 'I'm OK, you're OK', 'Become who you are', 'Sensitivity training', 'Growth weekend' and 'Encounter' all come from the humanistic approach to psychology.

Two leading representatives of this school will be referred to in this section, namely Carl Rogers and Abraham Maslow. Carl Rogers spent two years studying agriculture, before deciding to become a priest. After a number of years he left the seminary to work with children, paying his way through college where he studied psychology. Rogers was influenced by the ideas of Freud and by the behavioural approach, which, with its strictly scientific and objective principles, was very much in vogue during Rogers' time as a student in the U.S.

Rogers eventually reacted against Freud, however, and against Pavlov and Skinner. According to Rogers, the most important thing for a person is his perception of his own world, not the unconscious impulses which gave rise to this, nor the social circumstances which led to certain behaviour through conditioning processes. Rogers believes that people are not victims of their desires, nor of their social circumstances. The individual can direct his own destiny and is responsible for the way in which he lives his life.

Rogers' first important idea is that of *self-actualisation*. Each person, he argues, seeks to achieve self-actualization, by which he means that each person seeks to make optimum use of his own potential. Human nature causes each of us to strive towards adulthood and socialization. Each person is basically good, and each person wishes to actualize this goodness. It is true that people sometimes function in an irrational and aggressive manner towards themselves and others, but this, according to Rogers, is because they are frightened and are not functioning as fully developed people. The reader will not be surprised to learn that Rogers' views on this point have been strongly attacked in certain quarters.

Rogers' theory emphasizes change. Stress is laid upon self-actualization in the sense of changing from simple to complex, from dependent to independent, from rigid to flexible.

A second important concept in humanistic psychology is the 'self-concept', also called the 'self-image' or even shorter, the 'self'. Self refers to everything which someone thinks of himself, his opinion of himself, his own opinion of his characteristics and potential, his values and standards. In short: the answers to questions like 'Who am I, what am I, and what am I capable of?'.

The *self-concept* largely determines a person's outlook on life and the behaviour which he displays. If someone sees himself as 'weak, sickly and pathetic' (we call this a negatively-charged self-concept) he will have a bleaker than normal outlook on life, nor will he find it easy to change his life-style. It is quite different for someone who feels happy in himself, and 'ready to take on the world' (we call this a positively-charged self-concept). For a person like this, no mountain is too high, and no obstacle too difficult to overcome.

A person's self-concept is not just a chance mood. It is the underlying tone against which the whole of life is judged. Your self-concept is your perception of yourself and the importance which you attach to that perception. The self-image, although not the same as a person's daily mood, nevertheless appears to be changeable. Despite this changeability, it functions as a coherent, organised whole. The self is not like a little person inside us, it does not 'do' anything. It is a combination of experiences of which we are generally aware.

According to Rogers, we humans function in such a way that there is agreement or *congruence* between our different perceptions and between the self and the person's experiences. *Incongruence* occurs when there is a difference between the self and the actual experience. For example: if you see yourself as a person who has no feelings of hate, and you experience hate towards someone, then you are in a state of incongruence. This is a state of tension and confusion, and can lead to anxiety. If this happens, the person will respond by defending himself, he will try to deny the experience, or to change it in such a way that it corresponds with his self-image. Sometimes this doesn't work. The humanistic psychologist then rightly points out that the self-image need not correspond with reality. It is quite possible that someone actually achieves a lot, but because he always looks at his own actions in a sombre light (due to a negatively-charged self-image) he has the idea that none of it means anything. The achievements are not incorporated in the self-image; he doesn't recognise himself in them.

A concept related to that of the self is *the ideal self*. The ideal self is the self-image which the person would like to have, the image of himself which the person would most like to see. 'I wish I were an assertive woman, not afraid to say what I think in public', might, for instance, be

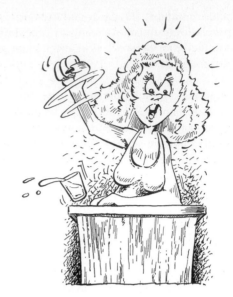

Assertive and attractive

the essence of a particular person's ideal self-image. People strive to achieve congruence between their self-image and their ideal self-image. Perception of a difference between the self-image and the ideal self-image, especially when this is a large difference, can be painful, and can arouse anxiety.

According to Rogers, every one of us needs a positive attitude from others, including warmth, respect, sympathy and acceptance. If a child can accept himself as he is, and is also accepted by his parents as he is, the self will develop in a healthy manner, even if the parents disapprove of certain behaviour on the part of the child. However, if this positive attitude on the part of the parents, or other people important to him, ceases to be unconditional, but dependent upon certain behaviour, developmental problems can arise. The child will then try to deny those experiences which do not lead to the love of his parents, that is, he will not incorporate them in his self-concept.

Rogers illustrated this point using the example of urinating. The emptying of the bladder when this is under pressure is associated with a pleasant sensation of relief. You are not, however, supposed to carry out this process in company, and with one or two exceptions, you are not supposed to talk about this sense of relief. The child tells his parents about this fine sensation of relief, but they do not accept the message. In response, the child will deny the experience and not include it in his self-concept. If a child notices that he only receives his parents' love when he is being nice, he will conceal all negative feelings. Anger, aggression, the urge to fight and jealousy – none of these are admitted to the self; the child will not accept them as being part of himself. Nevertheless, the child will experience them. This is an illustration of incongruence between the self and actual experiences.

There are, therefore, two possible differences: between reality and self-image and between self-image and the ideal self. Therapy based on humanistic psychology is geared towards reducing the differences between reality and the self-image, and between self-image and ideal self-image. This form of psychotherapy is called client-centred therapy. According to Rogers (1951), this means that the person who seeks help is not viewed as a dependent patient, but as a responsible client. Rogers does not use a medical model, that is the patient dependent on and accepting the diagnosis and treatment prescribed by the doctor, but the model of a person who wishes to grow, and a therapy which is geared towards removing any obstacles which stand in the way of that growth.

A healthy person can incorporate experiences in his self-image. Congruence is then seen to exist between the self and experience and there is no defensive attitude. A maladjusted person denies experiences. Experiences which are incongruent with the self are perceived as a threat, and are denied or interfered with.

The most important component of client-centred therapy is the therapeutic climate. Change will only occur if the therapist can provide three values: honesty, an unconditionally positive attitude, and empathy.

Honesty means that the therapist is himself, that he doesn't present a facade, but is open. In this way, he gives confidence to the client. The therapist tells the client what he feels, even when those feelings are negative.

An *unconditionally positive attitude* means that

the therapist conveys a deep and sincere concern to the client.

Empathy entails that the therapist is capable of perceiving the feelings and experiences of the client, and their significance to him. This requires active listening and sympathy with the client.

The therapist in client-centred therapy is directive to as limited an extent as possible – that is, he avoids steering the therapy to the best of his ability. He does not try to interpret what the client says, but listens to him, accepts what he says and then repeats it in different words. The therapist is, as it were, a mirror for the client. The idea is that this will lead to a process of change in the client.

Rogers' three conditions (honesty, unconditionally positive attitude and empathy) have become a basic attitude for every psychologist – and for other welfare workers – irrespective of their therapeutic school. If you are not honest towards a patient or client, if you do not accept him and cannot empathize with him, you will generally be incapable of helping him.

These three conditions form the basis for many courses on communication skills. Module 5 of this book could not have been written without this background.

The difference between self-image and ideal image is often encountered in somatic health care. A significant part of how you feel about yourself relates to how you feel about your body, how it functions, what it looks like, and so on. The feeling of being strong, being able to take life on, is also often based upon the idea that your body is strong, and that you are fit. What you think of your own body is sometimes referred to as your body-concept, body-image or body-idea. *Body-image* is an essential part of the self-concept (figure 1.2.8).

People who have no confidence in the functioning of their own body consult their doctor about every trifle; they have a negatively-charged body-image, and because the body-image is part of the self-image, they have a negative self-image. They are quick to become anxious about unusual physical sensations; in other words, they are hypochondriacal. People are hypochondriacal when medical examination reveals that the body is actually functioning properly. The reduction of the discrepancy between the hypochondriac self-image ('I'm ill, the doctor can say there's nothing wrong till he's blue in the face, but it's my body, I can tell') and reality is a difficult matter for the patient.

Patients with a real physical complaint have to deal with a comparable problem. The reality: 'My body is ill, it works painfully and badly' results in a discrepancy between body-image and self-image. Part of the self-image, namely the body-image, is exercising an influence which has a negative effect upon the self-image in its totality. 'I was always a man who could move mountains, now I'm lying here like a physical wreck!', quickly becomes 'I'm a wreck, I'm worthless, what kind of a father am I now?' This patient has to learn to split the physical reality from the body-image and self-image based upon it. In so doing, he can solve the emotional problems with which he is contending: 'My body is sick, it's functioning painfully and badly, and is not worth much at the moment. But that doesn't mean I'm worthless.' This point does, of course, apply to an even greater extent to chronically ill and handicapped patients.

We also see the impact of the body-idea on the self-concept at another level. If you have the idea that a particular part of your body has an unattractive appearance, this thought, which forms part of your body-image, can 'infect' your entire self-concept. A thought like: 'My hair is terrible, I can't do a thing with it', can turn into 'It's obvious that they're talking about it behind my back', and ultimately to 'I'm worthless too.' If, viewed objectively, part of the body really is proportioned in an unusual way, a reaction of this type will be considered understandable by many people.

The situation is different where another person would disagree that the feature is unnaturally proportioned, such as a supposedly big nose, protruding chin, breasts which are too large or too small or squinty eyes. Rogers talks of the person's own experience as the relevant starting point – what other people think is a secondary matter. In cases where the person feels that they look physically abnormal, we are dealing with an 'infected' self-image. The self-image has been 'infected' by a negatively-charged body-image. Because the body-image is part of the self-concept, the self-concept itself has thus now become negatively-charged.

One possible way of solving this problem is to adjust the actual physical proportions. The adjustment of physical proportions in accordance with the patient's wishes may entail cosmetic surgery. Research has shown that changing the size of the breasts in cases where the woman in question was extremely unhappy about her bust,

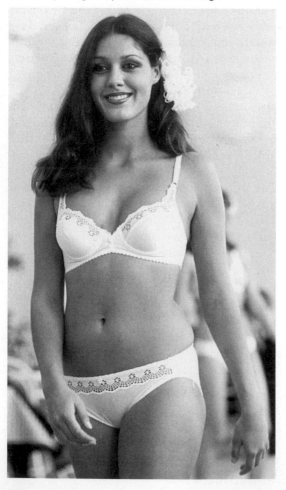

Figure 1.2.8
The 'body-image' is part of the 'self-image'

generally leads to positive results. By this we mean positive in both the surgical sense but above all in the sense of self-perception. The charge of the body-image shifted from (extremely) negative before the operation to (moderately) positive afterwards. As Rogers would predict, the patients' behaviour underwent a marked change, from shy and uncommunicative before to happy afterwards (in most cases), they began to take part in social life again, and felt able – in some cases literally – to show themselves once more. The 'infection' of the self-image by the body-image was cured.

Finally, the attitude that patients who undergo cosmetic surgery must be mentally ill is incorrect. This too was apparent from the aforementioned research. The women in question did not want a film-star's bust, they simply did not wish to stand out any longer in a negative manner because of their breasts.

The second representative of the humanistic approach whom we will discuss rather more briefly than Rogers, is Abraham Maslow. He is viewed as the leading theoretician of the humanistic movement. It was Maslow who described humanistic psychology as 'the third force in American psychology'. He criticised the two other forces, the psychoanalytical and the behavioural schools, for their negative view of people. Like Rogers, he argued that people are essentially good, and that the will to grow is present in all of us. Mental problems are the result of this essential human characteristic having been frustrated. Society is often the cause of this frustration.

Maslow is particularly well-known for his presentation of a hierarchy of human needs in the form of a pyramid (Maslow, 1954) (diagram 1.2.3). At the base of the pyramid we find the fundamental, physiological needs like food, air, water and sex. Higher up is the need for security, love and esteem, rising to the highest need, which is for self-actualisation.

People organize their lives around these needs, and try to satisfy each one. When all of the lower needs have been satisfied, the higher needs begin to make themselves felt. At each level, the failure to satisfy a need gives rise to conflict. As long as this conflict is not dealt with, the person will not proceed to the next level. If the satisfaction of lower needs ceases, the person drops back to that lower level until the needs in question have been met once again.

The first need which has to be satisfied is for food. When this has been satisfied, the person shifts to the need for security. Then comes the

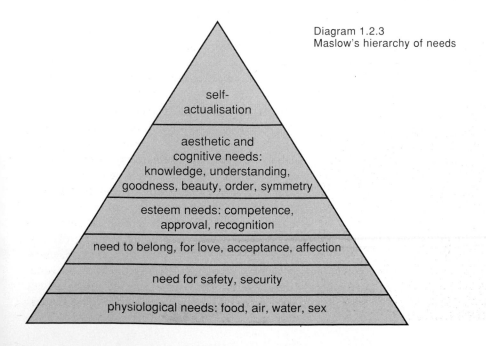

Diagram 1.2.3
Maslow's hierarchy of needs

need for love, affection and to belong some-where. The person feels the lack of friends, a partner and/or children. This need can be very intense, and growth towards the next level, that of the need for esteem, will only occur when love and affection are present. If the person has achieved competence, approval and recognition, he will develop further towards the satisfaction of aesthetic and cognitive needs. These needs relate to the search for knowledge, understanding, justice, beauty, order and symmetry. Finally, at the apex of the pyramid, the needs of self-actualization and self-fulfillment arise: the desire to be more than you are, to achieve everything of which you are capable.

In his later work, Maslow (1968, 1971) identified a further process within self-actualization, which he termed transcendence. This is a sense of wholeness or complete unity with the environment in which the person experiences a higher sense of peace and being. If you are interested, a library search on the topics of transpersonal psychology and transcendental meditation may prove fruitful.

As with other theories where stages are identified there is a danger of assuming that full satisfaction in each lower stage is necessary before movement to the next stage occurs. This is not so. It is not necessary to fully satisfy a need at one level before starting to satisfy a need at the next higher level. At any one time a person may have partially satisfied needs at more than one level. The important factor is that the person has satisfied the needs at the lower levels sufficiently for the present situation.

Maslow carried out an extensive study of healthy, self-actualizing people, in both the past and present. He studied individuals like Spinoza, Abraham Lincoln, Einstein and Eleanor Roosevelt.

This led him to conclude that such people have the following characteristics:
- they accept themselves and others as they are;
- they are concerned about themselves, but also recognize the needs and wishes of others;
- they can respond to the uniqueness of people and situations and do not react in a stereotypical or mechanical way;

- they can enter into deep, intimate relationships with a few people;
- they can be spontaneous and creative;
- they can rebel against conformity and act in their own interest, while still meeting the requirements of reality.

Maslow believes that every person has the potential to develop into an individual of this nature.

Study activities

  7. **a.** Study the case of Diane on page 30.
     b. Describe how this psychological movement would explain, diagnose and treat Diane's depression.

  8. Consider whether or not one or more schools of psychology fit within a holistic vision of nursing. Explain your answer.

  9. State which psychological school you would favour, and carefully support this choice.

8. Summary

This chapter has presented a description of the five main movements in psychology:
- neurobiological;
- behavioural;
- cognitive;
- psychoanalytical;
- humanistic (phenomenological).

It is apparent from the description of the different psychological schools that reality can be explained and predicted in a variety of ways.

No explicit preference has been made in this chapter for one particular psychological school.

A final word. The movements we have discussed in this chapter and the general introduction in Chapter 1 deal with the main currents in psychological thinking which stress the study of the individual. Some psychologists, while still concerned with the individual, are interested in psychology in the group context, that is, how group influences act on the individual, the functioning of human groups, etc. This is the field of *social psychology* and we will be addressing this perspective in Module 5.

Final test Module 1

Instructions

- This section comprises 44 yes/no questions.
- Each proposition, claim, statement, etc. may be *true* or *false,* either *yes* or *no.* There is no middle way: you must make a choice.
- Your assessment of whether items are true or false should be based on your reading of the book.
- The questions are arranged in order relating to subject or chapter.
- Check that all questions have been answered.
- Finally, mark the test yourself. You will find the answers at the end of the book.

1. Psychology is limited to the study of human behaviour.
2. The psychologist tries to discover rules in behaviour.
3. Introspection is a reliable method for discerning rules in behaviour.
4. Introspection is a form of self-observation.
5. The common terrain of the clinical psychologist and the psychiatrist is that of psychotherapy and psychopathology.
6. The title of 'chartered psychologist' is legally protected.
7. Objectivity is the effort to achieve minimal intersubjectivity.
8. Parsimony is a requirement which can be imposed upon a theory.
9. Compatibility is a requirement which can be imposed upon a theory.
10. The individual's score in a psychological test is compared with the scores achieved by a standard group.

11. A phobia can best be treated by means of a psychodynamically-oriented therapy.
12. The neurobiological approach is based on the premise that behaviour is primarily explained by the existence of objectivised birth-traumas.
13. A characteristic of the behavioural approach in psychology is the notion that (virtually) all behaviour is learned.
14. A characteristic of the behavioural approach in psychology is the notion that scientific research is less relevant.
15. A certain level of maturation and growth are important preconditions which have to be satisfied before behaviour can be learned.
16. Pavlov earned his fame by studying operant conditioning.
17. Association is a key concept in classical conditioning.
18. Extinction is the unlearning of a response.
19. Extinction is used in operant conditioning as a punishment for unlearning undesirable behaviour.
20. According to Skinner, behaviour develops in a particular direction because a reinforcing consequence follows.
21. Punishment is the infliction of a negative consequence.
22. Bandura used the cognitive factor in the explanation of the development of new behaviour.
23. This cognitive factor is referred to as a component of the O-factor.
24. The cognitive approach arose as a reaction to the humanistic school of psychology.
25. Expectations are cognitions.

26. Reaction formation is a cognitive process.
27. Piaget's theory relates to cognitive development.
28. 'Catharsis' is a sense of liberation arising from the free expression of emotions and the associated reliving of an emotional experience.
29. According to Freud, the human mind is an interaction between conscious and unconscious impulses.
30. According to Freud, the personality is built up of three important systems: id, ego and superego.
31. The id is the most primitive form of the personality.
32. The superego mediates between the desires of the id and the requirements of the ego.
33. According to Freud, repression is a defence against a threat.
34. The repression of needs and desires is a characteristic of mental illness.
35. Defence mechanisms are unconscious functions of the ego.
36. Intellectualisation is the attribution of logical and socially desirable reasons to something you do.
37. Erikson developed his theory on the basis of the Freudian tradition.
38. Erikson spoke of psychosexual stages.
39. According to the supporters of the humanistic approach, it is the objective experiences of the individual which are of particular importance.
40. The term humanistic refers to the fact that psychology is concerned with the characteristic features of people.
41. According to Rogers, people are victims of their passions.
42. The quest for self-actualization is at the centre of Rogers' work.
43. An unconditionally positive attitude on the part of the therapist is, according to Rogers, an important precondition for the success of the therapy.
44. A person who is very insecure can experience self-actualization.

References

Atkinson, R.L., Atkinson, R.C., Smith, E.E. and Hilgard, E.R. (1987). *Introduction to Psychology*, Orlando, Florida, Harcourt Brace Jovanovich.

Bandura, A. (1977). *Social Learning Theory*, Englewood Cliffs, N.J. Prentice Hall.

Deutekom, E.J., Philipsen, H. and Hoor, P. ten (1991). Plate waste producing situations on nursing wards, *International Journal of Nursing Studies*, 28 (2), 163–174.

Erikson, E.H. (1950). *Childhood and Society*, New York, (2nd ed.), Norton.

Freud, S., (1975). *Beyond the Pleasure Principal*, New York, Norton.

Groot, A.D. de (1961). *Methodologie*, Den Haag, Mouton.

Hall, J. (1982). *Psychology for Nurses and Health Visitors*. Leicester, The British Psychological Society.

Köhler, W. (1925). *The Mentality of Apes*, New York, Harcourt Brac. (Reprint ed., 1976), Liveright.

Marriner, A., (1983). *The Nursing Process: A scientific approach to care*, St. Louis, Missouri, C.V. Mosby.

Maslow, A. (1954). *Motivation and Personality*, New York, Harper & Row.

Maslow, A. (1969). *Toward a Psychology Of Being*, New York, Van Nostrand.

Maslow, A. (1971). *The Farther Reaches Of Human Nature*, New York, Viking.

Open University, (1984). *A Systematic Approach to Nursing Care: An Introduction* (p. 553), Milton Keynes, Open University Press.

Pavlov, I.P. (1927). *Conditioned Reflexes*, New York, Oxford University Press.

Piaget, J. (1952). *The Origins of Intelligence in Children*, New York, International Universities Press.

Rachman, S. (1979). Towards a new medical psychology. In Rachman, S. (Ed.), *Contributions To Medical Psychology*, vol. 1, Oxford, Pergamon Press.

Rogers, C. R. (1959). A Theory of therapy, personality and interpersonal relationships as developed in the client-centred approach. In Koch, S. (Ed.), *Psychology: A Study Of Science*, New York, McGraw-Hill.

Skinner, B.F. (1938). *The Behaviour of Organisms*, New York, Appleton-Century-Crofts.

Skinner, B.F. (1972). *Beyond Freedom and Dignity*, (UK ed.) London, Cape.

Stafford-Clark, D. (1965). *What Freud Really Said*, Harmondsword, Penguin.

Tolman, E.C. (1932). *Purposive Behaviour in Animals and Men*, New York, Appleton-Century-Crofts, (Reprint ed., Irvington, New York, 1967)

Watson, J.B. (1913). Psychology as the behaviorist views it, *Psychology Review*, 20: 158–77.

Watson, J.B. (1950). *Behaviourism*, New York, Norton.

Module 2

DEVELOPMENTAL PSYCHOLOGY

Introduction to Module 2

In your lifetime you meet a great many people, all of whom differ from each other, not only in appearance, but also in behaviour. That behaviour is partly determined by the circumstances prevailing at the time and the involvement in them of other people.

This module focuses on the development of the individual. What caused you to develop into the person who behaves as you do now? How could others have developed into the people who behave as they do now?

As a nurse, in a profession where you continually have to deal with other people, you need to know how behaviour develops, your own as well as other people's. Developmental psychology studies the order in which that development occurs and the factors influencing it.

In the first place we will discuss the concept of *development*.

This raises questions such as *'What is development?'*, *'At what point in a life cycle does that development start?'*, and *'When does development cease?'*. Psychologists offer various answers to these questions, and in this module human development will be considered from a number of different angles.

Psychological development is considered as a continuous process, starting at conception and ending at death. During that process of development the nature of the factors influencing it changes; moreover, people react differently to the same factors. There are four ways of approaching these issues:

- *The neurobiological approach* assumes that psychological development is determined mainly by heredity and innate characteristics. Development is therefore chiefly a process of waiting for what is already present 'in the bud', but not yet visible.
- *The learning theory or behavioural approach* emphasizes the influence of environmental factors on the development of an individual. Development is seen as a process of learning. This implies that development is strongly influenced by external factors.
- *The psychoanalytical approach* ascribes most influence to those bringing up children (therefore often their parents) during certain important stages of childhood. These stages are biologically predetermined. Aptitudes and environment are both important. The environment, however, (personified in those bringing up the children) leaves a particular mark on the early years of childhood.

– *The cognitive approach* directs attention to the development of knowledge and thought. This enables an individual to get to grips with his environment. Major biologically determined events are also important in the development of knowledge and thought.

A correlation of these different approaches presents the process of psychological development as an interaction of factors relating both to innate characteristics and to environment. We can call this the *interactive approach*.

Secondly, we will describe how the development process takes place during the life cycle of the individual. In this life cycle a number of phases can be distinguished which, in this book, are related to important problems an individual has to solve during various stages of his life.

When discussing the phases of development there is a need to identify periods. These periods may be identified in terms of age ranges and/or descriptions (e.g. pre-school child, adolescent). In this text we give both age ranges and descriptions. The age ranges attached to development phases are approximations and are more likely to receive general agreement in the earlier phases discussed than in the later ones. We accept this point and give the ages as *suggestions* for the staging of development and not as being *specifically* indicative of the particular phase.

1

Human development

1. Introduction

People are continually changing. Spectacular changes occur especially during the first few years of human life. Those changes which are age-related in particular can be assumed to be progressive. The concept of development therefore applies here too; the changes continually raise a human being to a higher and more complex level of performance.

In this chapter the psychological development of the individual is discussed from the point of view of:
– physical development;
– social and emotional development;
– cognitive development.

Psychological development is examined on the basis of four of the psychological approaches described in Module 1:
– neurobiological;
– psychoanalytical;
– learning theory (behavioural);
– cognitive.

None of these four approaches is identified in this module as being better than the others.

It is an accepted fact that an individual develops as a result of the continuous interaction of innate characteristics and environment. It will be shown that the relative importance attached to either innate characteristics or the environment determines the preference for one of these psychological approaches.

It is a mistake to think that developmental psychology is important only in paediatric nursing. In fact, human development is a process which continuous throughout the entire life cycle. In order to achieve a personal approach to a patient it is essential to have an understanding of the specific processes of development in the various stages of human life.

Learning outcomes

After studying this chapter the student should be able to:
- name and describe four features of the concept of development;
- indicate the subject matter of the study of developmental psychology;
- distinguish between three aspects of psychological development and subdivide the whole process of human development into ten phases;
- describe the central problem of development in each phase and name three features of this division of phases;
- list four approaches to the process of development and indicate the essentials of each approach;
- indicate what is meant by the interactive approach to the development process.

2. Characteristics of psychological development

You are working as a nurse in a hospital ward. In one of the rooms there are two patients, both of them seventy-five years old. One of them was born in a town, the other in the country. They have had a different education and worked at different jobs. One has been married for fifty years and has five children. The other has had a number of relationships, but no children. It is striking how two men of the same age can be so different from each other. One wants to leave hospital as quickly as possible, is cheerful, optimistic and full of interest for everything that goes on in the world. The other is silent and resigned, can see nothing to look forward to, and makes heavy work of his rehabilitation.

After reading this short case study, with its stereotyped examples, you can ask yourself several questions. How is it that people are as they are? How did they get like that? What course did the process take? Were there specific events which gave their life that particular direction? How much have they themselves influenced this development? What other factors have played a part? Were their different origins a factor? What was the role of their upbringing? Or was it through friends, more or less chance-met, that their paths took certain turns? Or did the women they knew have a great influence? Is it possible to determine at all what has moulded them into what they are?

It is, of course, impossible to give a concrete answer to all these questions. But that is not the crux of the matter. What is important is that by asking such questions you begin to wonder what factors play a role in human development. The concept of *psychological development* has not been around for very long. Only in the last three centuries has a difference been made between an adult and a child, from a psychological point of view. Before that there was only one view: that of an adult. From a social and emotional viewpoint, small children were treated like

Figure 2.1.1
Dressed like an adult, treated like an adult

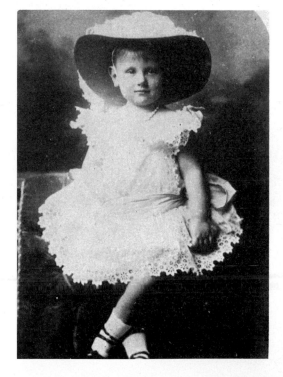

adults, albeit physically immature ones (figure 2.1.1). Children shared completely in adult life. They were involved in all aspects of daily life and nothing was kept hidden from them.

Gradually it was realized that the road to maturity was one of development, and that different phases could be discerned in that development. For example, for a young child aged between one and four, becoming toilet-trained (social and emotional development) is very important; the child learns to speak (cognitive development) during the same phase.
The pre-school child begins to leave her familiar environment and learns to associate with other children and adults. She has to learn to adapt to others (social and emotional development); she also learns to think rather more logically than the younger child (cognitive development).

In the last few decades the prevailing view has been that development does not stop in adults, but continues up to an advanced age. Whether it is still possible to call it development, in the sense of progress, is sometimes questionable. In the last phases of the life cycle there can be a painful break-down of mental functions, as, for instance, in dementia. But it is also possible for an individual to gain in emotional maturity and understanding of human relations until a very advanced age.

Study activity
 1. Describe the most important characteristics of the concept of development, basing your response on your own psychological development.

The most important characteristics of the development concept are:
a. Increasing complexity
   The result of a step forward in development is always more complicated than the situation existing before that step. When a child has learnt to read at school, she has progressed further in a cognitive sense than before she could read.
   In the course of her life, an individual's behaviour therefore shows ever-increasing complexity.

b. Irreversibility
   Once a certain stage of development has been reached, it cannot be reversed, except in very exceptional circumstances. It is not possible to go back to an earlier stage. Once you have learnt to read, you can no longer go back to the stage of 'not being able to read'.
   Equally, we are not really able to imagine how we would have faced a stay in hospital at the age of three. We can try, but to think in the same way as we did as a three-year-old is impossible. Irreversibility of development means that the changes taking place are permanent.

Study activity
 2 **a.** Give examples of changes in behaviour which can no longer be reversed, and which therefore fit into the concept of development formulated here.
   b. Give examples of changes which can be reversed, and therefore do not fit into this concept.
   c. What influence do changes of this second kind have on an individual's development?

c. The development process moves in phases
   Most theories of developmental psychology recognize moments in human development when important steps forward are made. By steps forward we mean the transition from a lower level of development to a higher level. These steps can occur at irregular intervals, and this is described as development proceeding by stages. The various approaches do not agree about the points at which these irregular advances are made. Characteristics of a development proceeding in stages are:
   – Every individual goes through the stages in the same order. You are never first an adolescent and then a toddler. What does vary is the speed at which you pass through the various phases. Moreover, a temporary relapse in development can occur in certain circumstances.
   – Within each phase itself there is at first a kind of supplementary development. This means that an individual always develops

horizontally first; she increases her knowledge and skills on the same level. Only when she has acquired sufficient knowledge and skills at that level is she able to move on to the next step. She is then ready to go on to integrate her new knowledge and skills: she develops vertically.

Study activity
3. It is argued in paragraph b above that the irreversibility of changes is an important characteristic of development. In paragraph c it is stated that a relapse is, after all, possible in certain circumstances. Explain this apparent contradiction and illustrate your explanation with an example.

d. Development consists of several processes
Three processes play an important part in development: growth, maturity and learning. *Growth* relates to the increase of purely physical qualities in people. They grow taller, stronger, they learn better muscle control. *Maturity*, on the other hand, refers to the increased potential for behaviour as a result of growth. They can only learn to walk when their motor skills have developed sufficiently. Finally, *learning* relates to the influence upon them of the environment. Clearly, these three processes are inextricably bound up with each other. On the one hand, a child whose vocal chords have not yet developed sufficiently cannot learn to speak; on the other hand, a child who has never been spoken to by anyone, will never learn to speak of her own accord.

Study activity
4. Describe the relationship between growth, maturity and learning in four different phases of someone's life.

These characteristics of development lead us to the following definition of developmental psychology. Developmental psychology is that field of study within psychology that is concerned with the development of human behaviour. In this definition development is considered to be an irreversible process that starts at conception and progresses in stages until death.

Within development there is an increasing complexity in the way humans function, as a result of growth, maturity and learning.

The phrase developmental psychology is normally only used for the period up to adulthood. This is also the part of the life cycle where most research has been done. In this book however, the psychological development of the adult is also studied from the commencement of adulthood through to the ageing years.
Human behaviour covers a large area. We therefore wish to distinguish three aspects of it and the development of each of these is discussed separately in this module.
- Physical development
  This covers such matters as physical growth, sensory perception, motor skills, development of the nervous system and sexual development. These points are, of course, interconnected, just as there is a connection between this aspect of development and the other two.
- Social and emotional development
  Under this heading we discuss such questions as the development of a relationship with parents and carers, the origins and development of self-awareness and identity, and relationships with other people.
- Cognitive development
  This aspect of development describes the development of skills such as thinking, perception and communication.

Study activity
5. Give an example of the links between the development of various elements within each of these aspects, and of the links between the three aspects.

Critical periods
A well-known concept, originating from ethology, and one which can be used to explain certain processes of development, is the critical period. The critical period is a particular short timespan in life during which the individual is sensitive to specific environmental influences. There are obviously several critical periods in a lifetime.

In the psychoanalytical approach, for instance, it is assumed that a child can learn how to associate with members of her own sex during a particular phase of development. If, for any reason, this does not happen during that phase, then it will not be easy to make up for this lost opportunity. Establishing and maintaining relations with members of the same sex will always remain a problem for such a person.

In ethology the critical period is that limited timespan in which a specific pattern of behaviour in an animal is aroused by the appropriate stimulus. The best known example was given by the ethologist Konrad Lorenz (figure 2.1.2). A new-born gosling will always follow the first moving object it sees when it is hatched. Usually this is its mother and then all is well. On one occasion Lorenz put himself in the place of the mother goose when her eggs hatched, with the results that the goslings followed him wherever he went (Lorenz, 1965).

In human development, too, several critical periods can be distinguished. For example, there is a theory that people can learn a language best between the ages of two and twelve. The human brain is thought to be most receptive to language information at that time. Later, of course, you can still learn a language, but it takes far more effort.

It is sometimes argued that a human being should receive specific stimuli at particular times, especially in the area of social and emotional development (see above for an example from the psychoanalytical approach). For instance, a child should acquire a sense of trust and security in other people at a very young age. If this does not happen, she will be basically distrustful of other people in later life and feel insecure in their presence. This attitude to other people can, of course, have a very strong influence on her behaviour towards them.

Study activity

6. If you agree with this reasoning about the relationship between the time at which things happen and their influence on the causes of problems, this can have an important bearing on the provision of help for people with these problems.
   Can you explain how?

Figure 2.1.2
Konrad Lorenz and
his geese

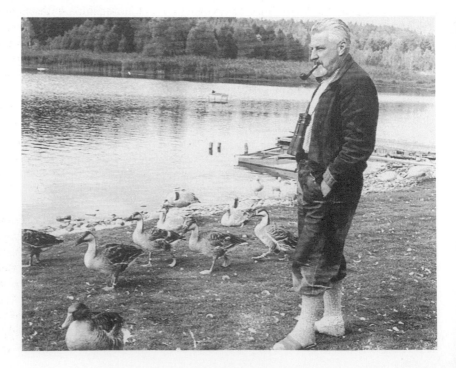

Classification of phases

Our classification of phases is based on the particular social problems confronting people at different phases of their life. Development in the sense of transition from one phase to another means 'having more or less solved or coped with the problems occurring in the previous phase'. This approach leads to the following classification:

– *The prenatal period*

This phase starts at conception and ends at birth. During this period attention is focused on the physical growth of the unborn child.

– *The postnatal period*

This phase starts at birth and ends six weeks later. The focus is on the child's entry into the world and her reception in her environment.

– *The first year*

The first year of life is dominated by dependence on the social environment.

– *The young child*

This phase, which lasts until about the fourth year, is dominated by the acquisition of a relative independence and identity (that is to say: having some idea of who you are yourself) in a restricted and protective environment. The young child acquires basic skills to enable her to function with some degree of independence outside her own protective environment.

– *The pre-school child*

In this phase the child begins to leave her familiar, restricted and secure environment. It is a period of transition from being a little child to becoming a schoolchild.

– *The schoolchild*

During this phase, lasting up to about the age of twelve, the child gains extensive knowledge of the world around her.

– *The adolescent*

This is the phase of identity formation; its duration tends to vary from person to person and is dependent on a large number of factors. In several areas the adolescent has to take decisions which determine the course of the rest of her life.

– *The young adult*

This phase lasts until about the age of forty. The young adult's task in life is to find her place in society. Some of the decisions made during adolescence give direction to this quest.

– *The older adult*

From about the age of forty the dominant feature in the life of an individual is stability. This stability, however, is one partly enforced by society.

– *The ageing years*

This phase, which starts around the age of sixty-five, heralds a period of reorientation for the individual in society, while there are also clear physical, social and emotional, and cognitive changes.

In determining these phases of psychological development, it is important to keep three points in mind. First, this division is not strictly tied to age groups. The moment of transition from one phase to another depends on the individual life cycle. In the early phases from birth to twelve years there are probably greater similarities in timespan and the beginning and end of phases among children, than in the later phases. This results particularly from the fact that young people's lives are more strongly governed by factors which are outside their own control, than is the case with older people. Older people are more self-sufficient and independent than children when it comes to making vital decisions.

It should also be remembered that a certain amount of time is needed to move from one phase to another. No-one moves from childhood to adolescence overnight.

Secondly, this particular classification of phases has both temporal and cultural parameters. It is based on the social aspects of the life of individuals. At certain times society makes certain demands on people which they then must try to comply with. However, society changes in the course of time; the demands it makes are therefore continually changing.

Society also differs from culture to culture. A classification of phases for people living in Africa will clearly differ from ours, which has been based on our western society. Situations could even be imagined where within the same community individual classifications would have to be employed for various groups, if these groups were sufficiently different from each other.

Study activity

7. Assuming that a classification of phases has temporal and cultural parameters, what phases could you suggest for:
   - someone living in the third world;
   - a child in London who has been homeless since the age of twelve;
   - yourself?

A third characteristic of this classification is that the phases always have to follow the same sequence. In each phase problems confronting the individual in society have to be solved. Only after that will the problems of the next stage become apparent. The way in which problems are solved in one phase, often determines the course of the next one.

3. Approaches to the development process

In Module 1, Chapter 2, five different approaches to psychology were described in detail. The four that take a clear-cut view of the development process are summarized here. Each of these approaches attaches importance to specific factors, or groups of factors, influencing the development process.

Study activity

8. Indicate which groups of factors are especially important to the following approaches:
   - the neurobiological;
   - the psychoanalytical;
   - the learning theory (behavioural);
   - the cognitive.

a. The neurobiological approach

This approach holds that psychological development is determined by an individual's innate characteristics. Heredity plays a role here, but also events during pregnancy. If a pregnant woman smokes, drinks or uses medication this can have an influence on the unborn child. Development therefore is more than a matter of growth. Whether someone is clever or stupid, active or passive, lazy or hard-working is determined by her innate characteristics. This is not really a matter of personal choice or contri-

bution. The environment only offers the individual the opportunity to exploit the properties and qualities which are already present 'in the bud'. You would, for instance, never be able to teach a mentally handicapped child to read a difficult book on mathematics. On the other hand it is quite possible for a normal, intelligent child never to learn to read. If such a child never attends a school or sees a book, she will never acquire the ability to read.

The neurobiological approach attempts to show that there is a close relationship between biological and psychological processes. One of the consequences of this approach is that a psychological property such as temperament is determined by heredity. Temperament covers, among other things, the level of an individual's activity. How active is she in her environment, how quickly does she react to stimuli? A fast reaction would be a feature of her nervous system. Temperament is thought to play a role in the development of thought. Active, temperamental children will acquire knowledge from

Figure 2.1.3
Susan is old enough for potty-training

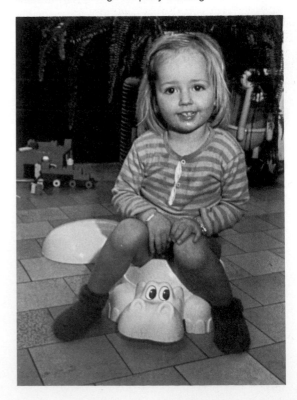

their environment faster and earlier than passive children, because they react to the stimuli from their environment faster. Research suggests more and more that dominance is an inherent characteristic. In summary, it could be stated that in theory a number of aspects of human behaviour are predetermined, or at least that there is a pre-existing foundation for those aspects.

The extreme conclusion of this approach, that all psychological qualities of an individual are determined biologically, is not currently accepted. Influenced by social developments in recent decades, this approach became less popular, but is now coming back into favour. Based on research in physiological psychology and socio-biology, the idea that individuals possess innate characteristics is again gaining ground (see Eysenck, 1987).

Study activity

9. Indicate the social consequences of taking the neurobiological approach to its logical conclusion. Also indicate the consequences of such ideas for the practice of nursing.

b. The psychoanalytical approach

Three features of the psychoanalytical theory are emphasized which can be of particular importance in understanding development processes.

- The basis of personality and therefore of later behaviour is formed in early childhood. In this period the way in which children express themselves is determined mainly biologically. The parents' handling of these expressions determine the behaviour and personality shown later.
- The individual and in particular the child seeks to satisfy her desires. The need for satisfaction is aroused by drives of a biological nature.
- The individual does not always understand the 'why' of some of her behaviour. This is known as the principle of the subconscious.

These three points determine the development and functioning of the psychological structure of the individual. This psychological structure is three-fold.

- The unreasoning id, primarily directed towards satisfaction of the senses.
- The reasoning ego, which takes into account reality and tries to compromise between the needs of the id and the demands of the superego.
- The superego, which represents in the individual society's norms, values and ideals.

The concrete experiences of the early childhood years, and during some of the important phases after that, determine the psychological development of the individual. Earlier theories within this approach set an end to development after what was called the puberty phase. Later theories, among them Erikson's (1950) well-known theory of developmental psychology, also recognize development processes among adults and older people. Major events occuring during the various developmental phases give this process direction. The approach is normative, that is to say, it distinguishes between good and bad development. In other words, the psychoanalytical approach prescribes what a healthy psychical development should be like. In a psychically healthy person the id has the upper hand in the psychological structure. The ego should determine the concrete behaviour of a human being, taking into account the needs of the id and the demands of the superego. Within developmental psychology this approach plays an important role. Its emphasis on social and emotional aspects of the behaviour of those caring for the child in the first years of life is especially valuable.

c. The learning theory approach

The learning theory or behavioural approach starts from the assumption that almost all human behaviour is learnt. The neonate's development is influenced by factors in his environment. This process follows fixed rules: the principles of learning.

First something about learning. By learning we mean far more than the kind of learning that goes on at school. It is a process in which behaviour changes as a result of experience. John Watson, one of the first supporters of the learning theory approach, claimed: 'Give me a dozen healthy infants. Let me rear them myself in my environ-

Figure 2.1.4
Playing and learning at
the same time

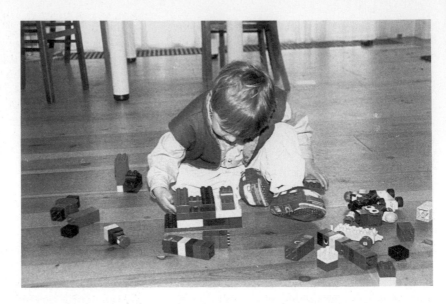

ment. I assure you, that I will bring them up to be doctors, lawyers, artists, beggars, merchants or thieves, as I choose' (Watson, 1950). Watson assumes that, if you control someone's environment, you control her behaviour and her development. He does not attach much value to the influence of innate characteristics or to all the physical properties making up the individual. Innate characteristics only indicate the parameters for the potential behaviour of the individual.

The supporters of the learning theory approach have, however, become convinced of the influence of an individual's physical capabilities on learning behaviour. Everyone realizes that the ability to control bladder and bowels is an important condition before starting on toilet training. Equally, it is not possible to train someone who is totally colour blind as a telephone fitter, because she would never be able to distinguish the differently coloured wires. However, within the limits set by the physical capabilities of the individual, the influence of environmental factors is decisive.

In this context, the environment has to be interpreted very widely. It can consist of physical circumstances, such as the climate and area where you live, the air you breathe, your pattern of nourishment, and so on. Psychological and social circumstances (such as specific events, the friends you make, the way your parents bring you up, and so on) are also part of it.

Within this approach, development is seen as a process involving a continuous interaction between the growing organism and its physical, psychological and social environment.

Learning can take place in various ways. The best known are:
– *Classical conditioning*, by means of which, for instance, a child learns to be frightened of the dark.
– *Operant conditioning*, by which, for instance, a child learns to beg for sweets.
– *Vicarious learning*, by which, for instance, a child learns specific gestures.

Within the developmental process these three ways of learning complement each other (for a further elaboration of these see Module 1, Chapter 2).

Study activity
10. Is patient-oriented nursing possible if the nurse adopts the principles of classical or operant conditioning for learning and unlearning behaviour? The patient is in that case surely no longer free to choose ... or is he? Explain your answer.

Within this approach, development is seen as a continuous process which is influenced by the environment. This could therefore mean that events in society demand a sudden adaptation of behaviour, such as, for instance, having to go to school at the age of five. Development also goes on throughout life and its results are also dependent on variations in the environment.

d. The cognitive approach

You might think that your behaviour is in part determined by what you know, or think you know. In that case you are taking a cognitive approach to your behaviour. In this approach the elements are the cognitions with which an individual works. Cognitions are impressions, interpretations, thoughts and knowledge acquired when we make contact with our environment. In this context your cognitions *vis-à-vis* yourself and other people, i.e. your social cognitions, are particularly important. For example, you can see yourself as being stronger or better than other people. In particular, the origin of cognitions is of primary importance.

All these elements can be described and categorized into structures of a higher order. This happens by means of certain organization processes. The cognitive approach to development holds that these organizational processes determine the process of the individual's development.

Through organization of her cognitions, an individual can get to grips with her physical and social environment and cope with that environment. The process of development then consists of achieving ever higher levels of these organizational processes. Eventually an individual acquires certain strategies, which she uses to organize her environment, so that she can cope with it. This organizational process can be fitted into a classification by phases. Jean Piaget, the Swiss biologist and psychologist, produced a very well-known system of phases to describe the cognitive development process (Piaget, 1952).

The cognitive approach to development should, however, be clearly distinguished from cognitive development. Every human being goes through a cognitive development in his life. A four-year-old child will assimilate information differently from an adult of twenty-five. This difference will be explained in turn in the light of each of the approaches discussed so far.

Cognitive development is just one aspect of development.

The controversy between nature and nurture

For several decades the controversy between nature and nurture has been a major element in discussions on developmental psychology. Is an individual the product of heredity and innate characteristics, or of the environment in which she grew up? We will explain this controversy by the example of human intelligence.

The nature concept of intelligence presupposes that heredity is largely responsible for the differences observable between individuals. A. Jensen, the psychologist and well-known advocate of this theory, held as an axiom that 80% of intelligence is determined by nature. This means that intelligence is a human quality, which develops almost completely independently of the influences of the environment or personal input (Jensen, 1969).

Research with rats demonstrated that it was possible to breed 'clever' and 'stupid' rats. Cleverness and stupidity were assessed by the rat's ability to learn the way through a maze. The 'clever' rats learnt faster than the 'stupid' rats.

Research with identical (monozigotic) and fraternal (dizigotic) twins and adopted children also indicates that heredity plays an important part in the development of intelligence. The similarity in the IQ of both members of a set of identical twins who were reared in different families was larger than that of fraternal twins who were reared in one family. In IQ scores, adopted children resembled their biological parents more than their adopted parents (figure 2.1.5).

Not every follower of the nature theory agrees with Jensen's figure of 80%, although they do agree that in the development of intelligence, greater importance should be ascribed to nature than to nurture.

In most cases they refer to the same research, but differ in the interpretation of the results.

Study activity
11. Analyse critically the nature concept of intelligence. Justify your analysis with arguments and examples.

Psychologists supporting the nature concept maintain that there is a relationship between heredity and aspects of personality such as temperament, dominance, and being introvert or extrovert (Eysenck, 1965).

The main problem in this kind of research is the difficulty of comparing like with like, because definitions of personal qualities are so diverse.

The nurture concept of intelligence, with supporters mainly among the learning theorists, holds that intelligence is determined by a number of very diverse environmental factors. These factors are already present during pregnancy in the shape of nourishment, medication or possible oxygen shortage, but especially after the child's birth, her environment, in the widest sense of the word, is very important. Research shows that such matters as upbringing, education and social milieu have a great influence on the development of intelligence.

Baby biographies of children in extreme conditions show how far they have adapted themselves to those conditions. The examples of the so-called 'wild' children, who grew up amongst animals (apes and wolves) and adopted animal behaviour are well known.

Study activity
12. Critically examine the nurture concept of intelligence. Justify your analysis with arguments and examples.

In contrast to the psychologists supporting the nature theory, who limit their argument to only a few human characteristics, those psychologists supporting the nurture theory hold that nearly all aspects of personality are formed through contact with the environment.

Figure 2.1.5
Results are based on 52 investigations of 99 groups. The greater the correlation coefficient (from .00 to 1.00), the stronger the link between genotype relationship and IQ

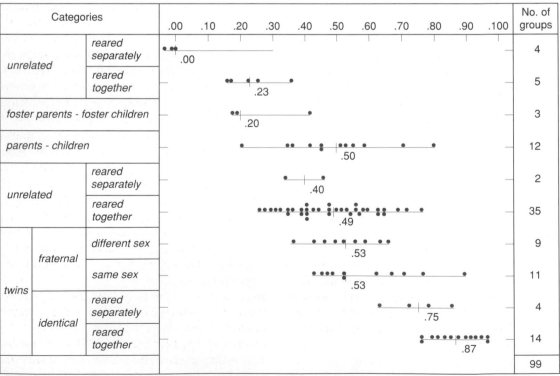

The correlation coefficients of each group are shown by red dots, the median for each range is shown by a vertical stripe (data collected by Erlenmeyer-Kimling and Jarvic in 1963)

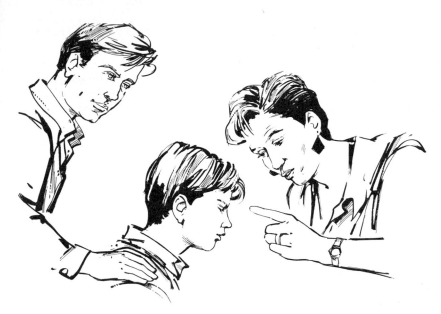

Figure 2.1.6
Painful, instructive,
loving: but what do
they mean?

Current research methods cannot resolve the controversy between nature and nurture.
At the moment most psychologists do not assume 'either/or', but prefer an approach combining both theories. Both nature and nurture influence the development process. The danger of the combination theory is, however, that nature and nurture are seen as functioning independently from each other. Nature would be exclusively responsible for the development of one trait, whereas nurture would be exclusively responsible for another. All behaviour could then be categorized in terms of 'caused by nature or nurture'.

e. The interactive approach

All the approaches discussed so far contain a core of truth. Separately they cannot explain all developmental processes, but only sections or parts of certain processes.
We therefore prefer an approach in which all these different theories have their place. This can be called the interactive approach, because it integrates the classical approaches and removes their contradictions, resulting in a theory of a higher order.

The development process is said to be approached interactively if a variety of factors play a part in that process. These factors can complement each other, or act in parallel, but they can also occur in a highly complex interaction. In short, if you want to explain someone's psychological development, you can never refer to any one event, one quality, or the influence of one person; which is exactly what the approaches mentioned earlier do. However, you can explain development by looking at the interplay of different possible factors. The words 'possible factors' are used advisedly here, because it is never possible to say with complete certainty exactly what role is played by which factors. The interactive approach certainly makes it more difficult to explain the development of an individual. The interplay of different factors has to be taken into account. A psychologist with a psychoanalytical orientation would explain bedwetting by a seven-year-old as regression. An interactionist psychologist would also take into account any changes in the child's circumstances and her parents' reactions to the bedwetting.
Interaction of several different factors does not mean, for instance, that the child's innate characteristics are responsible for 30% of this behaviour, and the parents for 70%. Interaction means that, given a child of this personality, the particular behaviour of the parents in these specific circumstances led to her particular behaviour. If

any of these factors changes, for example, the child's personality, her parents' behaviour or the circumstances, then the resulting behaviour may also change.

Study activity

13. Describe in outline how you have arrived at your present behaviour in your current phase of life, choosing any three of the approaches named: the biological, the psychoanalytical, the learning theory, the cognitive and the interactive.

4. Summary

In this chapter the concept of psychological development has been outlined.

Development has the following characteristics:
- the individual becomes more complex during the course of her life;
- a return to an earlier stage of development is impossible, except in exceptional circumstances;
- different stages can be recognized in development, characterized by particular problems;
- development is based on three processes: growth, maturity and learning.

On the basis of these four characteristics we have divided the human development process into the following phases and allocated a developmental characteristic to each phase, as shown in the following table:

1. The prenatal phase	until birth	physical growth
2. The postnatal phase	0–6 weeks	entering the world
3. The first year	6 wks–1 year	dependency on carers
4. The young child	1– 4 years	acquiring independence in a protective environment
5. The pre-school child	4– 6 years	leaving the protective environment
6. The schoolchild	6–12 years	acquiring knowledge of the environment
7. The adolescent	12–22 years	identity formation
8. The young adult	22–40 years	acquiring a place in society
9. The older adults	40–65 years	achievement of stability
10. The ageing years	until death	reorientation in society

The prenatal phase: the period up to birth

2

1. Introduction

In this chapter the prenatal phase is discussed, starting with conception and ending with the birth of the child.

The prenatal phase, the period in which the fetus is in the womb, can be subdivided into the following stages:
- the ovum period (the first two weeks after conception);
- the embryo period (the second until the eighth week);
- the fetal period (up to the birth of the child).

The discussion will cover successively:
- physical development;
- social and emotional development;
- cognitive development.

Cognitive development includes a comprehensive treatment of perception.

Learning outcomes

After studying this chapter the student should be able to:
- subdivide the prenatal phase into three periods;
- indicate what growth processes take place in each period;
- indicate the most important developments in each aspect of development;
- describe three factors, which can influence a woman's experience of pregnancy;
- indicate the influence the prenatal phase could have on later social and emotional behaviour;
- indicate which two systems develop that are important for cognitive development;
- list three categories of senses;
- distinguish between five stages in the perception process;
- indicate which five laws are recognized by the Gestalt school of psychology in the perception process;
- list six factors influencing perception.

2. The prenatal phase; a brief overview

In psychology the first phase of human development is regarded as starting with conception, which thus becomes the beginning of the prenatal phase, which ends with birth. This phase is subdivided into three periods:

- *The ovum period*, covering the first two weeks after conception. During these fourteen days the cluster of cells attaches itself to the uterine wall. This is also the period in which, according to some scientists, among them geneticists and gynaecologists, experimental research may still be done on the cluster of cells, because there would not yet be any question of the presence of human life.

Study activity

1. **a.** List the various views held in our society on whether or not human life is present during the ovum period.
   b. Decide where you stand on this question.
   c. Discuss your decision and those of the others in your group.

- *The embryo period*, lasting from the second until the eighth week. During this period the cluster of cells develops very rapidly to a tiny human being approximately 3 cm long. All anatomical structures and organs are in theory already present at this stage.
- *The fetal period*, ending with the birth of the child. From the second month the anatomical structures and organs develop into those present at birth. From approximately six and a half months onwards the fetus is capable, with special care, of remaining alive outside the womb.

In developmental psychology relatively little is yet known about the prenatal phase, because it is not clear what social, emotional, and cognitive processes take place in it. Moreover, it is not known what influence this phase has on the child's later potential behaviour. Far more is known about physical development. This is why its growth within a highly protective environment, with very little personal input, is seen as the central developmental problem – if it can be called a problem, when the child itself contributes little to its solution.

Case study: Carole

During the sixth month of her pregnancy Carole suddenly had to be admitted to hospital, because she showed symptoms of labour. The doctor told her that it would be a considerable time before she could be discharged, and she might have to stay in until the baby was born. Meanwhile labour-inhibiting medication was constantly administered. This led to high blood pressure, which, together with the fact that she had to lie still for so long, did not do her any good. She became rather agitated and restless, and also worried about the influence of all this on her child. Would he notice that she was restless? She had heard that babies react to signals from outside while still in the womb; if she was so agitated, perhaps the baby was, too. She asked the doctor about this, but he just said she need not worry, and the only alternative was that the baby would be born far too early. It was all very well for him to say so.

Figure 2.2.1
So small, and yet recognizable

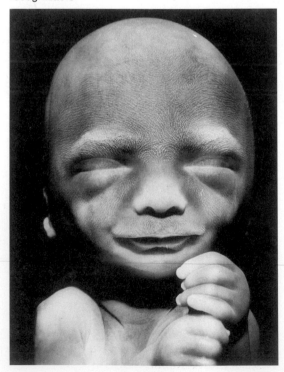

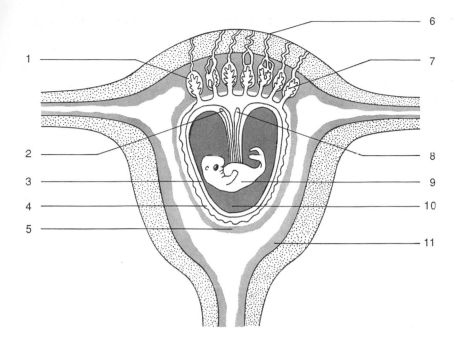

Figure 2.2.2
Relationship between
uterus, membrane and
embryo

1. Space filled with
   maternal blood
2. Umbilical vesicle
3. Amnion
4. Chorion
5. Inner membrane
   enveloping the
   embryo
6. Uterine blood vessel
7. Chorionic villi
8. Yolk sac
9. Embryo
10. Amnion containing
    amniotic fluid
11. Outer membrane
    enveloping the
    embryo

Study activity

2. **a.** Compile an information folder, with other students if possible, for pregnant women, with the aim of clearing up the many misunderstandings which exist about the influence of life-style, food, etc. on the health of the fetus.

   b. As a nurse, how would you be able to help Carole?

3. Physical development

During the prenatal phase a human being develops from a small cluster of cells to a tiny individual weighing approximately 3.5 kg, and about 50 cm long.

The embryo divides itself into three layers, from which eventually the various anatomical systems and organs are formed. These three layers are:

- the ectoderm, from which, *inter alia*, the outer layer of skin and the nervous system will develop;
- the mesoderm, from which, *inter alia*, the skeleton, the muscular, circulatory and excretory systems will develop;
- the endoderm, from which, *inter alia*, the gastrointestinal system and the respiratory organs will develop.

The embryo is attached to the placenta, which forms the connection between the protective membranes and the wall of the uterus, by means of the umbilical cord.

Substances from the mother's blood can be transferred to the blood of the embryo or fetus through the placenta. In reverse, the child returns his waste matter to the mother's bloodstream via the placenta.

Compared to the physical growth in the fetal period, the embryo, between the second and eighth week, grows extremely fast. After eight weeks even the fingers and the beginnings of genitalia can be distinguished; at the same time the basis of the nervous system is established. As will be shown later on, this is a very critical period in a pregnancy for the child's physical development.

During the fetal period, the structures and organs develop further. After four months the child's movements can be felt by the mother. There are then also outward visible signs that the mother is pregnant. At around twenty-six weeks the fetus is capable of sustaining life – albeit with specialized care – outside the protective environment of the uterus. The nervous system and respiratory organs are then developed to such an extent that they can function with assistance. Most senses can then also respond to stimuli.

Premature births

Neonates with a birth weight of less than 2500 grammes, who are born before the thirty-seventh week of pregnancy, are considered to be premature (figure 2.2.3).

We will now compare the situation of a child born after a pregnancy of twenty-seven weeks and a birth weight of 800 grammes with that of a full-term child with a birth weight of 3500 grammes.

At the moment of birth, the premature child probably has a backlog in his development when compared to the full-term child. That is not surprising, because he is in fact twelve to thirteen weeks younger. This disadvantage is usually made up within a year.

The environment in which both infants find themselves after birth is very different. The premature child will certainly have to spend some weeks or even months in an incubator. The incubator may be vital, but it is not the most ideal environment to grow up in. There is usually too much light and noise, and on top of that the child has to be drip fed. The question is how much the child is aware of all this. It is certainly true that some of his senses are already functioning.

The full-term infant is already in his own cradle and can sustain life without technical aids. Moreover, regular physical contact with his carers is possible, not only during feeding. In the premature child such contact with carers will have to take place through the ports in the incubator. An alternative which has recently reached us from the third world is the kangaroo method. In the absence of high-tech equipment, the premature child is carried around all day strapped to the body. These children have been proved to develop successfully without technical aid.

An important difference between these babies is the parental attitude. In the case of a premature baby the parents are probably still afraid of losing their child. The possibility exists and is a very real one. This birth is not a 'happy event' immediately. The infant also has to be separated for a time from his carers. How these carers cope with this situation is important, as is also whether they are capable of establishing a relationship with the infant. A full-term child normally means a 'happy event', which influences the carers' behaviour and attitude towards the child. The differences described here grow less as the period of pregnancy and the birth weight come closer to the ideal.

Because of the less than perfect situation accompanying the birth of premature chil-

Figure 2.2.3
Too small to live independently and without special care

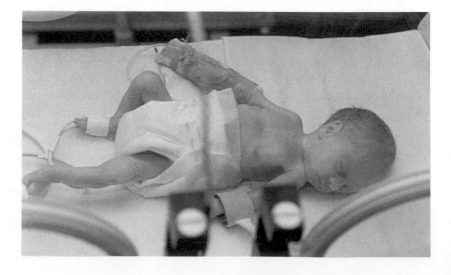

dren, the possibility of developmental problems increases. These problems can be in the areas of social and emotional, or cognitive development. There could, for instance, be relationship and learning problems. So far, research has not shown any clear results, partly because these problems only occur later in life; it is then very difficult to relate the cause to the premature birth.

In most hospitals there is an active support group for the parents of incubator babies. These groups offer parents with problems in this area the opportunity of working them out.

In the last twelve weeks of pregnancy the child prepares itself for the birth by, for example, the formation of subcutaneous fatty tissue as a protection against temperature changes, and by assuming a suitable position in the womb.

For some women pregnancy ends earlier without a living child being born. The human body often aborts an imperfect foetus spontaneously.

Study activity
   3. Suppose that you, or your partner, become pregnant. In what way would you change your life-style in order to have as healthy a child as possible? Is there a difference between intentions and actual behaviour?

4. Social and emotional development

Little is known so far about social and emotional development during the prenatal phase. The child is not yet capable of social behaviour, unless you regard his interaction with his mother by kicking in her womb as social behaviour. There is also no certainty whether the child reacts, for instance, to his mother's voice or to any other behaviour on her part. Research is currently trying to establish this.

We may, however, assume that the prenatal phase is hypothetically very important for social and emotional development.

At the very least the foundations are laid for some aspects of personality, such as temperament. These aspects or qualities play an important role in the development of the child's later social behaviour.

Apart from this, outward appearance also plays a part in social behaviour, and that appearance is formed during the prenatal phase.

In addition to heredity, which may perhaps determine aspects of personality, the following factors are also important:
   – An unwanted or undesirable pregnancy, which can cause feelings of great anxiety in a woman.
   Anxiety raises the adrenalin in the mother's blood. This adrenalin will also be absorbed into the child's blood.
   If a woman is unable to bring up her child herself, this will create a large degree of insecurity. This insecurity affects the way in which she experiences the pregnancy.
   Feelings of ambivalence and revulsion can lead to damage to the expectant mother's health and therefore also to that of the growing child.
   – The conventions and values of society.
   Society determines how a pregnant woman should behave. Consider, for instance, all the sound, and often also the very unsound advice, given to a pregnant woman.

Study activity
   4. Give actual examples of how a mother's poor health, as a result of an unhealthy life-style, can affect the development of the child's personality.

5. Cognitive development

Towards the end of the embryo period the foundations of the nervous system have been laid. The sensory system, too, begins to develop during this period. The brain – clearly vital for cognitive functioning – develops very rapidly during the second month of pregnancy. The process of maturation continues very gradually during the remainder of the pregnancy. It has been shown that babies are aware of stimuli from their environment before birth. It is even possible, apparently, to condition unborn children to certain sound stimuli. This implies that these stimuli are communicated to the brain, in a very basic form of cognitive functioning. It is, however, not likely that unborn children can perceive these stimuli. Perception implies not only an awareness of the stimuli, but also their classification and interpretation.

A fetus presumably cannot yet compare its awareness of a stimulus with an earlier awareness. The extent to which an unborn baby perceives from within its very protected environment is thus unclear.

Perception

Perception is an extremely important human function. Through perception a human being is able to absorb information from his environment. This information will influence him, so that he develops further; at the same time he is also capable of influencing that environment by making use of information acquired earlier.

We will limit our discussion here to the perceptual process itself, without considering its role in the developmental process.

Perception is a very active, and therefore subjective, process. On the one hand physiology plays a large and very important part. This aspect of the perceptual process, however, must be studied in books on anatomy and physiology.

On the other hand, perception is a function which cannot be explained without a large input from psychology. In psychology the importance of an active input by the individual during perception is emphasized.

Individual factors are responsible for the fact that people often perceive one and the same event in different ways.

In the perceptual process a large number of human senses play a role. These senses can be classified in three ways:
- The exteroceptive senses, such as:
  - sight;
  - hearing;
  - smell;
  - taste;
  - the various tactile senses, such as sensations of pressure, pain, heat and cold.
- The proprioceptive senses, such as:
  - sense of balance;
  - motor senses.
- The interoceptive senses, such as:
  - the awareness of one's own body and organs.

Through all these senses, stimuli from the environment and from the individual himself can penetrate to his consciousness. In this perceptual process the following stages can be distinguished:
- *Detection*

  In the first place the stimulus to be perceived has to be detected. Something has to be heard, seen or smelt. Whether the stimulus is detected depends on:
  - the properties of the stimulus. A noise has to be loud enough to be heard, the pressure on one's hand has to be sufficient to be felt. In psycho-physics each sense has been given so-called perception thresholds. For example, a human being can only perceive light from the visible spectrum, and not from the infrared spectrum, unlike, for instance, bees, which can. A human can also only hear vibrations with a wavelength of between approximately 20 and 20,000 Herz, while dogs can perceive sounds with a higher wavelength. A perception threshold is the minimal strength needed by a stimulus to be detected by a human being;
  - the condition of the sense. The structure and functioning of the sense naturally play an important part in the detection of the stimulus. This differs from person to person. One man's nose is more sensitive than another's, so that one man can distinguish a particular smell quicker than another. Women can see colours better than men.
- *Discrimination or distinction*

  When a stimulus has been noticed, it still has to be distinguished from other stimuli. If you listen to music, you have to be able to distinguish between the various notes. If you can not do this, as is sometimes the case with people who are partially deaf, the music sounds very flat. This stage, along with *detection* could more appropriately be called awareness rather than perception. Something still needs to be done with the incoming stimuli. In subsequent stages the stimulus reaches the central nervous system via the senses. This is where a human being processes the stimuli, albeit unconsciously, and only then can it be called perception.

– *Recognition*
In the recognition stage the incoming stimulus is compared with the information already stored in memory. Memory stores information which has come in from the various senses. Faces can be recognized, as can smells or a particular kind of stomach ache.

– *Selection*
Not all the stimuli encountered are used in perception. They are not all equally important or clear. Consider what stimuli you are subjected to through all your senses at this moment. You are only aware of a few of them. It is highly important for an individual to select from all incoming information only those stimuli which are important to him. If he did not do this, the world would become very complicated for him. This selection process is, however, not always a conscious activity. Selection is very largely determined by the factors summarized below. This process is called selective perception.

– *Interpretation and classification*
Finally, the incoming information has to be interpreted and classified. Some significance must be attached to it, or it must be linked to an emotion, and eventually it has to be named. If in the past, when you were a child, your tonsils were removed, this was probably an unpleasant experience for you, and you will particularly remember the smell of the anaesthetic used. For this reason the typical 'hospital' smell may still cause feelings of unpleasantness.

Particularly in the last three stages, recognition, selection and interpretation, a number of subjective factors are involved, especially with respect to the physical condition and the personality of the observer.

– *Sensory defects*
Sensory defects of various kinds determine whether information is assimilated and what kind of information is assimilated. Sight, for instance might be impaired. In blindness no information is transferred from the environment through the eyes. This can lead to a more extensive use of the other senses. It would certainly influence the impression one has of other people, because it would not be possible to perceive facial expressions. If you are colour blind, some information comes through, but something is missing from it. Certain colours in the spectrum cannot be distinguished from other colours. That, too, can lead to complications. A football player who can't tell green from red, will have difficulty in a match where his own team is wearing green, and the opposition, red.

– *Attention*
This factor determines whether a stimulus is noticed or not. If you are reading this with great concentration, you will not notice a number of stimuli from your environment, for instance, the sound of a passing car, or your own breathing. But if you direct your attention to these sounds, then you suddenly notice them. There are two factors involved in attention. First is the level of awareness of the observer. Someone feeling sleepy or tired, will have more difficulty in paying attention than someone alert and fit. Second, the stimuli may be so strong that they attract attention. However tired you may be, if something very exciting suddenly happens on television, you are at once wide awake and focus your attention on the screen.

– *The observer's personal attitude*
If you have a certain attitude to a situation, then that attitude will influence your perception. You can, for instance, prepare yourself for the fact that there are a great many traffic lights on a certain road. You will then not easily miss the traffic lights that are actually there. This could be called an expectation rather than an attitude. If you go to a party expecting it to be boring, you will probably find the behaviour of other people there boring. It should be understood that in this case perception is more a question of interpretation. You interpret their behaviour as boring.

– *Experience*
Knowledge or experience of something or someone influences perception of them. You can read the contents of this book, but how does a four-year-old regard it: it may as well be double Dutch. A pre-school child might hold it upside down, because he does not know what to do about those silly squiggles on the paper. By learning to read, the letters begin to mean something. Experience is important in perception, because on the strength of it many stimuli in the environment do not continually have to be re-examined from scratch. You can build on your experience and so develop a style of perception which strongly influences the whole cognitive process.

– *Frame of reference*
The background to someone's perception always plays a part in interpreting incoming stimuli. If you are working as a nurse in a ward, you will view the running of that ward differently from the patients in it.
As a nurse you have a different frame of reference than as a patient. You might consider your colleagues' laughter in the corridor to be cheerful, whereas, if you were a patient, you might call it intrusive. Even so, the same behaviour would be involved in each case.

– *Needs*
Human needs play an important role in the perceptual process. On the one hand, needs can influence perception. Someone who is hungry, will, when walking through a town, tend to notice restaurants, which he would not see if he were feeling well fed. On the other hand, perception can also influence needs. Just look for a while at TV advertisements for food, and you will be guaranteed to feel a great need for something nice to eat.

Apart from the importance given to these subjective factors, it is believed that the perceptual process is governed by a certain number of laws. These laws are the basic principles by which an individual organizes incoming information. These organized

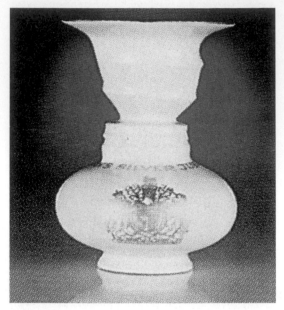

Figure 2.2.4
Form or background?

principles are known as 'Gestalt laws' – the German term 'Gestalt' meaning 'form' or 'pattern'. The main postulation of Gestalt psychology is that the whole of what is perceived is more than simply the sum of its parts. A house is more than an assembly of bricks, sand, cement, some wooden planks and a bit of glazing. We see a house, not its parts. Gestalt psychologists also maintain that an important condition of the perceptual process is that a human being always distinguishes between a shape and its background. That this is not always easy can be seen from figure 2.2.4.

The Gestalt laws of perception are rules which determine this process:
– the law of proximity;
– the law of similarity;
– the law of the 'good form';
– the law of closure;
– the law of common direction.

In all, it can be said that perception is a highly complicated cognitive process, which plays an important part in human development. A human being has a number of senses at his disposal which supply him with information about his environment and about himself. Assimilating and processing this information takes place according to certain rules, but is at the same time influenced by a number of subjective factors.

During the prenatal phase therefore, cognitive development is first and foremost a maturation process. This maturation process, however, does not always proceed without a hitch.

Study activities

5. List five factors influencing the developmental process in this phase of life.

6. List three ways in which carers can prepare themselves during the period of pregnancy to take measures to stimulate the child's cognitive development after birth.

6. Summary

From this discussion of the prenatal phase it is clear that much remains to be discovered.
It is by no means certain which factors in the mother's life-style, for instance, will positively stimulate the development of the child's personality.
In the last ten years scientific knowledge of the prenatal phase has indeed improved tremendously. However, the credit for this goes to other disciplines such as genetics rather than psychology.
In conclusion, this chapter also focuses the attention on perception as an aspect of cognitive development.

3
The postnatal phase: from birth to six weeks

1. Introduction

The postnatal phase begins with the birth of the child, not entirely a happy beginning, at least not from the child's viewpoint.

In physical development, the child's relatively diverse powers of perception are a striking feature.

In social and emotional development the pattern of interaction between child and carer is the focal point.

Special attention is also given to attachment and separation, because of the great significance attached to this phenomenon.

Finally, cognitive development during the postnatal phase is discussed.

Learning outcomes

After studying this chapter the student should be able to:
- describe the extent to which the senses are already functioning;
- indicate what differences are already clearly noticeable between babies;
- describe the role a newly-born child can play in the parent/child relationship;
- indicate the behaviour potential of a newly-born child;
- indicate what is meant by the concept of attachment;
- indicate what is meant by synchronized behaviour and the significance of this for contact between parent and child;
- define the concept of egocentricity applied to a baby's behaviour;
- describe the concept of a mental schema;
- indicate in what way a newly-born baby assimilates new impressions;
- indicate the significance of a newly-born child's smile;
- indicate the significance of crying as a means of communication.

2. The postnatal phase; a brief overview

Contractions start in the 39th or 40th week of pregnancy. They herald the end of the period of pregnancy and the start of the postnatal phase. The birth of a child is in fact the most important step in human life. It is the beginning of a life in a society – a typical characteristic of humanity. The process of birth must be a nerve-shattering experience for most people. Unfortunately you will not be able to remember how you yourself felt or what you thought; understandably so, because you had as yet no words to describe thoughts and feelings. Sounds, smells and touch would have penetrated to you, but would not yet be stored in your memory.

For babies, birth is probably not a pleasant event. The transition from the warm, protective en-

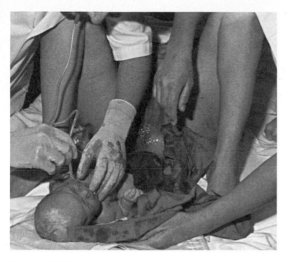

Figure 2.3.1
Birth, a traumatic event?

These two lines of conduct are central to the postnatal phase. In many countries the importance of the period around birth is recognized by government, too. Working women are given extended paid leave by their employers. In some countries this leave is longer than in others, possibly an indication of their differing views on the importance of the mother-child relationship. The postnatal phase lasts for about six weeks. By the end of this phase there will have been some stabilization of the process of interaction between parent and child and the child will have found herself a place in her environment.

In those six weeks all her senses will have started functioning, the child will have adopted a certain feeding pattern and her carers will have adapted their way of life to accommodate her needs.

Study activity

1. Describe as exactly as possible how a child might experience birth and the first few days after birth.

3. Physical development

When a child is born, the doctor assesses her condition by means of the Apgar score. A number of reflexes, such as the Babinski-reflex and the Moro-reflex are tested to see if the child's neurological development is normal. The child will already have shown certain very basic reflexes: she can breathe, blink her eyes, and suck when something is pushed into her mouth.

In general it can be said that at the time of birth all exteroceptive senses are functioning. The eyes function fairly well; the child can already distinguish different colours and variations in brightness. The ability to focus (accomodation) will not yet have developed so well; at first the child can only see objects clearly at a distance of 20 to 30 cm. This distance will gradually increase.

The child could already hear sounds when still inside her mother's womb, and will then already have become used to some extent to her voice. She can also already feel, smell and taste differences in stimuli. The sense of smell, in particular, is supposed to be fairly well developed at the

vironment of the womb to an enforced, independent existence in an alien world outside occurs suddenly and painfully. Up till now the senses have been able to develop quietly. There was little variation in the stimuli offered them: a few muffled noises, a constant temperature, the same sensations of touch and smell. But suddenly these senses are confronted with very intense and continually changing stimuli. Nearby, there is talking, crying, shouting and laughter, sometimes bright light, colours, movement and new smells. Baby is grabbed, her bottom is smacked and her throat is cleared. The tie she has with her mother is literally severed as a mark of her future independence. From now on she will have to learn to 'stand on her own two feet'.

For the people who have been expecting her, an important stage now begins. They have in their own ways prepared for the arrival of their child, and had their dreams for her. Sometimes they have already had to give up a great deal for her, or suffered pain for her.

In psychology nowadays much importance is attached to the period immediately after birth. This plays an important preparatory role for the future development of the child. Two interlocking lines of conduct are of vital importance:
– the parents' reactions to the child;
– the child's reactions to her environment, of which her parents are a part.

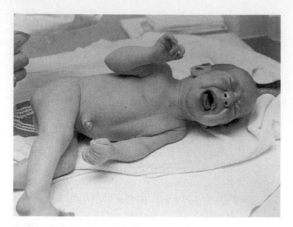

Figure 2.3.2
Not much fun, but you haven't much choice

time of birth; it is sometimes said that the first memories of an individual are memories of smell. The ability to register pain develops quickly during the first few days after birth.

In the first six weeks after birth the child grows very fast. This growth rate continues during the first year.

After birth you can already clearly establish that there are great differences between babies in their level of activity. Although a child will sleep for a large part of the day, she can be very active during her waking period: she moves, cries and looks around her (figure 2.3.2). To the distress of her carers, the child does not yet distinguish between night and day in her rhythm of sleeping and waking.

Study activity
2. List five factors which can influence development in this phase.

4. Social and emotional development

From the moment of birth, everyone engages in human relationships. Until recently, the very young child was thought by psychologists to play a passive role in building up these relationships. Communication between parent and child was thought to be one-way, implying that there would be no question of interaction in a real sense. However, nowadays it is thought that a new-born baby is far from being so passive. On the contrary, very young children have a whole armoury of movements, facial expressions and

sounds with which to provoke reactions from their parents (Korner, 1973). For evidence of this you only need to watch a baby and her parents together. We have also remarked earlier that children by nature possess different temperaments. Their temperament partly determines their activities. This temperament of the baby often persists to some degree throughout childhood (Thomas and Chess, 1977).

Study activity
3. **a.** What kind of caring behaviour is inspired by a one-month-old baby, who rarely cries, feeds peacefully and moves little?
   Describe three possible forms of behaviour.
   b. What kind of caring behaviour is inspired by a one-month-old baby, who cries often, feeds fitfully and moves about a lot?
   Describe three possible forms of behaviour.
   c. What differences are there in the forms of behaviour described under a. and b. above displayed by a nurse and, for instance, the child's mother? Illustrate your answer.

It can therefore be assumed that from birth there is a real pattern of interaction between carer and child. Bowlby (1973) even maintains that the interaction between carer and child must posses a specific quality, for which he uses the word *attachment*. By attachment he means the strong emotional ties existing between parent and child. In concrete terms this means: child and parent enjoy being physically close to each other, and make sure that they are together as much as possible. The child is selective in the people to whom she wants to become attached. During our lifetime we become attached to many people, and sometimes to animals and objects. According to Bowlby the basis for this attachment behaviour is established in the first weeks after birth. In those first weeks the child and her parents learn to tune in their behaviour to each other. This is called synchronisation. Synchronized behaviour gives pleasure to both parties and will, following the principles of learning theory, also then be repeated. As a result the child feels secure, gains confidence and builds a degree of regularity into her social behaviour. Relationships which people enter into later in life are influenced by these early experiences.

The principle of 'rooming-in' often used in hospitals in paediatric wards, is based on the assumption that the physical closeness of child and carer is good for the well-being of both.

Study activity

4. Describe from your own experience what separation feels like, when, for instance, leaving home, losing a friend or leaving a ward where you enjoyed working.

What happens if there is no attachment?

It is possible that a child may not be able to make social contacts at all, or only to a limited extent, immediately after birth. This could be because she was placed in a home, or because her carers paid her no attention at all. According to Bowlby's theory, one would have to conclude that the chances of such children entering into 'normal' relationships at a later date would be strongly diminished. Is that the case? And if so, what can be done to correct this 'negative' development?

Among the most important research into this subject is Harlow's (1959) study of the effects of social isolation on monkeys (figure 2.3.3). He separated newly-born rhesus monkeys from their natural mother and placed them in cages with two kinds of artificial mother. One was made of wire, with a nipple attached to its breast from which the young monkey could obtain its food by sucking. The other was covered with soft material but had no nipple so that the young monkey could not get its food from it. The young monkeys spent most of their time with the soft material mother and only went to the wire mother when they were hungry. If they were frightened they would also run to the soft mother figure.

In another experiment Harlow investigated the effect of complete isolation. The young monkeys were put in a cage by themselves, but were otherwise well looked after physically. The results after a few months were dramatic. The monkeys displayed a very peculiar kind of behaviour that varied from complete panic at the sight of other monkeys to inflicting injury on themselves. In the long term these monkeys were incapable of normal social and sexual behaviour. It was, however, possible to correct this behaviour by subjecting them to certain programmes of monkey therapy. This showed that the first few months after birth were a critical period for their social and emotional development. Research in this area on children shows that social isolation for a short period is detrimental to their development; it can result in a lag in physical and cognitive potential.

Social behaviour, too, was influenced unfavourably, just as it was with the monkeys. It transpired, however, that the adverse effect of long term social isolation on people can be corrected by various special measures. We must not lose sight of the fact that research situations are often not representative of reality. There are very few children who after a bad start in life end up in an ideal supportive situation. Their environment often reinforces the consequences of social isolation.

Study activity

5. Describe possible adverse effects on a child who has to stay in hospital for three months after her birth.

   Indicate, too, what you might be able to do as a nurse to minimize these consequences.

Figure 2.3.3
Harlow's monkey

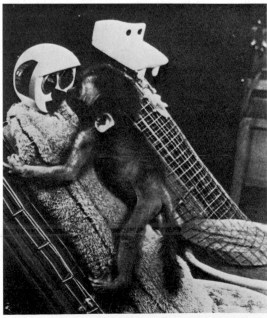

A child is very egocentric at this stage, despite her need for social contact. She demands exclusive attention and care. She is probably completely unaware that there is any difference between herself and other people. A small child looks at her hand in the same way as she looks at her rattle. Only through interaction with her environment does she develop a self-awareness, becoming aware of a distinction between herself and her environment.

Study activities
  6. Identify the difference between egocentric and egoistic behaviour.

  7. List five factors which can influence the social and emotional development of this age group.

5. Cognitive development

In the postnatal phase the child's brain is still growing. This process continues during the first year, but the rate of growth slows down. After birth the senses have to cope continually with more impressions. It appears that children can distinguish patterns of visual stimuli immediately after birth. They even display a preference for certain patterns, which include people's faces. During the first few weeks after birth the child begins to assimilate all those things that she sees regularly into mental patterns or schemata. Obviously these schemata are very simple at first and become more complicated as the child gets older. A four-week-old baby sees mainly the outlines of a face. Only when she gets older will a mouth and a nose come into her scheme (Haith, Bergman and Moore, 1977). A neonate will therefore not be quick to distinguish between people she knows and strangers by their appearance. She only does this if their appearance differs very markedly. One should not forget, that the child does not have a classification system at her disposal in which to store her experiences. A newly-born child makes completely new discoveries every day; she has hardly any past experience. Her classification system is built up only very slowly on the basis of her experiences.

Children can start to learn immediately after birth. It has been found that both classical and operant conditioning can affect them in this phase. A child will very soon make sucking movements when she sees a bottle.

Shortly after birth babies will smile at their parents. Many parents, however, are disappointed to learn that this smile should not be seen as a sign of recognition, but more as a mark of satisfaction at the pattern they see. They will also smile if you show them a piece of paper with dots on it.

Neonates have been shown to be already sensitive to a human voice, with infants as young as three days showing preference for their mother's voice against other woman (De Casper and Fifer, 1980). They may possibly have been conditioned to this during the prenatal phase.

Crying is one of the few means a baby has to show her parents how she feels. She has a variety of crying sounds, and her parents usually recognize after a while what the child means by her crying: she is hungry, feels a pain, or wants attention.

Small children can, however, also cry because they find the sound rather interesting. Later the child also learns to make sounds of satisfaction.

Study activity
  8. List five factors which can influence cognitive development in this phase.

6. Summary

'Getting acquainted' dominates the development phase immediately after birth, the first introduction of carers and child to each other.

During this phase the child is completely dependent on her carers. She is capable of only a few independent conscious actions, but she can elicit reactions from her carers by her behaviour. The interaction between both sides starts the development process. This period forms the foundation for further development.

The carers in their turn have to rearrange their lives. The newcomer has to be cared for, and demands time and attention.

The first year: from six weeks to one year

4

1. Introduction

The birth of a child is a joyous event in our society and an occasion for celebration. After the momentous event of the birth itself life goes on, and it then appears that the parents are very often just not properly prepared for the start of this new phase in their lives.

The reality of looking after the baby with its attendant hard work and responsibilities may not equate with the high expectations the parents had of parenthood. The new situation demands continuous readjustment, gaining new experience and learning new behaviour. Moreover, the parents are conscious that they are responsible for a child who is, temporarily at least, completely dependent on them.

After a brief overview the first year is described in terms of:
– physical development;
– social and emotional development;
– cognitive development.

Learning outcomes

After studying this chapter the student should be able to:
– list the six most important characteristics of physical development;
– list three factors which are important for the social and emotional development of the child, and give examples of them;
– describe and give examples of the concept of separation anxiety;
– describe four cognitive processes taking place in the first year of life;
– explain what is meant by 'memory' and define the following aspects of it:
  • memory functions;
  • sensory memory;
  • short-term memory;
  • long-term memory.

2. The first year; a brief overview

Some weeks after the birth the period of getting acquainted is over. Both parents and baby have acquired some kind of regular pattern in their daily lives. The child still sleeps through most of the day. The main occupation of the parents is changing nappies and feeding their child.

To begin with the child is still completely dependent on his parents. Any independence in his behaviour is still mostly a matter of reflexes and some instinctive sounds.

During the first year the behaviour of both parents and child is increasingly coloured by experience. The child goes through a period of vigorous growth. His muscular system gets stronger, but most of all, his ability to control his muscles increases. At some point the child can sit, then crawl and after that stand, and finally, by the end of the first year, he can walk with assistance.

There is also development from a cognitive point of view. The child's schematic perception becomes increasingly more capable of differentiation. He experiences many new things and has to assimilate them. His world is not yet very extensive; his social contacts are usually limited to his parents, but this small world is certainly as complex for the child as the big world is for us adults.

If you had to pick out a typical feature of that first year, it would be that development is within dependence. The child is dependent on his parents. They offer him an environment and experiences about which he has to do something, dependent on his nature. To the small child dependency also means protection. His

Figure 2.4.1
A small but complex world

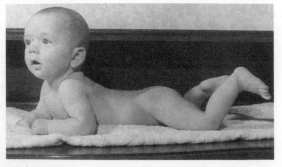

environment still takes full account of his limited capabilities and gives him the chance to allow his potential to come to maturity. The negative side of this dependency is that the child is also left to the mercies of his parents, however tender or not they may be. Dependency in the first year of life is a natural dependency, in contrast, for example, to an adult making himself dependent on others.

Case study: Nick and Betty
About six months ago Betty bore a healthy son, who was called Nick after his father.
Little Nick does not, however, distinguish between the concepts of night and day as accepted in our culture.
In the daytime he is an endearing, cuddly baby who is enjoying a well-earned rest from his nights, because at night his nibs carries on like a banshee! Indescribable ... He screams as if his lungs will burst. Things are slowly but steadily becoming quite intolerable for Nick and Betty. They are literally worn out, on edge, and see no prospect of a solution. Leave him to cry ... it doesn't help! Take him into bed with them ... the result is no better! Feed him as soon as he cries ... a disaster. The doctor thinks it will cure itself.

Study activity
1. a. List the possibilities and limitations, facing parents who have to cope with such a situation.
   b. How would you tackle this problem yourself?

3. Physical development

In his first year the child goes through a period of very rapid physical development. By the end of a year he weighs three times his birth weight and is one and a half time as tall as at birth. His physical proportions change noticeably. His legs grow very quickly, while his head, which is comparatively large at birth, becomes smaller in relation to the rest of his body. The conspicuous flexibility of his body slowly decreases, because his frame becomes more solid. After six weeks his movements, too, start to become somewhat less helpless. It is mainly his gross motor abilities that increase, as can be seen from the table on this page. It should be borne in mind that there can be considerable differences in individual performance between children. The Denver developmental screening test (Frankenberg and Dodds, 1967) is normally used to check children's behaviour at specific ages, which will show if there is a question of retarded development (figure 2.4.2).

Study activity

2. **a.** Describe the importance of the Denver development test or a similar instrument for the professional carer.
   b. What hypothetical dangers or disadvantages might be involved in such a test being applied by an amateur?

Figure 2.4.2
Physical development and co-ordination

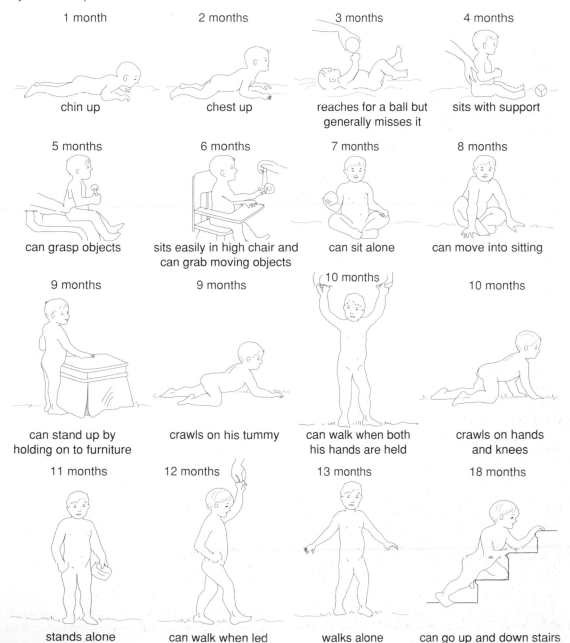

| 1 month | 2 months | 3 months | 4 months |
| chin up | chest up | reaches for a ball but generally misses it | sits with support |

| 5 months | 6 months | 7 months | 8 months |
| can grasp objects | sits easily in high chair and can grab moving objects | can sit alone | can move into sitting |

| 9 months | 9 months | 10 months | 10 months |
| can stand up by holding on to furniture | crawls on his tummy | can walk when both his hands are held | crawls on hands and knees |

| 11 months | 12 months | 13 months | 18 months |
| stands alone | can walk when led | walks alone | can go up and down stairs |

Activity	age (50% of all children)	age (90% of all children)
Sits with support	2.9 months	4.2 months
Sits without support	5.5 months	7.8 months
Stands up with help	5.8 months	10.0 months
Walks with help	9.2 months	12.7 months
Stands steadily	11.5 months	13.9 months
Walks well	12.5 months	14.3 months

Table 2.4.1 Children's behaviour potential

In general, however, research into children's behaviour potential, when related to age, shows widely differing results as table 2.4.1 indicates.

The table is based on research in America (Shaffer, 1985), and it shows that whilst 50% of children could already walk well at 12.5 months it is not until 14.3 months of age that 90% of all children can achieve this.

At first a small child can grasp objects by pressing his fingers against the palm of his hand. Only after nine months does he start to hold things with his fingers. Co-ordination of hand and eye, and fine motor system development play an important role in this. For children of 4.5 months, grasping something is a hit-and-miss affair. Later they have more sense of direction, because the child can control the movements of his hand by information received through his eyes. At approximately six months his first teeth come through.

The brain has an important function in most aspects of this physical development. It is the centre by which all movements are co-ordinated and from which orders are sent to the muscles. The brain develops very rapidly during the first year of life. At birth, it is only 25% of its final adult weight, but by the end of the first year this has already increased to 66%. The average body weight (10 kg.) is then only 14% of the adult weight (75 kg.).

Study activity
3. List five factors influencing physical development in this phase.

4. Social and emotional development

The future social and emotional behaviour of the child is for a large part determined in the first year. Important features are:
– his relationship with his parents
– his assimilation of a number of emotions

These two aspects should not of course be seen as separate issues and, particularly in the second, cognitive development plays an important part as well.

In this phase the child is mainly dependent on his parents for the fulfilment of his needs and his behaviour potential, and consequently the child develops feelings of trust and security. In the previous chapter this behaviour, linking parents and child, was called 'attachment'. Parents usually also have an idealized image of a child and try to realize that image in their own baby.
Their idealized picture can vary from that of 'an obedient, docile child' to one of an 'individualistic, independent child' or from a 'naturally naughty child' to a 'naturally good child'. Obviously these differing ideals lead to very different kinds of behaviour on the part of the parents.
The child is still egocentric. Only between the first and fourth month does he begin to realize that there is a difference between him and his environment. The realization that he is an individual comes slowly: he develops self-awareness, the beginnings of a self-image. He will not be able to recognize himself yet; if you hold a mirror to his face, he will look beside or behind the mirror for the person in it, just as a dog or a cat would.
From the age of four months a baby will also react to other babies. He will touch them or look at them, but otherwise ignore them.
From two months children develop what is called a 'social' smile. They smile at other people, because they enjoy seeing them. This is an important event in their development: people appreciate it when a child smiles at them. In their

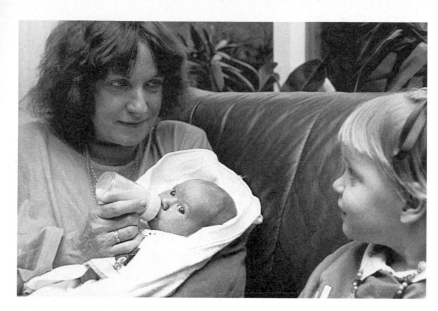

Figure 2.4.3
Attachment

turn, they will be inclined to react to the child and so increase the social contact. From six months the child's smiles become deliberate. He only smiles at certain people, usually his parents to whom he is attached. A child can become attached to more people, usually to two or three, who do not *per se* have to be his parents. They give him a sense of safety, from which the child can explore the world around him (figure 2.4.3). Two features of his parents' behaviour are important for the development of attachment in the child:
– reciprocal feelings;
– warmth.

Study activity
4. Give your opinion on the following two points and explain your point of view:
   a. Only a mother can bring up a child properly, because there is a natural tie between the two.
   b. A child will get less attention in a crèche, when both parents continue working, than at home.

The emotions shown by a child from birth up to the age of three to four months, are often related to changes in his environment and to physical experiences. If he feels well-fed, he will look satisfied and pleased, and if a large, strange object is put near him, he will cry.

After the fourth month, however, new and totally different emotions arise. These involve people in the child's environment. Usually at around six months children develop a fear of strangers. If they are approached by anyone other than their 'attachment figures' they will start to cry. The way in which a stranger approaches the child is important here. If it happens gradually and in a friendly manner, the child will often not be fearful. Compare this fearful behaviour on the part of a child with that of a dog approached by a stranger. This fearful behaviour reaches its peak around the age of one, and has nearly vanished by the age of two.

Fear of strangers has to be distinguished from separation anxiety, which starts at around eight months. The child becomes distressed when left alone by a parent. This behaviour is even more pronounced if the child is in strange surroundings or when there are strangers present. Separation anxiety reaches its peak at around fifteen months and will then gradually disappear. It is striking that fear of strangers as well as separation anxiety occurs at around the same age in most cultures. Finally, from about the eighth month a variety of fears appear, with children becoming frightened of specific things, such as dark places or some noises. After a while these fears disappear as fast as they arose. A general explanation for them may be found in the child's cognitive functioning at this age. We will examine this explanation in more depth in the next section.

Another explanation for these fears might be that situations where children are separated from their attachment figures are unusual and therefore the child feels insecure. While these people are there, the child feels at ease. The absence of familiar faces, or the too prominent presence of strangers, is associated with unease and is therefore threatening.

You can help children to forget these fears by playing games with them, such as peekaboo, and by explaining what is happening, as far as is possible at the child's cognitive level. This last is, however, not quite so feasible for children in this phase, as their language ability is still minimal.

Study activities

5. List five factors influencing social and emotional development in this phase.

6. Search your memory for examples of separation anxiety in your own experience.

5. Cognitive development

The development of cognitive functions in the first year is still mainly a process of maturing, in which reflexes and instincts still play an important part. In Section 3 we have already seen that the brain significantly increases in weight and that the nervous system develops substantially. During this year children have to assimilate a large number of impressions, and it is important to realize, that these impressions often involve things that are totally new and unknown. In a very short space of time, a child will see a large number of things for the first time in his life. He will also, albeit at his own level, very quickly start to compare new impressions with knowledge already acquired. Overall, the following cognitive processes take place during the first year:

– Children receive impressions from their environment through their senses. They will convert them into images and turn these into schemata. A three-months-old baby will therefore see a face as a circle with two small lines (the eyes) in it. It does not matter exactly

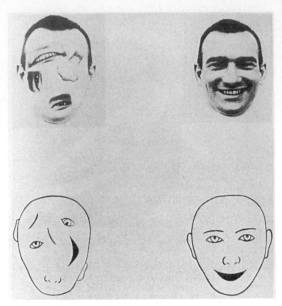

Figure 2.4.4
Schematic perception

where the lines are. Nearly every new face fits into this schema or configuration.

It can be assumed that the baby at this stage would not be able to differentiate between the faces on the left of figure 2.4.4 from those on the right. All would be as pleasing.

– As more impressions accumulate, children will begin to add finer detail. Their impressions, and therefore their schemata, are more refined. The face now becomes a face with two ovals (the eyes), a vertical line (the nose), and a wide horizontal line (the mouth) in a definite place.

At this stage the child would start to respond only to the correctly organized faces in figure 2.4.4.

– After this they form categories of impressions with the same characteristics. There is a classification of 'faces', and also one of 'warm soft hands'.

– In addition, they will also remember more impressions and for longer; in other words, memory is beginning to form.

Memory

Memory is a human function which lets you down when you most need it, and sometimes performs excellently when you do not want it to. While sitting an examination you cannot think of the right answer, even if you have just read through your notes. At the same time you cannot put out of your mind that you failed the same exam last time for the same examiner, and that knowledge makes you nervous. It is worth having a closer look at the way memory functions. It plays an important role in remembering and forgetting information which reaches us through our senses. This means, then, that not only words and images are stored in it: we also remember the smell of our parental home or the taste of asparagus. It is not yet clear exactly how incoming information is stored in the memory. For example, the DNA has a memory function because genetical information is stored in it. But information is also stored in the muscular system, because if someone who has not done any swimming for twenty years falls into the water, he will automatically make the swimming movements learnt in the past. It is probable that both neurological and biochemical processes play a part in the storage.

When information reaches our senses, it still has a long way to go before it is properly stored.

– In the first place, information reaches the *immediate* or *sensory memory*. This kind of memory holds information for a moment (approximately 0.5–4 seconds) without converting it. The capacity of this immediate memory is very limited.

– When the unconverted information has reached the immediate memory, it can be channelled on to the *short-term memory*. In this memory, which has a timespan of about 30 seconds, the information is processed and interpreted. This processing is governed by the same factors which influence perception. The short-term memory also has a limited capacity. This capacity has been demonstrated as being for 7 ± 2 items (i.e. between 5 and 9 items) which may be digits, letters or words (Miller, 1956). Information is stored in a coded form and this area of memory seems to prefer the acoustic code (e.g. the sounds of the names of the digits being remembered) although a visual code may be used when non-verbal information is being stored.

– New information entering short-term memory can upset the processing of stored information either through *displacement* or *interference*. Displacement is when more than the 7 ± 2 items are required to be stored so that some items are lost. Interference is when the coding of items is similar in the acoustic code and so the items interfere with each other causing confusion in storing. Information may also be lost due to decay, that is, as information is held only for a limited time, if we do not do anything with it, the trace of that information fades away. To keep information in short-term memory, it is necessary to re-enter (rehearse) it. When you look up a telephone number it is usual to repeat the number to yourself (rehearse), until you have dialled it. Equally, if you tell someone the way somewhere, he will remember only a limited number of left or right turns. For this reason you should never give your patient too much information at once, because it will just not fit into his short-term memory.

– Once the information has been processed, it can finally be stored permanently in the *long-term memory*. The capacity of this memory is unlimited, or at least so large that there is room for all the information absorbed by an individual in his lifetime. You may also take it for granted, however odd that may seem when you have just failed your human biology exam, that once information is in your memory, it can only be erased with the greatest difficulty. This erasure is known as forgetting. Despite this observation, it is true to say that we all have problems remembering information. Remembering turns out to be more difficult in practice than channelling information through from short-term to long-term memory. The reason why it is so difficult to remember things can be understood if the various memory processes are examined more closely.

– The efficiency of memory is affected by the processes of encoding, storage and retrieval. We have already identified that sensory memory and short-term memory are easily overloaded, and that, as far as acoustically coded information is concerned, interference from similar sounding information can disrupt the encoding and storage processes. Once information is in long-term memory then overloading does not seem to be an issue. As we said previously this memory is sufficient for all the information we are likely to receive in our lifetime.

The encoding of information for its storage is however important. Research on the recall of lists of words and sentences has shown that the preferred code of the long-term memory for verbal information is meaning, (Sachs, 1967, Kintsch and Buschke, 1969), whilst other modalites will have their own preferred codes. Other evidence for meaning as the preferred code comes from the examining of who said what to whom in real life social and political situations as cited by Neisser (1982). When encoding verbal information we often find that what we have to remember is meaningful. When this is not the case, such as when learning the names of the cranial nerves, then adding meaningful connections can improve recall (Bower, 1972). The more we elaborate this meaning the easier it becomes to recall.

− Once information is encoded and stored there may be difficulties in recalling it. The 'tip-of-the-tongue' phenomenon is one example of difficulty in recall. That we may be able to recall this information if we have the right 'recall cue(s)', or the information may simply 'pop up' when we are least expecting it even after we have strained unsuccessfully to find it, points to many of these failures to recall being related to retrieval difficulty and not loss of the information. It seems that the most important factor in the impairment of retrieval is interference. If we have associated different items with the same retrieval cue then use of that cue to retrieve one of the items may lead to the other item being recalled and so interfere with the recall of the one we want. One annoying example is when you consistently spell a word incorrectly. After learning the correct spelling, the use of the cue for that word may recall one or both forms of spelling; if both are recalled we may not be able to distinguish the correct one.

The above points to an interaction between encoding and retriceving. We have already considered adding meaning as an aid to remembering. Two other factors which aid remembering are organization and context. The more we organize information at the time of encoding the easier it is to recall and the less chance there is of interference affecting recall (Smith et al., 1978). It is also easier to recall a particular eposode if you are in the same context as that in which you encoded it (Estes, 1972). Context need not be an external factor. Our internal state at the time of encoding the information is also part of the context (Eich et al., 1975). Recalling the emotion at the time an event occurred has been shown to improve recall of the event (Bower, 1981).

Factors affecting storage of information do play a part in our ability to remember things. In the first place disturbances, such as concussion, can upset the filing processes. In that case information stored in the first two types of memory is lost, and you cannot remember what happened during or before your accident. This is known as retrograde amnesia.

In the second place problems may arise while the information is in long-term memory storage. The long-term memory appears to be subject to some kind of process of wear, which causes some stored information to be lost (Loftus and Loftus, 1980). Specific evidence for loss from storage comes from the investigation of people who receive electro-convulsive shock as a form of treatment. These people suffer loss of memory for events which occurred in the months prior to the shock but not of earlier events (Squire and Fox, 1980). It is considered that the shock disrupts the storage processes that consolidate new memories over a period of months or longer. The hippocampus (a structure located below the cerebral cortex) has been shown to be involved in this consolidation process but not to be the place for memory storage which is almost certainly the cerebral cortex (Squire at al., 1984).

An example of serious wear is dementia, in which, the latest acquired information gradually slips from the memory.

Finally, when recalling information, suppression or repression can also occur. This means that information you do not want to be reminded of, cannot be recalled. At the time you *consciously* suppress or *unconsciously* repress the unpleasant information. There is then a psychical block. Conversely, unpleasant events may make such an impression that they can never be erased from one's memory.

Through these processes a child assimilates new experiences and so acquires a better insight into the world around him and the events taking place in it. His schemata become more refined, partly because his senses are still developing and partly because he is still gathering new experiences. Moreover, you will also find that children are intensely interested in new things. Parents can encourage this interest by, for instance, choosing the kind of toys that will stimulate their child. You will soon find out whether a toy is too simple or too difficult. The child will turn away from it, and not play with it, or play with it but only for a very short time. This does not mean that this particular toy will always be suitable for one specific age. Children of the same age can differ on the cognitive level. As a carer you have to observe closely how a child reacts to a toy. If your choice of toy is governed by this observation, the child will be stimulated in his development.

Some psychologists distinguish specific important stages in cognitive development. The first to do so was Piaget. Between these stages there is a clear transition from one cognitive level to another. In the first year, the fourth month is such an important stage. Maturation of the nervous system results in a cognitive reorganization. This reorganization is also used to explain the various anxieties which arise from the sixth month. For example, a child becomes afraid of strangers, because he is able to see the difference between the face of a stranger and the schema he has formed of his parents. Separation anxiety, too, is explained in this way. The children has schemata for when their parents are away. In an unfamiliar situation they cannot use these schemata, and they become distressed. One might say that at this stage the child is only just becoming capable of recalling images from his memory to compare with the new situation. When the differences between old and new are too large, they lead to feelings of anxiety.

In the development of perception, the capacity to interpret increases steadily. In addition to the maturing of the senses and the child's innate characteristics, his experiences and the social context play a larger role: the child develops a style of perception and gradually learns what is important in his environment.

Language behaviour is, of course, important in this process. Psychologists see the first year as a pre-linguistic stage: the child is not yet able to express himself in language.

The first utterances which a child can make are crying and cooing. From the fourth month he begins to babble. At first this babbling has no particular meaning in the sense that the child wants to express something with it. Children who are born deaf also babble. From the sixth month there is a change in the babbling. Whilst at first the child simply took great pleasure in making noises, he now begins to suit his babbling to a particular situation, so his babbling probably begins to mean something. Eventually this leads, towards the end of his first year, to his pronouncing his first word. The child will, however, have been able to understand quite a few words spoken by his parents from as early as the seventh month.

The learning skills of a child increase, too. At first he will learn by means of classical conditioning. As he gets older, rewards and punishments, and therefore operant conditioning, become ever more important. There is still little question of learning by observation in the first year, because the behavioural abilities of the child are still too limited to imitate the complete behaviour of the parents.

Study activities

7. List five factors which influence cognitive development in this phase.

8. Indicate how you would act as a nurse, if the child in the case study (page 96), 'little Nick', was admitted to a ward with eight other children, and displayed the behaviour described in the case study.

6. Summary

During the first year the child is dependent on his parents for all he wants and does. They can make sure that the child feels safe and protected during this period and so builds up a solid foundation for his further development. The child's abilities, both physical and cognitive, increase, so that he will be able to cope with the problems that will face him in the next phase of his life. At the end of the first year a child is able to move around without the help of others.

He can speak one or two words, and tries to attract attention and make contact with people. However, he still needs his familiar social environment for this. From this he will try to acquire a sense of self-awareness and independence. His parents will play an important role in this, too.

The young child: from one to four years

5

1. Introduction

Parents often find the period from one to four years highly enjoyable. The children relate strongly to the parents, they are active, they like to explore, they are naughty ... All the same, during this period the child is slowly but surely being prepared to function more or less independently among her contemporaries, in the crèche and at nursery school.

Apart from the fact that parents can enjoy this phase of the young child's life enormously, the endless repetition of what was at first an amusing activity, can also drive them to distraction.

Bringing up children often causes feelings of guilt in parents. They sometimes feel afterwards that they have not succeeded in doing all they should to bring the child up 'properly'. The mixed feelings they have towards the child, of love and aggression, are often hard to digest.

The way in which a young child interacts with her parents is the subject of discussion in this chapter.

Learning outcomes

After studying this chapter the student should be able to:
- describe and explain the physical development of the young child;
- list and explain three processes which are important in the social and emotional development of the young child;
- describe in general terms the cognitive development of the young child.

2. The young child; a brief overview

At the end of the first year the child begins to stand on her own two feet – particularly in a literal sense. Even so, she feels most comfortable if her parents are near her, because strange situations involving unknown people still frighten her.

The child already knows how to indicate to outsiders what she wants and how she feels. But her radius of activity is still small and she lacks the fine motor skills to explore her world. She cannot feed herself yet and is not yet potty-trained, although her vocabulary is increasing fast, giving her improved communication skills.

In her encounters with all the demands made on her, and all the obstacles she finds in her path, the young child acquires a sense of self-reliance and a need for independence. She develops a will of her own, and exercises that will in her contacts with her parents.

A battle of wills ensues: their 'yes' is her 'no', and vice versa.

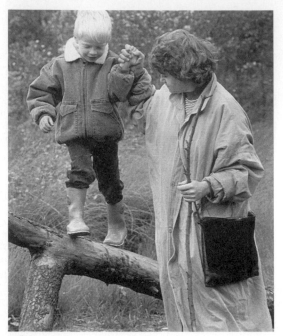

Figure 2.5.1
Learning to stand on his own feet

Play is very important in a young child's life. It is not just a pleasant occupation, but more particularly a means of learning. During this phase playing evolves from a solitary occupation to forms of play that can involve other children, too.

Social behaviour also develops in much the same way. The child develops from a highly egocentric creature to a little individual, who can recognize feelings and thoughts in others and who will even begin to take these into account.

Very many parents consider this phase of a child's life to be the most enjoyable, but at the same time it is also also the most time-consuming phase: from the age of one to four years old a child is a real tie. She wants to explore, move about, climb, offer resistance, do her own thing, but in fact needs her parents' attention for everything she does, because she is not yet able to assess her own abilities and recognize the dangers in her environment (figure 2.5.1).

Study activity

1. Describe in detail what would in your opinion be the right lines along which to bring up a young child.

3. Physical development

The extremely rapid physical growth characterizing the first year slows down to a more gradual growth. A striking feature of this gradual growth is that it does not affect all parts of the body at the same rate. The trunk grows, and then the limbs. However, during this phase the body is as yet far from achieving the proportions of an adult.

The uncertain, staggering gait of the one-year-old turns into the sure, almost adult walk of the four-year-old. Walking is an extremely interesting activity for a young child, one in which she has great scope for experiment. Fortunately it does not hurt too much when she falls, and if she falls she gets a comforting cuddle from her parents. Her legs can also take her to all kinds of places worth exploring. Hospitalization in this phase can therefore not only have a negative effect on her motor development, but can also be responsible for delaying other aspects of development, because the child misses out on some potentially stimulating situations.

Figure 2.5.2
Learning to climb the stairs

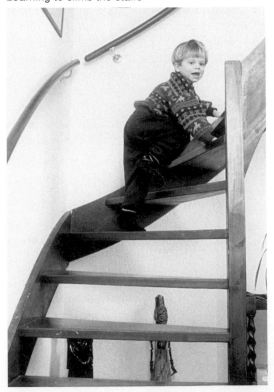

Study activity

2. Observe how children of different ages go up and down stairs. Describe the ways in which they do this (figure 2.5.2).

During this phase children begin to draw, thanks to a marked improvement in the co-ordination of hand and eye. Even so, noticeable differences can be seen in drawing skills (figure 2.5.3). Some children aged four still scratch all over the whole sheet of paper, pencil clasped in their closed fist, whereas others at the age of three can already draw crude figures, holding their crayon between thumb and index finger. Finer movements are still difficult for three-year-olds, which is clear from the trouble they have in doing up buttons, and tying up shoelaces. Even older children still sometimes have difficulties with this, to the dismay of schoolteachers in the bottom classes of the primary school.

Development of the brain, which at the age of two has reached 75% of its eventual weight (a two-year-old's weight is on average 20% of his adult weight), affects particularly those parts concerned with language and speech.

Because of the fact that motor skills have developed substantially, a child also has a great need for physical activity. She is extremely mobile and, moreover, loves movement. Children gradually learn a variety of skills through movement, too.

Study activities

3. List five motor skills which children learn in this phase of life.

Figure 2.5.3
No complete motor control yet

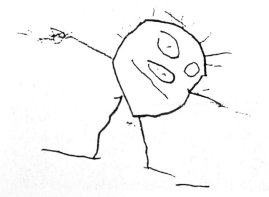

4. List five factors influencing physical development in this phase.

4. Social and emotional development

During this phase some very important things happen from a social and emotional point of view. Just as was true of attachment behaviour during the first year, it can be said that developments in this phase too are extremely important and determine factors for social and emotional behaviour in later years.

We will discuss the most important aspects.

The anxieties which determined the child's social behaviour during the first year, play an ever decreasing part. This means that other people, apart from the parents, can occupy an important place in the child's life. It should, however, be borne in mind that in this phase a child's life is still centred mainly on her parents and that strangers only play a marginal role.

The nature of her contacts, including those with the parents, is of course influenced by the child's increasing communication skills. She learns to express herself verbally, a uniquely human skill.

As the child gets older, the number of her contacts with other people, such as brothers, sisters, relatives and neighbouring children, increases.

We have earlier argued that in this phase the central problem of development lies in the acquisition of self-reliance and independence. Two processes play an essential part in this.

First comes toilet-training. At around fifteen months children can control their sphincters. Until then the excretory organs functioned reflexively. When the bladder or the bowels were full, the sphincters opened.

This is the start of a testing time for the interaction between parent and child. Her parents will try to persuade their child to relieve herself, at first only her bowels, but later also her bladder, in a specific place, usually a potty. To achieve that objective different methods can be used, labelled as potty-training, or toilet-training. This training can be done by coercion, using, for example, punishment or threats, but the child may also be allowed complete freedom to decide her own behaviour. It will be clear, that as the child is beginning to be aware of her own will and her capability for independent action, the methods of training used will have a strong influence on these developments.

Study activity

5. **a.** Describe three possible ways of training to help a child to become potty-trained. Indicate what the possible consequences of these methods could be for the social and emotional development of the child.

b. How would you, as a (paediatric) nurse, try to potty-train a child who has to spend a long spell in hospital? Explain your answer.

The child will often use toilet-training as a ploy to show her own will. This usually leads to the first clashes between parent and child. The best result of this conflict is for the child to become toilet-trained with her sense of independence and self-reliance remaining intact.

Another feature of this period is the battle of wills between parent and child, which occurs between eighteen months and three years old, and which partly coincides with the period of toilet-training: the obstinate stage. During this stage the child's behaviour is characterized by opposition to every demand or request made of her by the parent. Her behaviour is usually automatically negative and aggressive. Some children have frequent temper tantrums with which they hope to impose their will on their carers.

The obstinate stage results from the totally egocentric behaviour of the child during this phase. From birth the child is extremely egocentric in all she does, thinks and feels. By this we mean she always starts from her own central position and is not capable of putting herself in someone else's place. There are, incidentally, some indications that this egocentric behaviour does not occur in all children, but is culturally determined. The often-heard argument that the obstinate stage is essential to the development of personality would therefore be open to question. The battle of wills is fought particularly about everyday matters, such as eating, sleeping, and calls of nature.

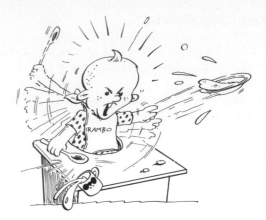

The obstinate phase

Parents play a central role in the process of learning to become self-reliant and independent. From their point of view, the child, once so sweet and dependent, has become a small individual who lets them know that she can and wants to do some things herself. She will try to impose her will on others. She often still has an enormous drive for activity and wants to investigate everything, preferably in her own way. Her parents will have to decide on their own behaviour in this process. Do they adopt a restrictive stance, that is to say, do they limit the child's capabilities to those they consider right and admissable? Or are they permissive, allowing the child to carry on as much as possible in her own way, and only protecting her from her most serious mistakes?

Study activity

6. For both of the above behaviour strategies, consider what possible consequences there might be for the social and emotional development of the child and the life of the carer.

In general it could be said that children in this phase of life need to know where they stand. This means that parents must always be consistent in their behaviour, however difficult this might often be. The way in which this consistency is shown, whether restrictively or permissively, depends on the image and the expectations they have of the child and her upbringing. In any case a child is not yet capable of coping with inconsistent behaviour and uncertainty.

Case study: James

James: 'I'll only eat peas today.'

Mother: 'Today? And all other days of the week, too. That's silly. Today you're going to eat cauliflower.'

James: 'Cauliflower ...! Ugh. It's horrid. Ugh ... very horrid. I like peas.'

Mother: 'James, I won't stand for this any longer. Either cauliflower, or nothing.'

James: 'Peas.'

James goes off, leaving his mother bewildered. In the past three months that boy has eaten nothing but peas. His insides must be green. He refuses to eat any other vegetables, whether I use force by punishing him, holding his nose and stuffing it into his mouth ... nothing helps.

Study activities

7. What would you do, if you were in James's mother's place. Explain your answer.

8. How would you as a nurse cope with James? Justify your treatment.

Besides these two processes, there are other developments.

As this phase of life progresses, the child's egocentric behaviour is replaced by behaviour typified by her ability to enter into the thoughts, feelings and actions of others: taking on a role, or role-playing behaviour. The child is increasingly able to look at her environment from someone else's perspective.

This development is clearly illustrated by the way she plays. Play is important in a child's life. It is sometimes described as a voluntary and spontaneous activity which is enjoyable and has no other purpose than the play in itself. Play also requires an active attitude on the part of the child. Different kinds of play activities can be distinguished.

- In exploratory play a child can be free to satisfy her urge to investigate things.
- Constructive play is instructive.
- In symbolic play a child can relieve her needs and emotions.

It is also possible to make distinctions in the way a child plays her games (Sylva and Lunt, 1982). Solitary play in her first year makes way for parallel play in the current phase (figure 2.5.4). Children will, in fact, look at each other during play, and, for instance, telephone each other, but so far there is little in the way of really playing

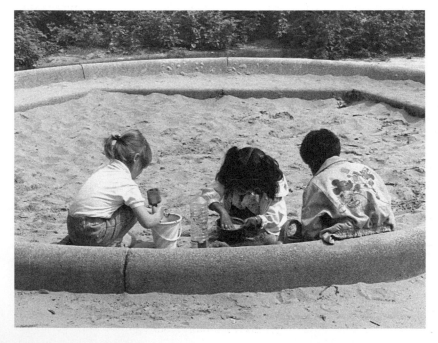

Figure 2.5.4
Parallel play

together (cooperative play). Playing together only starts during the third year and is connected with the disappearance of egocentric behaviour. At this stage two or three children will play together to achieve a common aim such as putting a toy together.

The changes are well illustrated in terms of play development, social interaction and the beginning of an elementary conscience by the following statements:

2 years: 'What's mine is mine; what's yours is mine.'

3 years: 'What's mine is mine; what's yours is yours.'

4 years: 'What's mine is mine; but you can play with it sometimes.'

5 years: 'What's mine is mine; you can have it anytime I don't want it.'
    (Kaluger and Kaluger, 1979)

Social behaviour increases strongly during this phase. Children will seek the company of adults and other children more and more. The way in which attachment to the parents took place during babyhood is one of the factors influencing the extent and quality of social behaviour in which there are often great differences between individual children. One child may be dominant and have a great deal of initiative, another may be docile and passive. At the competitive level, too, there will be differences. One child will be particularly keen to achieve something for herself, another is more intent on social objectives. Friendships evident in play at this age appear to be based on proximity and the shared aim, and are not necessarily lasting (Livesley and Bromley, 1973).

Study activity
 9. List five factors influencing social and emotional development in this phase of life.

5. Cognitive development

A factor with an important influence on the cognitive development of a young child, is her progress in the use of language. At the same time, this progress is part of her cognitive development. As already mentioned, a young child

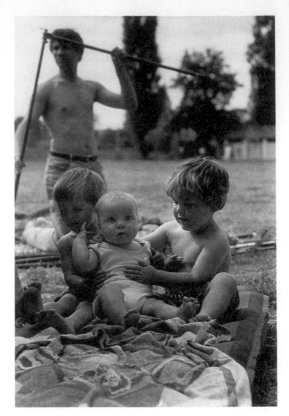

Figure 2.5.5
Taking notice

will start pronouncing her first real words around her first birthday. At eighteen months her vocabulary will contain on average fifty words and will expand to 180 words by the age of two. However, not only does the size of her vocabulary increase, but her use of language also becomes more complex. From about eighteen months the child can construct two-word sentences, such as 'see grandpa' or 'daddy car'. Linked with her social and emotional development, a child will also start using such words as 'I' and 'me'. From the age of two-and-a-half words like 'a lot', 'some', 'big', or 'little', appear, but they have no real meaning yet. In language development, motor skills, the manipulating of objects and cognitive development are closely associated.

Study activity
10. Indicate the difference between language development and cognitive development.

Another facet of cognitive development is perception. A child's perception changes in that more and more environmental factors play a role in it. These are in particular:
- *Physical environment.*
  The child gets used to particular shapes in her environment and will recognize them. They begin to mean something to her and will occupy a place in her mental world. For example, a child who observes the world from a supine position will develop a different image from a child who can walk around and touch everything.
- *Social environment.*
  The child learns to perceive things which are important to her. This is not limited to people themselves, but also relates to their behaviour. The child's perception becomes selective; she will increasingly abstract information important to her from her environment.
- *Upbringing.*
  According to the psychologist Witkin (1954), field dependency or independency is an important characteristic in human perception. By this he means the extent to which someone's perceptive judgement is influenced by her environment. The degree to which parents guide their child in her behaviour or leave her free will influence her perception.

As a last facet of cognitive development we will discuss the thought processes. To begin with, a young child uses symbolic schemata, although not yet efficiently. Concrete objects like a cuddly toy, a domestic cat and a canary, for instance, are all known as 'dog'. In her thinking the child manipulates the concept of 'dog' for all these objects. This is clearly seen from the child's play, in which objects can portray various different things. Fantasy is a very important aspect of childish thinking and playing. A young child still makes little distinction between reality and fantasy.

Human thought
To begin with a child will think that everything around her has the same properties as she has herself. From her own ego the child ascribes feelings and thoughts to things, toys and imaginary beings. This is called animist thinking. This kind of thinking is sometimes still encountered in races who believe that there are spirits in rocks or trees.

From the age of two this animist thinking changes into magical thinking. The child is not yet able to distinguish between cause and effect, and she often connects events which happen at the same time. In the first place this is the result of her limited cognitive ability and in the second place of her ignorance of the world around her. For example, if a child breaks a leg in a fall, she might think that this is a punishment because she was walking somewhere her mother had forbidden her to go.

It is important to keep the child's way of thinking and her perception of her environment in mind, especially in situations that might seem threatening to a child, like hospitalization. At the end of this phase children gradually learn to distinguish the cause and effect of events, and this heralds logical thinking.

A young child's way of thinking is preoperational and takes place mainly in one dimension (see also pages 44, 45). Piaget's conservation experiment explains this best (figure 2.5.6).

In judging the content of the glass a child will use only one dimension. Usually this is height: the tallest glass contains most water. She will not yet be able to understand that the content is also determined by width and depth.

Figure 2.5.6
Two glasses with the same liquid volume

Two identical glasses with the same liquid level

 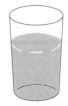

Liquid in two glasses of equal content, but different shape

Study activities

11. The child also has a one-dimensional view of behaviour. Describe the difference from a child's point of view between a one-dimensional and a multi-dimensional interpretation of:
    - being sent to bed by her parents, when it is so nice in the living room;
    - not being allowed to eat as many sweets as she wants;
    - her parents leaving at the end of visiting time in the hospital.

12. List five factors influencing cognitive development in this phase of life.

6. Summary

At the end of her third year a child will be reasonably independent. During this phase her motor development has advanced to the extent that her basic motor skills are essentially equal to those of an adult. Co-ordination of movements and balance are not yet fully developed, but the child is nevertheless able to move well within her world without the help of others. That is just as well, because after this phase of life contact with her parents decreases. Her social world will in future become more extensive and in the phase that lies behind her she will have acquired the skills to tackle the new situation. Confrontation with her parents, and coping with the conflicts arising from that, will have given the child a sense of self-reliance and independence. This self-reliance turns out to be incomplete, however. When essential restrictions are imposed on her, she knows that if need be, she will almost always be protected by her permanent carers. The restrictions are imposed by means of direct methods: rewards and punishment.

In the next phase of life a new problem awaits her. The child will then leave her trusted environment at regular intervals, her sphere of action will expand, and her parents will not always be in her immediate environment. She will have to rely on herself more and more, which also includes establishing the parameters of her actions. At the same time the child will experience clear typing as a 'he' or 'she', the discovery that there are boys and girls. These are all problems she will have to learn to cope with as a pre-school child.

The pre-school child: from four to six years

6

1. Introduction

The concept of the pre-school child is quite a vague one. He is no longer a playful toddler, but often not yet a 'learning' child. The pre-school child's main task is therefore the expansion of his world.
Hesitantly, step by step, and usually with parental support, his narrow protected world is abandoned. Contact is made with other children of the same age, and with adults he has not known before, a hesitant beginning, but a clear basis on which to be able to function independently as a schoolchild.
The pre-school phase is described from the point of view of:
- physical development;
- social and emotional development;
- cognitive development.

Learning outcomes

After studying this chapter the student should be able to:
- describe physical development in general terms;
- name and illustrate two skills which the pre-school child acquires to resolve social and emotional problems;
- give a rough description of role-playing (according to Selman);
- describe the following concepts:
  - socialization;
  - identification;
  - conscience;
  - sense of values;
- explain the cognitive development of the pre-school child;
- in general terms, explain what is meant by sexual identity.

2. The pre-school child; a brief overview

In many western societies children are given the opportunity of spending part of the day outside their familiar home surroundings from their fourth birthday. A child can then go into a playschool or a nursery unit at an infant school. Clearly society credits the pre-school child with the skills to be able to spend a part of the day outside his secure surroundings. Compulsory attendance at school, however, only starts when the child reaches the age of five. In a way this means that a trial period has been built in for the

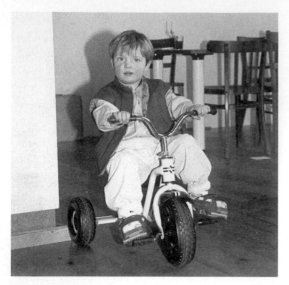

Figure 2.6.1
'Look what I can do!'

child, in which he can make a gradual switch from home to a more independent existence without his parents. It is possible that this also acts as a trial period for parents who want to keep their child longer in their care.

When he reaches the age of four, the child starts on a lengthy exploration of the outside world. The pre-school child quite instinctively acquires social cognition.

The expansion of his world is the central problem a child must resolve in the pre-school phase. In general he will no longer model himself exclusively on adults, but more and more on his contemporaries.

In addition to the fact that the pre-school child leaves his secure surroundings and extends his environment, two other important developments take place in this phase. Though children may have already learnt that they are either boys or girls, in this phase they acquire more understanding of what this means for their individual behaviour. In some specific respects the child also escapes from direct control by his parents. Instead he comes up against other means which ensure that he keeps to the rules of society. Up till now his parents' rewards and punishments have ensured that the child keeps to the rules. At this age a sense of values is developing.

In summary it can said that the pre-school phase marks a period of transition from the small, still

very playful young child, to the bigger, more questioning child. The pre-school period is a kind of childhood adolescence. Many adults find it hard to know how to approach pre-school children. What demands can you make of them? Can you hold them responsible for their behaviour, or is the child still playful, with little understanding yet of the consequences of what he does?

Whether the pre-school period is really a separate stage of development is a moot point. This can be seen from the constant reorganization of educational systems in some western countries. Along with the increase in the number of families where both parents are employed there has been a marked growth in the provision of day nurseries and play groups. In a situation like this it is possible that the concept of the pre-school child will disappear from current use.

Taking this into account it can be seen that a child's stages of development are very much a matter of social definition.

Study activity
1. **a.** Discuss whether the 'pre-school' stage of development also applies in the third world.
   b. List the advantages and disadvantages of specific attention being paid to the 'pre-school' stage.
   c. Why is it of great importance in paediatric nursing to pay specific attention to this phase of life? Illustrate your answer by examples.

3. Physical development

As the child gets older, the importance of physical development as an explanation of behaviour is continually increasing. In the pre-school phase the child is acquiring the appearance, externally at least, which will characterize him as an adult individual.

Childish characteristics, sometimes to the parents' distress, disappear; the child starts growing up. He begins to resemble an adult in his movements (figure 2.6.2). He can run, jump, hop and ride a bicycle, mainly as a result of an increasing sense of balance. In contrast to a toddler, the pre-school child is no longer so top-heavy; this is because he loses his baby fat and

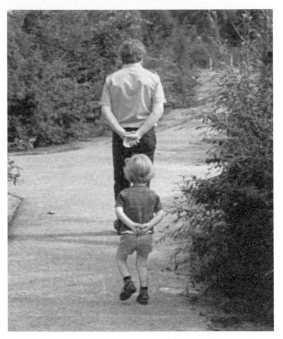

Figure 2.6.2
You can learn by
imitation, too

his centre of gravity alters. There is also more co-ordination in his various movements. Although pre-school children are still clumsy and their movements are not very refined, they can usually do up all their buttons, and trace or draw shapes on paper. Learning activities in the first classes in an infant school are therefore directed towards refining and expanding these kinds of skills.

A change also occurs in sexual development in the pre-school phase. While a baby will have reflex reactions to stimulation of the genital organs – one-year-old boys can, for example, get an erection – touching their genital organs also gives pre-school children pleasurable sensations. These feelings can best be interpreted as feelings of purely physical pleasure. You should not, however, equate them with the feelings experienced by adults, which are usually focused on other people. It is not clear whether pre-school children are already conscious of the sexual nature of their feelings. We will return to the psychological importance of sexual development in the section on development of a sexual identity (page 117).

During the pre-school stage the brain reaches nearly its adult weight. This heralds the end of the strong influence of physical maturing processes on cognitive development. From now on cognitive development will be primarily determined by environmental factors: the physical basis to it has been established.

At the end of the pre-school phase, growth in physique also begins to increase. The pre-school child is therefore stronger and is capable of hitting out quite hard; he does not yet control the application of his physical strength.

There is also an important development during this phase in the area of perception. The development of perception reaches a peak on the physiological level. In practical terms this means that the pre-school child is fully capable of perceiving details. Attention naturally has an important role to play here. The child's power of concentration begins to grow as a consequence of improvement in the functioning of the *formatio reticularis* (the filter in the brainstem that controls the attentive processes). From the pre-school phase onwards, recognition, a cognitive activity of perception, plays an ever more important part. There are very few further changes from the physiological point of view.

Study activity
2. List five factors which can influence physical development in this stage of life.

4. Social and emotional development

The child's development problems are primarily social and emotional in nature. If he gets into an argument about a toy, he must now sort it out for himself. At infant school he must listen to people who are not his parents. He may at first be distressed, or feel abandoned, without his parents to comfort him. The pre-school child needs to acquire some skills to be able to solve or handle these problems.

He acquires better means of communication. This enables him to broaden his social contacts and increases his knowledge of other people: a pre-school child undergoes substantial cognitive development at the social level, which enlarges on the skills in role-playing with which he had already begun to experiment as a three-year-old.

– At the same time there are developments in the area of cognition, to which we shall return in Section 5. They enable the pre-school child to understand what goes on in people's minds, and to be aware of the interaction between people. This is conditional on a decrease in egocentric thinking and behaviour, so characteristic of the child in earlier phases. Although Piaget maintains that egocentric behaviour only starts to disappear at the age of seven, other researchers suggest that this is already happening at the end of the young child stage. The pre-school child is already capable of putting himself in someone else's place – this is called role playing. Selman (1980) distinguishes the following stages in the development of role-playing:

- 4–6 years old. A pre-school child thinks that his interpretation of social behaviour is the only right one. He sees his parents being angry with his sister, and he assumes that they are right. He is not capable of imagining other interpretations of what is happening. He is still demonstrating behaviour which is somewhat egocentric, but this is only the first stage of this development.

- 6–8 years old. A child can imagine that other people have a different opinion about the reasons for the argument from the opinion that he has himself. He will hear from his sister that his parents were wrong when they were angry with her, and whilst he may not disbelieve her, he will not change his point of view.

- 8–10 years old. A child can imagine that other people are capable of expressing the thoughts and feelings of the opposing parties.

- 10–12 years old. A child is capable of putting himself in someone else's place, and looking at the quarrel from the other person's viewpoint. He can now understand his sister's point of view.

- 12–15 years old. A child is capable of imagining that the quarrel can be looked at from a neutral point of view, and that there can be several ways of looking at it. For instance, 12–15 year olds may realize that pacifists and professional soldiers can each have a different view of a conflict.

It will be appreciated, therefore, that development of role-playing runs more or less in parallel with the development of thinking, and proceeds from the concrete to the abstract.

The pre-school child pays attention to the feelings and emotions of other people. For example, he sees that his parents are distressed if he goes into hospital. So the pre-school child is capable of interpreting social behaviour in terms of the feelings of the persons involved, though informed with his own point of view. This is a great step forward in social and emotional development. It makes the pre-school child capable of taking account of other people's feelings in his actions.

In forming opinions of other children the pre-school child uses different criteria from those of older children or adults. Where these take more account of personal characteristics, the pre-school child judges on the basis of external features, such as the other child's physical characteristics, clothes, or toys. He will, for example, admire another pre-school child because he has such nice toys.

The pre-school child also differs from older children in the way he explains other people's behaviour. He sees the reasons for behaviour primarily in situational factors. Thus he will ascribe a nurses's cross face in the first instance to her having to get up early, and not to her unfriendly nature. In theory, pre-school children are capable of giving explanations of behaviour based on personality. However, they are not capable of explaining it in combination with situational factors, so that they tend to give priority to the latter category.

The social world of pre-school children is expanding substantially. In western societies many four-year-olds go to infant school for the first time. A number of children have already had some social experience before this in nursery play groups. The main feature of an infant school is that contact with other children of their own age becomes more intensive. Class-mates and adults increasingly become their models. Adults do not usually remember the names of play group leaders, but remember those of their infant school teachers. The probable explanation of this is that infant school teachers are identification figures. Above all, pre-school children imitate the behaviour of other children of the same age and sex. However, in play and in their choice of friends they do not yet make much distinction between sexes.

In infant school the child has to cope with more and more rules of behaviour, and the exercises and games are designed to develop the child's skills, including social skills. This last statement brings us to another important point of social and emotional development. Together with social and cognitive development, socialization processes (see also Module 3, Chapter 5) play an important role.

If we define socialization roughly as 'adopting norms and values from society', we can see that there has, of course, already been some degree of socialization in the earlier phases. Up to the pre-school stage, however, socialization was primarily based on authority. A younger child keeps to the rules because he is rewarded for doing so or – if he 'ducks out' of them – is punished. In the pre-school stage the socialization process acquires a new basis, as the process of identification comes to play an important part.

Identification is important for:
- the development of sexual identity: the awareness of being a boy or a girl;
- the development of a sense of values or conscience: an understanding of good and bad, of what is right or not right.

In this section the first of these, sexual identity, is dealt with; the process of formation of a sense of values is discussed in the section on cognitive development.

The pre-school child is aware of his genital organs. He appreciates that there is a difference between boys and girls, and that as a boy he cannot occasionally be a girl or vice versa: you can't change your sex, though you can sometimes put on the clothes of someone of the other sex. He also notices that he is like one of his parents and differs from the other. Most pre-school children now gradually acquire the idea

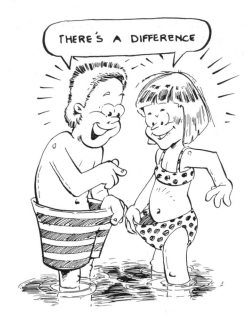

that he or she is either a boy or a girl. Each of the various approaches has its own explanation of how this process takes place. The psycho-analytical approach claims that there is identification with the parent of the same sex at the end of a period of conflict with that parent.

The learning theory approach holds that a process of social theory learning occurs, through observation and operant conditioning. In this learning process boys acquire a male identification from their father, and girls a female one from their mother. Clearly society plays an important part in the definition of that identity (Block, 1980).

The cognitive approach holds that pre-school children gradually acquire their sexual role behaviour through their general cognitive development.

Finally, the biological approach simply accepts that boys will display male behaviour and girls female. If any problems arise, the reasons are genetic.

Sexual identity
From this description of the acquisition of sexual identity you could conclude that humanity consists of people who are either male or female. There should be a clearly

noticeable difference between the two sexes in behaviour, and the expression of sexual feelings should be directed at members of the opposite sex.

General observation, however, will soon show that in reality sexuality is much more complex. Superman and Superwoman do not exist. In every individual, 'male' and 'female' characteristics make up a diverse whole. In general, men possess more male and women more female characteristics, but the proportions of these characteristics vary from individual to individual. The term androgyny is used for this complex presentation of sex typing.

There are also a very large number of variations in sexual behaviour. We will not discuss all these variations here, but will look briefly at the choice of the object of sexual behaviour: who chooses whom as sexual partner. Broadly there are two possibilities. On the one hand are the people who satisfy their sexuality with someone of the opposite sex. This is called heterosexual. On the other hand there are those who look for a partner among their own sex. This is called homosexual. These two extremes define a sliding scale of sexual preferences, on which an individual can be placed. Midway in that scale is the bisexual person, whose sexual behaviour shows no specific preference for either sex.

There are various opinions about the way in which sexual preference comes about. The views of Jung are worth mentioning. At the turn of the century he put forward the idea that everyone is in theory bisexual. Depending upon their experiences, they then develop into hetero or homosexuals.

So far, various kinds of therapy designed to alter people's sexual preferences have had little enduring success.

It is certainly plain that pre-school children are very interested in their own and other children's sex organs. Adults have often been embarassed in their bath by the frank interest of their pre-school child in their genital organs. Children also experiment with their ideas of sexuality and

sexual identity in playing at 'mummies and daddies' or 'doctors and nurses'.

During the acquisition of sexual identity the pre-school child adopts much of the behaviour of the adult with which he or she identifies. In this respect, therefore, socialization occurs through identification.

Study activities

3. List five factors influencing social and emotional development in this phase of life.

4. What will you as a nurse do about pre-school children in the same ward who are exploring each others genital organs in play? Give reasons for your answer.

5. Cognitive development

The pre-school child begins to organize his thoughts more. He can no longer get by with the magical way of thinking he employed in his previous stages of development. All kinds of new events force him to organize his thinking differently. He will gradually begin to distinguish between cause and effect when something happens, and he will be able to apply this knowledge to similar events. In other words, the pre-school child begins to think logically. He wants to know the ins and outs of everything, which demands considerable tact and patience from those around him, who have to provide answers to all his questions 'why?'. Through his curiosity the pre-school child also learns to solve problems better. When he has found a solution to a problem, he is able to apply the strategy for solving it to other similar problems. The 'trial and error' behaviour of earlier stages recedes even further.

In addition, speech increasingly accompanies action. When you watch young pre-school children, you can hear that they often say what they are going to do, so that actual events are expressed in speech.

This thinking aloud gradually disappears and changes into real thinking. This is a very important aspect of cognitive development. In the next stage of development this will eventually lead to the capacity for abstract thought.

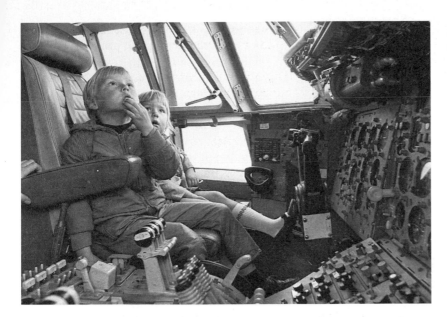

Figure 2.6.3
We've got a lot
to learn yet

The pre-school child knows the names of a great many things in his environment. The construction of his sentences can already be very intricate. Yet the pre-school child often makes mistakes in his speech because he does not yet know properly what the words mean. For instance, the four-year-old from next door regularly asks me where my mummy is, when he means my wife. He knows the word mummy, but applies it to all women, because he does not yet know properly what the word means.

The pre-school child also still has problems with the concept of time. He already has some awareness of time, but still confuses the words used to indicate it. He is, for instance, capable of saying that he was at granny's tomorrow, instead of yesterday.

The development of a sense of time also comes into play in the ideas pre-school children have about death. In general it is safe to say that you can talk about death with pre-school children, because they can already envisage to some extent what can happen in the future. But they are not usually capable of realizing that death is something irreversible. Grandpa may be dead, and may have gone away for a bit, but he will be back soon – this is what they usually think. Death is regarded as a kind of sleep where people go on living in some other way. Later in

the pre-school stage this idea changes and death is seen as final.

Together with his cognitive development there is also an essential change in the pre-school child's sense of values. Many psychologists, both psychoanalytical and cognitive, hold that the development of a conscience begins in the pre-school stage. They define conscience as an internal system of norms and values, on which an individual bases his actions.

The development of moral judgement is a part of this growth of a sense of values and a conscience. Moral judgement forms the base on which behaviour is evaluated. Kohlberg (1969) advanced a model to distinguish the development of moral judgement. This model identifies three levels, each with two stages. It must be noted however that Kohlberg (1984) now considers the final stage (stage 6) not to be a normally expected outcome.

Level I – *Preconventional morality* – up to 10 yrs. Within this level orientation moves from *Punishment* (stage 1), where the child obeys rules to avoid punishment; to *Reward* (stage 2), where the child conforms to rules to obtain rewards or have favours returned. According to Kohlberg some criminals never progress past this phase.

Level II – *Conventional Morality* – up to 16 yrs. Movement in this level is from the *Good-boy/ Good-girl orientation* (stage 3), where the child conforms to avoid the disapproval of others; to *Authority orientation* (stage 4), where the child upholds laws and social rules to avoid conflict with authorities and feelings of self guilt. Again according to Kohlberg many individuals do not progress past this level.

Level III – *Postconventional Morality* – 16 years plus. As indicated above, people who reach this level may not achieve both stages. Those who do achieve both stages move from a *Social contract orientation* (stage 5), where actions are guided by principles commonly agreed on as essential to the public welfare and which are linked to the individual's feelings of self-respect; to an *Ethical principle orientation* (stage 6), where actions are guided by self-chosen ethical principles based on justice, dignity and equality linked to a need to avoid self-condemnation.

Up to the pre-school stage a child's actions were determined by the rewards or punishments resulting from them. The young child does not judge behaviour in terms of good or evil. The pre-school child will begin to do this, though in an absolute sense, with no grey areas. He often bases his opinion of what is good or bad on the judgement of adults in his environment. They can be his parents, but may also be the infant school teacher. The pre-school child is very absolute in his judgements; complicated concepts like the meaning of other people's behaviour, do not yet affect his judgement of that behaviour. He still always looks at the consequences of behaviour, and bases his judgements on that. So, when you knock over a medicine bottle on the child's bedside table while you are trying to stroke his head, in his view you are always wrong; you knocked something over, and that is wrong, even though you meant well.

Study activities

5. List five factors which can influence cognitive development at this stage of life.

6. a. Imagine that a four-year-old child with terminal leukaemia is admitted to hospital. Describe the processes you follow, as a nurse, in deciding whether, and if so how, to inform the child of his approaching death.

b. Explain the advantages for the child in thinking that death is the same as going to sleep.

c. Explain how you can best describe death to a pre-school child in normal circumstances, in other words, when he is quite healthy.

6. Summary

The pre-school child already has the most important skills he needs for his task – learning to exist without the direct protection of his parents. He can communicate adequately, and his cognitive development enables him to solve the problems posed by his environment, and to acquire important new skills. These skills make it possible for him to operate better, particularly at the social level.

In the first place he learns to evaluate other people's behaviour better; his social cognition increases.

Next, children in this phase of life begin to type themselves as either boys or girls, and at the same time they begin to lose their baby appearance.

This creates a situation in which adults will take them more seriously in the next stage of their life. The schoolboy or girl has become a small individual who demands to be taken into account.

Finally the child begins to identify with adults as well. He is also expected to behave more and more in the way adults want him to behave. He adopts these expectations and in this way a pre-school child acquires a certain sense of values. This makes him capable at a later stage of acting in a way that makes him acceptable to his social environment.

The acquisition of these skills, whose development has for that matter only just started, makes the child capable of coping with the tasks awaiting him in his next phase of life.

The schoolchild must learn how the world works. He can then prepare himself to take up a specific place in it. He acquires his knowledge from the adults in his environment. A condition of acquiring this knowledge is that the adults also accept the child as someone to whom they can pass on their knowledge.

One mistake which must not be made – and this is a problem which arises from the pre-school stage onwards, because pre-school children have to deal with adults who are strangers to them – is to assume a child's psychological maturity from his physical appearance. Children who are bigger than average for their age sometimes come up against behaviour that is not tailored to their age. They are often taken to be more mature, psychologically, than children of the same age but of average size.

7

The schoolchild: from six to twelve years

1. Introduction

Who can forget their first day at school? The uncertain steps towards the classroom? The worry at being separated from home for too long a stretch? But who does not at the same time remember their very rich and varied experience with other children? Exciting games, competition, fellowship, quarrels – they are all part of it.

Many of one's experiences as a schoolchild stay in the memory. That is no coincidence. The transition from pre-school child to schoolchild is a big one, however many preparations may have been made for it.

This chapter explains how the schoolchild develops from the point of view of psychological development. Special attention will be paid to the child's ideas about sickness.

Learning outcomes

After studying this chapter the student should be able to:
- describe physical development in general terms;
- describe and explain three stages of the way in which a child conducts her friendships;
- explain Barenboim's model of personal perception;
- in general terms list and explain five factors which determine the way in which a schoolchild acquires ideas about sickness;
- describe in outline the schoolchild's cognitive development.

2. The schoolchild; a brief overview

In developmental psychology the schoolchild phase has for long been a neglected area. Freud even called it 'the latent period', the stage in which the driving force of development, sexuality, lies latent. In general this phase is characterized as quiet, in comparison with the other stages of development. The schoolchild phase, though it lasts longer, is less productive than the pre-school phase when the child developed a wide range of skills within a period of about two years. This does not mean, however, that this phase can be missed out. We will consider what important development processes take place in it. At about the age of six, when the child reaches the last year in the infant school, she takes an important step forward. Playful babyish behaviour is still acceptable in the pre-school child. She is also not yet considered to be responsible for her behaviour, and she cannot as yet take important decisions on her own. School, too, still makes allowances for her tremendous need for activity, and the rules are not too strict so far. The schoolchild, however, is faced with an entirely different pattern of expectations. She is

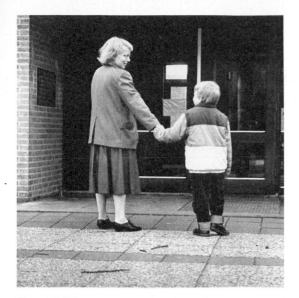

Figure 2.7.1
The first day at school;
it's hard to say goodbye

The ultimate consequence of this is that she acquires a complex image of herself. She is already turning into an identifiable personality. At the same time the schoolchild's knowledge of the world around her increases considerably. Her cognitive development enables her to acquire this knowledge, while society supplies it to her through education.

Society is also responsible for the fact that certain qualities like a competitive spirit and altruism, which are highly valued in society, begin to develop in the schoolchild.

All in all this is hardly a phase in which nothing happens. In our opinion there is certainly no question of a 'latent' period. The schoolchild is faced with an important task: she must acquire understanding of the world about her. She has already acquired the skills needed for this, or she will master them during this phase. The development process involved here is not as hectic as in the previous phases. The schoolchild's world is steadily becoming more complex and she needs more time to take in all the aspects of it.

already regarded much more as a full member of society. She is no longer so free to behave as she likes as the pre-school child. She is expected to produce results, and she is thought to be capable of doing so. At school she must keep to the rules, while she herself would prefer to play and get into mischief. In children's television news broadcasts she is confronted with disasters, and people's resultant distress. She is also considered mature enough to be a full member of her church and learns her catechism or receives religious instruction.

The child should certainly know the general norms of society. One of these norms is to tell the truth, which presupposes that she can distinguish fantasy and reality from each other. She must also behave politely. Faced with this pattern of expectations the schoolchild, within a period of some six years, undergoes a development in which we can distinguish the following important processes.

While she becomes less dependent upon members of her family, other people begin to assume an important place in her life. These are principally other children of the same age, with whom the child for the first time in her life forms firm friendships. Through these friendships she also gradually acquires a better image of herself, by comparing herself with her friends.

Figure 2.7.2
Reward for achievement

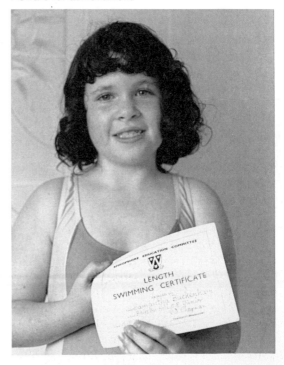

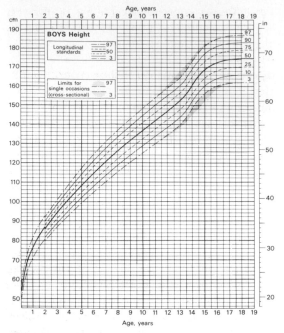

Figure 2.7.3a
Height standard chart
for boys aged 0–19 years
(Castlemead Publications Chart No. GDB11A)

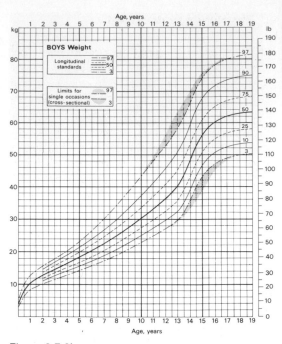

Figure 2.7.3b
Weight standard chart
for boys aged 0–19 years
(Castlemead Publications Chart No. GDB11A)

Figure 2.7.3c
Height standard chart
for girls aged 0–19 years
(Castlemead Publications Chart No. GDG12A)

Figure 2.7.3d
Weight standard chart
for girls aged 0–19 years
(Castlemead Publications Chart No. GDG12A)

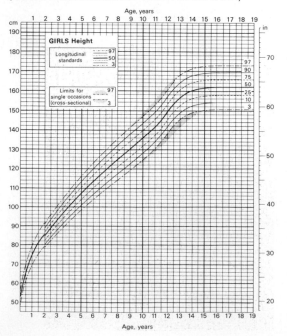

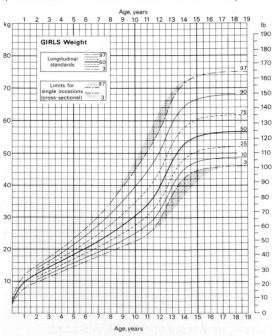

3. Physical development

Although physical growth is rather slower than before, it progresses gradually until the beginning of puberty, in about the twelfth year. The child already has in general lines the appearance which she will have as an adult. Partly as a result of the increase in muscular tissue, she has become stronger and more robust. Children of school age are also more distinguishable from each other. Whereas you will still have difficulty in telling one pre-school child from another, this will hardly cause any problems with schoolchildren. You can now identify a child better by her appearance; a schoolchild is much more of a personality, too.

The fact that a child's growth is mostly gradual does not mean that all parts of the body grow at the same rate. Arms and legs usually grow fastest, with the rest of the body following behind. You can easily tell seven and eight-year-olds by their matchstick-like legs with rather prominent knee joints.

In the course of this phase the proportions of the various parts of the body revert more or less to normal. It sometimes looks as if schoolchildren are playing very dangerously. They climb, crawl and tumble so wildly, that you would expect them to break something. Unlike pre-school children, they now have a fully developed sense of balance, and the strength to perform these acrobatics. Besides, they are still flexible enough in their joints to limit the damage from any fall to some grazes.

Most children in this phase choose to practise some sport. Their co-ordination is such that they are capable of manipulating a ball or any other object. Their movements are still in general rather crude, but well controlled. At first the young schoolchild will still have difficulty playing as a member of a team, or in concentrating on the game. These social and cognitive skills are, after all, only just beginning to develop.

Study activities

1. Describe briefly five factors influencing physical development in this phase.

2. Describe your own experience of physical development in this phase. What was or was not important?

4. Social and emotional development

As we have seen in Chapter 6, Section 4, pre-school children begin to acquire an understanding of social relationships. Their characteristic egocentricity begins to decline, and they begin to regard their social world differently. In practice, however, their own social relationships, if somewhat deeper, are primarily with adults: parents, other members of the family and teachers at school.

In the case of the schoolchild there is less dependence on the family. Part of her upbringing is taken over by other adults, but, much more importantly, relationships begin with her contemporaries. Friendships with other children become closer, and last longer. Through them the child gains greater understanding of how people relate to each other. She also acquires a clearer image of herself by comparing herself with them. We can distinguish three stages in the way in which children conduct their friendships.

Figure 2.7.4
The same age, but that is all they have in common

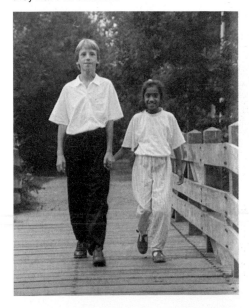

– From five to seven years old, their friends come mainly from their own form at school or from the neighbourhood. A child of this age appears to adults to be very casual about her friendships. They are ended just as quickly as they started, and feelings of distress about friendships breaking up are generally of short duration, particularly if she has already found a new friend. One explanation of this could be that friendships are not yet based on personality traits, but more on things like happening to live next door, or possessing some special toy. The social world is still very limited, but the same applies for many adults. Consider the saying: a good neighbour is better than a distant friend.

– From eight years old, children start taking an interest in who their friend is as a person, and superficial matters like toys or where they live play a less important role. There is often some kind of mutual trust in their friendships.
It is also very important that friends should do the same things together. You often see friends having the same interests and the same hobbies, or being members of the same sports club.

– From twelve years old, friendships usually become rather more stable than previously. Friends share emotions and swap secrets; friendships are now deeper, moreso perhaps among girls than among boys. Friends are also ready to help each other with their problems; the development of social skills like sympathy and ability to listen play an important part in this.

Study activity

3. Describe three of your own friendships and show which of the three stages described above they fit into.

The development of friendships runs in parallel with the development of the way in which the schoolchild forms an opinion of other children. If you ask a schoolchild to describe herself, she will not do so in terms of character traits, but mainly in terms of external features like name, address, hobbies, skills, and so on. This is how she regards other children, too. The psychol-

ogist Barenboim's 1981 model of personal perception illustrates this.

– The behaviour comparison stage (six to eight years old).
The child describes her impressions of another in terms of actual behaviour. For instance, she will say that the other child is very good at sums, or wears very nice clothes.

– The stage of psychological constructs (eight to ten years old).
Other children are described in terms of psychological characteristics. He works hard at school, or she is always nice.

– The stage of psychological comparisons (ten to twelve years old).
Whereas her impression of other children up to now has been an absolute one, the schoolchild now begins to build in some relativities. She begins to compare other children with each other. She is nicer than he is. The ability to see relativities is the result of the development of the schoolchild's cognitive skills. We will refer to this again in the next section.

The popularity of the schoolchild among her peers is usually not yet based on personality traits. What matters is whether you are doing well at school or have lots of friends.

How does a child regard illness?

We adults generally have a fairly clear idea of what is meant by illness and death. We know that we can become ill, and we can assess the significance of that illness on our lives. Sometimes we even know what made us ill. Depending on our beliefs, we may think that when we die, that is final, or we may believe that after death the soul or the spirit lives on. However, our behaviour does not always match our knowledge; emotion, for example, has its role, and influences our behaviour. We sometimes ask ourselves, against our better knowledge, odd questions, or we take peculiar measures when we are ill. 'Might I have become ill because I have been deceiving my wife?', or: 'If I now lead a very regular life and keep to a strict diet, then I will perhaps get rid of this terminal tumour.' Some people go on pilgrimage to pray for a cure for their disease from some particular saint. It also sometimes

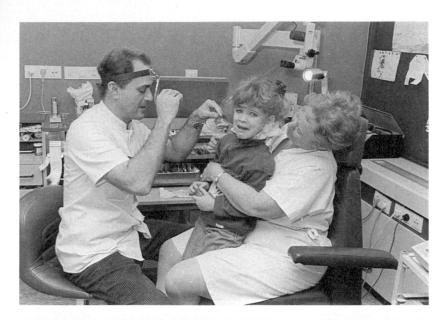

Figure 2.7.5
Why is this necessary?

happens that people personalize their disease and give their tumour a name. All these forms of behaviour or thoughts, which are only occasionally found among adults, are normal among children. Children's behaviour of this sort can usually be ascribed fairly easily to one of the stages in their cognitive development. They do not yet think like adults. Besides, they do not yet know so much about their own body, something we should not forget. It is therefore useful to discuss briefly how children regard illness.

Study activity
4. At what age should you:
   – let a child go to her grandmother's funeral?
   – let her see her dead grandfather?
   – explain death fully?
   Give reasons for your answers.

These observations apply particularly to children from pre-school age onwards. These children already react to information about illness and physical discomfort. They can tell you where they feel pain, and what sort of pain it is, whereas in the earlier phases of life sick children react primarily to the comforting presence of their parents.
We have said earlier that children of school age are beginning to learn about their own bodies. Their ideas in this regard are based on the body's outward appearance and the bodily functions. These ideas are to some extent determined by reactions from their environment. It is obvious that illness can have a great influence on the image that they have constructed of their bodies, particularly if there are physical changes as a result of a disease. A boy whose leg has been amputated as a result of bone cancer will have a different idea of his body to one who can use his body to run and climb.
Children's knowledge of their insides, and their internal workings, is very limited. A fairly simple physiological process, like the intake of food and its excretion, is only properly understood by most children in adolescence. Young schoolchildren can have very varying ideas about these processes. There are children who think that the inside of their bodies is made up entirely of food, or that food only comes out of it through vomiting. The number of organs that the young schoolchild knows is very limited too. Those known by most children are the brain and the heart, followed by the stomach and the lungs. They often do not know what they do or how they work.
From the age of nine, however, knowledge of their bodies increases quickly, as many researchers have shown. Children of this age

know many more organs and know more about how they work. For instance, a nine-year-old may be able to make a connection between the intake of food and the excretory processes, but how this process works is usually still a mystery, though she does know there is a link.

Knowledge of the functions and location of organs like kidneys, liver, etc. is almost non-existent among children of school age, unless they themselves have had a disease of one of these organs. Very little is also known about the functions of the genital organs before the adolescent phase. Think back a little to your own sex education. It is none the less generally thought important to inform children properly about their illnesses and about how their bodies work. Children notice that something is going on, and a good explanation helps to limit unreal fantasies and fears. Besides, children seem to cope much better with knowledge of a serious illness than people have always thought. It is important to strike the right note in telling them about it, so that the child understands something of what is happening. However, sound information does not solve the emotional problems of a disease.

When children become ill, this can have important consequences for their lives, such as:
– not being able to play any more;
– falling behind at school;
– being separated from parents or friends;
– having to change their eating habits;
– becoming dependent again, whereas they were previously beginning to become less dependent on parents;
– getting more attention from parents;
– not having to go to school any more;
– getting lots of presents.

Study activity
5. a. Say what positive and negative aspects can be linked to the following illnesses for a schoolchild:
    – influenza;
    – a lengthy attack of pneumonia;
    – a complex fracture of the pelvis.
   b. What was your own experience of illness as a child?

A child's attitude towards her illness can be influenced by a variety of factors, of which the most important are:
– age (cognitive development);
– her own experience of her illness;
– her family's reaction to her illness;
– the nature and seriousness of her illness;
– the restrictions her illness imposes on her;
– the medical and nursing treatment which her illness demands;
– the prognosis of the illness.

Depending on their age, the following factors always play an important role with children.

Young children (though this can also occur with older children) often think of their illness as a punishment for forbidden thoughts or actions. Fantasy plays an important part in this.

For older children, who are already beginning to care about what others think of them – and they judge this, as we saw earlier, primarily from external appearances – the effects of illness on their appearance are very important. The illness can be a direct assault upon their body image.

Finally, illnesses which are accompanied by clearly visible symptoms, like vomiting, a rash or diarrhoea, are more easily accepted by children than illnesses whose consequences are not so obvious.

Case study: Margo
Margo is nine years old and is in hospital because of an unexplained high temperature. No diagnosis is expected for the moment. Margo has recently been transferred from the local hospital to a specialist children's unit, about 50 miles from her home.

Her temperature fluctuates widely and leaves her completely exhausted. At the peaks of the fever she suffers from serious delirium. She then talks nonsense. After the fever diminishes, she has no memory of it. Margo completely fails to understand that she is ill. There has never been anything wrong with her and her parents are also quite healthy. Besides, she has never been naughty ...

Study activity

6. a. Describe in as much detail as possible how you think Margo feels about her illness.

b. Are her feelings compatible with her stage of development or not? Explain your answer.

c. Develop a personal nursing care plan for Margo, built round keeping her informed.

School is a true instrument of socialization. By the manifold contacts with other children of the same age, the schoolchild is informed of her behaviour. These include such things as caring for others, being a success, behaving aggressively or being popular.

All these developments eventually result in the schoolchild obtaining a very complex image of herself. Her social experiences have given her some knowledge of her capabilities and she also knows to which social group she belongs.

If you want to belong to a particular group, she thinks, you must also make that clear to the outside world. Older schoolchildren are already beginning to make sure that their clothing is fashionable and that their hair is cut in the right style. Their appearance is important to them and they attach great significance to the opinions of their peers.

Schoolchildren are also very aware of being either a boy or a girl. Occasionally they are not quite sure how to behave as a result, but they quickly find out under the influence of friends of both sexes and of parents.

Study activity

7. Describe briefly five factors which influence social and emotional development in this phase of life.

Child abuse

One of the more popular subjects in the media in recent years has been child abuse. The word 'popular' is grossly misleading here, since the problem is a fundamental and serious one.

The term 'child abuse' appeared for the first time in the literature in the early 1960s, but we can assume that the phenomenon existed much earlier. Writing and reading about this subject involves not only the provision and acquisition of information about it, but also the evocation of feelings of incomprehension and revulsion. For many people child abuse, like incest and rape, belongs to the 'not people like us' category. Everyone has heard of it, but never had a close encounter with it. Yet the figures show that child abuse occurs increasingly in our society. In the 1980s there was a significant increase in the number of known cases.

If it is assumed that not all cases are recognized and/or reported, it could be argued that one to two percent of the child population (up to 15 years old) have had to cope with child abuse in their life. This percentage is probably even greater if you make the definition of abuse as wide as we shall do below. Statistics often only report active physical and sexual abuse, and take no account of psychological or physical neglect and emotional abuse.

It is therefore important that we define the concept of child abuse clearly, since, by doing so, people, who occasionally slap their child when she is naughty, avoid being wrongly accused of abuse. A definition will also prevent the phenomenon being underestimated.

Child abuse is defined as *'any form of physical, emotional or sexual violence which children suffer, not by accident, but by the agency or negligence of their parents or other adults, causing, or threatening to cause, injuries of a physical or psychic nature. This implies that the behaviour referred to of the parents or other adults must occur repeatedly, and with some degree of regularity, and that there is no question of the parents providing comfort for the child after the behaviour displayed.'*

In applying this definition, it must be borne in mind that culture plays an important role in the evaluation of abusive behaviour. Contact with children is prescribed by culture, and what would be called abuse here, might elsewhere belong among the normal package of child-rearing measures.

In practice three types of abuse, occurring in both active and passive forms, can be distinguished.

- • *Physical abuse*, implying causing physical harm to the child by, for example, hitting or kicking.
  • *Physical neglect*, implying depriving the child of the most essential means for a healthy life.
  This can mean giving the child nothing to eat or drink, not preventing the child when she wants to run into a road full of heavy traffic, or not looking after her when she is ill.
- • *Emotional abuse*, implying passing on negative feelings to the child with the intention of doing her some harm. This can be by swearing at her, but can also occur by having such great overt expectations of the child that she can never achieve them.
  • *Emotional neglect*, implying depriving the child of the most elementary emotional support, by ignoring her or withholding anything nice from her.
- • *Sexual abuse*, implying allowing or forcing the child, to perform sexual acts with, or in submission to, an adult.
  • *Sexual neglect*, implying debarring the child from any natural physical contact. This can be by punishing the child for touching her own body, or from portraying sexuality as sinful or bad.

Giving an explanation for child abuse is a complex task. Everyone will assert in the first instance that he or she would never be capable of it, but reality shows that there are in fact a number of people in all social classes who are.
Several factors usually play a part, interacting with each other, such as:
- the abuser's past history, where it is often the case that they were themselves abused;
- the failure of the behaviour or capabilities of the child to come up to the expectations of her parents;
- problems in the parents' lives, such as unemployment, financial difficulties;
- problems of relationships, which are sometimes worked out on the weakest member of the family.

To what extent, abuse affects the child depends on:
- the degree of abuse;
- the ability of the child to endure it;
- the degree to which the child is given comfort or support from elsewhere, or later in life.

In assessing the effect on the child we must distinguish between direct physical consequences and indirect, usually more far reaching, psychological consequences.
A bruise usually disappears quite fast, but a negative image of oneself lasts longer. We must not make the mistake of underestimating the influence on the self of serious physical abuse. It can have serious and long-lasting consequences and can also, for example, cause fear of certain situations or people.

By the nature of their work – involving close contacts with parents and children – nurses are often the obvious people to detect child abuse and have an important role to play in its identification (Dingwall, 1983). The detection and recognition of any indications of it through careful observation is important but even more important is to know how to react in these situations. Because the indications are in themselves no proof of child abuse, any suggestion of the parents being guilty must be avoided. The indications must therefore serve the nurse as a guiding light enabling her to observe correctly, and to try to acquire further information.

Indications from parents can be:
- lack of interest in the child: for example, parents not coming at visiting times, or not asking how the child is getting on;
- conspicuous nervousness or tension in the presence of nurses;
- keeping themselves separate from other parents who may be there;
- a sudden change of doctor or hospital.

Indications from children can be:
- abnormalities in their physical condition, such as the state of their skin, bad hygiene and/or retarded growth;

- abnormal behaviour, such as extreme reactions like aggressiveness, apathy, fear, withdrawal and/or not wanting to play;
- changes for the worse in behaviour in the presence of their parents;
- not wanting to be touched or undressed;
- sleeping problems.

Many other indications of this kind could be listed. In themselves they have no great diagnostic value, in that they are also normal reactions to going into hospital. The combination of several of them gives reason to suspect that there might be a case of child abuse. Consultation with colleagues is indicated if child abuse is suspected.

Study activity

8. If you establish that a child is being abused, how would you approach the problem:
   - as one of the child's carers;
   - as a friend;
   - as a nurse.

5. Cognitive development

Quite a lot is expected of the schoolchild on the cognitive level. Certainly in this society the child must acquire a great deal of knowledge if she wishes to get on in the world. While the acquisition of knowledge or learning has until now been done effortlessly and at random, it now becomes systematic and purposeful. The child must learn skills like counting and the use of language, but she also has to learn that the world, as she knows it, is only a small part of a large and complicated whole. There is, of course, a reason why the systematic introduction of the child to learning, in this but also in most other societies, begins at about the age of five or six.

In the first place this is because at about this age most children are able to give their full concentration to following instruction. They have to be able to sit still for a while and concentrate on something.

In the second place they must be capable of assimilating a great many new experiences,

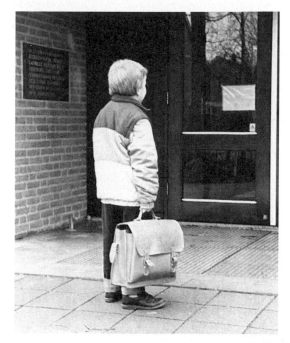

Figure 2.7.6
Life is getting more difficult

facts and skills. Assimilating includes being able to understand events around them and putting them into a logical order.

We have seen that in the pre-school stage the child is already beginning to think logically. This logical thinking develops further in the schoolchild stage, though still on a material level. Thus an eight-year-old child will be able to understand racial discrimination, an abstract concept, more easily if she is given an example: for instance, that the black children in her class might not be welcome in the local shop. She will at that stage have difficulty handling the concept in some other situation, clearly different from the one she knows, but where the same concept is involved. She will also have difficulty in imagining what it is like to be discriminated against.

In the context of the situation with which she is familiar she can apply reason about cause and effect. So you will find that if you tell schoolchildren that they must obey the rules of hygiene, and must therefore wash their hands before meals, they will do so. You should not expect them automatically to apply the same concept of hygiene when they go to the toilet.

Functional symptoms in children

Below is part of a letter from an eleven-year-old girl, who was reported to have various physical symptoms. She wrote the letter at the end of her treatment.

I am doing fine with reading and writing. Now I will tell you something and (....) I will start at the beginning.

My father and mother had a bit of a quarrel, and I thought to myself that perhaps it would get so bad that they would get divorced. Imagine that! (...) I thought to myself, if I pretend that I can't write, they will think more about me than about quarrelling. So that's what I did, and my father and mother realized that I couldn't read or write, and the next day the quarrel was over. I was very pleased the quarrel was over, but I was stuck with that reading and writing. I could not immediately pretend it was all right, that would have looked too odd. So I kept it up, that thing about reading and writing. And one day I had to go to to the psychologist (....) and so I pretended that I could not do it. That was easy. And when I had to write you a letter on paper I pretended that I couldn't and then I started to cry. I cried, not because I couldn't do it, but because I had been so stupid as to think: 'I'll pretend I can't do it'. One step further and I was in hospital and I just pretended that I couldn't do it. But in the end that isn't easy, you know!. I finally gave it up and I shall think hard before I do anything (....) I hope you are not angry with me for doing it. And my punishment was writing and reading.'

This girl was in the first instance reported to have a mild form of epilepsy. After remedial treatment she soon afterwards became incontinent. This disappeared spontaneously when she went to hospital. Next she had serious learning problems. By this stage the child had long lost any control and was no longer capable of handling the situation. At this stage the neurologist called in the psychologist, because from his point of view he could not affirm that all the symptoms, taking the rest of her behaviour into account, were nervous ones. Thanks to the perspicacity of the neurologist the first step could be made towards an investigation of factors other than somatic ones.

After various observations, psychological investigation and various interviews with the patient and her parents, the mystery of her symptoms could be exposed. The letter which she sent at the end of her treatment shows better than any theory how symptoms can be functional.

Symptoms like the ones referred to above, are known as functional symptoms. There are many different definitions of this concept in the literature. Some definitions allow no organic abnormalities while others do not exclude them.

All, however, have one thing in common, that there must be some asomatic reason for the symptom.

A widely known example of a group of functional symptoms is known as 'school sickness'. This usually means that a child does not want to go to school because she does not like it or is afraid to go. This is shown by some physical symptom. These can be faked, for instance, by complaining about a headache when in fact there is none. Children seem to be very creative in making an illness look very real in this way.

Research by Bender (1988) in the Netherlands showed that half of 92 pupils investigated in the first form of their secondary school had at some time pretended to be ill to achieve some particular objective. In nearly 70% of cases the child's parents had taken their child's illness seriously. Thirteen of the children were seen by the family doctor and were treated by him. Moreover, in some cases things went further and there was a possibility of them being admitted to hospital.

There are dramatic examples of children who have had to endure a variety of investigations and interventions when there was no organic abnormality causing their condition. However, one should not always blame the doctors for the long time it takes to diagnose a symptom as functional. A symptom can often look plainly functional when in fact it is not. Obviously no doctor wants to run the risk of ignoring a potential somatic cause that may really be there.

During this phase there is development in thought, in that concrete thinking gradually changes into the abstract thoughts of the adolescent.

Another feature of cognitive development is an increase in the use of differing dimensions or points of view with regard to the same subject. Pre-school children are still quite absolute in their judgments. The nurse giving them an injection is not nice. A schoolchild looks at this kind of situation differently. The nurse giving her an injection may hurt her a bit, but otherwise she thinks she is very nice.

It is sometimes said that the environment begins to get more complex for the schoolchild on the cognitive level. You might also say, though it is not quite the same thing, that the schoolchild begins to qualify her judgements. A cognitive skill on which much emphasis is placed in our society is forward thinking. It is important to realize that you can obtain a substantial gain in the long term by foregoing small gains in the short term. This kind of thinking is particularly important in education. Because a long time passes between starting and finishing education, the goal can easily be lost sight of, and people often choose to give up in the middle. Thinking ahead is also a necessary skill for completing other protracted activities. School plays an important role in its acquisition.

Study activity
9. Describe briefly five factors influencing cognitive development in this phase.

6. Summary

Reaching adolescence, at about twelve years old, marks the end of an important period in life. Real childhood is left behind. So much has been experienced as a schoolchild, that now, as an adolescent, she can prepare for life as an adult, which measured in years will be the longest stage of her life. In other words, during childhood a number of basic skills have been ac-

quired, so that it becomes possible to make a start on the serious business of life. These skills are in various areas.

Physically the schoolchild has gradually grown up into a clearly identifiable individual. She has the features which will soon characterize her as an adult. She has grown in height and weight to the extent that she can literally receive the shocks to which she will be subjected in the turbulent times to come. Her body has in any case reached the stage where full physical development can take place. A number of children, particularly girls, already have the first indications of physical maturity, such as the development of breasts, and their first menstruation, by the end of their primary school period. Socially and emotionally, the schoolchild has had her first experiences outside the familiar pattern of family relationships. She has formed relationships for the first time with other children of the same age so that people other than her parents have become important to her. She has formed judgements about them, and by doing so has achieved some degree of self-assessment. She will soon have to convert her judgements of herself into a more complex understanding: into her identity, who she is, and how others see her.

8

The adolescent: from twelve to twenty-two years

1. Introduction

Adolescence: a period many parents do not look forward to. This is, of course, a social and cultural phenomenon. Fortunately most adolescents have no objection at all to this phase. Usually it cannot come soon enough for them, the hankering after adulthood ... for independence. But for his growth into adulthood the adolescent must also pay an obvious price: he swings from high peaks of happiness to the depths of despair and loneliness.

This is apparently the price that everyone must pay for seeking and finding their adult identity.

This can be a difficult phase for parents, because the adolescent's choices of behaviour are made independently of them. Parents lose their control over 'their child', who is on the road to adulthood.

How developmental psychologists interpret this stage of life is discussed in this chapter under the headings of:
– physical development;
– social and emotional development;
– cognitive development.

Learning outcomes

After studying this chapter the student should be able to:
– describe in general terms the physical developments in adolescence;
– define the concept of identity and describe what Erikson means in this context by:
  • continuity and stability;
  • congruence.
– describe and give examples of the social and emotional development of adolescents;
– describe in general terms the cognitive development of an adolescent.

2. The adolescent; a brief overview

At about the age of twelve a period starts for a human being in which he and the world do not know how to cope with each other. He is no longer a child, but not yet an adult. This feature is the essence of adolescence as a phase of development. It commences at about 12 years and ends somewhere between 16 to 22 years. The task of the adolescent is the formation of a clear identity, so that he has a foundation for beginning his life as an adult, and mastering an adult's problems.

The development of identity is accompanied by

some degree of insecurity. This insecurity is particularly evident at the beginning of adolescence, when the adolescent is going through major physical and sexual changes. These changes are only part of the process of forming an identity.

Another cause of great insecurity is the changes in the social and emotional area which are important in forming aspects of identity. In addition to breaking free to some extent from his existing relationships, the adolescent must also learn to make new ones. This involves not only the search for a partner, but also relationships at work and in society generally. The process often involves conflict.

A very distinctive aspect of someone's identity is his sense of values, or rather, his pattern of norms and values. Together with, and as a consequence of, processes in cognitive development, the adolescent makes substantial developments in this area. He leaves his familiar world for good, and encounters a host of new things. In this period he developes his own pattern of norms and values.

Inherent in this pattern is taking decisions about important aspects of his life. According to Erikson (1963), the adolescent phase is still a

Figure 2.8.1
Child or adult?

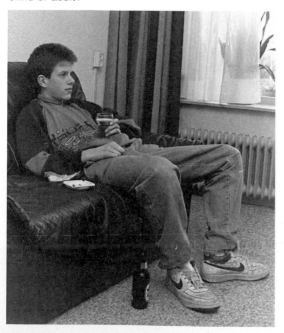

moratorium, a trial period, in which final decisions do not yet have to be made. The adolescent must be able to experiment in coping with events in his life, without this having irreversible consequences for him in society. Particularly in our society, which is so complex, and offers so many possibilities, the individual must have the opportunity to find his own way. This is also why adolescence lasts for such a long time in western society. In less complex societies, or for that matter in specific areas of our own society, the adolescent phase is much shorter, and people are regarded as being adult earlier. Think, for instance, of the initiation rites which in some cultures mark the change from childhood to adulthood. They sometimes only last for one day, after which the child is completely familiar with the adult world, and has acquired his place in it.

How the adolescent takes his decisions, but also the nature of the decisions he takes, finally give form to his identity. It will be obvious that the differences between individuals increase steadily from the start of this phase of life. It is also increasingly difficult for the psychologist to discover any regular pattern in the process of development. The whole process becomes more involved, partly because more and more factors have a role to play, and partly because reactions to these factors become more and more diverse. Finally one last introductory comment about adolescence. It is also a phase in which quite a lot can go wrong. Because the influence of established authority, like parents and teachers diminishes, adolescents sometimes take decisions which are not seen as desirable in our society. This problem is well illustrated by the content of two textbooks on adolescence. Conger and Petersen (1983) has chapters on drugs, criminality, truancy and psychiatric problems like attempted suicide and abnormal eating. Herbert (1987) has chapters on unemployment, alcohol and drug abuse, sexual activity, and defiance. To all intents and purposes, these kinds of subjects were absent from the earlier stages of development.

Many parents are not exactly overjoyed when their children reach adolescence. They are not only worried about their upbringing, but they are also afraid of the harmful influences which may be brought to bear on their children. They must accept the independence of their child as well, since society expects that he will soon be able to stand on his own two feet.

3. Physical development

The beginning of adolescence is particularly noticeable because of a number of physical developments.

At about the age of eleven for girls, and thirteen for boys, their bodies suddenly start to grow fast, especially in height. Early adolescents can be recognized by the length of their arms and legs which are out of proportion to their bodies. Their weight increases too, as their bones get heavier, and there is more fatty tissue.

There are also various physical and sexual changes. This stage of sexual maturation is called puberty. It is a process of growth on which the environment has little influence (with the exception of abnormally heavy physical stress, like strict physical training for sport, or eating problems like anorexia).

In boys the first indications of puberty are growth of the testes, the scrotum and pubic hair. About a year after these initial indications the penis grows larger. Next they grow hair on their face, chest and in the armpits, after which their voice gets deeper – their voice 'breaks'.

In girls puberty begins with the growth of pubic hair. Sometimes the breasts also start to be noticeable. These changes are followed by growth of the uterus and vagina.

In boys the changes finally lead to the first ejaculation, and in girls to the menarche, the first menstruation.

A logical consequence of these changes is that soon after the beginning of this phase the adolescent is physically capable of bearing or begetting children.

We must also not lose sight of the fact that within this group, among both boys and girls, there is a wide spread in the age at which these changes begin and end. The age at which a boy becomes sexually mature varies from thirteen to seventeen. In girls the menarche can start between the ninth and seventeenth year.

It is particularly important to be aware of this, because the processes of mutual acceptance among adolescents tend to be associated with the outward and visible signs of sexual maturity. It should be no problem to have had no ejaculation by the age of fifteen, or not yet to have had a period, let alone a lack of visible signs like the growth of facial hair or breasts; however, their environment will soon raise these problems for them.

Compared with other aspects of adolescence, the physical aspects of development have the most direct connection with the central problem of development, the formation of identity. Important characteristics of identity are continuity and stability, and physically these have no place in adolescence. The adolescent undergoes great changes in a short time, so that his image of himself must be changing continually.

This may explain why adolescents have such strong attachments to their idols, such as pop groups and sporting heroes, based on appearances. They often model themselves in appearance and behaviour on these examples, and this gives them something to hold on to in coping with their own changes.

Study activity

1. Search your memory for your heroes or heroines when you were fifteen. Analyse what you did to imitate them, and why.

Acceptance and discrimination based on clothes, make-up, hairstyle and other external characteristics are nowhere more important than among adolescents. Consider the groups of young people like punks, skinheads, casuals, and so on, each of which have their own uniform. Their outward appearance shows clearly who they are, provides something to hold on to, and in the long run it gives them self-confidence, too. For most adolescents acne is a real disaster; they are very sensitive to criticism of their appearance.

Physical and sexual changes are another problem in themselves. On the one hand they can bring about anxiety and confusion, on the other, they are something to which a child often looks forward. They are the signs of approaching adulthood. The way that adolescents finally cope with these changes is often determined by their view of themselves and of their environment: in brief, whether they regard them as something positive, something desirable, or as something negative and dangerous.

Study activity
2. Describe five factors which can influence physical development in this phase of life.

4. Social and emotional development

Many adults will assure you that they had most problems with their children during adolescence. If you then ask them what the precise difficulty was, they will tell you that you never know where you are with an adolescent.

The concept of identity
'Each individual is unique' is a phrase you will be familiar with. Nonetheless, one of the aims of psychology is to formulate general laws or explanations of human behaviour. It tries to explain the 'unique' behaviour of individuals by these general laws. Does this mean that people are not unique at all, because they behave according to general laws?

Yes and no; both answers are true to some degree. The operation of the general laws is, however, so subject to the influence of various factors that every human being has the opportunity of distinguishing himself from other people and in this way expressing his 'uniqueness'.

The uniqueness of any individual is expressed primarily by his identity. It is by his identity that he distinguishes himself from other people, and by it he is identifiable to others. Possibly some of you may by now be thinking of the concept of personality. There is, however, a difference between identity and personality. Personality applies primarily to the sum of individual characteristics and qualities, and their continuity in a diversity of situations. Identity applies more to someone's social identification, his personality in a social context.

Erikson (1963) states that the concept of identity only applies when someone's behaviour is characterized by:

– *Continuity and stability*
  He himself must have the feeling of always being the same person in spite of the changing situation in which he finds himself. There should be a feeling of consistency in thoughts, emotions, and actions. He must be identifiable and unique in his own eyes.
– *Congruence*
  There must be agreement between the picture he has of himself and the picture other people have of him. He must be identifiable and unique in the eyes of others.

According to this interpretation, identity is a dynamic principle of organization. It has less to do with who you are than with how you approach your problems, and how you get on in social situations, your intelligence, social skills, etc. This dynamic situation also means that someone's identity can change. A child often has no identity as yet. Children can behave in a completely unexpected and unrecognizable way in one situation compared to another. Identity develops in adolescence, but it can change during the course of life under the influence of experience. Naturally this influence becomes less over the years, because the identity becomes more stable. You change less easily as you get older.

Continuity and stability

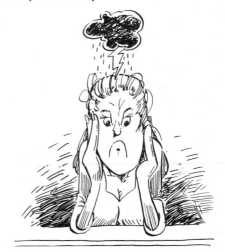

It is also true that during adolescence continuity and stability in behaviour is difficult to maintain. Another specialist term used to typify the behaviour of adolescents is *lability* (the tendency to change). Goethe characterizes this period very elegantly: *'Himmelhoch jauchzend, zum Tode betrübt'*, exultant one moment, despairing the next.

Identity results from interaction with other people. At the same time it implies self-reliance and independence. Its acquisition involves principally two areas.

– The adolescent has to break free from the traditional authority of parents and teachers to strive for independence. This usually leads to conflicts, because he does not yet possess the skills to do so without giving offence. In addition, the adolescent is still to a large extent dependent upon these authorities: he is often still being educated, and living at home. The process of learning to stand on his own feet is marked principally by negative behaviour, like opposition, without offering any positive alternatives to offset it. The adolescent is still caught between opposing interests, and must start by trying to find the proper balance between them.

In this respect the role played by the authorities is certainly important. Do they try to maintain their position of authority, or do they recognize the adolescent's need for independence? There was a comparable problem earlier, during the obstinate stage of the young child. The difference between then and now is that the adolescent comes much better equipped for the conflict. He is more mature, stronger, and more intelligent than the young child.

The need for independence is also closely linked to the culture and the times. There has always been a conflict of generations, as it is sometimes called. For several decades, however, this conflict has been fought out much more publicly, partly because official authorities have also been involved. Today's adolescent also has more opportunity of escaping from the conflict at an early stage, because society recognizes more readily the right of the young to lead an independent life.

Moreover, changes in society, around which this conflict is really based, nowadays occur so fast that it would be better not to talk of a conflict of generations so much as of a conflict of decades.

– The second area where the adolescent must prove himself is in his decisions. After the period of opposition comes the period of exploration. Eventually his decisions, which he makes in a variety of areas, contribute to the completion of his identity.

The partner

The adolescent goes out to look for a partner. For one thing, he needs one, because he is getting all kinds of sensations and urges for which a partner is desirable. For another, in his environment he sees nothing but adults, admittedly in a variety of ways, preferring to live together in pairs to living alone. He has to cope with feelings of love and affection which are rather more insistent than the feelings he has had up till now.

Choice of partner: the search for happiness?

Looking for a partner is an activity highly regarded by humanity. The emotion that should be displayed in this activity is probably the dominant subject in the world's literature, and is responsible for important events in world history: it is love. Not to have a partner or be able to acquire one is a disadvantage in our society. 'Loners' are penalized by our tax system, have to pay more for their holidays and find it difficult to mix with people living in a partnership. Self-help groups for single people can certainly list a whole catalogue of ways in which they are disadvantaged.

In the United Kingdom the vast majority of all adults live, or have lived, in some kind of way, with a partner. The rest of this account therefore applies to this category of couples. We will assume that when we talk of relationships these must be, to some extent, of a lasting nature.

The foundations on which the search for a partner is based can differ enormously. You may, of course, believe in love at first sight.

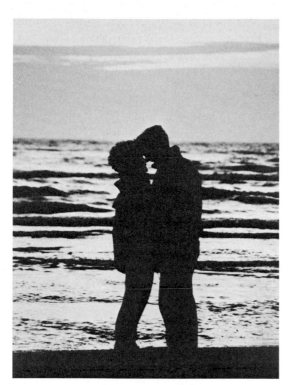

Figure 2.8.2
Romantic love:
many people's ideal

This is often interpreted as: there is only one person in the world who is meant for you. It is in that case a remarkable coincidence that this one person often lives quite close to you, since most people find their partner within a ten-mile radius of their own home. You can also have a much more complex idea of love, as a process in which needs, similarities and coincidences play a great part. This can also include the possibility of several people being suitable partners for anyone. You are likely to be shocked at such a suggestion if you are at the moment very much in love, and certainly not looking for other possible partners. In reality, love by itself appears to be a very shaky foundation for a lasting relationship. Look at the number of divorces in society. A large number of those involved were probably very much in love with each other, but in most relationships the condition of passionate love changes into a situation in which other emotions come to play an important part.

Not so long ago people used to get married for economic reasons. Today, too, one often hears that someone has hooked a rich partner. Nor does it appear to be the weakest basis for a lasting relationship, considering that there used to be much fewer divorces in the past.

Bear in mind that we are taking no account of the quality of the relationship here.

An important part of the process of choosing a partner is the reason why. Why do people feel attracted to each other? As we have said earlier, we start here from the idea that love, which in our society is irrevocably linked with the formation of this relationship, is something very complex.

Psychoanalysts express a clear opinion about the reason why. Basing their reasoning on the Oedipus and Electra complexes they claim that all adolescents and adults are searching for a continuation of their relationship with their father or their mother. Therefore they see their new partner as a replacement for the lost parental love, and their partner should therefore resemble their father or mother, or possibly some other important identification model.

Research in social psychology supports two main streams of thought about the formation of relationships: similarity and contrast. The similarity stream says that people are attracted to each other because they have a number of things in common, like similar interests, coming from the same class, doing the same kind of work, etc. The contrast stream says that people, on the basis of experiencing a lack in themselves, seek to make up this lack in their partner. The partner is therefore the opposite of oneself, at least in some aspects.

In reality the formation of relationships is probably a very complicated affair, as we can see if we look at ourselves and our environment.

Study activities
3. Describe the relationship of three couples who you know are good friends, and who have long-standing relationships, in the light of the discussion above.

4. Discuss how you yourself came to make your choices of friends, of your partner, and of your profession.

One final comment. Traupmann and Hatfield (1981) state that people who have a partner to share their ideas, feelings and problems with are happier and healthier than those who do not.
In this connection, however, remember that the category of people without partners is a very diverse one. They may consciously choose to live alone, but it is also possible that they have no partner (or no longer have one) because of pressures beyond their control.

Adolescents can experiment with relationships. To have a boyfriend or girlfriend need not be definitive, and many people will advise them to play the field and not to tie themselves down too quickly to a permanent partner. Flirtations allow them to try out what it means to have a relationship with someone, whichever person suits them best, and what emotions, both positive and negative, can exist between two people. This experimentation with relationships includes making decisions on whether to engage in sexual activity. The views held in society about all manner of sexual activity are probably more liberal than at any time in previous history, although views on promiscuity are probably changing due to the publication of the dangers of HIV/AIDS infection. Access to birth control methods and abortion have also played a part in this change by reducing the fear of pregnancy. At the same time behaviour guidelines have become less clear, leading to conflict for the individual in defining his own behaviour. Early research showed that about 18 percent of females and about 40 percent of males had experienced sexual intercourse by the age of 20 (Kinsey et al., 1948 and 1953). More recent estimates put the current figures at over half of all males and females having experienced sexual intercourse by the age of 20 years (Mori, 1991). Despite the accessibility and wide variety of contraceptive methods available, about 45 per 1000 teenage female population become pregnant, 15 of these being terminated by abortion. Reasons given for these pregnancies include erroneous beliefs about the likelihood of becoming pregnant, the unplanned nature of intercourse, and negative views towards contraceptive methods which are seen to interfere with the enjoyment of sex (Morrison, 1985). Further, it seems that adolescent girls prefer to be 'swept off their feet' and not be seen planning for sexual activity especially if they are not sure of their own standing on sexual behaviour.

The group
In adolescence in particular, you learn what it

Figure 2.8.3
The group is important
for the adolescent

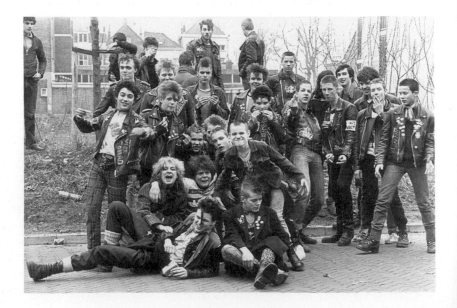

means to belong to a group. The adolescent is characterized by extreme conformity of behaviour among members of the same group and age group, two categories which often embrace each other. Just as he sets himself against authority, so he adapts himself to his peer group. This conformity is expressed in a special kind of language, in definite opinions and ideas he holds, and in the way he dresses.

The group often offers the adolescent the security which he lacks so much in his private life.

Career

Generally an adolescent makes preparatory decisions with an eye to the career he will later follow. After primary school, where most children still have no real career expectations, he goes on to secondary school. The choice of a type of education sometimes determines the parameters within which his eventual career will fall. If you choose technical subjects, then you are unlikely to become a lawyer.

The adolescent also registers great progress in the area of social cognition. His understanding of other people's thoughts and feelings, and of their motives, continues to improve. This development runs in parallel with his cognitive development.

Study activity

   5. List five factors which influence social and emotional development in this phase of life.

5. Cognitive development

Two streams can be distinguished in the cognitive development of an adolescent. In the first place there is the development of thought itself, in which remarkable changes can take place. In the second place there are the changes in the sense of values, or pattern of norms and values, which accompanies the development of thought. There is a quantitative change in thought. An adolescent can think more quickly and efficiently than a schoolchild. This is because as he goes through life he acquires more experiences in the area of problem solving and he gradually learns to make better use of these experiences. If you define intelligence as 'the capability of profiting from experience, and of

learning quickly from new ideas and behaviour', you can describe someone's potential intelligence in adolescence as being 'more identifiable'.

The IQ (Intelligence Quotient – a measure of intelligence) becomes more stable, and corresponds better with later intellectual performance, demonstrating a change in the cognitive processes. Thought also changes qualitatively. There is a different approach to problems: adolescents not only think more quickly and efficiently, but also differently, indicating a change in the cognitive structure.

The concrete thinking of the schoolchild is gradually replaced by the abstract thinking (the formal operational stage of Piaget) of the adolescent. It would, however, be more correct to say that abstract thinking is potential, because it is quite possible for someone never to learn abstract thinking, even when he becomes an adult. Abstract thinking is considered to be the final stage in the development of thought. It involves thoughts no longer being linked to material facts, events or objects, but all assembled into one general category or concept. If an adolescent uses the concept of racial discrimination, this can refer to many different situations in which general rules of discrimination are applied. He would even be capable of including non-existent, but imaginable situations, such as Martians being discriminated against by Earthmen.

Development of a sense of values is on the one hand strongly influenced by the capacity for abstract thought. On the other, his environment also imposes high expectations on the adolescent in this respect. While the schoolchild still enjoys reasonable freedom on the issue of norms and values, the adolescent is expected to know how to behave.

Initially attempts are made to pass on to the adolescent the pattern of norms and values of his parents, or as an extension of them, of the school. In this respect he is already considered an adult at an early stage. In his confrontation with his environment, which is often far more complex than that of the schoolchild, the adolescent, who is already insecure as a result of his physical development, starts to have doubts.

Is the familiar pattern of norms and values right? It is obviously not the only pattern. Many adolescents react to this doubt by setting themselves against what is familiar and generally accepted. That does not mean that they have anything new to put in its place. From their initial opposition most of them later develop their own pattern of norms and values, that need not *per se* be based upon the existing ones, and can also hark back to earlier patterns. Thus many parents who grew up in the turbulent period of the 1960s and 1970s, when they adopted a fairly progressive pattern of norms and values, are currently faced with the fact that their children, now in the same phase as they used to be, are developing a conservative pattern.

The adolescent's sense of values is generally an absolute one. He still brings very few qualifications to his norms and values, which is also understandable. The world is so complex, that when the still hesitant adolescent starts to introduce qualifications, he cannot see the wood for the trees. There is plenty of scope for him to develop his own pattern of norms and values. Besides, thanks to a multitude of communication channels, everyone is informed of a variety of alternative patterns. For the adolescent, salvation lies in being absolute.

Whatever values an adolescent adopts, definite streams can still be distinguished in their pattern of values.

- In his opposition to the familiar, he will at first conform fairly closely to his age group. Individual interests are subordinated to the interests of the group, and this guideline directs his behaviour.
- This leads eventually to the development of general principles for himself, when he is no longer linked to the group. In this way he acquires something to go by when he meets similar situations. At first he applies these principles very consistently.
  Adolescents at this stage often complain about the world being unfair: adults, in their opinion, are too flexible in their principles.
- Finally, these general principles acquire a somewhat more logical base as a result of his experiences as an adult.

An important characteristic of the development particularly of values in adolescence is that they become steadily more consistent. Values do not change quickly, and are interconnected within his whole pattern of values. It will be obvious that the development of a sense of values, as it has just been described above, takes up a considerable time, and is certainly not completed in adolescence. Often the process lasts through the whole of life. Values form an integral part of identity, and determine many of the essential decisions which have to be made during adolescence. This has been discussed in Section 4 of this chapter. Values are linked to the times, and changes in the dominant pattern of values can be identified in history.

Study activity

6. List five factors that influence cognitive development in this phase of life.

Case study: Jerry

Last night Jerry was taken to hospital after attempting suicide. His parents are shocked. They can't understand it. Their son ..., Jerry, slashing his wrists. But why?

On second thoughts, Jerry, eighteen last month, was rather quieter than usual. Well, that had happened before. And his girlfriend had just left him. But that seemed to be more of a relief to him. Or was it? His parents are in despair and can't understand it at all.

The next morning, when Jerry is in the ward, he hardly speaks. He tells the nurse that he does not want to see his parents. No appeals will make him talk to a psychiatrist or a psychologist.

The only person to whom Jerry will say at least something is Jane – the student nurse who started her course three months ago. Jane, as it later turns out, was in the same class with him at school.

Study activities

7. **a.** Suggest reasons why Jerry does not want to speak to his parents.

   b. Is it justifiable, as a nurse, to agree to Jerry's demands not to see his parents? Explain your answer.

8. a. Is it sensible to leave Jerry's case to Jane? Give reasons for your answer.
b. Give your opinion on the question of whether it is professional for students, who may themselves still be adolescent, to be given the charge of an adolescent. List the pros and cons.

9. Draw up a nursing plan for Jerry's treatment, covering problems, objectives and implementation in the interests of his general welfare.

6. Summary

Adolescence is a period during which the differences between individuals grow steadily greater. The development of the adolescent is therefore more difficult to sum up in general terms than human development in the earlier stages. Although the adolescent's central problem is the formation of an identity, we should not imagine that this problem is resolved by the end of this phase. On the contrary. It can, in fact, be claimed that only the outlines of his identity are sketched in at this stage. The adolescent has made only preliminary decisions in various areas. The adolescent will also be able to describe his pattern of norms and values, and express them in his behaviour. Society has given him the opportunity to develop all this with a certain degree of freedom.

From now on, however, life becomes more serious. In his encounter with the adult world, it will become apparent how much he will be able to realize his decisions. He will now have to prove himself, and in doing so will no longer enjoy the freedom he had earlier. More responsibility is put on him, and the question is whether, now that he is an adult, he can cope with it.

9

The young adult:
from twenty-two to forty years

1. Introduction

The young adult is in the prime of his life. Many older people look back on their young adulthood with nostalgia. This is a period which they would often happily repeat.

In the previous chapter we looked at various situations which presented the adolescent with opportunities for experimentation with his behaviour and attitudes. Now these situations (the choice of partner, of further study, of a career, etc.) are, for the young adult serious matters of great import, where far reaching decisions have to be made.

One of the requirements for dealing effectively with these situations is a great deal of energy and in this respect the young adult is better equipped, both physically and emotionally, in comparison with other phases of his life. The vitality of the young adult is an essential attribute if he is to bring all the tasks of development to completion.

How the young adult functions is described in this chapter following the pattern of the previous chapters.

Learning outcomes

After studying this chapter the student should be able to:
- describe and explain in general terms the young adult's physical development;
- describe the most important aspects of social and emotional development from the point of view of:
  • work;
  • relationships;
  • attitude to life.
- describe in general terms the young adult's cognitive development.

2. The young adult; a brief overview

True adulthood begins in this phase of life. The study of the psychology of this phase is a recent development because it was assumed until recently that there was no more psychological development after becoming adult. Psychology could therefore be limited to establishing a few rules of human behaviour, without having to worry about any processes of development. Nowadays the general opinion is that adults have their own development problems, which can be studied. This is in fact the subject covered by life cycle psychology.

It is difficult to define adulthood. When does an individual become an adult? The question must first be considered from the point of view of society. In the United Kingdom, for example, society calls someone adult when they have reached the age of eighteen. They can then vote in elections; they can also sign official documents without having to have their parents' consent.

On the other hand a sixteen-year-old is considered an adult sexually, while eighteen is the age for the contraction of marriage without parental consent.

Psychology has no absolute criteria for adulthood. It also makes no sense to consider adulthood as a limit to be reached, or a threshold to be crossed. It should be regarded as a dynamic process, in which a process of development can be perceived. Adulthood is also never complete as long as there are areas where there can still be development. A father can often be heard wondering when his twenty-three-year old son will ever behave like an adult. At the same time grandfather, aged seventy, will be saying the same thing about his son of forty-five!

The problem the young adult has to solve is 'achieving a more or less definitive place in society'. She achieves this place by bringing to realization a number of decisions for which she prepared herself as an adolescent. These decisions affect various areas of her life, like her relationships, her work, and her attitude to life. Her occupation with these decisions is a sign of her being an adult.

Adulthood is a
relative concept

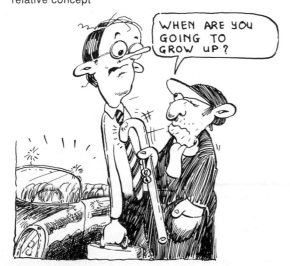

Case study: Peter and Kevin

Peter and Kevin will celebrate their twenty-first birthdays tomorrow. They both feel fully adult already. Peter still lives at home and his parents are giving him all Beethoven's symphonies on compact disc. His main hobby is classical music. This is his final year at the polytechnic, and after that he will begin professional training to become an accountant. He has not yet got a steady girlfriend. He has certainly thought about it, and about what it would be like to have a family, but going steady, no, not yet!

Kevin's wife gives him a set of tools, so that he can make toys for his eighteen-month-old son. When his girlfriend fell pregnant, two years ago, he gave up his training as a physiotherapist. Now he works for a temping agency, because he needs the money. That does not worry him much, because he was never really that interested in study. He has no clear plans for the future. He is all right financially, because his parents regularly subsidize him. Life is very pleasant for him as it is.

Study activities

1. Who is behaving in a more adult way, Kevin or Peter?

2. Draw up a list of criteria on the basis of which you could establish that someone was behaving like an adult.

Try to discover which of these two shows the most adult behaviour. Arguing theoretically, that will not be easy. From the theoretical point of view, the young adult phase is a difficult one. In the first place development has become such a complex process that it is more difficult to analyse the three aspects of development separately. You will also find, much more often than previously, that a description of one aspect of development might apply equally to all the others. Entering into a relationship will serve as an example; there is both a social and emotional, and a physical side. In the second place there is such diversity among individuals, that it is difficult to distinguish general lines of development. At this stage the process of human development can be compared with the expanding universe. From a common origin a large number of entities have evolved in the course of time, ever moving further apart and differing from each other, but held together by the same forces, and subject to the same laws. The idea that such forces and laws also exist in the life of adults helps to describe adulthood.

3. Physical development

The young adult is in the prime of life. At the start of this phase of life an individual reaches the peak of physical development. Only in the second half of the phase, do her physical powers, albeit slowly and gradually, start to diminish.

This is evident from the age at which various sporting champions deliver their best perform-ances. In individual sports like swimming or athletics, which make heavy demands on the body, standards are set by fifteen to twenty-five year olds. A few athletes over the age of twenty-five can keep at the top for a time, but they are usually finished by the time they reach their thirties.

In team sports, equally demanding on the body, but where people are also very dependent upon the contribution of others, and in which experi-ence is very important, the top is not usually reached until after the age of twenty-five. There is then a gradual decline after the age of twenty-

seven or twenty-eight, which can usually still be offset to some extent by experience.

Case study: Tom

Tom has a busy life. He is twenty-three, has a steady girlfriend, and has been working for a year, nursing in hospital. He is also a very keen long-distance runner. He trains every day for at least an hour and a half, and often competes at weekends. In addition he is busy doing up a house, because he wants to get married fairly soon. He sometimes asks himself where he gets all the energy; he sees his father collapse in front of the television every evening. His father used to be a very keen sportsman too, thinks Tom.

It would be safe to assume that the first half of young adulthood is characterized by maximum physical performance. The brain works well and fast, the muscles are resilient, the joints strong and flexible, the skin supple and unwrinkled, and energy seems to be boundless. In the second half of this phase, from about thirty, a slow decline begins. There is an increase in fatty tissue, greater efforts are needed to keep your weight down, you move more slowly, your re-actions are slower and you need longer to re-cover from your efforts. The first signs of age can also be seen in your appearance. Men can

Figure 2.9.1
At the dawning of adult-hood this image still seems very distant

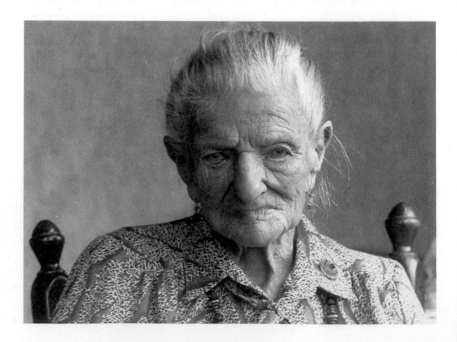

start growing bald and grey, women get their first wrinkles round the eyes, and their skin becomes less supple. In the case of women, pregnancy also plays a part in physical development; this is why women can sometimes age more quickly physically.

The brain, too, stops growing. Cells which die are no longer replaced, and after the age of thirty-five it may become noticeable that the memory begins to be less reliable.

From this age on, people also have more problems with their health. Aches and pains increase, and the likelihood of serious illness is greater.

From the sexual point of view there are also obvious changes. Men reach their highest sexual capacity around the age of twenty, and women at about twenty-five. After the age of twenty-five the possibility of her having children very slowly declines and after thirty-five the likelihood of her having a handicapped child is great enough for many couples to decide against it.

From a physical point of view, this phase can be said to enable people to realize the hopes and ambitions of their adolescence. They have enough energy and physical strength to achieve their objectives.

Study activity
  3. List five factors which can influence physical development at this stage of life.

4. Social and emotional development

As was explained earlier, young adults develop at different rates and in diverse ways. It is therefore difficult to give a general description of the processes of social and emotional development. It is difficult to forecast how a young adult will develop, because of the enormous number of factors which can affect this development.

At best we can assume that in a young adult's process of development a few central themes play a leading role. Everyone comes up against these themes in this period of their lives. The extent to which they determine an adult's life is, however, dependent upon her culture and her times. For example, many young adults are currently going through a crisis of belief, which

would not have been the case in this country forty years ago, or in Islamic countries now.

Three important themes of life can be distinguished in our society, as follows:
– work;
– relationships;
– attitude to life.

The importance of these themes, and their influence on the life of the young adult, is illustrated by the following case study.

Case study: Marion and Charles
Marion is twenty-eight. She is married to Charles. Both work at the hospital, he as a junior doctor, she as a radiographer, so you can say that they have a comfortable income. They buy new clothes regularly, they eat out at least once a week, and don't worry too much about the bill. It has never occurred to them that there are some things they can't afford. Marion begins to get the idea that she would like a family. In a few years she may be too late. She does not want her children, while they are still young, to be saddled with ageing parents. Besides, it is better not to be too old when you are pregnant. However, having a family has its disadvantages: Charles still has at least three years before he can become a consultant. Besides, it is not certain whether, after that, he will find an established post as a paediatrician somewhere. If they have children, she wants to stop working at once. After seven years in one and the same department, she has had enough.

Study activity
  4. Go over the reasons for having or not having a family from your own point of view.

a. Work

In our society work is considered as one of the most important activities for a young adult. To count for anything, you must have a job and your status in society is measured by the job you do. 'How do you do?' is in effect replaced by 'What do you do?'

Work not only gives status, but above all an income as well, at any rate more income than if you did not have a job. The income in its turn ensures that you can function better as a member of society. You can pay the rent, eat, buy clothes, do exciting things, and also practise your hobby or give money to good causes.

For many people work supplies a meaningful content for their lives. Imagine for a moment what it would mean for you if you had no job and you had to start every day by thinking of something to do. If you had plenty of money, it might be less of a problem, but money comes as a reward for work. The Marxist system of social philosophy is in fact based entirely on people's work or labour. It regards work as the most important factor in human life.

Study activity
5. Describe briefly how important it is to you to have a job, and how you would organize your life without work.

Each individual decides how important work really is. For some people work is their 'all'. They have built their life round their jobs. These workaholics are addicted to their work to such an extent that they don't know what to do with leisure time, for their work is an end in itself. You may, however, think that work is not an end in itself, but just a means of maintaining your quality of life.

In our society, for most young adults, work is one of the three important themes of life. The basis for this has usually been laid in adolescence, when people make decisions affecting their eventual choice of occupation, and when they also acquire their personal attitude to work. Work can satisfy various needs of the young adult, such as those below, listed in the sequence

The workaholic

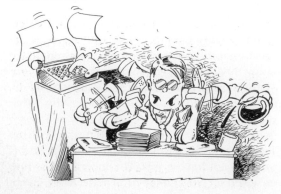

of Maslow's (1954) hierarchy of needs (see diagram 1.2.3):
- *Financial security*

  Work provides an income that in general guarantees provision of the basic needs of a family. There is, of course, a complicated package of provisions to provide a basic income for people without work. These provisions are only made possible because people in work surrender part of their income.

  If you have a job and your financial security is guaranteed, it is also easier to enjoy various other facilities society has to offer. You can buy a house or arrange a loan, go on holiday, and so on. In other words, work creates a pattern of living and a pattern of needs. These patterns in their turn ensure that you are dependent upon your job, because you cannot do without the money.
- *Need for social contacts*

  For most people their work is the place where they are most likely to meet other people; their colleagues are important to them. Apart from their work related contacts they often make and maintain friendships there.
- *Need for achievement*

  The need for achievement and for status relative to other people can be satisfied through work. In western societies the need to achieve is usually considered an essential quality. In addition, the need for achievement includes an element of competition: achieving more than other people. Schooling and sport introduce these ideas to the attention at quite a young age.
- *Self-actualization*

  Of course, purely individual needs can also be fulfilled through work. You can make use of your talents and skills. You can achieve fulfilment in your job. Work often gives a feeling of your own worth and self-confidence.

Study activity
6. You have made a decision to spend your life working as a nurse. Discuss, with other students, which of the motives listed above played a part, to a greater or lesser degree, in your choice.

Many adults nowadays decide not to implement their choice in this area for a longer or shorter time. In other words, they do not get a paid job, or they drop out of work.

Unemployment figures of around nine percent (with regional variations) are not exceptional at the moment. This means that a substantial proportion of adults cannot take their part in one of the three themes of life. Moreover, you should bear in mind that the three themes are not independent of each other, and that the issues listed above can thus also influence the other two areas of life.

There are various reasons for this difficulty. In the first place, of course, is the economic situation, and the number of jobs available. Political decisions have a great influence here. Then there are a number of personal factors influencing it, as, for example, the choice you made of your area of study, your attitude to getting a job, personal qualities, and so on.

Unemployment can lead to a number of problems, such as:
- being labelled 'unemployed' with all its consequences;
- coming to the conclusion that you have chosen the wrong course of study;
- being less acceptable socially;
- social isolation;
- financial insecurity;
- having to put off planned activities, like starting a family;
- in the long term finding it steadily more difficult to find a job; the skills you have acquired may now be out of date;
- looking for an escape in less acceptable forms of behaviour, like alcohol, drugs or crime.

b. Relationships

It is generally expected of young adults that they will realize their need for human contact by entering into a relationship with a partner. Living with a partner is the standard pattern on which our society is based. Most laws, types of housing, restaurants and shops are made not for the individual, but for the individual with a partner, and best of all with children, too. For example, solitary diners get the worst places in a restaurant, and in shops single people find that pre-packed vegetables are in family-sized packs. Most young adults have themselves grown up within this standard pattern and do not appreciate that other forms of living together could also satisfy their needs for social contacts, affection, intimacy and sexuality.

In this phase of life they enter into a relationship, whether short or long term, and whether or not officially blessed. They have usually had some experience of forming a relationship in their adolescent period. Now as young adults they capitalize on this experience. In the process of forming and maintaining a relationship the following stages can be distinguished.

Looking for a partner and sealing the relationship

Human beings need affection and intimacy, and look for a way of satisfying this need. The form this takes is determined by society. What used to be an obvious matter has nowadays become a problem, or is made into a problem: how can you formalize your relationship with your partner? Every adolescent or adult is confronted with this question sooner or later. Whereas previously it was quite clear to everyone that when you grew up you got married and started a family, or else you stayed single, nowadays there is a choice of several possibilities, at times limited by public opinion. For some people cohabitation has already become something quite normal, sometimes as a kind of trial marriage, sometimes in what seems a permanent arrangement. Many people are also familiar with the LAT relationship (living apart together) and with communal living, and having children has for a long time not been circumscribed by the marriage relationship.

Most people still feel that there should be an intention of making the relationship permanent, that is to say, one that lasts as long as possible. In the United Kingdom, for example, the vast majority of people still marry at least once in their lives.

Marriage is very popular. You may ask why? Does marriage provide the best solution for a number of human needs? Is social pressure so great that most people conform to the norm? Or does marriage offer the best financial or legal arrangements for people? The work of Traupmann and Hatfield (1981) indicated that married people are in general happier, or feel happier, than unmarried ones. At the time of writing, just under 80% of British people living in private households lived in married couple families.

The figures below taken from official statistics published in 1986 show the situation then (table 2.9.1).

Marriage is still very popular among younger people, as the research shows. About 80% consider it the form of partnership which they would wish to enter into in the long run.

Marriage, however, also carries with it rights and obligations *vis-à-vis* the partner, children and society.

Study activity

7. **a.** List five obligations to your partner, your children and society, which you take on when you get married.

   b. List five legal rights with respect to your partner, children and society which you acquire on marriage.

The existence of many alternative forms of relationship suggests that marriage does not satisfy all human needs, or even hinders the satisfaction of some of them.

In addition to the problem of the form of the relationship, it is also important to consider what you put into the relationship. It is certainly not an established fact that the form of the relationship also determines its content. Thus

Table 2.9.1

I Structure of population aged 16 and over by form of cohabitation

	Unmarried	Married	Widowed	Divorced
Men 1984	28.8%	63.4%	3.7%	4.1%
Women 1984	21.9%	58.8%	14.4%	4.9%

II Households

	1971	1984
Single individual	18%	25%
Two or more people	82%	75%
Total no. of households	18.32 million	19.5 million

III Marriage, birth, divorce

	1971	1981	1984
Marriages (thousands)			
First marriages	369	263	259
Remarriages	90	135	136
Divorces (thousands)	80	157	158

	1981	1983	1984
Live births (thousands)			
legitimate	554	530	526
illegitimate	81	99	110

some people in LAT relationships allow each other less freedom than others would in a marriage. In the end you work out with your partner the rules governing your life within a relationship. These rules governing your life can cover:
– allocation of jobs;
– allocation of responsibilities;
– rules of the game for sex;
– planning for the future;
– management of finances.

It is obvious, when you look at the figures for divorce in the United Kingdom, that to give both a satisfactory form and content to a relationship is no easy task.

Currently one out of every three marriages ends in divorce, and it is expected that this ratio will increase in the future to one in two. So far we have said nothing about the quality of those relationships which endure. The investment by the partners in a relationship to keep it in being can be heavy, and can often be at the expense of individual happiness. The alternative, divorce and a new relationship, is often very unattractive financially, and involves enormous emotional problems.

To have children or not

Every couple, and nowadays many single individuals too, ask themselves this question. Not so long ago the answer was self-evident. If you had a firm, officially blessed relationship, then children were a part of it.

Nowadays it is all much more complicated, for the following reasons:
– It is socially acceptable for people, whether living alone or together, to take advantage of their potentiality for reproduction. You need therefore no longer be married *per se* in order to have children.
– The decision to have no children is socially acceptable, and moreover easier to achieve because there is a whole range of contraceptives available. About one tenth of British couples choose not to have children.
– Adults who are not capable of having children (about 10% of the British population) because some factor impedes the reproductive processes either of the man or the woman, are nowadays offered a whole range of methods for removing these impediments.

The availability of all these possibilities faces the young adult with a difficult decision. For most adults having children or not is a fundamental decision whose consequences are irreversible; children are for life. We list below some of the consequences for a relationship of the decision to have children.
– Consequences for both partners:
  • change in the pattern of life;
  • change in responsibilities;
  • changes in the pattern of expenditure;
  • changes in the feelings each partner has for the other;
  • changes in their value systems.
– Consequences specific to the woman:
  • bringing a pregnancy to term, and experiencing a confinement;
  • the woman is no longer just a daughter, but becomes a mother;
  • a change in her status in society;
  • having to share her attentions between her partner and her child;
  • having to give up (temporarily) her job or career;
– Consequences specific to the man:
  • living through the woman's pregnancy;
  • being a father;
  • less attention from his partner;
  • increased responsibilities.

Study activity
8. **a.** Give a concrete example of each of the consequences of becoming a parent.
b. Describe the differences for a couple without children, taking the general consequences of parenthood as your starting point.

The decision to have children also entails the parents having to turn their minds to bringing them up. Parental responsibility also includes teaching the child to behave as a full member of society. Bringing up their children is one of the most important occupations for young adults. The problems involved in this have already been described in detail in the chapters on the various phases of the child's development.

c. Attitudes to life

It has already been said that the young adult tries to realize a number of fundamental decisions

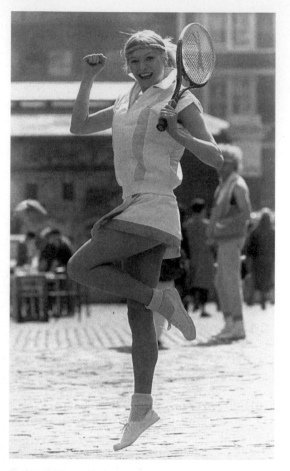

Figure 2.9.2
Young, active, attractive
and sports-loving: society's ideal

In this connection one can think of:
- the way you dress, furnish your house, and how mobile you are;
- your interest in culture, your taste in music, and the time you spend watching television;
- your hobbies, and the money and effort you devote to them;
- your eating and drinking habits;
- your contacts with your family.

Norms and values system

Young adults will often discover that their expectations do not correspond with reality. In the areas of morality, ethics and religion they are confronted with specific situations which often throw a new light on their norms and values. They are in fact being forced to make qualifications because reality is shown to be more complex than they thought, particularly when it comes to realizing their ambitions.

Thus, in adolescence they may have chosen nursing as a career because of all kinds of idealistic motives. Later in life they will find that income is important, too, because children, for example, are expensive. So they work for a managerial post, pushing their original idealism into the background.

Ambitions from adolescence, when they would put the whole world to rights, are changed by the adult into political activities, because they see that that is where real power is exercised. Or they go out to a developing country and try to implement their dreams there – even if they have to adapt them a little. Personality naturally also has a part to play here. One person is more prepared to fight for her ideals, and to uphold her norms and values, than another.

Reaction to potential crises in life

Naturally things can also go wrong in a young adult's life. Increasing age brings with it a greater chance of events occuring which can be traumatic, and which can give a different direction to life. Crises in the lives of young adults usually involve unravelling the decisions made at various earlier phases of life. The arrival of such crises is all the harder to cope with, because they were not expected in this phase, which is typically a constructive one.

taken in adolescence, and prepared for during that phase. How this was done in regard to work and relationships has been discussed above. However, there is much more in the young adult's life than work and maintaining relationships. This 'much more' is covered by the phrase 'attitude to life'. Attitude to life includes very ordinary things like having a hobby (admittedly not an ordinary thing for some people), but also serious matters like practising one's religion, the achievement of political office, or doing charitable work. Some examples are analysed below.

Life-style

Young adults stand on their own feet and can develop their own life-styles. Advertising makes grateful use of the need of many adults to keep up a life-style of their own.

The most important crises in this phase of life are:
– Crises in working life, such as:
  • not being able to find a job after you have trained for one. Expectations which had been aroused are not fulfilled, and plans for the future cannot be carried out;
  • losing your job, which in its turn can lead to financial problems, particularly if you have already taken on specific obligations;
  • the onset of illness or an accident, causing you to become incapable of working. There are in our society measures to support those falling by the wayside, but none the less they do not compensate for personal disappointment.
– Crises in relationships, such as:
  • the death of a partner and/or a child, as a result of illness or an accident;
  • separation from your partner and/or children;
  • having a handicapped child or one in poor health;
  • the death of your own parents;
  • not being able to have children;
  • problems arising from your children's decisions.
– Crises in attitude to life, such as:
  • an illness which causes you to make fundamental changes to your life-style;
  • financial problems resulting from your life-style;
  • factors in society affecting your life-style, like environmental pollution or economic recession.

Study activity
  9. List five factors which influence social and emotional development in this phase of life.

5. Cognitive development

Up to this phase of life, cognitive development was mainly structural in nature. By this we mean that the principal changes occurred in the process of thinking and perception. By the end of adolescence cognitive development had reached its peak in this respect.

The content of the adolescents' thoughts and their process of thinking were seen as being different from those of children and older people. The interaction between the content and process of thoughts and the special concerns of adolescents, contributes to the way they think. In the case of young adults the situation is completely different. There is little change now in the process of thought; but the development in its content is all the greater.
These developments are explained in more detail below.

a. The cognitive process

The young adult has usually reached the stage where she is capable of abstract thought. Her memory is functioning at its optimum, and she can store incoming information properly. She thinks quickly. In short, from the cognitive point of view the young adult is at her peak.
Scientists in areas where pure thought is important, like mathematics and physics, often produce their best achievements at a young age. For instance, Einstein was only twenty-six when he published his theory of relativity. He had indeed had the idea on which the theory was based several years earlier.
As a young adult there is still, however, one thing lacking, and that is sufficient experience or knowledge of the world: the content of thought. This is perhaps an advantage for the mathematical sciences, but for the life sciences, like psychology and philosophy, it is an obvious disadvantage. These scientists usually produce their greatest achievements when they are older. Their thought processes are perhaps no longer at their peak, but that defect is abundantly compensated for by their experience of life.
In the second half of the young adult period, the human capacity for thought slowly starts to decline. The memory becomes less keen, and it is more difficult to remember names or telephone numbers, and such matters. Learning new things also becomes more difficult, and it takes longer. This is not a dramatic change, but it is noticeable. This does not mean that overall ability diminishes. The adult is still capable of solving problems, perhaps even better than before, because she can make more use of experience.

b. The content of thought

In the previous section several references have already been made to 'experience'. Starting in the young adult phase, and continuing in subsequent phases of life, there is a clear cognitive development in respect of the content of thinking. An adult's thought could be said to become deeper. Because she undergoes many and, above all, fresh experiences, her outlook on things alters. Many young adults will have noticed that the ideas they had in adolescence, most of which were matters of principle, are gradually changing. They start to look at things from another point of view, they see the relativity of that point of view and therefore become less rigid in their thinking.

The experiences which are encountered as a young adult penetrate strongly into the personality and influence thoughts and perception fundamentally. Consider for a moment the influence the birth of a child can have on the parents: the world looks quite different when you have responsibility for a new citizen of it. Crises in life, too, bring home to you the relative nature of many things about which you thought you had well-founded and fixed opinions. If you suddenly become seriously ill, the concept of health takes on another dimension.

This new outlook on the world might be regarded as a change in your value system. The value system of an individual is not a fixed entity which remains unaffected in adulthood. Values are dynamic elements linked in a specific way. A change in one of its elements disturbs the connecting links, too.

Case study: Christine

Christine suddenly had very heavy menstrual bleeding. Her family doctor sent her straight to a gynaecologist. A major operation was necessary, as there was a suspicion of cervical cancer. Christine, a strong, brisk woman of thirty-five, had up till then always enjoyed life. Suddenly she had a completely different outlook. At the moment she was seriously ill, and only saw problems in the future. She had postponed having children, because she did not want to give up working yet. Now she could never have any. She suddenly realized that all kinds of unpleasant things, which always happened to other people,

could happen to her, too. She also realized suddenly that her parents had meantime reached an age when they might get ill and die.

Study activities

10. **a.** On the basis of Christine's case, explain her outlook on death at the cognitive level.
    b. Describe the differences in Christine's cognitive perception in all the previous phases of her life.

11. List five factors which influence cognitive development in this phase of life.

6. Summary

The period of young adulthood is a very active period in human life. Young adults are expected to develop initiatives in areas such as work, relationships, and attitude to life. The young adult is in the prime of her life, has great energy, and is in general not yet frustrated by the lack of time to do all she wants to do. She has, certainly in our society, still enough time to recover from any mistakes, setbacks or disappointments. If she loses her job she can look for a new one, or retrain, and after a separation she can find a new partner. In the area of her norms and values, too, there are plenty of alternatives available in our complex society.

The young adult has a great many opportunities. The world offers her an enormous choice from which to take her pick. She is not yet old, her behaviour throughout this phase of life can be youthful, and she holds her life in her own hands. It is a period during which an individual probably most often thinks that she controls her own life, and makes conscious decisions in which she allows herself great freedom.

The older adult: from forty to sixty-five years

10

1. Introduction

The older adult: a phase which seems a long way off for most students, and one which, from the social point of view, can often be influenced by the mid-life crisis for both men and women.

Obviously it is a difficult phase in human development. People have to face the challenge of achieving the stability essential for the second half of life. Moreover, the older adult knows only too well that this second half is the final half.

In our society the position of the older adult is a changing one. The image we have of older people is shifting, especially where the forty to sixty-five age group is concerned. With their wisdom and experience of life, they are still often in the midst of life, and still giving it good service.

This chapter also describes how the process of development in this phase does not always run smoothly.

Learning outcomes

After studying this chapter the student should be able to:
- describe in general terms the physical development of the older adult;
- describe the social and emotional development of the older adult in respect of:
  - work;
  - relationships;
  - attitude to life;
- describe the cognitive development of the older adult in respect of:
  - thought processes;
  - thought content.

2. The older adult; a brief overview

At around the age of forty many adults get to the stage of asking themselves: 'What am I doing?' or 'Is this all there is?' They feel that progress in the three main aspects of development has come to a halt. Physically there is the beginning of an obvious decline. In the social and emotional area a number of decisions have been realized, others have proved too ambitious or have gone wrong. In the cognitive area wear and tear is also beginning to be apparent.

The world has not much new to offer them. The adult has reached a watershed in his life, a point that, perhaps not accidentally, coincides with the start of the second half of his life. Crossing this watershed heralds the dawning of a new phase in life.

The typical characteristic of the older adult is stability. We should, however, only refer to stability with reservations, because it depends on the way in which the watershed is crossed. For some adults a serious crisis marks the start of this phase of life. After this crisis, stability can usually be achieved. Not everyone succeeds in this, and the consequences of that will be discussed below. The crisis arises because the adult is faced with a very fundamental new decision. Will he carry on as he has done so far, or will he make an entirely fresh start, in which he can put right or avoid his earlier mistakes? This fundamental decision is particularly relevant for the three themes of life.

Although the last paragraph sets it out in very general terms, it must be appreciated that there is an enormous difference in the way different people experience this crisis; in fact not everyone would call it a crisis. While it is possible for some people not to consider this period as one of transition, others may need help to overcome their crisis. This help may be available in self-help groups for women and men which aim to assist them to cope with this change of life. The fact that there are separate organizations for women and men, shows that women experience the crisis in a different way from men; this is confirmed by their titles: the man's crisis is called 'mid-life crisis', whereas in women it is the 'change of life' or 'menopause'.

However, once the crisis is over, a period generally dawns for the older adult in which life is typified by its stability. He knows that his current circumstances are unlikely to change in any significant way. Even if he has chosen a fundamental new direction for his life, he knows that he has a considerable distance to go along it, unless life forces new changes upon him.

The older adult is conscious of having a position in society, and he knows the ways in which society values him. He is also too young for society to brush him aside. He has helped to build up this society, and is now occupied in maintaining it. The older adult is very actively engaged in this in various areas, such as his work, political parties, societies, and also in his family. He possesses energy and experience, which he no longer has to expend on his own behalf alone.

3. Physical development

The decline in the physical area, which had already begun to be noticeable towards the end of the young adult period, is now clearly evident. This also means that physical development again becomes a significant factor in the total development process.

Some of the phenomena with which the older adult has to cope are listed below:
– declining mobility;
– declining strength;
– diminishing reaction time;
– an increase in subcutaneous fat, particularly in the abdominal region;
– wrinkles;
– greying of the hair, and – particularly in men – baldness;
– a decline in sight, leading to the need for reading glasses;
– a decline in hearing;
– a decline in the man's sexual potency;
– the cessation of menstruation, along with a change in the hormone balance.

Case study: Bill

Bill is a PE teacher in a big comprehensive school. He prided himself on the fact that hardly any of his pupils could beat him in the various sports he practises, and that in spite of the fact that he is already forty-five. However, he has recently had to accept that he has been beaten

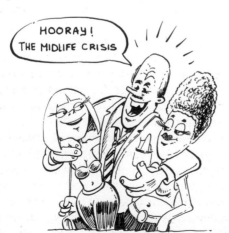

HOORAY! THE MIDLIFE CRISIS

on several occasions, and that the winners were not always real athletes.

Last week he was asked to turn out for the veterans' team. He, the key player for the senior second team!

At first he was insulted by the request, but after a time he thought it was justified, after all. He could not really compete with all those seventeen-year-olds any more. Besides, he had to constantly contend with muscular injuries, and they were beginning to complain about that at the school. His wife had also pointed out to him that he should adapt his conduct more to his age. Otherwise he might even have a heart attack.

Not all older adults, however, will show all these signs of ageing at the same age or to the same degree. In the first place these physical changes do not all occur at once. You can have grey hair, and still have a beautifully smooth skin, and

Figure 2.10.1
'Being old' depends on culture, too

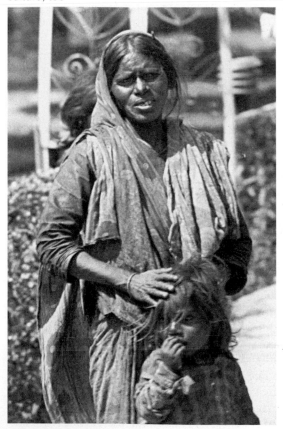

bald men do not necessarily have to have a more generous waistline.

In the second place the ages at which these phenomena occur can be very different. Some women begin the menopause when they are forty, others still have a child in their fifties. The innate characteristics of the individual obviously play an significant part in the physical changes, but also the lives people have led may have an important role to play. Repeated pregnancies, at brief intervals, can leave their traces on the female body, like stretch marks, or a weakened abdominal wall. And men who have carried out heavy manual labour in the open air for years, have a tanned, wrinkled skin. The differences between people of different cultures are even greater. While the older adult in our society may still be in the prime of his life, his contemporary in India, where the average expectation of life is only forty-five, is already well advanced in age. Physical development in this phase of life is, for all that, not an autonomous process; you can influence it to a large extent yourself by your behaviour. You can keep your physical condition up to the mark by sport or by slimming. The cosmetics industry takes advantage of the human need to go on looking young by flooding the market with camouflage products. Beauty specialists too earn a good living from people's fear of getting old.

Research has, however, shown that the physical ageing process cannot in fact be halted. One man in three at this stage of life is faced with an increasing loss of hair. Baldness is something many men have anxiety about and methods of solving this problem are constantly being advertised.

The woman's crisis in this phase of life, the menopause, is principally a physical one, and this aspect of it is discussed in this section. It should not, however, be forgotten that there is also a social side to this crisis, and this is discussed in the next section.

As a consequence of hormonal changes a woman loses her capacity to bear children at around the age of forty-five. This process begins with irregular menstruation, accompanied with various other physical problems, such as fatigue, hot flushes, headaches and listlessness; finally menstruation ceases entirely. This is a traumatic event, since menstruation, with all its problems, has been part of the woman's life since the beginning of adolescence. Most women do not look forward with any pleasure to this happening, as they are then obviously made aware that the fertile period of their life has ended. Their self-image, or their image of themselves as a woman, in which the possibility of becoming pregnant has always had an important place, has to be adapted. At the same time it can also be a relief for those same women that they no longer are going to have periods. Perhaps, prior to the menopause, some women were afraid of becoming pregnant, being well aware that the risks to the health of mother and child are greater than at a younger age. Now it is a relief to be rid of these anxieties. Contraceptive measures – sometimes so cumbersome – are now not needed any more. Often women's sexual lives blossom. They can enjoy sex again without having to worry.

Study activity
1. List five factors which can influence physical development during this phase of life.

4. Social and emotional development

From the social and emotional point of view this phase of life has a very turbulent start. It brings to an end a phase in which people expended great energy on achieving their position in society. In doing so they were able to bring to fruition – some more than others – a number of decisions on the three themes of life. That this was no easy task can be seen by the fact that this phase lasted just as long – almost twenty years – as all the preceding phases put together.

Moreover, according to statistics, the adult has half his life behind him. In short, this is a moment for reflection; the adult has reached a turning point in his life. He looks back on a crowded period, in which he really had too little time for reflection. He is conscious, too, that he still has half his life to come, and that if he still wants to change anything in it, he must do so now. Moreover, he can see that in his environment further development would be difficult in a number of areas.

This taking stock, and this realization, may have

as its result that the adult is faced with a crisis. In women this crisis is still further heightened by the physical changes accompanying the menopause. The older adult can begin to have doubts about the decisions he made previously. He stands before a new, fundamental decision: to carry on in the same old way, or to make a fresh start in one or more of the themes of life.

He will eventually achieve a new equilibrium as his life goes on. He usually accepts his existing situation, and continues forward, albeit with a few adaptations, along the same road. Sometimes, however, he makes a radical break with the old ways, and starts off along new ones.

How this crisis is successfully resolved depends on such factors as:
- personality, including the ability to withstand stress;
- situation in life;
- relationships;
- the availability of alternatives.

It will again be obvious that there are great differences between individuals in respect of these factors. It is, however, precisely the possibility of turning aside from the lowest common denominator which characterizes the process of development after reaching adulthood.

In the next section the development process of the older adult is analysed further along the three themes of life.

Case study: Anne

'Well, there we are,' thinks Anne. She has just taken her youngest son to the hospital's residential quarters. He is commencing his career as a nurse, and they decided that he should move into the living quarters; all his friends have already left home.

On the way home Anne begins to realize that the house will be very quiet now. Not at weekends, because that is when all the children come home. But the days will be very long during the week. Running the house will take up less time, and she sometimes wonders about taking a job, not for the money as her husband earns more than enough, but to get out among people a bit. But there may be little chance of getting a teaching job now. Besides, if she did, she would be depriving someone younger of the chance of a job. On the other hand, she surely has the right to a job too, and with a refresher course she may well get one. Perhaps she might get a reception class, but could she still cope with young children? She doesn't know what to do. But she does not want to sit at home until her husband retires. She will have to discuss things thoroughly with her husband.

Study activity

2. Is it possible for Anne or other women to prepare themselves for this vacuum? And if so, how?

a. Work

In theory the experience of older adults in this area would apply to both sexes. In our present-day society it is unfortunately still the case that at this phase of life the theme of 'work' is relevant to most men, and to significantly fewer women. This does not mean that the development of women outside paid employment is not influenced by this aspect of life. Most non-working women have a relationship with a man who does work, and experience through his agency the consequences of 'having work to do'.

The older adult is conscious that the scope for further development in the area of his work is diminishing. His career opportunities grow less; in job advertisements you very rarely see anyone looking for people over the age of forty-five.

The older worker sees that younger employees are catching up and even overtaking him. It is a difficult moment when he has to accept a younger man as his boss. He then realizes all too well that he has got as far as he is going to go; there is not much more in store for him. Of course, there are also jobs where you only reach the top later in life though very few in our society are in the running for them. This particular small group of older adults really have got to the top, both in business and in politics.

To accept such a situation is certainly not always easy, as can be seen from the number of people who, through all sorts of social provisions like early retirement and disability pensions, retire before the age of sixty-five. Early retirement is usually a positive choice; people want to enjoy

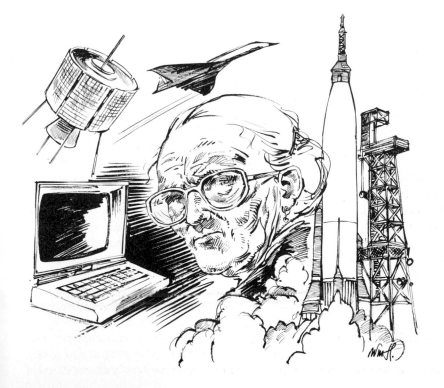

Figure 2.10.2
How do you keep up with it all?

their leisure time or to make room for younger workers who cannot find a job. Disability pensions often force a decision where one is given no choice.

As far as these provisions are concerned, we are living, for the moment, in a time of luxury. There are, however, indications that the existing provisions will be changed again. There have been forecasts that more people will have to work at least until they are sixty-five. For example, the health care industry has a growing need for labour, because of the increasing numbers of older people, resulting precisely from the past success of health care.

Another problem facing the older worker in his job is his diminishing flexibility. Reorganizations, innovations, and technical developments take most of their victims from among the older employees. They often have difficulty adapting to these changes, and it costs them extra effort to keep up with technical developments.

When taking stock of what has been achieved so far, there is also the realization that opportunities have been missed. Missed educational opportunities sometimes leave people dissatisfied with the work they are doing. Our society has endeavoured to fill this gap with adult education.

As we said earlier, these problems are relevant for most of the employed population. In addition, women still have to cope with their own specific problems.

Study activity

3. List as comprehensively as possible the specific problems which can be encountered by working women.

As people get older, so the number of problems, both for men and women, increase. Stability is only finally achieved by those who know how to resolve these problems or those who can accept the situation as it is. Thus stability does not automatically result from reaching this phase of life.

b. Relationships

For many people this phase also starts with a crisis in their relationships. This crisis can occur in the following areas.

The relationship with their partner

In their relationship with their partner this can be a period of stocktaking. As adults, they have always been kept busy looking after their children or at work, with the result that they have given less attention to their partner. This changes in this phase of life. They have more time for each other again, and that is by no means always easy. If we assume that most people marry around the age of twenty-five, then by the beginning of the time they are older adults most partners know each other through and through. This also usually means that the exciting, passionate nature of the relationship is over. There is little that is not familiar to both of them. The true value of the relationship is now revealed. In earlier phases, potential breakdowns in the relationship were camouflaged by both partners' busy occupations.

That this is a difficult problem is shown by the increasing number of relationships falling apart after twenty to twenty-five years of marriage, influenced by the spirit of our times, though such situations have probably existed for as long as marriages have been contracted. Children are often the reason that people, in spite of great problems in their relationship, stay together. When the children can stand on their own feet, the need for staying together goes too.

Most relationships are, however, strong enough to overcome these kinds of problems, and can develop in this phase into relationships in which mutual respect and trust take the place of the earlier passion.

Part of the problem of relationships is also the acceptance of each other's physical decline. The image people have of each other at the start of the relationship disappears, and compared to that former image, the outward appearance has now become less attractive. It is all the more difficult in this case if physical attraction was an important element in the original relationship.

Together with one's appearance, one's sexual life also changes. In the first place there are physical changes, such as the man's diminished potency, and for a considerable time, irregular periods for the woman. Secondly a new and different attitude to their relationship may now be needed due to these physical changes. At this stage in their lives, however, they may find it difficult to adapt to this changed situation. For their part, women can feel themselves liberated from the burden of possible pregnancy, because they no longer have to use any contraceptives. They can therefore be more liberated in their sexual behaviour, making a man possibly feel uncomfortable, because he is not used to this behaviour in his wife, and has difficulty accepting it.

The relationship with children

The older adult has to cope with the 'empty nest syndrome'. Most relationships in our society result in children, and in this phase of life the time is ripe for the grown-up children to leave the parental home. After a period of conflict, another more balanced and friendlier relationship often evolves. The adult knows from the moment that he decides to have children that this conflict will occur, in its own time. He has, after all, also been a child, and has in fact experienced it. It is a difficult moment for many parents when their first child shows signs of wanting to stand on his own two feet. It is even more difficult when the last child leaves the family. The day-to-day life of the family changes completely, particularly for the person who always looked after the children. There is less activity and fewer friends and acquaintances calling in.

It must be accepted that many variations are possible on this theme. So far we have assumed a relationship based upon two people. Currently, however, in the United Kingdom one in every four families is a one-parent family. We have also been assuming that there are children in the family. We must not forget, however, that ten percent of adults living together can, for a variety of reasons, have no children, and that another ten percent do not want any children. It is also important to take into account that currently many people only have children when they are in their thirties. That means that these parents will only encounter the problems described above when they are well into this phase of life. Obviously this affects the way in which they cope with these problems.

c. Attitude to life

The older adult also develops in his attitude to life. For most people a clear shift occurs in their pattern of interests. This shift is to some extent determined by experiences in work and relationships: their system of norms and values changes in parallel to it.

Some aspects of this development are discussed in more detail below.

Life-style

The older adult has started on the second half of his life. Although you may see dating advertisements referring to 'a young man of 52', society, and particularly the younger section of it, regards the older adult as already 'old'. That also means that there is a pattern of expectations governing his behaviour and life-style, expressed in such things as:
- the clothes they should or should not wear: a fifty-year-old woman should not wear a mini-skirt, unless she is an attractive pop star;
- the places where they meet their peers: an older adult does not fit in at a disco;
- preferences for music: people think it unusual if a man of fifty likes hard rock;
- being fixed in one's habits;
- the social pattern of which they are part;
- the things which give them pleasure, like their house, or a nice carpet.

An important factor affecting life-style is the increase in the older adult's financial means. A young adult may have a great many plans which cannot be carried out because of lack of money or the pressure of other priorities. An older adult often has the money, but no longer the energy to carry out his plans.

System of norms and values

It is sometimes said that one's sense of responsibility increases as one gets older and that the older adult also becomes accustomed to bearing responsibility. All this influences his pattern of norms and values to the extent that he can now be considered as a rational socially responsible individual. Society's conventions have become his, and he is no longer going to be quick to display very unorthodox behaviour. He will be less ready to support major changes, because they put at risk what he has built up, and he also feels responsible for the way the society in which he lives functions.

He will also, more often than before, find himself shaking his head when watching the activities of younger people. It is difficult for him to imagine that he, too, when he was young himself, wanted to turn the whole world upside down.

The older adult's pattern of norms and values can best be described as conservative. He knows from experience that principles cannot be taken to their logical conclusion and that you often have to abandon your own principles. The older adult could be said to have achieved wisdom through experience – or perhaps through learning the hard way.

His pattern of norms and values is naturally also influenced by the experience he has undergone. As he gets older, he can, of course, call on his experience of life. He has done a great deal in various areas of life, and it would be a pity to waste this experience. The older adult's pattern of norms and values is therefore more mature, more soundly based.

Coping with possible crises in life

The older adult copes with the crises of life differently from the young adult in two respects.

In the first place there is a greater likelihood of encountering a crisis of life. The older adult is more likely to come up against the deaths of people in his environment, such as his parents. His children are reaching the stage in life where they have to take important decisions, with all the consequences that these can bring, such as interrupted education, failed relationships, and so on. The probability of him or his partner contracting a serious illness increases.

If he loses his job, it is more difficult to find a new one. Moreover, the older adult knows that these things can happen; they are part of this phase of his life.

These are not pleasant things, and they will make him stop and think, and realize that he is getting older.

In the second place his ability to bend before life's crises diminishes. He has less energy to make a fresh start, and therefore fewer opportunities are open to him. A broken relationship cannot be replaced by a new one so easily, and

it is soon obvious that his value in the labour market has also gone down.

With an eye to these realities we can conclude that the older adult has to cope with a heavier load, but with less carrying capacity.

Study activity

4. List five factors which can influence social and emotional development in this phase of life.

5. Cognitive development

In this phase of life as in the previous ones we must distinguish, in cognitive development, between the structure or process of thought, and its content.

There are changes, albeit very slow ones, in the areas of both structure and content.

a. The process of thought

The main phenomenon with which the older adult has to cope, as time goes on, is a slowing down in his thinking. He needs more time to drag things from his memory, and to put his thoughts in order.

We must be careful here with the picture we are painting of the older adult. We should certainly not regard him as a computer that has crashed. The changes occur very gradually, but to the older adult himself they are clearly recognizable.

This slowing down has considerable consequences for the performance of tasks requiring great use of cognitive skills. Thus he will be slower in solving problems, and remembering names and telephone numbers becomes more difficult than it used to be.

From research into the pattern of older (aged forty and over) employees' capacity to learn, it appears that a substantial percentage of people think that they:
- do not want to learn;
- are less critical in what they learn;
- are made insecure by learning;
- learn more slowly;
- have too fixed ideas;
- have more difficulty in remembering.

However, these opinions are not, to a large

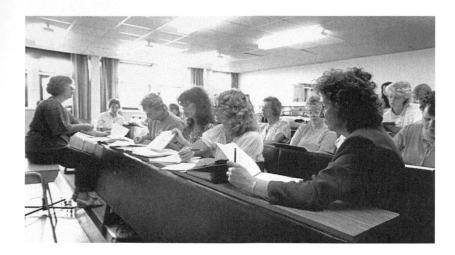

Figure 2.10.3
Adult education:
never too old to learn

degree, consonant with the facts. Older adults' capacity to learn is influenced by:
– their level of education, associated with the type of work they do. If manual skills are most important for their work, then their cognitive skills decline because they have no need to call on them. A high cognitive performance is not needed if you stand beside the assembly line in a factory. It may even be necessary to 'turn off your intelligence' in order to be able to do the job. If on the other hand the work demands cognitive performance, such as learning, remembering, reasoning, planning and so on, then the mind is kept active, and cognitive skills can be kept at their peak;
– their attitude to cognitive activities. They may enjoy learning new things, thinking over situations and problems, or they may hate it;
– experience, in the sense that older adults will more easily place new experiences into a familiar context with the advantage that the new experience then fits into the existing pattern;
– social environment, and particularly the expectations of that environment about older adults learning. Thus in some social classes it is often not acceptable for anyone in their fifties to start studying again. In this respect women are doubly handicapped; such an activity is not expected of them at all. They will constantly be asked: 'What is the point of it?'

Case study: John

John has always been very keen on art and music. However, as a lecturer in nursing studies, and the father of two growing children, he has never been able to study these subjects in more depth. On the occasion of his fiftieth birthday his wife has given him a most appropriate present: a course in art with the Open University. As a result, John nowadays spends three evenings a week swotting in his study. He has a general acquaintance with much of the material. He knows most of the jargon, but he finds it difficult to learn definitions by heart. He is conscious, during the workshops, that some of his younger fellow students read a book in half the time he takes. He notices with pleasure that he is not the only mature student. He is also pleased that his wife does not disapprove of this activity.
Various people in his environment had a completely negative reaction to the idea when he told them that he was going to take the course. 'What are you thinking of at your age?' and 'a waste of money' were among the milder comments.

b. The content of thought

The older adult has gained experience in, and is familiar with, many areas of life. His knowledge covers not only real, factual things, like the history of the last twenty years, literature and so on, but also social matters. He knows how he should behave, how he should react, and he also has a greater familiarity with the way in which other people are likely to behave. On the basis of the greater amount of his knowledge, both factual and social, the older adult is well placed to put things in perspective.

The ability to put things in perspective is, on the one hand, a positive one. He can see things in proportion, and has a better comprehension of specific situations. On the other hand, this can result in a cynical attitude, killing all initiatives at birth. The older adult does not find it easy in our complex society, characterized by very fast change in some of our basic assumptions. Existing knowledge is constantly being replaced by new developments particularly in the area of professional work. This causes problems for many older adults. They not only have to learn new tricks, but at the same time learn to forget their old ones.

Study activity

5. List five factors which can influence cognitive development in this stage of life.

6. Summary

We started this chapter by characterizing older adulthood as 'a period of stability'. In this summary we must add some glosses to this description.

In the first place this stability may be achieved only after going through a period of crisis, which is different in nature for women and men. In particular, the woman's crisis is associated with a significant physical change, the menopause. Both sexes must find a new orientation in respect of the three themes of life. Dependent upon their success in this, one can say that they have achieved stability. Physical developments proceed more slowly and this is evident both to the older adult and to those around him. From the cognitive point of view one cannot speak of a real decline; too many factors determine development in this area to be able to distinguish a general direction of development.

In the second place, it is much more difficult to establish general lines of psychological development, than it was in the previous young adult phase. In other words, the differences between individuals, as a consequence of factors in the course of their lives, are now so great, that it has become difficult to draw general conclusions. It is impossible to say in advance how older adults will react to what lies ahead of them.

The ageing years: from sixty-five till death

11

1. Introduction

Old age approaches us gradually with its many characteristic physical changes being easily recognized. These physical changes such as becoming over or underweight, going gray, or developing hyperpigmentation with all the effects on the individual's self-image that these imply, will be experienced by the elderly.

There is also a failing of the senses that elderly people have to adjust to. In a society such as ours where processing information through the senses is an increasingly important feature, this deterioration makes life more difficult.

The process of social and emotional, and of cognitive development in the elderly is a complicated one. A multitude of physical and mental processes influence each other. This means that physical and/or mental weaknesses can occur either independently or in association with each other.

Fortunately, at present a reassessment is being made of the quality of old age. This is very necessary, since the quality of a culture is determined, among other things, by the way it looks after its old people.

Learning outcomes

After studying this chapter the student should be able to:
– describe in outline the physical development of the elderly;
– describe the social and emotional development of the elderly, and explain them in terms of:
  • work;
  • relationships;
  • attitude to life;
– describe the cognitive development of the elderly.

2. The ageing years; a brief overview

Somewhere around the age of fifty-five most people begin to feel that they are getting older. They may have had this feeling even earlier, when they became grandparents, but that was then primarily a family affair. Now people around them begin to think of them as being old, and let them see it in a variety of ways. This attitude can be expressed positively, for example, by giving them more privileges, by consideration for them, by offering help; or negatively, for instance, by letting them see that they are not needed, and they are no longer capable of doing their job.

As an adult you know that the last phase of life

Figure 2.11.1
Why not?

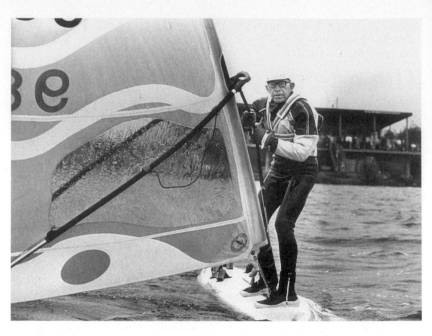

has dawned and that this final phase can go on for a long time. It is a phase which can have both positive and negative aspects. You know that both personally and socially a number of important changes will take place. Your capabilities, both physical and cognitive, become less. You have to cut down on your work and finally stop doing it. The likelihood of losing those dear to you increases. You acquire an ocean of free time, more leisure, and less responsibility. Your health will probably gradually deteriorate, and eventually you must expect to die.

How you experience and cope with this phase of life depends on your attitude to all these changes, and on your capabilities, physically, socially, cognitively, and in your community. The main developmental problem of the elderly is one of reorientation. The quality of their life depends upon the past life of the individual and there are therefore also great differences between elderly people.

For a long time the elderly phase of life was described by psychologists as a period of many negative and few positive aspects. However, this image of old age is now changing, at least in our society. The change was set in motion by three developments.

In the first place a new outlook was necessary, since the number of elderly people is increasing fast. The population is getting older, in part thanks to the high level of health care and the quality of our diet. It is forecast that in the next fifty years the average expectation of life will reach eighty-five (it is currently eighty-two). At present women when they reach the age of sixty-five, still have nineteen years to live on average. However, those who were born after the war, during the baby boom, will reach this stage of life just after the turn of the century, which will mean that the number of elderly people will rise sharply in absolute terms.

In the second place, the elderly segment of the population is changing in character. On the one hand is a group of elderly people who live at subsistence level, or who have little life force left. On the other is a group of the 'new' elderly, who have benefited from improved social care and pension provisions. This group has on average a higher level of education. They are more self-confident, have more interests; they stand up for themselves more and to better effect.

In the third place and finally, the increasing life span is blurring the image of the elderly. All things considered, a distinction should be made between the elderly of up to about seventy-five, who typically have great vitality, reasonable health and independence, and the aged, of seventy-five and more, who lack these characteristics.

There is no longer a typical senior citizen. So much variation in behaviour is possible in this phase of life that gerontology, the study of the old, has almost become a separate branch of learning within psychology.

3. Physical development

The physical development of older people again becomes very important in the context of the psychological development process. In the first place, age is particularly visible on the physical level. Although the body has clearly been getting older from about the age of thirty, from about fifty-five the process now picks up speed. A number of these changes are listed below:
– Changes in appearance:
  • Wrinkles and folds from a decrease in sub-cutaneous fatty tissue, and lowered elasticity; in advanced age the skin sometimes becomes like parchment;
  • hyperpigmentation;
  • thinning of the hair, and, particularly in men, baldness;
  • greying of the hair;

Figure 2.11.2
Mother and daughter;
in the same age group?

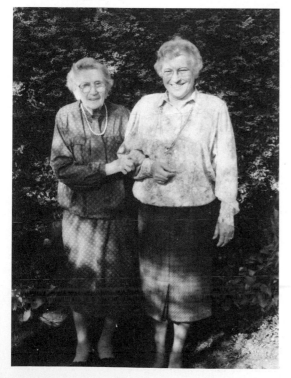

– a decrease in height as the cartilage in the joints shrinks; old people sometimes walk bent over.
– Sensory changes:
  • hearing deteriorates; in particular the perception of high notes can cause problems;
  • the power of sight decreases; many older people need reading glasses, and a good light to read by, and older people often suffer from night-blindness;
  • some loss of taste and smell.
– Internal changes:
  • blood pressure, breathing and cardiac functions deteriorate; as a consequence the general condition of the elderly person goes down, and efforts which could earlier be made very easily, are now much more laborious;
  • the size and elasticity of muscles decrease, causing a decline in strength; speed of movement thus also grows less;
  • the bones become more brittle, with a consequent greater risk of breaking: many old people therefore become more careful in their movements;
  • the joints become stiffer, so that changing position becomes more difficult, and actions become slower;
  • bladder and sphincters function less efficiently, so that people have to visit the lavatory more often, particularly at night, and the likelihood of stress incontinence increases;
  • changes in metabolism and circulation occur, so that many old people often feel cold;
  • the pattern of sleep changes, in that periods of deep sleep become shorter, and there is more need of short naps in between.
– Sexual changes:
  • men have more difficulty in achieving and maintaining an erection;
  • ejaculation takes longer, and it is longer before it can be repeated;
  • women are more likely to find sexual intercourse painful because of vaginal changes (less fluid discharge).

All these changes do not occur in all cases or to the same degree. Besides, not everyone sees them as being negative. Many older people find the slowing down in the tempo of life pleasant. Here, too, it is the case that their expectations govern how they experience those changes. The consequences of these changes can be very varied.

– Mobility can become less. When walking is an effort, then you are less inclined to go out visiting. When you have always driven, and because of physical failings can do so no more, then your freedom of movement is considerably limited. You can, of course, look for alternatives in public transport, but that again demands some reorientation. Mobility of itself need not grow less, as can be seen from the fact that many older people continue to practise sports, if only as veterans. Their performance probably costs more effort than when they were younger, but none the less it is possible to keep very active. Diminished mobility obviously has social consequences. These are discussed in the next section.

– Some activities can no longer be enjoyed. Consider cleaning the house or keeping up the garden; it is often more difficult to move furniture about or to mow the lawn. Moreover, hobbies needing strength, flexibility or keen senses can no longer be practised. At a later stage people can be so hampered by physical changes, that they can no longer look after themselves properly. This, too, has social consequences, to which we shall return in the next section.

Study activities

1. List five factors which can influence physical development in this phase of life.

2. **a.** Describe what your own attitude would be to the physical developments occurring in old age.
   b. Can they really be called 'developments'? Explain your answer.

4. Social and emotional development

The awareness of being old is central to the social and emotional development of the elderly. Physical deterioration is not the only reason for this awareness; other important factors are what they see happening to contemporaries around them and what they know about elderly people and about the social measures, like early retirement and pensions, which now apply to them, too. Nevertheless most elderly people assume that there is still a future for them, and that they can make something of it. They are confronted, however, with a number of changes which call for a reorientation within the three themes of life. The case study below shows that such a reorientation does not go easily for everyone.

Case study: Mrs Forrester

Mrs Forrester was sixty-five last month. She was not particularly pleased about it. It sounded so old: sixty-five! Her birthday was a real celebration. Naturally all her children and grandchildren called to wish her many happy returns. She had cleaned the whole house beforehand in one day, from top to bottom, and this had been a bad mistake. She couldn't bend down so well lately, and she took much longer than she used to over some jobs. She had also had some backache recently. Should her age really matter so much? To tell the truth, she had never thought about it much before. She had always kept a good home for her husband and her three children. The children had, of course, left home for some time, so that life was a bit quieter. The house seemed much bigger now, too. Perhaps they ought to think of moving to somewhere smaller and nearer to the shops.

Study activity

3. In general, how can a nurse help elderly people to reorient themselves?

Reorientation, settling into a new situation in life, demands some exertion from the people who have to make this change. And this exertion takes effort, just when the elderly person feels he needs some rest. He has exerted himself his whole life long, and his energy and vitality is beginning to fail. He has less resilience and flexibility to cope with changes in his situation in life. It depends then on his energy or vitality how his old age progresses.

Two things are important here.

– The personality of the elderly individual is more stable. When someone starts on the last phase of his life, he already has a whole career behind him. During that career he has coped with the problems and crises of life; for some these problems and crises have been more numerous, and more traumatic, than for others. These crises in life formed his identity. In general it is now possible to forecast reasonably well how he will react in specific situations. The elderly individual does not change as fast as he did when younger. Social changes, and certainly personal ones, will therefore be accepted with more difficulty, particularly if they conflict with what he is accustomed to. This principle applies all the more when these changes occur in those areas from which he has derived his identity or personality: work, relationships and attitude to life.

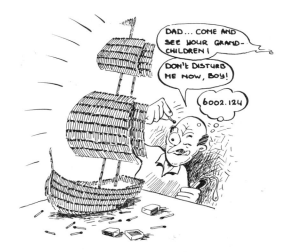

Being old: you don't have to sit still and do nothing

– Growing older is accompanied by the fact that the responsibilities he has always had to bear become less. These responsibilities always had to fit into specific parameters, such as hours of work, or dress regulations, looking after children, or even being polite to the boss when he did not feel like it. As he grows older, his freedom of action increases. He no longer has to meet his former boss, the children are independent now, and he can go on holiday whenever he likes.

Not all elderly people can free themselves of the feeling of responsibility. Their reactions to this feeling of responsibility, however, determine the significance of the changes for them. They can remain prisoners of their old pattern of behaviour, and so have a negative view of the changes, or accept the changes as they are and look at them positively.

Both factors are important in determining the likelihood of an enjoyable old age. They are responsible for how an individual is going to spend the time he has ahead of him, or how he will use the capacities that he still possesses. The changes experienced by most elderly people in the three life themes are analysed further below.

a. Work

Older people retire from their work when they are sixty or sixty-five, or nowadays often even

earlier. For some of them, approaching retirement is very significant in their last few years of work. In many cases people prepare themselves for it by gradually working less in this period. A separate and ever-increasing category includes unmarried working women, who have had a threefold task in their life: working, running a home, and coping with living by themselves. Work may have given them the opportunity to meet people and to make friends and consequently retirement can mean the loss of perhaps the only social activities that they have.

Eventually everyone receives an old age pension, sometimes supplemented by a private pension scheme. Most elderly people are pleased to have reached this age; work has often become a burden for them. It is difficult for them to maintain the pace, and to keep up with new developments. Many of them, unless they have heavy financial obligations, such as children who are still being educated, or a heavy mortgage, take advantage of the provisions for early retirement. They look forward positively to the time after their retirement, because they will at last have some time of their own. They can now lead their lives as they would like. They have time for their hobbies, for their children and grandchildren. They can organize their lives at their own speed. To take such a positive view of this period, a number of conditions must be fulfilled, such as:

– the children must respect the widened interests of their parents;
– they must have hobbies or at least some specific interests: many adults are kept so occupied with their work and their family that they have had no time for anything else;
– they must still possess the ability to exercise the hobby to which they had always looked forward – learning new skills usually presents problems for older people;
– they must still possess good health and plenty of vitality;
– they must have sufficient financial means. The old age pension on its own allows little scope for anything.

Others have always avoided facing the day when they would have to retire. Their work has been their life, and they do not want to leave it. They have often derived their identity from their work, and have therefore certainly not yet given any thought to, let alone made any preparations for, the time after their retirement. When therefore they are forced to give up working, they find this difficult to cope with. Everything which has given substance and direction to their lives has gone. They usually have no idea what to do with their free time, because they are not accustomed to doing anything except their work. Moreover, they do not know how to organize their lives without the guidelines provided by their hours of work. They feel that they have lost their identity, and they become insecure, apathetic, depressive, and withdraw into themselves. This is even more the case when all their social life was based upon their work; their social contacts have gone with their work. Age is a burden for these people, and reorientation a great problem for them.

One category of elderly people who have problems as a result of their partner's retiring, are women who have never worked themselves. They have always been their own boss at home; this was their 'kingdom', where they worked on their own without their partners breathing down their necks. This kingdom must now be shared. Their partner is at home much more than he used to be, and with much more opportunity of interfering in matters which he never had time for before.

Understanding this situation, and being prepared for it, can often prevent conflicts. Husbands can then make a really meaningful contribution to the housework, and relieve the burden on their wives.

Loss of work is a situation which every older person has to face. This new status can sometimes bring new financial problems and many people have to pull their horns in a bit. In the future, however, there will be a great many more old people, who will find themselves in a more comfortable financial position, which they have built up over the years. By doing so they have created more opportunities with which to fill their lives. Moreover, they sometimes possess talents of which society can make good use. The committees of many organizations are only too pleased to find people with plenty of time for voluntary work. These talents are also increasingly being used by organizations for the elderly themselves. The organizational level of the elderly is steadily growing, so that their influence in political and social life is also on the increase.

b. Relationships

Relationships – in the case of the elderly this aspect is better extended to include all social relationships – are also subject to substantial changes. By the time they start growing old most people who have had a family are on their own again: the last child has usually left home, and there are just the two partners together again. Singles and people without children are usually already reconciled to this situation, if they did not choose it deliberately. Partners usually know each other through and through, and are aware that their relationship will probably only be terminated by death. They are increasingly thrown into each other's company, partly because their social world is shrinking.
– Contact with children can grow less, because the children often have growing children themselves, and are increasingly occupied with their own lives. Many parents respect this, others on the other hand continue to make claims on their children. A breach can often arise between the grandchildren, who often have a special place in their affections, and the grandparents, as a result of the enor-

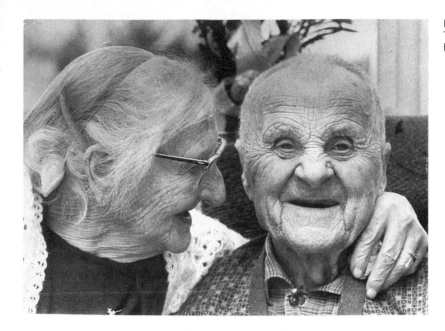

Figure 2.11.3
They still possess all
human qualities

mous gap in thought and behaviour between the two generations.

- The contacts kept up with people outside the family grow fewer. The word 'loneliness' is indeed often used as a label for the social situation of the elderly. In addition to the fact that the number of elderly people's social contacts is indeed reduced for practical reasons, we must not forget that loneliness is a general problem in our society. This problem, however, affects the elderly all the more because they have to cope with the actual disappearance of ever more members of their social circle. These are not only contemporaries who become frail and die. Many young people do not try to keep up their contacts with old people. The contacts between young and old are often professional ones in the sphere of social assistance, though this does not, of course, rule out normal human relationships. Besides, the elderly themselves start to take less initiatives towards social contacts, even with their contemporaries. Older people meet each other at festive occasions with their children and grandchildren and at funerals. Homes for the elderly, are usually particularly designed to be meeting places, yet you often see old people keeping to themselves and becoming lonely.

It is not, however, essential that you must give up all social contacts when your grow old. Of course, physical weakness and declining vitality play their part, but people also regain vitality from the social contacts themselves. The practical possibilities are often determined by the attitude of the individual. More and more elderly people who have lost their partner make new friendships and even remarry. The new situation brings them fresh vitality, and they regain a positive outlook on life.

Eventually, however, in advanced old age, many old people are on their own. Even their own children are sometimes dead, as are their brothers and sisters. Moreover, the very old can often no longer live independently, and become the responsibility of professional carers, such as nurses, who are often their only remaining social contacts.

c. Attitude to life

One of the consequences of age, and particularly advanced old age, is that a change becomes necessary in where and how one lives. When the children have left home, the house sometimes gets too big, not only in terms of space, but also in the effort needed for its upkeep. One is no longer always in physical shape for it, and it is necessary to call in the children or else expensive professional help. Only a small proportion of old people finally end up in an old people's home.

The so-called 'retirement homes', where elderly people look after themselves, and only make use of some of the common facilities of an old people's home, are a good compromise for many people. Also many more elderly people, when they can afford it, are beginning to live together while preserving their privacy. In this way they can help each other in emergencies, or combine to pay for professional help. Another section of the elderly lives with one of their children, and yet other old people manage to go on living on their own with the help of their children. Another group, categorized by major physical or mental problems, finally ends up in a hospital or nursing home. But the majority go on living on their own.

A change in where and how they live also has consequences for their perception of their environment and their behaviour. For example, it is a strange experience for someone of this age suddenly not having to get his meals any more. Many elderly people have great problems in accepting their new way of life. Whether these problems occur, often depends on whether the new situation was one of choice or was imposed upon them, either by some unavoidable factor like ill-health, or by the fact that the children found their parents too much of a burden.

Many elderly people have little contact with the world outside. They become increasingly withdrawn, and lose interest in what is going on around them. Material things like nice clothes or a new car lose their importance, and they can no longer keep up with new developments. This phenomenon is usually described by the word 'detachment'.

For many elderly people religion often occupies, or again occupies, an important place in their life. This may be the religion which they have practised all their lives, and about which their feelings are now more intense, but can also be a general belief in a hereafter, which has its origin in their inability to accept that there can be a final end to life.

Religion often gives old people the support to face their approaching death.

Study activity
4. List five factors which influence social and emotional development in this phase of life.

5. Cognitive development

There are many prejudices about cognitive development in elderly people. When you think of an elderly person, you often have a picture in your mind of someone who is absent-minded, slow in speech, not interested in anything except pictures of his grandchildren, and who immediately forgets everything you tell him. The words 'second childhood', 'dotage' and 'senile' come quickly to everyone's lips.

Case study: Granny Miller
Sunday afternoon, three o'clock. Granny Miller is woken by the doorbell. She has to think where she is, the room looks so unfamiliar. Oh yes, she lives in a flat for the elderly now. It was funny having to move out of her home after living in the same house for forty years. But it was high time, she had asked for it herself. There goes the bell again, she must get up. She is greeted by two happy children's voices: 'Hello, Granny, we've come to see you'. She has to think for a moment to remember the names of her grandchildren. She has sixteen, and the eldest already have their own children, her great-grandchildren. It becomes more and more difficult to remember all those different names.

Case study: Paul
Paul has been living for six months in a flat in the city centre. With five friends, three men and two women, he has bought a share in a block of flats and that suits them fine. They help each other as much as possible, and can get along for the moment without professional help. Each cooks in turn for the whole group. They regularly go, in a party, to concerts or the theatre. After the death of his wife, three years ago, Paul lived alone for a while in their old house, but that did not really suit him. This is an ideal solution for him.

He has recently been busy researching into his family tree; after coffee and reading his paper he often goes down to the Records Office. It takes up a lot of his time, but he finds it worthwhile. He meets so many other people there, surprisingly many older ones particularly, and that gives him an interest in life.

Study activity
5. Describe what you would consider the best form of living accommodation for yourself if you were seventy and in reasonably good physical and mental condition.

The stereotyped picture above does not often match reality. It is true that there is an increasing number of people suffering from senile dementia, but that is because many more people are reaching an ever greater age. And our failure to adapt ourselves to old people's slower pattern of thinking has something to do with our image of them.

If we look properly at the elderly, we will see people who, subject to some adaptations, can deliver the same cognitive performance that we can ourselves. They need a little more time to solve problems, and find it more difficult to draw on their memory, but the final result is the same as that produced by someone younger.

We will now again distinguish between the content the and process of thinking.

The thought process
In the process of thought the most common change is a slowing down in the speed of thinking. This change applies not only to the handling of the existing content of thought, but to the assimilation of new information, to learning. On the whole it takes longer to add new information to existing knowledge, and it is more difficult to concentrate on what one is doing. Older people also need more time to take in new facts. Their memory does not function as well as it did, so it can happen that they are no longer able to remember where they put their spectacles, or that they are confused when the furniture in their room is rearranged. Elderly people also more often become fixed in their habits, like a regular place at table, or the same nurse who comes to give them a bath. This gives them a feeling of safety and security in a fast-changing world. In the end there can be some cognitive deterio-

ration in old people, moreso in some than in others. In theory, however, the older person is capable of an excellent cognitive performance. Take as examples De Gaulle, Adenauer and Churchill, who coped with very complex political problems up to very advanced ages.

The content of thought
'The age of wisdom' is a familiar saying with some relevance to the changes in the content of older people's thought. It suggests that older people are credited with the ability to understand the deeper problems of life. Indeed, in many cultures the elderly function as counsellors for problems. This is, of course, because to acquire an understanding of the problems of life, you have to wrestle with them yourself, and that often takes time, much time. But to link wisdom to reaching an advanced age is another matter. Wisdom implies more than just giving solutions to the problems of life. It implies that these solutions are of an appropriate quality, and for this more is needed than just reaching a great age. Most of all it implies a certain ability to see things in perspective, and this is just what some old people cannot do.

For many 'wisdom' is then more a matter of being opinionated: of not being able to distance oneself from one's own point of view or opinion when there are good arguments against it.

Still, many old people, on the basis of their experience, and because they are no longer so bound by interest or status, are able to be less personally involved in important problems, and are therefore able to make an useful contribution to their solution. Think, for instance, of institutions like the upper houses of many legislatures, where places are reserved for elder statesmen.

The past and the future are in the forefront of older people's thoughts:
– Elderly people are aware that the greater part of their life is behind them. The most important things in their life have already happened; they have attended at births and deaths, experienced disappointment and happiness, and the future will only bring more of the same. The thoughts of the elderly are therefore directed less towards the future. The past has become important for them, and occupies

an ever greater proportion of their thoughts. This concentration does not mean 'a lament for the good old days', though this, too, is often typical of old people's thoughts, but it can result in a positive evaluation of the past. They ask themselves if they always acted rightly and made the right decisions. Sometimes they blame themselves for mistakes they made. But learning to accept the past in all its aspects, whether good or bad, is part of growing older. This acceptance will finally enable old people to achieve the peace of mind they need.

– The future of the elderly leads finally to an event already predetermined by their birth: their death. The concepts of life and death now take on a new reality for them. We have already established that a characteristic of the elderly person's changed attitude to life is an interest in religious or other beliefs. This interest certainly has something to do with the awareness that life is finite. The elderly person has more to do with contemporaries, who die, sometimes unexpectedly, sometimes after lengthy preparations. Central to thoughts about death is certainly the idea of life after death. He will ask himself whether life is limited to this period on earth, or whether there is something more. And he will ask what the nature of that something is.

Thoughts about death also means that the elderly individual is making preparations for it. These preparations can be of very different kinds. He can make a will, or draw up provisions to make sure that, whatever happens, the surviving partner will not be in financial difficulties. He can divide his possessions among his children and grandchildren. And there are even people who organize the details of their own funeral. Thinking about death implies nowadays much more thought about the manner of death. Many people are very afraid of a painful and long-drawn-out death. The ability of doctors to prolong life is also much greater. The 'emancipation' of the elderly includes their desire to have more say about the manner of their death.

In many cases the person with whom they then want to discuss these things is a nurse.

Study activity

6. List five factors which can influence cognitive development in this phase of life.

6. Summary

It is difficult to discuss the psychological development of the elderly if we stick to the criterion that development always involves an increasingly complex form of behaviour. For many elements of elderly behaviour, such as drawing upon experience, or their relationships with other people, this criterion is valid. For most of the elderly, however, it is not, and finally the curve dips down again to its nil value. Although everyone knows that this phase includes this final point, we have tried to show that it need not be so negative. In theory many kinds of behaviour are possible for the elderly. It depends upon their attitude to life how they make use of these possibilities. In this, of course, the social circumstances in which they live also play a role. Both factors eventually determine the quality of life in this phase.

At present there is an image of the elderly becoming more emancipated, in contrast to the traditional image of old age. We will return again to social and cultural considerations of the elderly in Chapter 4 of Module 3.

Final test Module 2

Instructions

- This section comprises 77 yes/no questions.
- Each proposition, claim, statement, etc. may be *true* or *false,* either *yes* or *no.* There is no middle way: you must make a choice.
- Your assessment of whether items are true or false should be based on your reading of the book.
- The questions are arranged in order relating to subject or chapters.
- Check that all questions have been answered.
- Finally, mark the test yourself. You will find the answers at the end of the book.

1. The most important characteristic of the concept of development is that it is irreversible.
2. Increasing complexity is evidence of the concept of growth.
3. Within each phase of the development process there is differentiation.
4. A critical period refers to a short time in which an individual is insensitive to external stimuli.
5. The division into phases within psychology is strictly tied to age groups.
6. Temperament is a psychological quality determined by heredity according to the neurobiological approach.
7. The psychoanalytical approach concentrates on a number of aspects relevant to growth.
8. In the learning theory interpretation some people have been convinced of the influence of physical factors on learning behaviour.
9. The nurture interpretation assumes that a great part of intelligence can be explained on the basis of heredity.

10. The nature/nurture controversy cannot be resolved by present-day research methodology.
11. The interaction approach is an integration of the traditional psychological approaches, and removes the contradictions of these theories resulting in a theory of a higher order.
12. The prenatal phase comprises the ovum and the fetal period.
13. In comparison with the fetus the embryo grows remarkably fast between the second and the eighth week.
14. A premature child is one with a birthweight of less than 2500 grammes and born before the thirty-second week of pregnancy.
15. Little is known about social and emotional development during the prenatal phase.

Items 16 to 19 inclusive are exteroceptive senses:
16. Hearing.
17. Awareness of one's own body and organs.
18. Smell.
19. Taste.

20. The postnatal phase has the function of stabilizing the process of interaction between parent and child.
21. In principle all interoceptive senses function from birth.
22. According to present-day psychological theories, there is also some interaction between child and parents in the postnatal phase.
23. Bowlby has formulated a theory of attachment, which has led, among other things, to 'rooming-in'.

24. According to Bowlby, social isolation can also have harmful consequences for cognitive and physical development.
25. In the postnatal phase the child is predominantly altruistic.
26. A four-week-old child cannot recognize a face because of the level of its cognitive structure.
27. That children in the postnatal phase are sensitive to voices is possibly the result of prenatal conditioning.
28. In the first year of life the interaction between parents and child is mainly determined by experience.
29. During physical growth in the first year of life the proportions change so much that the head becomes relatively smaller in relation to the rest of the body.
30. In the United Kingdom 90% of children can walk after 12 months.
31. From the age of two months the child also reacts to other babies.
32. The most important feature of the emergence of attachment behaviour is reciprocal feelings.
33. Fear of strangers is similar to separation anxiety.
34. The development of the cognitive functions in the first year of life is mainly based on growing more mature.
35. Memory develops in the first year of life.
36. In storing information biochemical processes probably play a predominant role.
37. Immediate memory has a timespan of 0.5 to 35 seconds.
38. The capacity of long-term memory is theoretically infinite.
39. During the fourth month of life there is a cognitive reorganization, which can explain the fears experienced at around six months.
40. During the first year of life the child develops from altruism into an existence that takes more account of its own interests.
41. Around the twelfth month of life most children can gain control of their bladder and bowels.
42. The child seizes upon potty training to show its self-will.
43. The obstinate stage is marked by the child's absolutely egocentric behaviour.
44. A child can sublimate his desires and emotions by exploratory play.
45. Field dependency refers to the way in which perceptive judgement is influenced by the environment.
46. From the second year magical thinking turns into animist thinking.
47. Role play is a social and cognitive skill.
48. The pre-school child acquires social understanding.
49. During the pre-school phase the influence of physical maturing processes on cognitive development comes to an end.
50. The pre-school child's powers of concentration increase as a result of the improved functioning of the filter in the brainstem.
51. The pre-school child begins to undergo a process of social and cognitive development.
52. Socialization is the absorption by the pre-school child of society's norms and values.
53. According to the learning theory approach the learning of behaviour occurs by means of observation.
54. An androgynous pre-school child is, for example, a boy with predominantly feminine characteristics, and vice versa.
55. During the acquisition of sexual identity socialization occurs on the basis of identification.
56. According to pre-school children death is an irreversible process.
57. In theory, the pre-school child has no more problems with a sense of time.
58. Seven and eight-year-olds are easy to recognize by their long thin legs.
59. The schoolchild acquires a clearer image of himself.
60. The stage of psychological constructs refers to the description of other children in terms of concrete behaviour.
61. From the age of twelve, a childs' knowledge of his own body increases.
62. Older schoolchildren cannot yet grasp abstract concepts.
63. Functional symptoms have an asomatic background.
64. Just as in pre-school children, the schoolchild's thinking is dominated by absolutes.

65. According to Erikson, the moratorium is a phase of development in which there are still opportunities for experimenting with behaviour.

66. The central problem of the adolescent is the formation of identity.

67. According to Erikson, congruence is an important characteristic of identity.

68. Consistency in thinking is an aspect of congruence in relation to the concept of identity.

69. The Electra complex as an explanation for choice of partner needs to be classed in the behavioural approach.

70. The adolescent's sense of values is generally still an absolute one.

71. The young adult is characterized physically by peak performance.

72. Crises in the lives of young adults usually involve the unravelling of decisions made earlier.

73. Cognitively the young adult is not yet at his peak.

74. Physical development is an autonomously progressing process in the older adult.

75. The older adult's ability to put things in proportion can also result in cynicism and the killing of any initiative.

76. The slowing down of the tempo of life is regarded as negative by older people.

77. It is difficult to discuss the psychological development of the elderly on the basis of a definition of development always involving more complex behaviour.

References

Barenboim (1981). The development of person perception in childhood and adolescence: From behavioral comparisons to psychological constructs to psychological comparisons. *Child Development*, 52(1):129–144.

Bender, H. (1988). *Functionele klachten van kinderen, psychologische diagnostiek en behandeling*, Lisse, Swets & Zeitlinger.

Block, J.H. (1980). Another look at sex differentiation in the socialization behaviour of mothers and fathers. In: Denmark, F.and Sherman, J. (eds.), *Psychology of Women: Future Directions of Research*. New York, Psychological Dimensions.

Bouchard, T.J. and McGule, M. (1981). Familial studies of intelligence: a review. *Science*, 212: 1055–59.

Bower, G.H. (1972). Mental imagery and associative learning. In: Gregg, L.W., (ed.), *Cognition in Learning and Memory*, New York, Wiley.

Bower, G.H. (1981). Mood and Memory. *American Psychologist*, 36: 129–48.

Bowlby, J. (1965). *Child care and the Growth of Love*, Middlesex, Penguin Books.

Bowlby, J. (1973). *Separation: Attachment and Loss*, vol. 2, New York, Basic Books.

Buckler, J.M.H. (1979). *A Reference Manual of Growth and Development*, Oxford, Blackwell Scientific Publications.

Central Statistical Office (1986). *'Social Trends 16'*, London, HMSO.

Coleman, J.C. (1988). *The Nature of Adolescence*, (2nd ed.), London, Methuen.

Conger, J.J. and Petersen, A.C. (1983). *Adolescence and Youth: Psychological Development in a Changing World*, (3rd ed.), New York, Harper & Row.

DeCasper, A.J. and Fifer, W.P. (1980). Of human bonding: newborns prefer their mother's voice. *Science*, 208: 1174–76.

Dingwall, R. (1983). Detecting child abuse. *Nursing Times*, 79 (15 June): 66,68–9.

Eich, J., Weingartner H., Stillnam R.C. and Gillian J.C. (1975). State-dependent accessibillity of retrieval cues in the retention of a categorised list. *Journal of Verbal Learning and Verbal Behavior*, 14: 408–17.

Erikson, E.H. (1963). *Childhood and Society* (2nd ed.), New York, Norton.

Erlenmeyer-Kimling, and Jarvic, L.F. (1963). Genetics and intelligence: a review. *Science,* 142, p.p. 1477–79.

Estes, W.K. (1972). An associative basis for coding and organization in memory. In: Melton, A.W., Martin, E. (ed.), *Coding Processes in Human Memory*, Washington, D.C., Winston.

Eysenck, H.J. (1987). The Myth of the Shared Environment. *Behavioural & Brain Sciences*, 10(1): 23–4.

Frankenberg, W.K. and Dodds, J.B. (1967). The Denver developmental screening test. *Journal of Paediatrics*, 71: 181–91.

Haith, M.M., Bergman T. and Moore, M.J. (1977). Eye contact and face scanning in early infancy. *Science*, 198: 853–55.

Harlow, H.F. (1959). Love in infant monkeys. *Scientific American*, 200: 68–74.

Herbert, M. (1987). *Living with Teenagers*, Oxford, Blackwell.

Jensen, A.R. (1969). How much can we boost I.Q. and scholastic achievement?. *Harvard Educational Review*, 39: 1–123.

Kaluger, G. and Kaluger, M.F. (1979). *Human Development: The Span of Life* (2nd ed.), London, Mosby.

Kinsey, A.C., Pomeroy, W.B. and Martin, C.E. (1948). *Sexual Behaviour in the Human Male*, Philadelphia, Saunders.

Kinsey, A.C., Pomeroy, W.B., Martin, C.E. and Gebhard, P.H. (1953). *Sexual Behaviour in the Human Female*, Philadelphia, Saunders.

Kintsch, W. and Buschke, H. (1969). Homophones and synonyms in short-term memory. *Journal of Experimental Psychology*, 80: 403–407.

Kohlberg, L. (1969). Stage and sequence: The cognitive-developmental approach to socialization. In: Goslin, D.A., (ed.), *Handbook of Socialization Theory and Research*, Chicago, Rand McNally.

Kohlberg, L. (1984). *The Psychology of Moral Development: Vol. 1, Moral Stages and the Life Cycle: Vol. 2. Essays on Moral Development*, New York, Harper & Row.

Korner, A.F. (1973). Individual differences at birth: Implications for early experience and later development. In: Westman, J.C., (ed.), *Individual Differences in Children*, New York, Wiley.

Lees, S. (1985). *Sexuality and Adolescent Girls*, London, Hutchinson.

Livesley, W.J. and Bromley, D.B. (1973). *Person Perception in Childhood and Adolescence*, Chichester, Wiley.

Loftus, E.F. and Loftus, G.R. (1980). On the permanence of stored information in the human brain. *American Psychology*, 35: 409–20.

Lorenz, K. (1965). *Evolution and Modification of Behavior*, Chicago, Chicago University Press.

Maslow, A.H. (1954). *Motivation and Personality*, New York, Harper & Row.

Maslow, A.H. (1968). *Towards a Pschology of Being*, New York, Van Nostrand Reinhold.

Maslow, A.H. (1971). *The Farther Reaches of Human Nature*, New York, Viking.

Miller, G.A. (1956). The magical number seven +2: Some limits on our capacity for processing information. *Psychological Review*, 63: 81-97.

MORI (1991). Teenagers 'risk unprotected sex'. *The Guardian*, p. 4, 14 August.

Morrison, D.M. (1985). Adolescent contraceptive behavior: A review. *Psychological Bulletin*, 98: 538–68.

Muller, D.J., Harris, P.J. and Wattley, L. (1986). *Nursing Children: Psychology Research and Practice*, London, Harper & Row.

Mussen, P.H., Conger, J.J. and Kagan, J. (1969). *Child Development and Personality*, 3th ed. New York, Harper & Row.

Mussen, P. H., Conger, J.J. and Kagan, J. (1984). *Child Development and Personality*, 6th ed. New York, Harper & Row.

Neisser, U. (ed.) (1982). *Memory Observed: Remembering in Natural Contexts*, San Fransisco, Freeman.

Piaget, J. (1952). *The Origins of Intelligence in Children*, New York, International Universities Press.

Rubin, Z. (1980). *Children's Friendships*, London, Fontana.

Rutter, M. (1990). *Maternal Deprivation Reassessed*, London, Penguin.

Sachs, J.D.S. (1967). Recognition memory for syntactic and semantic aspects of connected discourse. *Perception and Psychophysics*, 2: 437–42.

Selman, R.L. (1981). *Growth of interpersonal understanding: Development and clinical analyses*, New York, Academic Press.

Shaffer, D.R. (1985). *Developmental Psychology: Theory, Research and Application*, Belmont, Wadsworth.

Smith, E.E., Adams, N. and Schorr, D. (1978). Fact retrieval and the paradox of interference. *Cognitive Psychology*, 10: 438–64.

Smith, P. and Cowie, H. (1987). *Understanding Children's Development*, Oxford, Blackwell.

Squire, L.R. and Fox, M.M. (1980). Assessment of remote memory: Validation of the television test by repeated testing during a seven-day period. *Behavioural Research Methods and Instrumentation*, 12: 583–86.

Squire, L.R., Cohen, N.J. and Nadel, L. (1984). The medial temporal region and memory consolidations: A new hypothesis. In: Weingarten, H., Parker, E. (eds.), *Memory Consolidation*, Hillsdale, N.J., Erlbaum.

Sylva, K. and Lunt, I. (1982). *Child Development: A First Course*, Oxford, Blackwell.

Thomas, A. and Chess, S. (1977). *Temperament and Development*, New York, McGraw-Hill.

Traupmann, J. and Hatfield, E. (1981). Love and its effects on mental and physical health. In: Fogel, R.W., Hatfield, E., Kiesler, S.B. and Shanas, E., (eds.), *Aging: Stability and Change in the Family*, New York, Academic Press.

Watson, J.B. (1950). *Behaviorism*, New York, Norton.

Witkin, H.A. (1954). *Personality Through Perception*, New York, Harper & Bros.

Module 3

SOCIAL PSYCHOLOGY AND SOCIOLOGY

Introduction to Module 3

There are unlikely to be many days when we do not meet anyone at all. In fact, we usually meet many people every day, and a number of different kinds of meetings take place daily. The development of such contacts depends on a wide variety of factors.

In your profession as a nurse, you are in touch with a great many people. Your colleagues, patients and doctors make up the environment in a ward. On some occasions you are dealing with one person only, at others with several people at once. Co-operation is usually a vital feature of such contacts, since working in a ward requires teamwork. The ability to work with other people is therefore essential. When working alongside others in a team or a group, everyone has his or her own task. The various tasks depend on a person's position in a team. Working in conjunction with others therefore also implies that you must be able to associate with the people performing the various duties that occur within a group.
Social psychology and sociology are the two sciences mainly concerned with the various kinds of human relationship, and the subject matter of this module is therefore based mainly on those two branches of knowledge.
A knowledge of the concepts and processes employed in the two subjects will lead to a better understanding of your own world and that of others in your environment. A better understanding is a prerequisite for being able to function better in social situations.

Our starting-point in Chapter 1 is the individual. How are you 'trained' to deal with other people, and what kind of factors play a part in such contacts? The following concepts will be considered:
- relationship and interaction;
- involvement;
- norms and values;
- socialization;
- attitude;
- attributions.

Chapter 2 focuses on the group. We look at a number of social concepts and consider how they can be combined:
- the group;
- roles within a group;

– power and leadership;
– co-operation;
– conflicts;
– groups in relation to other groups.

In Chapter 3, we consider the concepts of health and sickness from a social point of view. We first provide a definition of the concept of health. On the basis of that definition, we may regard sickness as a disturbance of the balance between biological, psychological and social functioning.
The concept of sickness is then set in a broader social perspective. Social processes that are usually regarded primarily as positive contributions to society are reviewed. Such processes often have a less favourable aspect as well. Environmental pollution as a consequence of increasing prosperity provides an example. Even health care itself may constitute a threat to health: consider, for example, the side-effects of medicines. Two concepts will be dealt with in this context:
– clinical iatrogenesis;
– social iatrogenesis.

Finally, the concept of sickness is tied in with three sociological theories, i.e.:
– consensus theory;
– conflict theory;
   interactionist theory.

The object of considering these theories is to place the concept of sickness in a social context.

Chapter 4 focuses on particular social groupings which exist in society, in particular the community and the family. These important unit ideas or sociological concepts are explained in some detail as they relate to how the majority of people live in social settings.

In regard to community, Durkheim's description of mechanical and organic solidarity and Tönnies' description of gemeinschaft and gesellschaft social organizations are presented and compared. In regard to family, the ideas of nuclear, extended and symmetrical family structures are presented and related both to the social function of the family and to different types of communities.

Chapter 4 also includes a consideration of the elderly in the context of modern-day community and family structures. This supplements those considerations of children and adults in earlier chapters of Module 3 and in some of the psychology modules. In its final sections the chapter addresses the implications of community and family structures for health and health care.

After reading this module, you should be able to recognize various social concepts, social processes and social structures and their relation to health care.

1

People as social animals

1. Introduction

Human beings have relationships with other human beings throughout their lives. To put it briefly: people interact with others and with their environment and influence one another. Starting relationships is not a matter of free choice: in our complex society it is almost impossible to function without establishing contacts with other people.

The first part of this chapter therefore focuses on the concepts of relationship and interaction. Subsequently, all the aspects of relationships and interaction that are of importance to you and your professional work will be considered. They include:
– involvement;
– norms and values;
– socialization;
– attitude;
– attributions.

Learning outcomes

After studying this chapter the student should be able to:
– define the terms *social psychology* and *sociology*;
– give at least ten examples of topics in the area of health care which are, or might be, objects of study in these two branches of knowledge;
– define the two concepts, *relationship* and *interaction*;
– explain how relationships and the amount of involvement in them may vary;
– give a definition of the concept of socialization;
– indicate the difference between primary and secondary socialization;
– indicate what is meant by norms and values;
– explain the difference between formal and informal norms;
– distinguish between three kinds of norm in terms of validity;
– give a definition of the concept of social control;
– explain the meaning of positive and negative sanctions;
– give a descriptive account of attribution theory;
– give an example of an attribution error;
– give a descriptive account of dissonance theory.

2. Social psychology and sociology

Case study: Mrs Anderson

Mrs Anderson, aged eighty-one, has been in hospital for several months. A fall at her home, where she lived on her own, was the original reason for her admission. Fortunately, it turned out that she had not sustained any fractures. The only reason why she is still in hospital is a shortage of beds at the nursing home. It became apparent in hospital that she was suffering increasingly from dementia, so that it would be impossible for her to return home. Mrs Anderson is usually an easy patient. She has some regular habits and a number of favourite haunts. Sometimes, however, the pattern is disturbed, usually without any apparent reason. Occasionally she has been found in a different part of the hospital, in a somewhat desperate state.

One afternoon she could not be found in any of her usual haunts. This was discovered when tea was being served. No one knew how long ago she had disappeared. A search began immediately but proved unsuccessful. More and more people became involved. At first it was only the nurse who had brought round tea, but more and more nurses and even a few mobile patients joined in the search. The area where the search was taking place was extended further and further and within half an hour at least fifty people in various departments had been informed. Anxiety increased by the minute. Unexpressed thoughts about what might have happened created a noticeably tense atmosphere, especially in the ward.

Then, after about three quarters of an hour, someone entering the bathroom area heard a sound coming from the shower cubicle. The door was ajar and there was Mrs Anderson. Why she was there, nobody knew, but it was probably because she thought that she was to be given a shower and so she was waiting patiently for someone to come and help her.

Study activity

1. Consider what would be the effect on you as a student, in terms of your relationship with the team leader, if you had to tell her that Mrs Anderson had disappeared.

The case is interesting because of what the participants do together. Mrs Anderson's behaviour has a powerful effect on her environment and various processes can also be observed going on all around her: people are being organized and are influencing one another, as the increase in tension shows.

People 'do' things to their environment and the environment 'does' things to people. This relationship between people and their environment, as well as the processes that play a part in this, constitute the areas on which the attention of both social psychology and sociology is focused.

a. Definitions of concepts

Like psychology, social psychology and sociology are sciences which involve the study of people. What distinguishes social psychology and sociology from psychology is the degree of attention devoted to the human environment and the relationship between human beings and their environment. The fact that there is also a distinction between the two branches of sciences is apparent from the following definitions.

Social psychology is a science which studies how an individual's thoughts, emotions and behaviour are influenced by the presence of other people.

As you see, the individual as influenced by other people is at the centre of this definition. The actual physical presence of the other person is not always required. Thinking of someone – being present in thought – may also affect a person.

It is easy to realize that other people affect you if you compare the company of a good friend with your contacts with an unfamiliar patient. You will behave and feel differently in the two situations, and your thoughts about the two contacts will also differ.

Study activity

2. Indicate two different kinds of contact that you have had with people this week and describe the differences.

Sociology owes its name to the philosopher August Comte (1798–1857). He tried to gain a scientific understanding of society as it was in the nineteenth century. Living in chaotic times, Comte was concerned with social and political order and how this might be achieved in society. Although he adopted a narrow consensual interpretation of society – 'Order and Progress' was his motto – Comte gave us the title and field of study we today recognize as the wider discipline of sociology. Sociology may therefore be defined as follows:

Sociology is a branch of knowledge which studies the structures of people living in groups and the processes involved.

As you see, the subject focuses on the social environment rather than on the individual. The term 'structure' in the above definition may refer to society as a whole, but also to a hospital as an organization.

Since the area studied by sociology is so vast, a distinction is often made between *macro-*

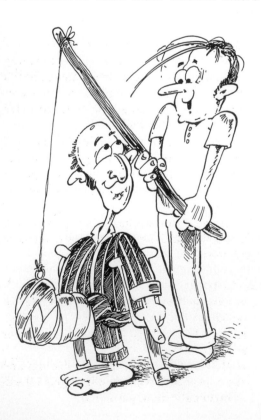

sociology and *microsociology*. The former is concerned with the major structures and processes such as society as a whole or the concept of culture. Microsociology is directed more towards smaller processes and structures, and how people experience their social worlds.

Study activity

3. Give five examples of structures or processes which are, or may be, the subject of sociological study.

If you compare the definitions of social psychology and sociology the definitions show that the two branches of knowledge have major similarities. Whether you are considering the way in which individuals are influenced by their environment (social psychology) or the way in which they themselves form the social environment (sociology), you will come across a large number of identical concepts. It is frequently impossible to differentiate between social psychology and sociology (particularly microsociology). The difference is essentially one of perspective in dealing with similar subject matter.

In the following sections and chapters it will only be indicated which of the two sciences was used as a source if that would be useful.

b. Health care

There are a great many topics in which both disciplines are interested and this applies not only when you are considering society as a whole, but also when you are studying its various components.

Health care in society is no exception. Sociology even includes an area of research especially concerned with health care, i.e. medical sociology. Initially medical sociology, one of the largest areas of sociological study today, concerned itself with *macrosociological structural-functionalist approaches*. That is, it addressed social structures such as social class, family structures, poverty, housing etc. and their influence on health and disease. Research tended to consist of large scale epidemiological surveys. This is indeed still the case in this

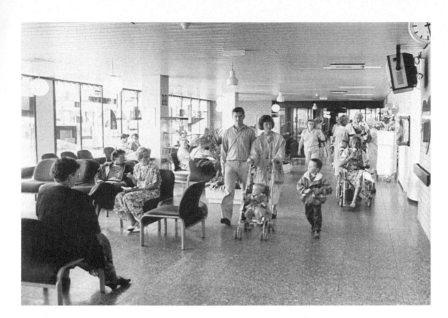

Figure 3.1.1
A hospital reception area. People react to one another even there and sometimes they co-operate

tradition. The Journal of Health and Social Behaviour which reflects this perspective is one of the most influential academic journals in the social sciences.

However, in recent years there has been an increasing concern with social processes and how health and illness become institutionalized in society. This alternative approach is *interactionist* rather than structuralist in its orientation and generally adopts a *microsociological* perspective. Topics such as labelling, life in health care institutions, how medicine may actually cause or 'construct' disease rather than treat it, are all examples of the concerns of this other type of sociology. It is perhaps better described as the Sociology of Health and Illness, the title of the academic journal introduced to reflect this perspective.

Study activity
  4. Try to describe as clearly as possible the field of studies in which medical sociology is engaged.

It is not difficult to give examples of health care topics which include socio-psychological or sociological aspects. Some examples are concerned exclusively with health care,

whereas others also apply to different areas of society. If you compare work in a hospital ward with that, say, in a local government office, there will be differences as well as similarities.

A number of examples are given below:
  – There are certain expectations about the way in which people working in the area of health care behave. There are expectations concerning the 'role' of patient, the 'role' of nurse and the 'role' of doctor.
  – It is possible to identify various groups and sub-groups of people working in a hospital;
  – In hospitals, some people have more power than others. Power is also exercised in different ways;
  – Norms and values change, even in health care. Think of examples such as euthanasia and abortion.

Study activity
  5. **a.** Give at least five specific examples of health care topics which are, or may be, suitable for study by social psychologists or sociologists.
  b. Explain the importance of sociology and social psychology to nursing in general and to practical care in particular.

3. The concepts of relationship and interaction

In the introduction to this chapter, we argued that living in a community is essential to human beings. Living in a community means starting relationships. In common parlance, the concept of a relationship is limited to people we know. The owner of a shop, for example, talks about a relationship when he is referring to a customer he knows well. You yourself probably talk about a relationship when referring to a friend. Outside the area of everyday speech, the concept is far wider. The people in a doctor's waiting room also have a relationship, even though they do not know one another.

We talk about a *relationship* when referring to any connection with another person or persons.

Much of what we do, think or feel is determined by the relationships we form, since there is interaction within the various relationships. The concepts of relationship and interaction are therefore closely linked. The term 'relationship' refers to the contacts that people have. The term 'interaction' refers to the process that takes place within such contacts.

Interaction is the process of mutual influence within a relationship.

Within a relationship there is always interaction or mutual influence. Its intensity is naturally not always the same and it is more easily identifiable on some occasions than on others.

Interaction also occurs in the above example of the doctor's waiting room even though no one says anything and no one knows anyone else. When Mr Jacobs goes into the doctor's consulting room after the buzzer has sounded, Mrs Nelson reacts to his departure, for instance by becoming slightly more nervous because it will be her turn next. In a waiting room of this kind, interaction becomes especially apparent if someone tries to jump the queue.

An example of interaction

Imagine that you, a student nurse, are going to work in a ward for the first time. If you have already experienced the situation, it will not be difficult to conjure up its memory. You may have felt nervous and insecure, and perhaps you even tried to avoid making contact with the patients. After all, they might have asked you questions that you could not answer yet. In short, a student nurse's first period of duty in a ward is not likely to leave him or her totally unaffected. Such emotions depend largely on what is happening all around you. Are you working with an experienced colleague who introduces you well? Are the patients easy to talk to and do they 'help' you when you are trying to make contact? Had you been given favourable or unfavourable information about the ward? All those factors as well as many others influence your first contacts with patients.

Patients, on the other hand, also react to the newcomer. They usually tell you less, since confidence has not yet been established. Sometimes, however, they tell you more because they hope you will have more time than other people. Here again it is true that patients react to your first appearance, but also to the uncertainty emanating from you more or less obviously on this first occasion.

Study activity
6. **a.** Try to describe the interactions in the above example as accurately as possible.
   b. In what way do you think that interaction with patients influences you when you start practical work for the first time?

The above example provides a good illustration of interaction or mutual influences. The example also makes it clear that there are many factors which affect the interaction process. The process of interaction does not exist solely at the time of one's first contacts with patients. It develops over time. It is true, however, that the factors that play a part in the process do not always remain the same. Your experience, for instance, begins to play its part.

Study activity
7. List as many general factors as possible that affect interactions.

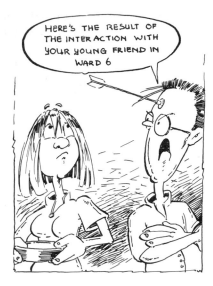

What has been said so far about the terms 're-lationship' and 'interaction' leads us to draw two important conclusions:

- there is always interaction in a relationship;
- there is something unique about every re-lationship.

The second conclusion stems from the remark made earlier on to the effect that the factors that play a part in the interaction process change. One of the circumstances that has not yet been mentioned concerns your own background. Your upbringing and everything that you have learnt play a part in the interaction process. Upbringing and experience vary from individual to individual in a number of ways. There are, of course, similarities as well. The contact that you have with a particular patient is just a little different from a colleague's relationship with the same patient. This kind of difference may be greater on some occasions and almost imperceptible on others.

Study activity

8. Two adjacent beds in a ward are occupied by:
   - an elderly man of eighty-two who is rather forgetful at times and tires easily;
   - a boy of nineteen, who is spontaneous and high spirited;

   Both are in hospital because of leg fractures and you are the person who has to look after

them both. Try to consider what differences there may be if you compare the relationship between you and each of the two patients.

People as social animals

You cannot read a single book about people without coming across the word 'social' at least several times. The present volume is no exception. It is usually accepted without argument that man is a social animal. But is it true?

Let us first look at the term *social* itself. It means literally: living with members of its kind. If, however, you come across the concept in specialist literature, it means something else as well. In that case, the term is usually based on the idea that people do not only live in communities but that living in communities is essential to man.

In Maslow's (1970) hierarchy of needs, de scribed in Module 1, social contacts come second in the category of basic needs, with physiological needs topping the list. This, too, emphasizes that social contacts are more than merely accidental happenings – in fact they represent basic needs.

When you say that social contacts are a necessity or a basic need, this means that humans depend on them for their existence. To demonstrate that man is indeed a social animal, two things need to be illustrated:

- firstly, it is necessary to indicate how people's interdependence is constituted;
- secondly, it is necessary to show that humans cannot relinquish ties with others without a risk.

A human being's conception is its first experience of dependence on someone else. Without the existence of two people, the creation of human beings would be impossible. Even after birth, humans remain dependent for a long time. It is interesting to consider how long their state of dependence lasts compared with that of animals. Animals can provide food for themselves much sooner than humans can.

Contacts with other people, however, serve more purposes than producing the next generation. You also depend on others for the way in which you look at yourself, for forming your own identity. The things you think are important or unimportant, your personal interests and the things that motivate you are formed in relationships with other people. Something has already been said about interaction in relationships above. Sociology's interaction theory (also sometimes termed symbolic interaction theory, or simply interactionist theory) will be dealt with in Chapter 3 of this module.

Another important area of dependence is one created by man himself. It is concerned with that which, for the sake of convenience, we shall call society. This means all the arrangements, structures and organizations which combine to create the picture of contemporary society. To be able to function in this society, each human being must possess a vast amount of knowledge. First of all, you have to learn a language so that you can communicate with other people. Besides that, you have to learn innumerable other things if you are to be capable of any kind of independent existence. Examples of this are managing money, operating the telephone, organizing health care, etc. There are two ways in which society's complexity creates interdependence between people.
- Firstly, all knowledge has to be acquired, and can only be acquired with the assistance of others who already possess knowledge.
- Secondly, the structure of society is so complex that certain purposes can be achieved only if we co-operate. A hospital is a good example of this. Not a single individual, however clever he or she may be, can carry out all tasks without the quality of care being affected. Co-operation and interdependence are therefore inevitable in a hospital.

Three major areas of human interdependence have been mentioned above, i.e.:
- preserving the human race;
- forming one's own identity;
- holding one's own in our complex society.

One can think of many other areas, sometimes individual ones, in which people feel a need to share with others. Consider the way in which many people experience their religion for example.

It has been mentioned already that if you wish to show that people are social animals, more needs to be proved than interdependence alone. It also has to be made credible that contact with other people cannot be avoided with impunity. In the case of babies, who are still totally dependent, this is obvious. But how about adults? What happens if someone is living in total isolation?

According to the *social isolation hypothesis*, there is a considerable risk of psychological abnormalities if people live in total isolation. You might also put it this way: to maintain a psychological balance, contact with other people is essential.
Donald Crowhurst's suicide provides a good illustration of this.

On July 10, 1969, a deserted yacht was found in the middle of the Atlantic. Although the vessel showed signs of having been at sea for a long time, she was undamaged and fully equipped. It turned out that the ship had belonged to Donald Crowhurst, a thirty-one-year-old Englishman who had been taking part in a solo round-the-world yacht race. The complete log led to the conclusion that Crowhurst had committed suicide after sailing on his own for 243 days. He had simply stepped overboard. Why?

When the Sunday Times announced a solo round-the-world yacht race, Crowhurst, an excellent marine yachtsman, decided to take part. His financial means were inadequate for building a yacht capable of such an achievement, but he managed to get several newspapers interested in starting an appeal for funding. As a result of the publicity, the BBC became involved as well. A nation-wide fund-raising appeal followed and the result was that Crowhurst was able to build his boat although he was pressed for time. According to the rules , October 31, 1968, was to be the final starting date. Crowhurst's yacht, 'Teignmouth Electron' was launched on September 23. The interval between the two dates, between five and six weeks, was far too short for sea trials and a period of rest. In spite of everything, Crowhurst set sail on 31st October 1968 and his departure was filmed by the BBC.

Almost immediately after his departure, the yacht appeared to be in serious trouble. It is uncertain when and where Crowhurst decided not to sail round the world at all and just to pretend that he was doing so. In any event, he began to make fraudulent entries in his log quite soon after his departure. Instead of sailing round South America and into the Pacific en route to Australia, Crowhurst continued to drift around in the South Atlantic. He wrote up his log in a way that would subsequently make it appear as though he had been in the Pacific and the Indian Ocean. He listened to the weather forecasts and noted the weather conditions in the areas where he ought to have been. Crowhurst avoided radio contact, and so his true position remained undiscovered. We can only guess at his motives for the deception. He was known to have a highly optimistic and narcissistic personality, and it is assumed that fear of the loss of face that would ensue if he were to return shortly after his departure, without having achieved anything, made him decide on his subsequent course of action.

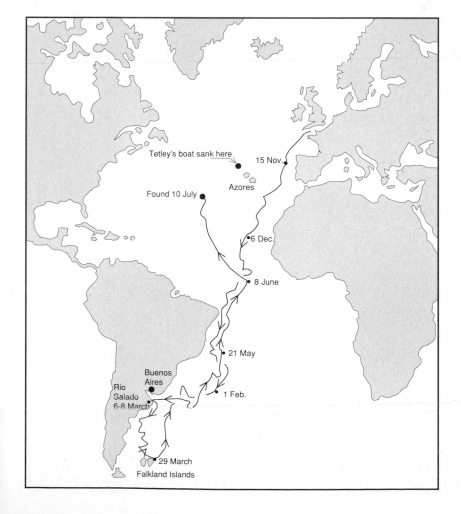

Figure 3.1.2
Donald Crowhurst's voyage. Start: Teignmouth, England, October 31, 1968. The yacht was found deserted on July 10, 1969. Position: latitude 33 11' North; longitude 40 28'West; distance covered: 16,591 nautical miles; length of voyage: 243 days

The course of the race suggests that Crowhurst had intended to mingle with the other solo yachtsmen as they passed the Cape of Good Hope on their return journey. He resumed radio contact with the organizers and reported his correct position. He did so at the time when two of his rivals were already well past the Cape. He was now, he thought, lying in third place. Coming third did not seem at all bad, although he had always insisted that he would win. He also assumed that the organizers would scrutinize his logbook far less minutely than that of the winner. Unfortunately, Crowhurst's assessment of the situation was incorrect.

The yachtsman who was lying first had sailed much earlier than Crowhurst and his position was of no interest for the purpose of the race. The yachtsman in second place, Nigel Tetley, was alarmed to find that Crowhurst was hot on his heels. Tetley's yacht was in a bad way, and he could only reach England by sailing slowly. Tetley took too many risks. On May 21, 1969 he could not manage to take in sail quickly enough when a sudden storm blew up near the Azores, and he went down with his yacht.

Crowhurst was now in a position that he had not wanted – in the lead. He knew that he was going to win and that he would be unmasked as a fraud in a few days when his logbook was checked.

In the course of the month, the log became oddly disjointed. Crowhurst spent a week writing a personal document addressed to the world at large and 25.000 words long. Among his writings was a kind of world history of the past 2000 years. He phrased it in a mixture of mathematical and religious sentences, with frequent references to Albert Einstein.

Meanwhile, pressure on the home front was mounting rapidly. Newspapers were anxious to interview him; BBC Television wanted a rendezvous at sea in order to film him; several ports were urging him to put in there.

Crowhurst refused almost all contacts, and his psychological collapse reached a climax on July 1, 1969. He wrote in his logbook,
'It is finished
It is finished
It is the mercy
... I have no need to prolong the game
It has been a good game that must be ended at the
I will play this game when I choose I will resign the game 11 20 40 There is
no reason for harmful...'

The page in the logbook was full. Crowhurst could have turned it over and continued writing, but he did not. He stepped overboard.

The account shows how someone who had been living in almost complete social isolation for a long time reacted to a problem. He solved the problem of 'loss of face' by resorting to deception and then made an incorrect assessment of the situation; he was about to win the race in spite of himself. The thought that his deceit would undoubtedly be revealed after an enthusiastic and festive reception, became unbearable. Of course it is very difficult to solve that kind of problem. Why did Crowhurst not withdraw from the race and, once back in England, move to a place where no-one knew him?

The psychologists and psychiatrists who have studied the log agree that Crowhurst's social isolation, combined with his personality , was the cause of his suicide. If he had been able to talk to other people, to his wife for instance, he would have found that although he was a fraud, his entire life was not in ruins. He would have realized that he still had plenty to live for, despite the great difficulties which now faced him.

Because of his self-imposed isolation, Crowhurst gradually lost touch with social reality. This led to complete psychological collapse. Crowhurst's death is a dramatic illustration of the fact that we humans live in groups, not only because we like it but because we cannot do otherwise.

a. Differences and similarities between relationships

The conclusion drawn earlier in this chapter was that there is something unique about each relationship. This was attributed to the various factors affecting the interaction process. The differences in relationships which bring about this uniqueness will be considered in further detail in this section.

Study activity

9. Compare you relationship with a patient whom you have been looking after for several days with your relationship with your mother.
   Try to indicate a few differences.

Differences between various relationships are often easier to indicate if you consider a number of criteria, including:
- purpose;
- form;
- the way in which the relationship is maintained;
- depth;
- the extent to which the relationship is voluntary;
- emotional content.

Every relationship can be studied on the basis of each of the above criteria, so that the differences and similarities between relationships can be indicated.

Not every relationship, for example, serves the same *purpose*. The purpose of a relationship with a fellow nurse differs from that of a relationship with someone with whom you go out in the evening. Work is the main object in the former situation, whereas enjoyment is the principal aim of the latter one.

Relationships also differ in *form*. Your relationship with the managers of a hospital where you are employed as a nurse will be recorded in a contract expressing some of the characteristics of the relationship. Such an official course would not be adopted for an evening out with friends where any arrangement would, as a rule, be made orally.

You receive your salary every month and you are expected to do your work as well as possible in return. This is one of the ways in which the relationship between employer and employee is *maintained*, even in a hospital. The bunch of flowers with which some men maintain their relationship with their wife is a classic example. Paying attention to each other is an important way of keeping up a relationship in many different kinds of circumstances. The way in which the attention is paid, differs from one relationship to another .

Case study: Mr McKee

In the surgical ward, Mr McKee has died. The patient celebrated his seventy second birthday a few weeks before his death. His heart failed as secondary cancers gained an increasing hold on his body. During those last few weeks, the nursing staff had come to know him and his family well. Sadness about his inevitable end had

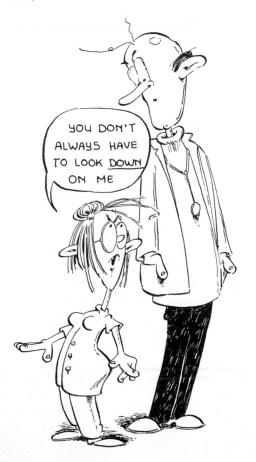

YOU DON'T ALWAYS HAVE TO LOOK DOWN ON ME

therefore not been limited to Mr McKee's family. The ward's regular nursing staff had also been affected by his death. Notices in the local press showed that at least five other people had died in the town on the same day. But none of these people were known to the nurses on the ward.

This is an everyday example, similar to what any nurse is likely to experience several times in the course of his or her career. Why does the death of one patient affect you more than that of another? Even if you know a person whose death is mentioned in a newspaper, there will be a difference in the intensity of your emotions. This difference depends on the depth of the relationship, which varies in each case. You soon feel a close bond with some people, whereas your relationship with others will remain superficial.

The idea of *depth* has a great deal to do with involvement in a relationship, and there are a number of factors which affect involvement. This will be considered in further detail in the next subsection.

Not every relationship is begun *voluntarily*. Your relationship with your parents is an example of a relationship which, in principle, is involuntary; you were, after all, unable to choose them. Membership of a sports club, however, is an example of a voluntary relationship. Most relationships are neither entirely voluntary nor totally involuntary. You do not choose your fellow nurses in a ward, but if you cannot get on with them you can always apply for a transfer or resign if need be.

Emotional content is another criterion which may vary in different relationships. One relationship may be regarded as being positive, whereas another is considered negative. Some teachers are entertaining, others send you to sleep. Some ward sisters are strict, others tolerant. Many other characteristics of this kind play a part in the emotional content of a relationship.

Study activity

10. Look at the previous study activity (9) and use the above criteria to indicate the simi-

larities and differences between the two relationships.

The purpose of your relationship with the hospital managers is your contribution towards the patient's recovery process. It takes the form of an employment contract and the quality of the work and the salary are among the aspects that maintain the relationship. If you substitute another word for 'hospital' and 'recovery process', the above will apply to most employment situations.

Although the various criteria have been dealt with separately, they cannot be totally dissociated from one another. It is improbable, for instance, that the depth of a relationship has no connection with its emotional content. A relationship with great depth usually has a positive emotional content as well. That does not always apply: during adolescence, for instance, people's relationship with their parents, which usually has great depth, is not infrequently accompanied by a negative emotional content.

b. Involvement

When J.F. Kennedy was assassinated in Dallas, a shock wave passed through humanity. The murder of the American president was to occupy people's minds throughout the world for many years. Books, newspaper articles and television programmes have been devoted to the event ever since it occurred. Even in 1992 one of the major new feature films of the year is the most recent account of the events surrounding JFK's assassination. It was also found that, many years later, people could still remember exactly where they were and what they were doing when they heard the news about the assassination. Many people were so shaken that the moment when the report came was, as it were, engraved on their memory.

The above account provides an example of an event with which everyone felt closely concerned at the time and perhaps they still do. Close involvement also occurred in the case of Mr McKee in the previous subsection. You may have a sense of involvement with events, people or situations.

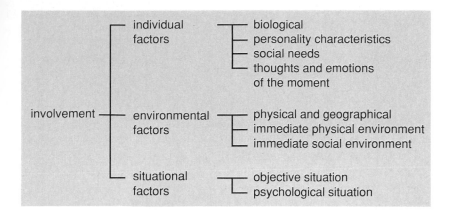

Diagram 3.1.1
Factors affecting
involvement in
situations, relationships
and events

What are the factors affecting involvement? They have been set out in Diagram 3.1.1. As you will see, involvement is quite a complex concept. It is not always possible to decide exactly on which factors the involvement is based.

In the case of Mr McKee, situational factors undoubtedly played a part, i.e. the factors concerning the psychological situation. This, however, also applies to environmental and individual factors. The same may be said of the assassination of J.F. Kennedy. It is important to be aware of this complexity in situations when you are surprised or caught off guard by your own involvement.

Individual factors

These may affect involvement in various ways. In contacts with others, physical attractiveness appears to be an important *biological* factor. Intelligence is another example of a biological factor which may influence involvement in a relationship.

There are many ways in which *personality characteristics* can play a part in relationships. You will probably realize that it is more difficult to feel involved with someone who contains his or her emotions than it is with someone who can talk about them.

Study activity

11. Consider what your reasons were for choosing to become a nurse.

When you have completed Study Activity 11 and compared your results with other people's, it will be apparent that there were a great many reasons to list. Many of the reasons for choosing nursing as a profession are based on *social needs* which differ from one person to the next. The need to work as part of a team is the principal reason for some people, whereas for others it is the need to make oneself useful. The degree of involvement in various situations will depend on the individual pattern of needs.

Imagine that it is morning. You have an appointment to see the ward sister and your nurse tutor in a couple of hours' time. The purpose of the interview is to discuss how well you have performed in the ward in recent months. You know that you have not done too badly on the whole, and yet...

The tension you feel on account of the interview affects your mood in the hours leading up to it. One of the consequences will be that you feel less involved than usual in what is going on around you. This is what is meant by the *thoughts and emotions of the moment* as shown in diagram 3.1.1.

Environmental factors

These constitute the next group of factors that affect involvement.

Towards the end of 1987, three nurses were arrested at a hospital in the Netherlands. They were supposed to have practised active

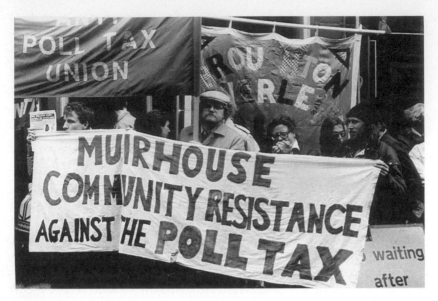

Figure 3.1.3
Group pressure: the impact on the social environment

euthanasia without the knowledge or consent of other people. For various reasons, the press was full of the event for days.

The above occurrence may help us to understand what is meant by *physical and geographical environment*. Concern about the happenings in 1987 was probably greatest among people working in hospitals themselves. If you form part of the health care 'environment', you are likely to feel more concerned about matters relating to health care. The geographical distance plays a part as well. If you imagine that the above events took place at the hospital where you are employed, you will feel more concerned than if they had happened in some remote city. The *social impact theory* described by Latane (1981) is perhaps a useful vehicle for understanding such influences. Where an individual is close to a social influence and this is of high social force or impact, there is a tendency to react strongly. This reaction is also likely to be influenced by how others, particularly influential others, react to the situation. Thus if concern or condemnation of these nurses was widespread in the hospital, the social impact on other nurses would be significant. Their level of arousal or anxiety would also be high and they might be influenced to join in the condemnation.

Social environment means the complex of norms and values that are important in a culture

at a particular time. The 1987 incident provides a good example of this as well. Euthanasia was a hotly debated issue at the time, just as it is now. There was no prospect of social consensus about what should, could, or could not be done, or about what was permissible. The consequence was that any incident in which euthanasia played a part immediately led to fierce discussions. In 1987, it was the actual lack of common norms and values that gave everyone a sense of being involved in the events.

Situational factors

A distinction is made here between the objective and the psychological situation. The objective situation means that which is perceptible to all. The psychological situation refers to the significance attached by someone to the situation, and therefore differs from individual to individual.

Study activity

12. Mrs Lawson, aged forty-two, is in a single room in the Gynaecological Department. What is the objective situation? What might the psychological situation be for:
    – you, as a nurse;
    – Mrs Lawson's nineteen-year-old daughter;
    – a man from the Maintenance Department who comes to her room to do some repair work?

Anyone can feel involved in an *objective situation*. An accident or an increase in salary are examples of objective situations in which one may feel involved to a varying degree.

The *psychological situation*, however, is the principal source of influence. The psychological situation depends on the background, in the widest sense of the word, that people attribute to the situation individually. Psychological situations are included in environmental factors, since the psychological situation is linked to the situation itself. If that were not the case, it would be a matter of one of the individual factors considered earlier on. In practice, however, it is often difficult to distinguish between the psychological situation and the individual factors.

People's involvement in a relationship, or at the time of a particular event or in certain circumstances, have been analysed in this subsection. In the case of relationships, this means that a highly complex process is taking place since, if two people feel involved with each other, the above factors affect each of them.

All this might create the impression that contacts between human beings are so complex that it is not actually feasible to study them. Fortu-nately, that is not true: contacts are governed by a whole range of social and psychological patterns, some of which which will be considered in this module. The issues of interaction and relationship are returned to in Module 5. Chapter 3 of that module in particular addresses how nurses interact with patients and the specific nature of the nurse-patient relationship.

4. Norms and values

The concepts of relationship and interaction at the centre of the previous subsection are of great importance in social psychology and sociology. The same is true of the concept of norms and values. Relationships with other people are, after all, bound by a number of rules and conditions. Those rules, in turn, are associated with whatever is considered to be important in a particular culture at a particular time.

Case study: Mrs Sadiq

Mrs Sadiq, a thirty-two year old Asian lady, has been admitted to the Neurological Ward. She came to the United Kingdom six months ago; before this she lived in Pakistan. Her stay in the ward has had its problems. She has made it clear in her broken English that she is not allowed to eat certain food on religious grounds and this

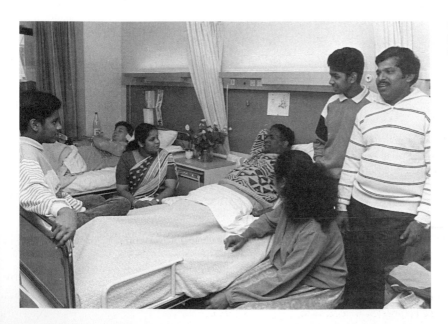

Figure 3.1.4
Norms and values are different in every culture

upsets some of her fellow patients. She also has serious qualms about being washed by a male nurse.

In the above example, there is a clash between the norms and values of two totally different cultures. In Mrs Sadiq's view, the food that she chooses to eat has a religious significance. In the view of some of the other patients she is being too fussy and is getting special treatment. Her objection to being washed by a male nurse is also due to cultural differences, although, in this case, patients' attitudes also vary in British culture.

Norms and values determine much of our behaviour and they also play a major part in the assessment of other people's conduct. The two concepts may be defined in the following way:

Norms are the written or unwritten rules of conduct on how to behave in a particular situation.

Values are opinions on what is right or wrong, proper or improper, important or unimportant, etc.

Norms are concerned with rules of conduct, whereas values tell us something about opinions. The two concepts are closely linked since behaviour does not exist without opinions on what is right and proper. Values, on the other hand, usually become apparent only as a result of someone's behaviour.

These links between rules of conduct and values

are highly important. The strength of valuing, that is, the strength of feeling attached to what is right and proper, determines the strength of social imperative to adhere to norms. In his now classical comment on culture, Sumner (1906) recognised the varying nature of this social imperative by dividing norms into folkways and mores. Sumner described *folkways* as common modes of behaviour recognised as generally acceptable and desirable by the social group, while *mores* are more significant, insisted-upon social rules.

Study activity

13. **a.** Give three examples of norms and values that play a part in contacts with patients.
    b. Give three concrete examples of a possible conflict between personal and professional values and norms.

Finally, to end this subsection, two important characteristics of norms and values as referred to above need to be restated:

– Norms and values are linked to a specific culture and may therefore differ from one culture to another. You might, for example, compare countries where it is usual for relatives to help look after a hospital patient with the totally different situation in our country.
– Norms and values are linked to a specific period. Changes may occur over the years. Views held thirty years ago, on patients' rights for example, have changed radically in recent years. Even ten years ago, patients in

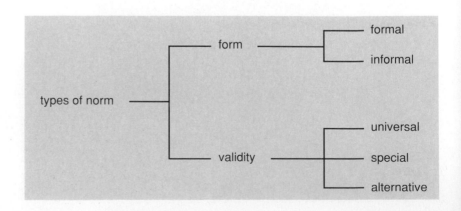

Diagram 3.1.2
Classification of norms according to form and validity

the United Kingdom were largely passive recipients of care. Now in our National Health Service we have a Patients Charter which clearly specifies the patient's rights and the carers obligations.

a. Types of norms and values

There are usually no rigid rules telling us that we must address patients, and older patients in particular, as 'Mr' or 'Mrs' or 'Miss' and that we may call fellow nurses by their first names. In some hospitals, however, the rules do demand that you wear uniform when you are on duty.

Despite the fact that there are often no fixed rules for the former situation but there usually are for the latter, we mostly keep to both rules of conduct. The most important of these are set out in diagram 3.1.2.

Formal norms are norms contained in laws, regulations or agreements. **Informal norms** mean the rules of conduct that everyone in a particular environment keeps to even though they have not been imposed officially.

Calling fellow nurses by their first names and addressing most patients as Mr or Mrs are examples of informal norms. The regulation about uniform is an example of a formal norm. Formal norms are to be found in laws, employment contracts, school rules, rules of play, information booklets, etc. At face value it may seem that formal norms and mores are the same while informal norms and folkways are the same. However, some formal norms e.g. not parking

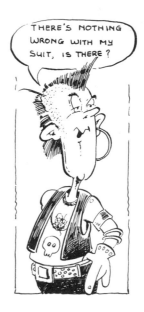

on a double yellow line are not held as social mores. There is often general agreement among many people in Britain that you *can* do this, but you try not to get a parking ticket! This is an example of a *formal* norm which falls within our *folkways*. Conversely, while it may be an *informal* norm to give your child a birthday present, it would be a major breach of social rules not to do this. The requirement is not formally required, there is no law demanding it, yet the social *mores* for conforming in this regard are very strong.

Study activity

14. Think of a formal and an informal norm with regard to touching a patient's body.

Diagram 3.1.3   Examples of types of norm

	Formal	Informal
Universal	The laws of the land	Table manners
Special	School rules	Football supporters' rival chants
Alternative	—	Copying a favourite pop star

As for the validity of norms, a distinction was made in diagram 3.1.2 between universal, special and alternative norms.

Universal norms apply to everyone in a particular area or in a particular culture. You might take traffic rules as an example.

Special norms apply to special groups only. The regulation that wearing uniform of a particular kind is compulsory is a norm which applies to a well-defined group only.

Alternative norms are norms which one may choose to adopt or ignore. There is a measure of freedom in deciding whether or not the norms are to be adopted. For example, you might decide whether or not you are going to have vegetarian food.

Universal and special norms may be either formal or informal. This does not apply to alternative norms, which are always informal. Diagram 3.1.3 gives an example of each combination.

Values can be categorized as universal, special and alternative. They can also be classified as:
– *minor values,* which have only a limited significance or refer to a small section of the population only;
– *central values,* very important values which concern everyone all the time and have a profound emotional significance for everyone in the community.

Some communities are built up entirely around

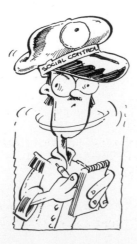

central values, and in that case we think in terms of ideologies rather than values.

Study activity
15. A strike or walkout by nurses is unlikely to occur in the case of a labour dispute. Consider the values relating to this. Are they minor or central values?

b. Social control
Norms are pointless unless people keep to them. Compliance with them is therefore checked, sometimes reciprocally, whereas at other times someone is specially appointed for the purpose.

Case study: Mr Vernon
Mr Vernon, aged fifty-two, has been admitted to the cardiological ward. He is a difficult patient and complains about most things : the food is awful; the other patients keep him awake; nurses do not respond to his call quickly enough, etc. He himself does not keep to ward rules: he is frequently away from the ward when he should be there, and he takes no notice of the agreed rest period. The ward sister has rebuked him and fellow patients ignore him as much as possible.

Study activity
16. What kinds of social control do you observe in this example?

Mr Vernon fails to keep to the established norms in a number of ways. He breaks ward rules, ignores arrangements and also flouts norms of social behaviour. Fellow patients as well as the nursing staff are aware of this and everyone, depending on his or her position, tries to do something about it. The ward sister tackles him on the subject and patients ignore him.
This brings us to the definition of social control.

Social control refers to monitoring and ensuring the observance of norms.

The above control is established by means of sanctions. In everyday speech, the term sanction usually has a negative connotation. It is important, however, to realize that sanctions may be either positive (rewarding) or negative (punitive).

In the case of *positive sanctions*, you might think in terms of promotion or an increase in salary. Extra attention might also be regarded as a positive sanction.

Positive sanctions are intended to stimulate desirable behaviour, whereas *negative sanctions* try to make undesirable behaviour unattractive or even impossible. Suspension, fines or, more seriously, dismissal or imprisonment are examples of negative sanctions.

Attention may also play a part in negative sanctions in the sense that a person is ignored as much as possible, as Mr Vernon was by the other patients.

Sometimes the two are combined, for instance if a father promises his child a sweet if all the toys are put away. The sweet appears to be a reward but if the toys are not put away properly and the reward is not given, it works as a punishment.

Study activity

17. Paying attention to someone or, alternatively, ignoring him or her, was referred to as a sanction. Consider how this works in the light of *operant conditioning* as described in Module 1.

Generally speaking, everyone is concerned with social control. This, however, does not mean that anyone is entitled to impose any kind of sanction. It depends on one's social position: only a police officer or the judiciary may impose a fine, and only a hospital ward sister is in a position to give a student nurse a good or poor assessment for practical work.

A measure of social control also occurs in respect of values. This certainly applies to communities where central values in the form of ideologies have been made into a source of inspiration to all. In that kind of community you are punished if you are suspected of having deviant views.

The situation is less extreme in our western culture. There is a reasonable amount of tolerance for different views, provided people keep more or less to the rules as far as behaviour is concerned.

If sanctions do occur, they often take the form of paying or withholding attention, in a sense because of the lack of alternatives.

c. Norms and values in health care

Throughout this section we have looked at a number of examples of norms and values relating to health care and you were asked to identify instances of these in the study activities. You will not find a complete list of health care norms and values but a few more examples are given below.

The case of Mr Vernon in the cardiological ward shows that there are norms for patients as well as for nurses and other hospital workers. Norms for patients are sometimes informal but quite frequently formal. The hospital's information leaflet issued to every patient is one of the sources where these formal norms are to be found. The following two quotations are taken from one such booklet.

'*Leaving the ward*.
You may only leave the ward with the consent of the senior nurse on duty. You are requested to remain in your own ward after 10 p.m. for the sake of keeping the hospital as quiet as possible.'

'*Departure*.
It is usual to leave hospital in the morning. Please do not embarrass staff by giving them presents or money. It is our job to provide good treatment and care.'

Study activity

18. **a.** Take a look at an information booklet for patients who are to be admitted to hospital. Give a few examples of the norms contained in them.
    b. Indicate five norms that you and your colleagues observe when dealing with patients.

Hospitals also provide examples of informal norms. Training schemes for nurses pay a lot of attention to informal norms relating to patients and fellow nurses. Concepts such as helpfulness, comradeship, care, respect and tolerance are linked to the nursing profession with varying degrees of conviction.

It was stated earlier that norms and values are products of their times. This is evident if you look at the values relating to various views of mankind. There are few modern nursing text books in which you are unlikely to find something about the holistic view of mankind. It is generally argued that such an approach is preferable to the more reductionist conceptions that prevailed previously, i.e. a patient-centred rather than task-centred approach is advocated.
It may be true that the holistic approach is accepted by most people these days. In practice, however, this value still has not been converted into norms. Training, lack of staff and the way in which hospitals are funded ensure that although thinking may be holistic, working methods may continue to be reductionist or task-centred as a rule.

5. Socialization

From the day of a child's birth, and to some extent even before then, interaction occurs between the baby and his or her environment. Initially, it is very primitive, but both child and parents learn how to adjust to one another's wishes through such interaction.

Parents soon learn from the way in which the baby is crying whether it is demanding attention, or whether it is hungry or in pain. The baby, in turn, learns how to make use of these differences.

Such interaction becomes less and less primitive as the child grows up. Parents – who, for good reason, are called 'educators' in some languages strive increasingly to teach the child norms, values and behaviour, e.g.:
– how to address people;
– how to thank people;
– how to eat 'properly'.

Others, official bodies as well as individuals, become increasingly involved in the growing-up process. Examples are: friends' parents, schools, television etc. Children also educate one another by means of games and true or fabricated stories.

During this interaction process, which begins in a child's very first years, people are, as it were, prepared for life in society. The process, however, is never complete. Changing norms and values, new contacts and environments are constantly forcing people to adapt.

Socialization is the sociological concept used to express the above process. It is a process in which the concepts of relationship, interaction, norms and values that were considered in previous sections converge.

The socialization process is not limited to what is usually called upbringing. Just as a child has to learn how to become independent, an elderly person is obliged to learn to adapt to circumstances and the other occupants of a warden-assisted flat. Socialization is therefore a never-ending process.

There is a close connection here with developmental psychology as described in Module 2. When reference is made to learning social behaviour in the present module, this is a description of the socialization process. In developmental psychology, this is linked to age or developmental phases. In the present module, the concept of socialization is always related to people or situations.

a. The concept of socialization

The above remarks should provide some idea of what is meant by the term socialization. The concept may be compared with the part that an actor has to learn for a film or a play. Just as learning a part is more than knowing the text, the socialization process is more than simply learning how to behave. The concept of socialization may be defined as follows:

Socialization is the interaction process in which the norms and values of a culture are learnt, whereby the individual learns to adapt his or her behaviour to that of a social group.

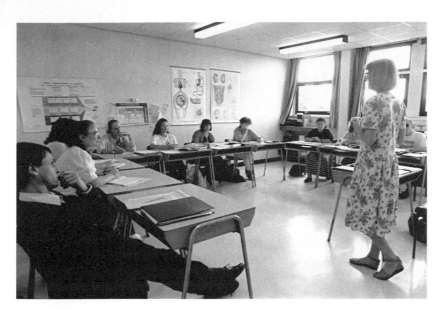

Figure 3.1.5
The process of
socialization is a
learning process

It is important to re-emphasize the concept of interaction in the above definition. Where there is interaction, influences are reciprocal and socialization is not merely a one-way process. Parents learn from children just as children do from their parents. In the same way, teachers learn from pupils, heads of departments from students, etc.

The socialization process is not limited to the simple social skills required in contacts with others. You can also think in terms of socialization:

– when you learn to adjust to your environment in the wider sense, for instance a hospital 'environment' or, as it is sometimes called, 'the hospital culture';
– when you learn as part of a group what is expected of you in the position you occupy, e.g. as a chairman, a nurse, or a patient, etc.

Within the concept of socialization, a distinction is made between primary socialization and secondary socialization. *Primary socialization* means the elementary learning that takes place mainly within the family circle. Learning the role behaviour of boys and girls is a good example of this. *Secondary socialization* takes place mainly outside the family circle. Learning

the role behaviour that is appropriate to a nurse is a good example of this and has been mentioned several times previously.

Sometimes secondary and primary socialization are in conflict. This may occur in situations where secondary socialization in peer groups may introduce the young adolescent to subcultural norms which are incompatible with norms presented in the family through primary socialization. However, often more fundamental socialization processes are carried through from primary socialization into secondary socialization. One such instance, pertinent to the profession of nursing, is gender socialization. Franzini et al., (1978) illustrate how modelling and conditioning influences are brought to bear on young people, both within the family (primary socialization) and the wider social milieu (secondary socialization). Boys and young men learn to be more dominant and aggressive, and aspire to 'male' occupations such as business, engineering and the sciences. Girls and young women learn to be more passive and nurturant, and aspire to 'female' occupations such as teaching, social work and nursing. This helps explain how nursing has come to be a female-dominated profession and how male recruitment to the profession continues to be a major problem.

Study activities

19. List a few things which form part of the socialization process of becoming a nurse.

20. Is there a link between the development of the nursing profession and the fact that the majority of nurses are women? Try to explain this in the light of the concept of socialization.

The fact that socialization is an interactive process has been mentioned already. This is very evident in health care in the case of a number of subjects for which there are no common norms and values as yet.
Examples include:
– euthanasia;
– abortion;
– terminal home care;
– economies;
– increasing opportunities for day-care.

Debate about these issues, heated at times, is taking place at all levels of society. Such discussions are no more than attempts to exert influence so that norms, values and behaviour are adapted to one another. The socialization process relating to these subjects is therefore still in progress.

b.   The socialization process

As should be evident from the above, the concept of socialization is closely linked to learning. Influencing, adapting and role-learning may give the impression that the socialization process is concerned mainly with imposing norms and values. Some writings on the subject include definitions which are certainly based on that. Such imposition, however, is merely one of the ways in which the concept of socialization is normally viewed. If you look at the various opinions, you will find that there are two extremes, with the others spaced out somewhere in between them.

The two extreme views may be defined in the following way:
– socialization as *a process of repression*. This expressly means the imposition of norms, values and behaviour;

– socialization as *an initiation ritual*. Socialization viewed from this angle means a process aimed at allowing the individual to benefit from his or her environment to the maximum possible extent.

In the socialization process that we experience in everyday life, we are usually somewhere in between these two extreme views. We sometimes feel under some compulsion, whereas at other times we want to know what kind of attitude is best to adopt.

Case study: Maria Gibson

Maria Gibson, aged twenty, is a first-year student. Becoming a nurse was a deliberate choice. The tales she had heard from an aunt, a former nurse, had not only stimulated her choice of occupation but also aroused expectations.

She began her preliminary training with a number of ideas on what was, or was not, important. In the course of that period, her expectations developed in the sense that some of them receded into the background and others were reinforced to some extent.
She first started work in a surgical ward. Because of staff shortages and frequently complex nursing tasks, not much came of Maria's ideals. As a student nurse, she also had a feeling that she herself had little influence on the way she performed. Hoping that her next ward would turn out more to her taste, she simply put up with the situation.
She was then sent to the maternity ward, quite a change from the one she had just left. There was more time to talk to people, it was all a little less technical and there were more discussions with colleagues.

Study activity

21. Try to outline the effect of practical assessments and theoretical tests in a student's socialization process.

If you look at Maria Gibson's expectations and ideals, you will find that she adjusted them several times. During various periods, she learnt to adapt her behaviour to her environment. Her norms and values probably changed as well.

Two learning processes play a part in social-ization, i.e. conforming and identifying. *Con-forming* means keeping to certain norms without necessarily adopting them. In the case of Maria, this was most apparent in the surgical ward. She behaved in the way she was expected to behave, but she kept her own norms and values to a large extent. In the case of *identification*, you identify with the norms and values you encounter, and so they become your own norms and values i.e. you eventually *internalize* them. Important people in your environment, often referred to as '*sig-nificant others*', play a major part in this. Before Maria took up nursing, her aunt played a part in the development of a number of expectations.

Conformity and identification quite frequently overlap. If your own norms and values are dif-ferent from those of people in your environment and there is no other option, you usually con-form at first. It may well be, however, that in the course of time some of the norms and values become your own norms and values. In that case it would be a matter of identification. We shall return to this matter when dealing with disson-ance theory in the next section.

c.   The concept of attitude

If you look up the word '*attitude*' in a dictionary you will find that the meaning provided there scarcely reflects the significance attached to it in sociology and social psychology. The term 'attitude' has been defined by social scientists in the following way:

Attitude is the predictable way in which a person thinks about social information, and how he evaluates it and behaves in regard to that social information.
The social information in this definition refers to people, groups, situations, circumstances, ob-jects etc.

A psychologist may use rather different termi-nology. He will speak of an enduring cluster of beliefs, feelings and behavioural tendencies re-lating to any person, group, object or issue. A person will believe something about a person or object. He will have positive or negative feel-ings or emotions toward that person or object.

His beliefs and feelings will influence how he behaves toward the person or object. However, if you compare this definition carefully with that above, you will find they are essentially saying the same thing, but from different perspectives.

Norms and values also play an important part in the concept of attitude. The word 'predictable' in the definition adds something to this, i.e. that an attitude has a more or less fixed character. This does not mean that the attitude cannot be changed, but it does mean that change takes place slowly and often with difficulty.

Study activity
22. Describe the attitude of an ideal nurse.

The concept of attitude is considered in this section on socialization since there is a clear link between the two ideas. Attitude, according to its definition, is after all the aim of the socialization process.

It is important not to confuse the concepts of socialization and attitude with the concept of role. The concept of role will not be dealt with in detail until the next chapter, but has already been mentioned in the past few sections. A brief characterization of the three concepts is there-fore provided below:
- socialization refers to the process of learning behaviour, norms and values;
- attitude is a more or less stable disposition towards persons, objects or ideas - resulting from the socialization process;
- a social role indicates the position occupied by someone in a group. An attitude formed by means of a process of socialization naturally goes with such a position.

d.   Conditions of socialization
Study activity
23. Before reading the following section, con-sider what factors may, in your opinion, have an effect on socialization processes.

Socialization consists of learning processes. As in any learning process, this also means that not nearly everyone completes such a process at the same pace. Elkin (1960) has researched the factors affecting the socialization processes of children. These factors also apply in part to adults.

– *A stable social environment.*

This means, above all, a clearly defined environment. A situation in which various norms and values clash with one another may inhibit the process of socialization and sometimes even block it. This is self-evident in the case of bringing up children.

Case study: Sister Baxter and Dr Rolston

In the Medical Ward, there has been a conflict between Ward Sister Baxter and Consultant Physician Dr Rolston for some time now. The latter takes the view that he should only give patients brief and limited information about their complaints and the further course of events. The rest, he feels, is up to the nursing staff. Sister Baxter thinks that he should spend much more time on giving information and guidance. This because, in her experience, much of the information is not properly understood by the patients. If the nursing staff try to rectify the incorrect notions, the patients firmly refer to what 'the doctor' said. This difference of opinion between Baxter and Rolston has never been talked through properly and a workable solution has not, therefore, been achieved.

Imagine that you are a student nurse in a ward like that. What are you allowed, or not allowed, to tell patients? You cannot expect much help from the ward sister, as she refers you to the consultant. The same applies the other way round. It is a confusing situation, not least for a student. It will therefore be difficult to find the right attitude or, in other words, socialization will be a more laborious process.

– *The ability to develop relationships which have some some depth.*

It is easiest to imagine what is meant by this if you consider a relationship with a good friend. You know each other well and so there are many situations, even new ones, in which you realize quickly what is expected of you. Even if you do not agree, it is easier to make that plain than if you are faced with a total stranger.

People vary when it comes to the degree of 'intimacy' that they are willing to allow in a relationship. In the case of people with a psychopathic personality, which may result from a very insensitive upbringing, that capacity may even be partly or totally lacking. This constitutes a powerful obstacle to any further socialization process.

– *Biological heritage.*

This includes intelligence. If your intelligence helps you to understand more quickly what is expected of you, it also makes it easier to decide on your attitude.

Your biological heritage does not consist of your intelligence alone. Physical defects such as speech impediments that hinder contacts with other people, may prove an obstacle to the socialization process.

6.   Social observation

When you make your first appearance in the ward as a nurse, you gain a lot of new impressions. In spite of all the theoretical preparation and discussions, much will be new to you at this stage. Whereas various syndromes were largely paper symptoms or case histories during your lessons, you now suddenly find yourself facing people made of flesh and blood.

Since people display a whole range of conduct in addition to their pathological behaviour, those first few days may be highly confusing, and certainly tiring. From the very first day, however, a process of *habituation* also begins to take place. Habituation – you might also call it routine – ensures that work becomes easier. You are no longer taken by surprise quite so much by all the new impressions.

The concept of socialization as considered in the previous section, plays an important part in this process of habituation. In practice, you learn to adapt your behaviour, norms and values to the ward in which you are working. If you compare your lessons and practical experience, you will find that there is an important difference as far as socialization is concerned. During lessons, you are usually told how you should behave, and you even practise a certain kind of behaviour at times. In practice, however, all this occurs far less explicitly. Interaction, and therefore the socialization process, between you and any patient takes place far less obviously than during lessons. What you think and the way in which you behave depend largely on how you observe and interpret the situation, as for example in the following study activity.

Study activity
24. You arrive on the ward and someone is groaning in his sleep. What do you do?

The solution in this case depends wholly on your interpretation of the situation. In other words, you will not be able to decide what to do until you have some idea of what is causing the patient's behaviour.

There is a phone call to the ward to say that Mr Johnston is downstairs in the reception area. How you respond to this information depends on your interpretation.
It may well be that you will think, 'Mr Johnston quite often goes off to have a cigarette without telling us', or, 'They probably phoned so that we don't have to hunt for him if he is wanted.' It is also possible that you are alarmed because you know that Mr Johnston is sometimes confused. The call would then be regarded as a warning, and you would therefore take action as quickly as possible.

Both in the task and in the case of Mr Johnston, certain behaviour is attributed to a cause. We attribute behaviour to causes whenever we observe behaviour, not only other people's but also our own. If you are in a bad mood and someone enquires about the reason, you can usually provide an explanation such as not being given the day off that you had applied for, shortage of staff, a quarrel with a friend or spouse etc.

There is a reason for attributing behaviour to causes. If we did not do so, we would get lost in all our isolated observations. Working in a ward would always seem just the same as it was on the day when you first started there. Socialization as described in the previous paragraph would be

quite impossible; no routine of any kind would develop.
Attributing causes to behaviour is intended to provide a structure for our observations. Such an interpretation, or attribution of causes, does not occur in a vacuum. Your views depend largely on your frame of reference, which means on the sum total of the knowledge, experience, norms and values that form part of yourself.

As was stated previously, socialization would be impossible if we did not attribute causes to our observations. Conversely, it is also true that the socialization process plays a part in the interpretation of these and of any further fresh observations.

a. The attribution theory

The attribution theory is an important theory concerning the interpretation of behaviour; it may be defined as follows:

The *attribution theory* is concerned with the way in which people are inclined to attribute their own and other people's behaviour to underlying causes.

The theory was propounded by F. Heider (1958) and was further developed by H.H. Kelley (1967). The latter also made a distinction between two kinds of attribution.

Internal attributions. These occur when the cause of the observed behaviour is to be sought in the person displaying the behaviour. If a colleague is in a happy frame of mind and you attribute that to his or her cheerful nature, that is an internal attribution.

External attributions. These occur when the explanation of the observed behaviour is based on the situation. If you attribute that same happy frame of mind to passing an end-of-year examination, that will be an external attribution.

Study activity
25. Mrs Simpson is complaining about painful spots where she has had several injections. Think of an internal and an external attribution.

If it is argued that the cause may be attributed either to the person concerned or to the environment, it is important to check how the choice is made.

In the case of a patient such as Mrs Simpson you are unlikely, in practice, to seek an internal as well as an external attribution.

According to Kelley there are three criteria for you to apply when deciding whether an external or an internal attribution would be appropriate. They are:
- differentiation;
- consensus;
- consistency.

Case study: Mr Gallacher and Mr Brown
Mr Gallagher and Mr Brown are in the same ward as a result of perforated appendices. They also have the same consultant. One of them complains about the medical treatment whereas the other is perfectly satisfied with it.

Because of the difference in their conduct it is likely that their behaviour will be attributed to their characters. In this case *differentiation* means that an internal attribution is given to their behaviour. In another situation, differentiation might mean that an external attribution was made.

Imagine that one of the two gentlemen is to be transferred to another ward and treated by a different consultant. If his behaviour changes it is likely that, because of the difference, his behaviour is given an external attribution.

Whereas differentiation is concerned with differences, the concepts of consensus and consistency refer to similarities.

Consensus occurs when two or more people attribute certain behaviour to the same cause. As the result of the consensus or agreement, an internal or external attribution is, as it were, reinforced.

You might also take another look at the example of Mr Gallagher and Mr Brown. If you attribute Mr Gallagher's dissatisfaction to his character

and your colleagues do the same, this reinforces the internal attribution that you made.

Mr Gallagher's recovery is proceeding slowly but satisfactorily. His elder brother had an operation for bowel cancer some years ago and now has a colostomy bag. When Mr Gallagher experienced the first signs of his appendicitis, his greatest fear was that he was suffering from the same disease as his brother. Even when it became apparent that the pain was caused by a perforated appendix, he could not quite manage to dismiss his fears.

In fact, these fears were at the root of his uncertainty about his examination and treatment. Had this information been available to you earlier on, it would have had certain consequences for the underlying cause that you attributed to Mr Gallagher's behaviour. You might still have decided on an internal attribution such as, 'his behaviour is caused by his nervous disposition.' It might equally well have been an external attribution, i.e. his elder brother's illness.

Because of the consensus that had occurred among your colleagues, you might say that an internal attribution of this kind becomes the 'spectacles' through which you continue to observe this patient. There is not much the patient can do about the situation; he cannot change the way in which people regard him.

The *consistency* criterion plays a part similar to that of consensus.

Study activity
26. Mrs Duncan, a patient herself, is deeply concerned about a patient in the bed next to her. When you see her again after you have been away on sick-leave for a few days she also enquires about the state of your health. Think of an internal attribution for Mrs Duncan's behaviour.

There is a good chance of your associating Mrs Duncan with an internal attribution of social-mindedness or something similar. Her behaviour was the same in two instances, i.e. one concerning the health of a fellow patient, and the other concerning yours. This similarity in observation is what is meant when we are referring to the consistency criterion. Here again, an attribution is reinforced.

It was noted in respect of the concepts of both consistency and consensus that they reinforced attributions that had already been made. This has further consequences for future attributions. Remember the 'spectacles' that were referred to previously.

Once an internal attribution has been found for someone, it is likely that the attribution will again be an internal one in the case of some future behaviour. The same applies to external attributions.

As stated previously, we make attributions in order to provide a structure. In this way, we acquire a greater grasp of what we observe. There is some similarity between carrying out scientific research and the process that leads to making attributions. They are both concerned with cause-and-effect relationships. There are major differences as well, however. If, in the course of day-to-day dealings with people, a cause is found, we are unlikely to look any further and possible alternative explanations will be disregarded. As the case of Mr Gallagher shows, not all the required information is available to us. In the case of scientific research, more time is spent on finding important data. Another difference

with scientific research is that in formulating attributions there is usually not enough time to spend too long on seeking causes.

It is important to realize that nothing has yet been said about whether the attributed causes are correct. This is because the attribution theory tells us something about the way in which we interpret our observations, but not about their correctness.

For the purposes of the theory, that is of minor importance. It is quite possible that different people will interpret the same behaviour differently. There is a very remote chance of everyone arriving at the same attribution in the study task set out below.

Study activity

27. What is going on in Figure 3.1.6? Compare your attributions with those made by other people.

Making attributions has a lot to do with differences in frames of reference. An important consequence of this is that attributions do not merely tell us something about observed behaviour, but also about the person making the attribution.

As will be evident by now, differences in making attributions are by no means exceptional. They do not only differ, they may also be wrong. Errors and differences may occur more or less

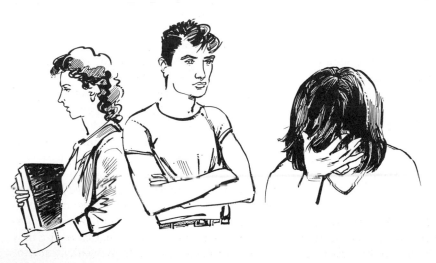

Figure 3.1.6
Attribution theory: we
can interpret behaviour
by our observations

accidentally, but they may also be based on a pattern. Two patterns of this kind form the subjects of the next subsection: the fundamental attribution error and the dissonance theory (also known as cognitive dissonance theory).

b.   The fundamental attribution error

Case study: Mr Waverley

Mr Waverley, aged forty-six, has been admitted to hospital because of a stomach ulcer. He is the managing director of a medium-sized printing works. Although he is in hospital, his mind is still occupied with his business for most of the time. He is afraid that everything will go wrong while he is not there. His bedside telephone helps him to keep in daily touch with developments. He even calls customers to discuss business matters. He does not actually want to do all this, but he simply does not dare to let go of the reins.

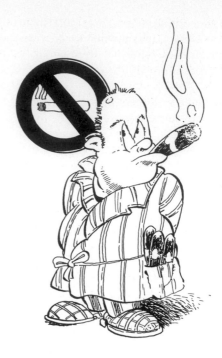

How is Mr Waverley likely to judge his own behaviour? The attribution theory, after all, is also about interpreting one's own behaviour. He will probably make an external attribution: his position at work which makes him indispensable.

How are the nursing staff likely to assess Mr Waverley's behaviour? It would be predictable for them to make an internal attribution, something in the nature of 'the workaholic'.

It is more or less predictable that the nurses will make an internal attribution and the patient himself an external one. This is because of what Ross (1977) has called the *fundamental attribution error*, which may be defined as follows:

If a person's behaviour is judged to be negative, there is a tendency for others to underestimate the external attributions and overestimate the internal ones. If a person's behaviour is regarded as positive, the reverse applies.

People are inclined to attribute their good deeds to themselves and their less favourable behaviour to the situation or to circumstances. Those observing the behaviour, the spectators, do precisely the opposite. People are often blamed personally for bad behaviour, whereas good behaviour is in many instances attributed partly to circumstances, e.g. 'He had an easy examination paper', or, 'She had plenty of time for it', etc.

c.   The dissonance theory

Why do you want to take up nursing? This is the question usually put to every applicant. Supposing your answer was that you liked working with people. Let us assume that this is the main reason for your wanting to become a nurse. In terms of the attribution theory you will therefore expect this internal attribution to provide the future explanation for your behaviour at work. Contact with other people, however, will rarely satisfy all your needs. Remember Maria Gibson in the surgical ward (Section 5b). There may be various reasons why your aspirations do not conform to the expectations other people may have of you.

In a situation like that, particularly if it continued for some time, you could obviously give up nursing and look for another job, hoping that it would come closer to satisfying your own aspirations. It is more likely, however, that you would go on nursing and find another attribution to fit your work behaviour. Examples of a new attribution might be: opportunities for promotion, a pleasant team, variety of duties, etc. These are examples in which the internal attribution is exchanged for external attributions. You might also choose a different internal attribution, for instance the need to complete something once you have started it.

Study activity
28. The need to contribute towards a patient's recovery process may be an important internal attribution for a nurse.
   To what extent can the same internal attribution be used for looking after a terminal patient? What other attributions might play a part in those circumstances?

The object of the study task and the exposition preceding it is to demonstrate that attributions may be changed to fit in with a situation. This is the most important process resulting from *cognitive dissonance* theory, a theory first propounded by Festinger (1957). Dissonance refers to matters which do not agree with or correspond to one another. In music, for example, a discordant note is a dissonant.

The dissonance theory may also be defined as follows:
The dissonance theory describes the process of changing attributions in situations where the original attribution is no longer compatible with the displayed behaviour. The motto of dissonance theorists is that "inconsistency hurts". Where one attribution is faced by another opposing one, or indeed when we are faced by opposing attitudes, a state of tension is often the result. This unpleasant tension is known as 'dissonance'. In the case of Maria above, she felt she should be able to spend more time talking to patients, but the busy schedules and workstyles did not allow for this. She could have reduced her tension or dissonance by two means. Firstly, by adding *consonant* elements. She could have held on to her personal views and justified behaving differently as a result of the staff shortages. This rationalization would allow her to behave in a way 'consonant' or in keeping with nursing behaviour on the ward while still holding onto her ideals. Secondly, she could have *changed* her ideals and adopted the ideals and

behaviour of nurses on the surgical ward. You may feel that nurses relinquish their ideals in this way too often.

7. Summary

This chapter began with the social sciences of social psychology and sociology. Particular attention was devoted to the question of whether and to what extent subjects and theories from those disciplines are recognizable in health care.

Two basic concepts, relationship and interaction, were then considered. The various kinds of relationship were described and the amount of involvement within a relationship was considered in further depth. Interaction in this context means the mutual influence that always occurs within relationships.

The basic concepts of norms and values were also considered. In the case of norms we made a distinction between form and validity. In the case of values the distinction was between minor values and central values. To maintain norms and values in a community, a measure of control is required. This kind of social control operates sanctions when people depart from existing norms and values. Sanctions may be either positive or negative. In the former case, there are rewards of various kinds; in the case of negative sanctions, punishment occurs.

The concept of socialization was dealt with next. This is the process in which we learn to adapt to people, situations and circumstances. The socialization process leads to attitudes, which are more or less stable.

The theory concerned with the attribution of underlying causes to the behaviour of others, is attribution theory. Here we made a distinction between internal attributions, i.e. causes rooted in the individual, and external attributions, i.e. causes provided by the situation.

Finally, two theories about differences in attributions and changing attributions were considered; they are called the fundamental attribution error and dissonance theory.

2

People in their environment

1. Introduction

The previous chapter focused mainly on the concepts of relationship and interaction. In the present chapter, the concept of the group is considered in all its aspects. Throughout their entire lives people operate in groups, starting with the family then the playgroup, the school class, the group of friends at work and so on. You might also think of examples such as a class of college students, a group in which you learn to work together, to experiment, to communicate, etc.

Co-operation plays an important part in the nursing profession; you work alongside:
– other students in a class;
– other nurses in a ward;
– doctors, psychologists and social workers;
– radiographers, physiotherapists, etc.

It is therefore hardly surprising that a substantial chapter in this module is devoted to the group. It is important for professional work and, not least, for yourself.

The final part of this chapter deals with theory. The skills required for being able to work in a group are described in Module 5.

Learning outcomes

After studying this chapter the student should be able to:
– give a definition of the concept of a group and describe the concept of a social network;
– distinguish between various kinds of groups;
– indicate what functions a group may have;
– give a definition of the concept of group cohesion and state what the consequences of cohesion are for a group;
– give a definition of the concept of role and indicate how roles are learnt;
– describe the concepts of role conflict and role strain;
– give a definition of power and name several kinds of power;
– describe the concept of status;

- distinguish between an autocratic, a democratic, and a laissez-faire leader;
- identify some consequences for groups with various styles of leadership;
- define the concepts of task process and group process, and also indicate the connection between them;
- describe what is meant by a pluriform society and by the concept of culture;
- distinguish between various groups concerned with health care and give at least two examples of differences in aims between these groups.

2. The group

Case study: John and Linda

Night duty in the Medical Ward ended as usual with the night staff handing over the care of patients to the day staff. It had been John Chapman's and Linda Pearson's last night on duty that week. On such occasions, it had become something of a tradition for nurses to go and have a coffee with their colleagues at a nearby sandwich bar, and today proved no exception.

Linda left after about half an hour as she had been offered a lift home. John stayed on rather longer than usual because of a heated discussion with some of the others about changes in the procedure for swapping shifts.

After a while he, too, went home, travelling in a bus which, by this time, was usually crammed with schoolchildren.

As mentioned previously, there is constant interaction between people and their environment. Just as in the case of John and Linda, such relationships are sometimes brief and sometimes lengthy. Sometimes several people are involved, at other times there is only one other person.

The total number of more or less permanent contacts that people have constitutes their social network. Linda and John are part of each other's social network. Their colleagues on day and night duty form part of both their social networks.

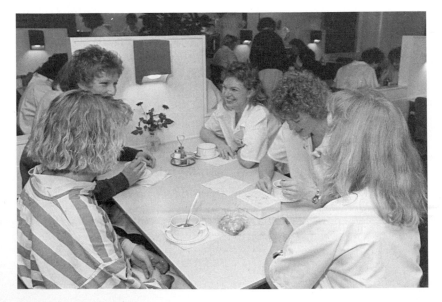

Figure 3.2.1
You form part of various groups

Diagram 3.2.1
Basic concepts for
distinguishing groups

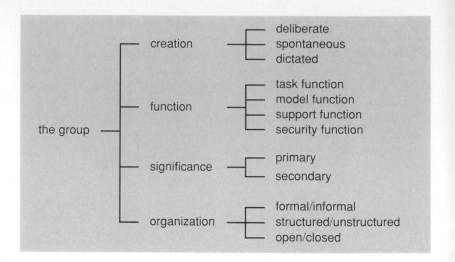

Many of our contacts with other people take place in groups. If, as appears from many definitions, two or more people form a group, all social contacts in fact take place in groups.

The example of John and Linda also makes it clear that the number of groups to which we belong at any particular time may be very large. The following groups occur in the example:
– John and Linda;
– the people on night duty combined with those on day duty;
– the group of people from the night shift who go out to have a coffee together;
– Linda and the person who is giving her a lift;
– John and the group of people with whom he is having a discussion;
– the people on the bus with John.

Study activity
1. Try to list as accurately as possible the groups of people with which you were in contact yesterday.

There has been a considerable amount of discussion among sociologists on the question of what precisely constitutes a group. People's involvement with one another is one of the important themes that has been considered. Not everyone is inclined to call arbitrary bus passengers a group, and how should one regard four people waiting to cross a road at a zebra crossing, or all dog owners?

The outcome of these discussions is that there are now many definitions for the term 'group'. This module is based on the broadest possible definition, the one given by L. Berkowitz (1975):

A *group* is a collection of people which can in some way be distinguished from its environment.

In the example of John and Linda, this definition was anticipated in the suggestion that even the two of them constituted a group. The passengers on John's bus were also called a group.

It is, however, usually accepted that the way such a collection of people is identified relates to their social interaction with each other. This is highlighted in Sprott's (1985) contention that a group is 'a plurality of persons who interact with each other in a given context *more* than they interact with anyone else'. This is very much in keeping with the classical definitive statement by Homans (1950) in his celebrated study of human groups. He suggested that:

'A group is defined by the interaction of its members. If we say that individuals A, B, C, D, E... form a group, this will mean that at least the following circumstances hold. Within a given period of time A interacts more with B, C, D, E... than he does with M, N, L, O, P... whom we choose to consider outsiders or members of other groups. B also interacts more often with A,

C. D, E... than he does with outsiders, and so on for the other members of the group. It is possible just by counting interactions to map out a group quantitatively distinct from others'.

The consequence of these definitions is that in the context of Berkowitz's definition you are a member of an infinite number of groups. The family into which you were born, your student class, your friends – they are all groups to which you belong. You also belong to the group made up of all British people, possibly to the group of people wearing spectacles, as well as to either the male or the female group. To be a member of a group it is therefore unnecessary to know the other members or even to have met them. However, in the sense suggested by Homans, you are in a *social* group only if you interact with other members in some way.

To recapitulate: you are a member of an almost innumerable number of groups which may differ from one another in various ways.

Study activity
  2. List as many differences as possible between the following two groups:
     – a class of students;
     – a group of patients chatting in a hospital reception area.

Because there are so many differences between groups, it is also possible to identify many different kinds of group. This chapter includes a selection of the possible criteria for a system of classification. Firstly, groups can be distinguished by the way in which they were created. The function of a group, its significance, the way in which it is organised are all potential bases for a system of classification. The creation of a group will be dealt with in the next subsection; the other three criteria will be considered in subsequent subsections. The various possibilities are set out in diagram 3.2.1.

a. The creation of a group

Groups may be created in various ways and for various reasons. They may be formed for business or emotional purposes but it is also possible that there are no apparent reasons for their existence.

Case study: Sally Simpson
Every day, a number of people seek one another's company in the dayroom of the surgical ward. The group is made up of a regular core of long-stay patients, but a varying number of others join them. The topics they like to talk about are television, their physical complaints, members of staff and any other matter that may crop up.

Figure 3.2.2
A group can be formed in all kinds of places

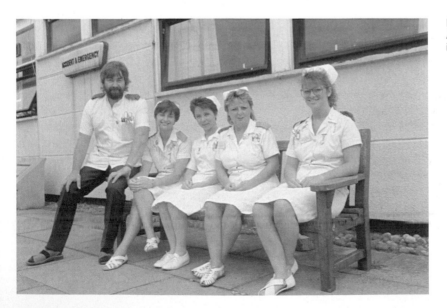

As a rule, it is all fairly light-hearted. One day, however, the mood was different. Two regular members of the group had been told off by Nurse Simpson in the morning. The reason was that they had taken themselves off to the hospital reception area without telling anyone. And, as if that were not enough, the same nurse had made some remark about one of the patients who had more than the two visitors allowed at any one time.

The dayroom group discussed both incidents grimly. They were particularly indignant about the way in which they, as adults, had been treated by a mere whippersnapper. During the discussion, people's irritation was directed increasingly at Nurse Simpson, particularly after other patients had also mentioned some minor incidents. The patients finally decided that a complaint should be made to the ward sister. One of them became the spokesperson and three of the others went along with him. They also decided to put the complaints in writing and to make an appointment to see the ward sister next day.

Study activity

3. Give at least five examples of groups that were created spontaneously.

The creation of a group is sometimes directly related to its function. At other times the function seems entirely separate. In the example, the function of the group of patients was primarily to enjoy one another's company and, perhaps, to some extent to support one another. The group was created spontaneously. People simply met in the dayroom, apparently without anyone actually organizing anything.

As a result of the various annoyances, the structure of the group changed. A small group was selected from the larger one to go and voice their complaints to the ward sister. This little group was created deliberately.

Diagram 3.2.1 shows three ways in which a group may be created:
- deliberately;
- spontaneously;
- dictated.

Groups are usually created deliberately because people either think or hope that they will achieve more jointly than they would as individuals. A group of nurses working in a ward is therefore a deliberately created group.

Study activity

4. Give at least five examples of groups that have been created deliberately.

As we saw in the example, groups can also be created spontaneously. Consider your circle of friends and acquaintances. Most friendships are created spontaneously, but it need not be so. A group of people who make up a team in a sports

Figure 3.2.3
A spontaneously
formed group

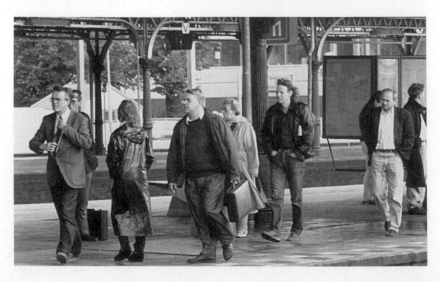

club and eventually become friends is a group which has been created deliberately. The group of patients in the surgical ward and the circle of friends make something else clear as well, i.e. that the reason for their creation may change over time. A group that was created spontaneously in the first instance, may be continued deliberately, or in a different form. The opposite may occur as well: the deliberately formed sports team may develop spontaneously into a group of friends. Usually this occurs as a result of a change in the group's function. This will be considered in further detail in the next subsection.

A number of people may also be viewed as a group, irrespective of whether or not they wish to be regarded as such. In that kind of situation groups of people are dictated. When you talk about 'the patients', you are indicating a group without considering whether people do or do not wish to belong to that group. There are three grounds upon which the creation of a group is usually dictated:
– external characteristics e.g. race, colour of hair, etc.);
– income (poor or rich);
– language and geography (Northerners, foreigners, etc.).

There is something forced about groups that have been dictated. Their members do not opt for membership. It may even be that members feel that they have had membership foisted upon them.
A clear example is that of a group of ex-psychiatric patients. If other people consider that one belongs to that kind of group, one may run the risk of being avoided or taken less seriously in daily life. Another example, and perhaps the most common dictated group, is the family.

Study activity
5. Give at least five examples of groups that have been dictated.

The family
Having and maintaining social contacts is one of humanity's basic needs. Besides being a need in itself, it also has a supportive function as a result of which problems in other areas may be neutralized. For example, you may be better able to put up with problems at work if you can rely on people with whom you have a good relationship.

Many, though not all, important relationships are created within the family. That is the reason for taking a closer look at the family and its development.

Sociologically, the *family* is an important group. This is where the norms and values that you will need if you are to survive in society, are first instilled in you. Other sociological concepts also play a part within the family, for instance role behaviour, power, primary socialization, etc.

The family has undergone a considerable amount of change in the course of time. Tasks that were once part of the family's responsibilities are no longer regarded as such, and others have completely changed their character.
A number of tasks are listed below. In the days of our ancestors, they were family tasks.
– The production of:
  • capital goods (buildings, tools)
  • consumer goods (food, clothing);
– the consumption of the produced goods;
– the partners' sexual relationship;
– procreation;
– the care of young children;
– the care of the sick;
– the care of the elderly;
– socialization (young children and youngsters);
– self-defence;
– entertainment or recreation.

If you compare this package of family tasks from the past with the functions performed by the family today, you will see that much has changed.

There were many functional changes, especially during the Industrial Revolution. To further economic interests to the greatest possible extent, it was essential to increase productivity. This meant that workers had

Figure 3.2.4
Involvement in the
family group

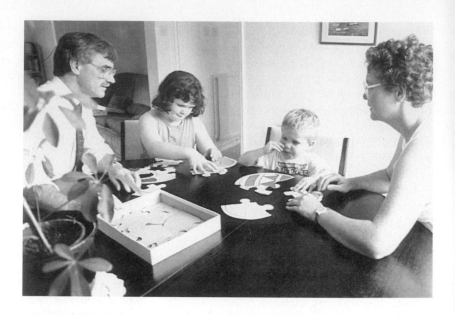

to produce as much as possible. Some tasks were therefore transferred to larger units such as factories, government bodies and institutions.

Self-defence is one of the family tasks that has disappeared. The care of the elderly and, to a large extent, the care of the sick is no longer a primary task for the family although many elderly and sick people – especially children – are still cared for by their families.

It is important to realize that, because of the economic and social changes in the 19th century, independent professions were created which previously did not exist at all, or not to the same extent. The nursing profession provides a good example. You may therefore argue that the Industrial Revolution cleared the way socially for the creation of the nursing profession.

Although some of its functions have disappeared, the present-day family has also retained a number of tasks. Their character, however, has often changed. One of the major differences with the past is the fact that today there is often no need for any particular task to be carried out *within* the family. People can choose to what extent other people are to be called upon to help

with, or take over, certain tasks. The tasks which are normally retained by the family appear to be concerned primarily with the interaction between members of the family. It is therefore said sometimes that the nature of a family has changed from a 'production family' to an 'emotional family'. In former days, production was a vital task, whereas members of a modern family are more emotionally involved with one another. Family is an important sociological concept and will be returned to again in Chapter 4.

b.　The functions of a group

Case study: Nancy Cook

A group of nursing students in a college's introductory course had just taken their first intermediate examination. People had been working very hard and, as usual, some of them had been obliged to put in far more effort than others. Some of them had joined forces before the examination in an attempt to prepare for it together.

When it was all over, someone suggested that they should all go out for a meal. After various discussions about who was to be invited, it was decided that friends were not to be included. Nancy Cook constituted a special problem. She had given up her training just before the examination, as she obviously could not manage to keep up. She was still in touch with a number of her former classmates, however, and they felt that in some way she still formed part of the group.

In this class, apparently, there is a need for more than just the performance of a task. That is not exceptional for a group. People are together because they are being taught together, but they also support one another if they have to prepare for the examination outside the organized lessons. Apart from work, there is also a need to enjoy themselves together.

Several functions were mentioned in diagram 3.2.1, i.e.:
– task function   – task aspect
– model function   }
– support function   } – bonding aspect
– security function   }

The first function, the task function, is also referred to as the task aspect. The three other functions combined are called the bonding aspect.

Most groups have more than one function. That was evident in the example of the nursing students above. Not infrequently, however, one

of the functions is the principal one. In many groups, that is the task function. That means that the group was formed primarily for a specific purpose. Such purposes can vary widely. A hospital unit, a police unit, a political party and a class of students primarily have a task function.

Another of the group's functions is to provide its members with models: the model function. The most obvious example is the family. Parents serve as models for their children. Ideally, they show children how to behave as adults and how to solve various problems. The model function, however, does not only occur in families. Individuals or groups who are trendsetters can also serve as models for other people's behaviour. Designer fashions and trendy lifestyles provide examples of this. To some extent, your tutors and supervisors may be regarded as officially appointed models.

Study activity
6. Consider whether there are any classmates on whose behaviour, in some area or other, you would like to model yours. Try to identify your reasons for this.

In the example of the introductory course students above, several people were studying

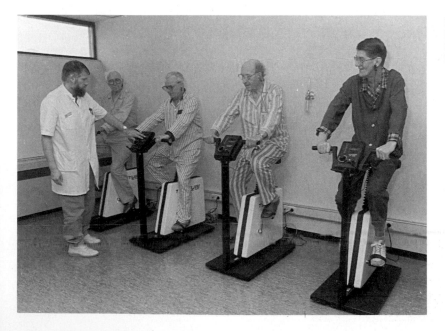

Figure 3.2.5
Example and support
for a group of patients
in rehabilitation

for the test together. It is likely that this was done partly to help maintain a certain amount of rhythm in their learning pattern. They were supporting one another in their studies. This is what is meant by the support function that a group may have. The support may relate to the task that needs to be performed, but it may also refer to other matters of concern for the individual or the group. The support function is sometimes a group's principal function; think of the various groups of women with experience of incest, or of meetings held by fugitives from a particular country.

The security function is a group function immediately connected with the above. Support, after all, is easier to accept if you feel safe or secure, especially if emotional matters are concerned.
If a group has a strong security function, it gives you the feeling that you can fall back on the group if problems arise.

This function is to some extent apparent in the discussions about Nancy Cook in the example. A group offering security does not, after all, immediately let go of someone who is falling by the wayside. Some people felt that Nancy was still part of the group although she was no longer involved in the task function. An evening out would provide a good opportunity for giving her a sense of security.

In this subsection, a positive view has been taken of the possible functions of a group. Naturally, not every member of the group may have this kind of experience. If, for instance, you are not accepted in a class for some reason or other, you will feel inhibited rather than supported. During adolescence, for example, not everyone is likely to have felt happy about being a member of his or her own particular family.

c.   The significance of a group

Groups may have different functions, and also a different *significance*. The two concepts seem closely connected. The concept of function refers to the group's benefit to you, whereas its significance is concerned with emotional involvement.

Study activity

7. Consider the remark, 'You are working badly', and compare the significance or value that you would attach to it if it were said by:
   - your parents;
   - a brother or sister;
   - a tutor;
   - a supervisor;
   - a sister;
   - a consultant;
   - someone visiting a patient.

It is likely that you will attribute a different emotional significance to each of the above situations. The remark would probably affect you more on some occasions than on others. This, of course, also applies to comments of a positive nature. You do not always attach the same value to compliments made by different people. Such differences are partly concerned with the distinction between *primary* and *secondary* groups, (see diagram 3.2.1.). The concepts may be defined in the following way:
- a *primary* group is a small group whose members know one another very well, are closely associated with one another, and strongly influence one another;
- a *secondary* group is any group not having close or primary ties, but with some goals and functions in common.

The terms primary group and secondary group represent extremes, which means that it is impossible to draw a distinct line between them. Examples of primary groups include the family into which you were born and the group of friends with whom you associate a great deal. A group of people queueing at a supermarket checkout, soldiers in an army regiment and members of a church congregation are clear examples of secondary groups.

What, however, should one say about your class, or the ward where you are working? Whether you regard those as primary or secondary groups will depend on a number of factors concerning your closeness or involvement with group members. To check up on these, you should turn back to Chapter 1, Section 3b, in this module.

Study activity

8. Give three examples each of primary and secondary groups to which you belong.

d. The organization of a group

In the previous sections, we considered the creation, the function, and the significance of a group. Like the *organization* of the group, those features relate primarily to the differences between groups. Organization, in this context, should be regarded as a broad concept. It does not merely concern organization within the group, but also organization in relation to the environment. The definitions of the various concepts will make this clear.

In diagram 3.2.1, the following distinctions were made:
- formal/informal;
- structured/unstructured;
- open/closed.

As you see, there are three sets of opposite concepts, representing the extreme forms that may characterize a group. It is important to realize that many groups are located somewhere in between those extremes. A group may be more or less formal, more or less structured and more or less open.

Just as in the case of the various potential functions of a group, the above concepts do not rule out one another. Something can be said about the formality, the structure and the openness of any group.

Case study: Dr Alder

The medical staff of a hospital has regular monthly meetings with management. Those attending include all consultants and, true to custom, other specialists such as the clinical psychologist, the pharmacist and the microbiologist. The medical staff is a recognized group at the hospital and has a number of fixed duties and responsibilities. The group's committee therefore has regular meetings with management.

On this occasion, and not for the first time, one of the items on the agenda is the provision of 24 additional beds for the hospital. Several special-

ists have previously let it be known that they could do with the extra space. The need for extra beds, however, exceeds the number to be provided. There have frequently been heated discussions, in which many different arguments were produced. Although the ultimate decision rests with the management, the recommendations of the medical staff are crucial.

The specialists Dr. Alder and Dr. Kirk are among the interested parties. Along with some others, they have therefore drawn up a proposal on how to allocate the beds. They had met in secrecy the week before the present meeting. The idea is that Dr Alder will put forward the scheme on behalf of the consultants and that the other doctors will agree. The divisions among the other members, and perhaps to some extent the element of surprise, will give the scheme a good chance of success.

Study activity

9. Think of an example of an attempt in a class of student nurses to influence a decision in a similar manner.

Two groups are mentioned in the above example, i.e. the multi-disciplinary group in its entirety and a group of specialists who have joined forces for a specific purpose. In organizational terms, the former is a formal group and the latter an informal one. The following definitions will make this clear.

A *formal group* is deliberately founded. It is usually recognizable to everyone as a group and arrangements are frequently made about the relationships between its members.

An *informal group* is usually created spontaneously and is not always recognizable as a group to other people. Frequently there are no clear arrangements about interrelationships or keeping the group intact.

In the example, the medical staff constitutes a formal group such as exists in every hospital. The medical staff has a set of rules in which mutual relations and relations *vis-a-vis* the hospital, as well as rights and responsibilities are laid down. All members of staff in a company may also be regarded as a formal group, since their rights, duties, etc. are laid down in a collective agreement or individual contracts of employment.

Finally, a class of students may also be seen as a formal group. It is quite clear who does or does not belong to the class, and each member is aware of his rights and duties. Mutual relations are also clear; the rights and duties apply to all students, so that there are no differences between them.

Study activity
10. Explain why, in the light of the case of the medical staff, an informal group may be important.

As indicated above, an informal group is a group that was not formed officially. In the example, that applied to a number of specialists led by Dr Alder and Dr Kirk. That kind of group does not have any official rules and, in this particular instance, there was merely a limited agreement on who was to be the spokesperson. A group of friends enjoying an evening out is another example of an informal group.

It often happens that informal groups exist within formal ones. Consider your own class. In addition to the class as a formal group , there are probably a few people who go around together more than they do with others. That kind of a sub-group is an example of an informal group. If you think about who actually belongs to it, it may happen that you are in doubt about several people. In the case of an informal group, that kind of thing is not always quite clear.

Another way in which you can look at a group is concerned with its structure. In a *structured group*, there are clear differences between the members' roles. People know who does what, and tasks are allocated to specific members. In an *unstructured group* it does not matter who does what as long as the job is done.

A hospital ward provides a clear example of a structured group. Each individual has a fixed 'role' as a nurse, a doctor, a patient, a sister, etc. Certain duties go with each role or position, and as a rule everyone knows what they are.

The terms formal/informal and structured/unstructured may appear somewhat confusing so it may therefore be useful to set out the concepts once again.

The characteristic quality of a structured group is the agreement and clear understanding among

Figure 3.2.6
A closed group

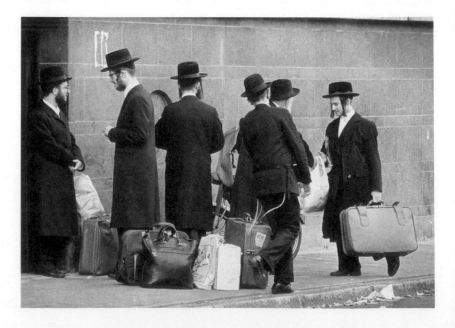

the members regarding the various roles or positions within the group. In the unstructured group there is no such clear definition.

The terms formal and informal refer to the way in which the group was *created*. The formal group was formed deliberately, the informal spontaneously.

Study activity
11. Give five examples of structured groups and mention a few functions that can be identified within them.

The terms open and closed are used to indicate the third aspect of organization referred to in this chapter. Again, it is a matter of extremes. An *open group* is a group which people are free to join or leave at will. A *closed group* is a group which does not admit any new members and which existing members cannot simply leave.

In the case of an open group, you might think in terms of shoppers in a department store on a particular day. People walk in and out of the store and all you need do to be admitted to this group is to go in at the door. When you leave the store you leave the group .

Membership of an exclusive golf-club is one example of a closed group. Often specific social and other conditions for joining must be met, an individual has to be proposed for membership and acceptance may be dependent on the outcome of a secret vote. A secret society is another example of a closed group, especially if resigning from it is prohibited on pain of death (e.g. the Mafia). As suggested earlier, the two concepts are extremes and most groups fit in somewhere between the two.

Case study: Mrs Groves
Mrs Groves, aged fifty-two, had been having trouble with her right knee for some time. Neither her visits to her GP and a physiotherapist nor various medicines had brought her any relief. On her own insistence, she was finally referred to the clinic run by Mr Brown, an orthopaedic surgeon. He examined her on several occasions and again tried to cure the trouble with medi-

cines. After some time had elapsed and several consultations had taken place, it was finally decided to admit Mrs Groves to hospital for an exploratory operation. A slight irregularity, which may have caused the trouble, was found and removed.

Both Mrs Groves and Mr Brown were satisfied with the way in which her recovery was proceeding. It looked as though the trouble had been remedied. A minor problem, however, arose at the end of her stay in hospital. Mrs Groves' eldest daughter was about to celebrate her silver wedding and Mrs Groves was very anxious to be at the party. Mr Brown, however, would have preferred her to remain in hospital for a few more days, but after further discussions and armed with all kinds of instructions Mrs Groves finally went home in time for the party.

Study activity
12. Consider co-operation between nurses in a hospital ward in terms of:
   – open/closed groups;
   – formal/informal groups.
   List some examples and discuss these with your fellow-students.

Before Mrs Groves joined the in-patients group, certain obstacles had to be overcome. Patients cannot simply walk into a hospital and be admitted when they feel like it. There are also certain conditions attached to leaving the group, in this case the hospital. In spite of all these conditions for being admitted to and leaving the group, there is no question here of a strictly closed group. New patients may join it and others are discharged; sometimes they even go against medical advice and discharge themselves.

Proposition:
A group of students is an example of a group which is partly open and partly closed.

Study activity
13. Discuss the above proposition with your fellow-students.

It was suggested at the beginning of this subsection that the terms formal/informal, structured/unstructured and open/closed were not mutually exclusive. In the case of a formal group, you might, for instance, be able to say something about its structure and the extent to which the group was open or closed.

A group of people waiting at a bus stop may be an example of an informal group, an unstructured group, and, at the same time, an open group.

Study activity

14. Describe the following groups in terms of the three aspects dealt with above:
  - a group of people in a waiting-room for out-patients;
  - a hospital's accounts department;
  - a group of patients sharing a ward;
  - members of a staff association.

e. Group dynamics and group cohesion

Case study: Mr Lamont

All the beds in Surgical Ward 15 have been occupied for a whole week, with three new patients being admitted within the space of 36 hours. The other beds have been occupied for a longer period and Mr Lamont has been in hospital longer than anyone else. People cautiously began to get to know each other. By way of topics such as occupations, the hospital, cars, politics, and, of course, ailments, they became increasingly well acquainted.

At first, Mr Lamont acted as a kind of mentor to the group, but that became less apparent after a day or two. People were on good terms on the whole, but Mr Birch was rather more reserved and kept himself somewhat apart from the group.

Then Mr Lamont had a mild myocardial infarction one night. The ensuing flurry of activity and Mr Lamont's removal to Intensive Care made a great impression on everyone. People were clearly tense and made sure that the nurses kept them informed about Mr Lamont's condition. Mr Birch was upset as well and shared the other patients' tension.

The above case study illustrates an important feature of groups, i.e. a group has dynamic rather than static qualities. In almost every group changes are happening, the group is evolving in its own way. In the above example although the members of the group remained almost the same, interaction within the group changed; there was a measure of development. The group ceased to be static and became dynamic.

That is the essence of the concept of group dynamics: *group dynamics* refers to the changes occurring within a group during its existence.

It is usual to distinguish phases in *group development*. In the above example, you might distinguish a phase of becoming acquainted and a phase of increasing involvement on the part of the members. A possible classification would be:
  - an introductory or initial phase;
  - a phase in which involvement within the group increases;
  - a phase in which the group presents itself more as a unit in its dealings with others;
  - a run-down or final phase.

Many groups are likely to experience the above phases, although the speed at which they occur may vary considerably. Events such as Mr Lamont's myocardial infarction may affect that. In a family, for example, people go through the first three phases quite quickly, whereas the final phase does not begin until the members begin to die.

Many groups pass through all four phases but occasionally one of them is skipped. A group that has been created for business reasons only is unlikely to spend much time, if any, in the increased involvement phase.

It is also important to note that there is not always a clear demarcation line between the various phases; it is possible for them to overlap.

That happens, for instance, when some far-reaching event occurs while the group is in the phase of presenting itself more as a unit. Involvement within the group will then increase and the second phase becomes important again.

Study activity

15. Try to evaluate your class in the light of the above phases. Mention any events affecting the various phases.

Not all groups will have the same degree of involvement. There is unlikely to be much involvement in the case of a random group of people talking in a hospital reception area. At the other extreme, however, there is a time just before a final examination when a class of students is likely to reach a measure of involvement which extends far beyond that of many other groups. That kind of involvement has a lot to do with the next concept to be considered, i.e. group cohesion.

The literal meaning of cohesion is 'sticking together', and that is perhaps the determining factor in the development of a group. The concept may be defined as follows:

– *Group cohesion*, sometimes called the 'us-feeling', refers to the extent to which the members of a group wish to retain their membership.

Involvement and the concept of group cohesion have a lot in common, as has been mentioned already, but they are not the same. Besides involvement, there are some other factors which affect cohesion, i.e.:

– the phase in which the group finds itself;
– the situation in which the group finds itself;
– members' personal attractiveness to one another;
– the regular achievement of group aims;
– the amount of tolerance for deviant opinions;
– the differences in power and status among the members of the group;
– the effort required to become a member of the group.

Depending on the above factors, a group may have a high or a low cohesion. A group with a high cohesion is usually characterized by an atmosphere of mutual trust and high degree of motivation among its members. Members of a group with a high degree of cohesion will always try to avoid harming other members.

In groups with a low cohesion, members usually take a casual view of their membership; motivation and the atmosphere among themselves are consequently less important themes.

Many groups will be situated in the area between a high and a low cohesion. This will depend partly on the phase in which the group finds itself, but will also be due in part to the extent to which members are trying to achieve greater group cohesion.

One of the reasons why the concept of group cohesion is so important is that it has certain consequences for the process of co-operation.

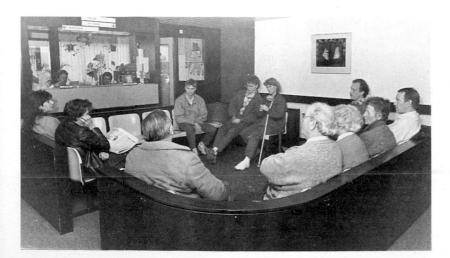

Figure 3.2.7
A group with low cohesion

Diagram 3.2.2
Sociogram: the
involvement of
individuals in a group,
with the sub-groups
circled

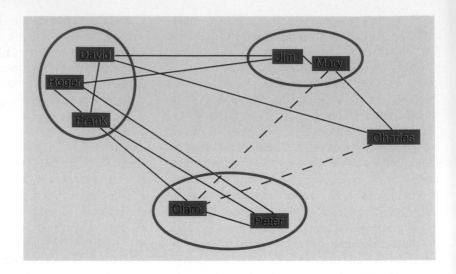

Motivation, mutual trust and comradeship are not only characteristics of cohesion, but the same factors affect the quality of whatever aims the group may have. A hospital ward or department with reasonably high group cohesion is likely to function better and more pleasantly than one with low group cohesion.

The various factors determining a group's cohesion can also be represented graphically, e.g. by means of a sociogram. A *sociogram* is a diagram showing the interactions or interrelationships between members of a group. It is a device used in sociometry, an approach devised by Jacob L Moreno (1953) for mapping the relationships of attraction and rejection among members of a group. The approach can be used to identify the most frequently interacted-with individual (the star), the least frequently interacted-with individual (the group isolate) and others in between. It can thus be very useful in identifying individuals who are frequently sought out by their fellow members and are important role models or '*relevant others*'. Interactions or interrelationships can be mapped out by external observers or by asking individual members to indicate these by making choices for or against other members of the group. One of the ways in which you can use a sociogram is to indicate the involvement of individual members in relation to one another by placing them at various distances from one another. An example is provided in diagram 3.2.2. A sociogram may represent various factors such as involvement, appeal, co-operation, etc.

Study activity

16. Draw a sociogram of your class. Its theme is: the ideal nurse, which is shown as a dot in the centre of the page. Now show the distance, from 1 to 10 cm, of each member of the class from this point.

A sociogram usually represents personal points of view. Your opinion of the class is likely to differ to some extent from the views of its other members, who, in turn, differ from one another. It would, of course, also be possible to produce a joint sociogram.

3. The role of the individual in the group

Case study: Ken Dalton

The staff association had been doing badly for several years. A poor turn-out at several events had considerably reduced any eagerness to put much effort into it in recent years.

This had been a source of annoyance to Ken Dalton for some time. He had been working in the hospital's maintenance department for a year and had been an active member of a flourishing staff association in his previous job.

When Ken was invited on to the committee of the present association, he decided to give it a new lease of life. This was made easier because he was elected chairman before long. Karin Vernon, a dietician, proved to be a good ally.

She, too, had wanted to liven up the association but had not had much support until Ken arrived on the scene.

One of Ken's first acts as chairman was to re-allocate various responsibilities. Karin was made treasurer and Joe Beck became secretary. Along with the rest of the committee, they drew up a list of activities to be organized that year. The work involved in organizing them was also shared out.

The previous section was concerned with the group, and the fact that a group may have a structure. That applies to the group in the above example: after Ken Dalton's arrival various tasks were shared out among the members of the group. The tasks or roles that a person may perform are the subject of this section.

A *social role* is what people expect from themselves or others in terms of behaviour and attitudes, on the basis of their respective positions in the group.

It is important not to confuse this concept with those of socialization and attitude referred to in Chapter 1. They are repeated here for clarity's sake:

Figure 3.2.8
The roles of patient
and nurse

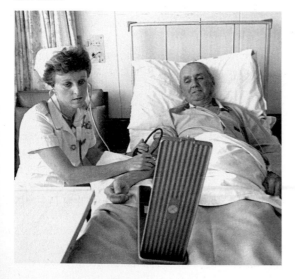

– socialization refers to the process of learning behaviour, norms and values;
– an attitude is a more or less stable disposition towards persons, objects or ideas - resulting from a socialization process;
– a social role refers to the position occupied by someone in a group.

In the example, Ken Dalton has the role of chairman, but another of his roles is that of encouraging everybody else. Two conclusions may be drawn from this. Firstly, that people perform several roles at a time, in this case the role of chairman, the role of a stimulator, the role of a male. Other groups provide other roles. Secondly, there are formal roles and informal roles. We encountered the two concepts when considering formal groups and informal groups. A formal role goes with a formal position or status, i.e. a person has been appointed to perform that role. At least, the role has been recognized officially. Ken's chairmanship, but also his job in the maintenance department, are formal roles. The fact that he stimulates the others, acts as a pace-setter, is an example of an informal role.

The roles that one plays come from many sources, e.g. occupation, gender, character, status, abode, etc. These starting-points will be considered in further detail in the next subsection. The role of a patient, an important one in this particular book, will be dealt with in the section on interaction theory in the next chapter.

Study activity
17. **a.** Give at least ten examples of your social roles.
    b. Give five examples of your various roles as a nurse.

a. Learning roles

A social role requires certain behaviour. Conversely, *role behaviour* makes it plain what role one is playing. The behaviour that goes with such a role is acquired; it is learnt through the socialization process.
Generally speaking, few people will have difficulty in accepting the statement that role behav-

iour is acquired behaviour. Not infrequently, however, this is forgotten. Take, for example, the role behaviour that goes with a man or a woman. This, too, is acquired, and not inborn, as some people think.

If a role is acquired, this means that the role behaviour may also change. As a nurse, you may teach yourself to behave differently to patients in future. Your role as a child in a family is another good example of changing role behaviour. As you grow up, different demands are made on you and your conduct as a child depends on your age.

Study activity
18. Select one example of a role you have acquired. Describe how this role developed and changed over time.

The terms conformity and identification were mentioned previously in the context of socialization (see page 205). These concepts also play an important part in role-learning.

When you start working in a ward as a student nurse, things are often quite different from what you had expected. The ward sister, fellow nurses and patients may also have expectations of you which differ slightly from your own. Since you are in a somewhat powerless and dependent position while you are still a student, you will often decide to behave in the way that the others would like. You will then be conforming to the role as other people see it, even though your own ideas may well be better. There is something slightly bogus about conforming: you act the part but without total conviction. *Conformity* is an important aspect of role behaviour: the way you behave and thereby reveal the role is one of the important criteria on which people base their assessment of you. Conformity also explains why people sometimes display extremely different behaviour in different roles. Take the paternal and understanding politician who turns out to be a domestic tyrant! Or, to give a more everyday example, many people have experienced a strict teacher, or a dour headmaster, who turns out to be pleasant company out of school hours.

It is important to be aware that conformity is not something that is contemptible or wrong. Behaviour, as expected in a particular role, has a further function in that it clarifies what people can and cannot expect from one another. A certain kind of role behaviour is expected of a nurse, irrespective of his or her personality. Extreme differences in role behaviour may cause confusion. Patients, too, will largely conform to their role as patients. If they do not, their recovery may even be affected.

Case study: Martin Croft
Martin Croft had always wanted to be a doctor. His father and grandfather had been members of the medical profession. Martin's idea of a doctor's role had therefore been formed during childhood. He had especially admired his dignified and rather stern grandfather. For years he had wanted to be a doctor like his grandfather, and although the image had faded to some extent, it continued to influence him.

You can hardly regard the above tale as an example of conformity. You would expect that the role of doctor had become part of Martin himself and that, as we have seen, is a matter of *identification*. In the case of identification, you acquire certain behavioural characteristics that go with a particular role. To put it rather more formally, this means that identification is the process leading to *internalization*; it becomes part of yourself. The acquisition of such characteristics is influenced by important people in your environment or by significant or relevant others.

In Martin's case, they were mainly his father and grandfather, but you might also think in terms of an uncle or aunt, an important secular or religious leader, your neighbour, etc.

The concept of 'significant other' requires further explanation. A *significant other* is a person with whom the individual has interacted frequently and has a close emotional relationship. The attitudes, behaviour and roles of this very important (to the individual) person are thus crucial to socialization. George Herbert Mead (1934) introduced this term to describe these early socialization influences. However, he suggested that as socialization proceeds the young person relates not only to 'significant others' but to the *generalized other* i.e. society or the social group at large. So important are the influences of other individuals and the social group at large in forming our behaviour and – ultimately – roles, that Mead introduced the now-famous term *taking the role of the other* to describe this interaction process. In essence, this means that we behave in line with how we *think* others expect us to behave. We take our role from the perceived expectations of others – especially those *significant others* who are highly important to us.

Significant others might also include well-known pop singers or film stars. Their clothes and behaviour are copied by many people, not because they are conforming, but because they themselves have begun to think that it is attractive or smart to dress and behave in the same way. It has thus become part of themselves i.e. they closely *identify* with and eventually *internalise* the ways of thinking and behaving. However, as the individual gets older, it is increasingly the social group as a whole – the "generalised other" which has a major influence on role formation.

Stereotypes sometimes assume the form of caricatures. In that case certain behavioural characteristics that go with a role tend to be presented in exaggerated and ridiculing terms , e.g. civil servants are idle, mothers are always kind, etc.

Study activity

19. **a.** Describe the role of an ideal nurse. Consider to what extent you measure up to that in reality.

b. What behavioural characteristics do you adopt in this role without their being part of yourself (conformity)? What behavioural characteristics are part of yourself (identification and internalization)?

As mentioned previously, roles also have a function relating to the clarity of co-operation. People know where they stand, so that they do not need to query all kinds of matters in their dealings with one another. In this way, roles also contribute to the attribution process (see Chapter 1, Section 6a). We have pointed out how we learn roles which are based on our impressions and assessments of other people. In addition to this there are several general factors on which roles are frequently based, i.e.:

– biological conditions, e.g. gender and age.
– social factors such as occupations or economic positions;
– political wishes; a good example is the preferential treatment which may be afforded to women these days when they apply for certain posts.

b. Role characteristics

The title of this subsection does not refer to the various kinds of behaviour that go with a particular role. It concerns statements about gen-

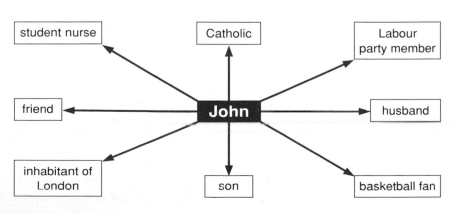

Diagram 3.2.3
Diagram of a limited number of John's roles

eral characteristics, which can be made because of the fact that roles exist.

– Everyone always has more than one role. You may be a daughter and a wife as well as a nurse. In Study activity 18, you probably managed to mention a number of your current roles. Diagram 3.2.3 provides an example of someone's various roles. A role is not therefore the sum total of a personality or individual. We in fact have *multiple roles* and some people simultaneously hold a large number which they act out, usually at different times.

Having more than one role does not usually present any problems, but there are exceptions. The role problems that you may encounter will be considered in the next subsection.

– Roles are usually *complementary*, which means that they complete one another. You might say that the role of student cannot exist without the role of teacher, and vice versa.

In addition, how a role is played out at any particular time depends on which one of these 'complementary' roles the individual is interacting with. The various roles a nurse interacts with may include those of doctor, patient, physiotherapist, relative, nursing colleague, ward sister and hospital chaplain. These are the nurse's *role set* i.e. the complementary roles with whom she interacts. She interacts *as a nurse* with all, but varies her behaviour according to which one she is interacting with. The role set (i.e. those with whom one interacts in one particular role) must not be confused with multiple roles (i.e. the various *different* roles one may occupy).

The role of nurse could not exist without the role of patient. The same applies to the role of doctor. To be admitted to hospital as a patient, you need the doctor's consent. (The issue here is not being ill, but assuming the role of patient.) It is also true that patients can be admitted by the doctor only if there are enough nurses.

Study activity
20. a. Take five roles and indicate the comp-

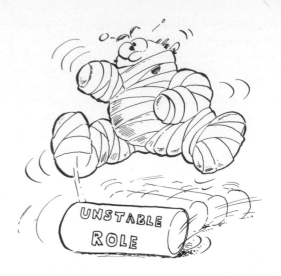

lementary roles (i.e. role sets) that go with them.
b. Repeat the task in a., but now with special reference to the situation in your professional environment.

– A role is often more *stable* than the individual. An example of this might might be a patient faced with a different nurse, one who is unknown to him. He will expect the new nurse's role behaviour to correspond to what he has seen in the case of other nurses. The function of roles in providing clarity in the area of co-operation or contact has been referred to already. From that point of view, the reasonable stability in respect of roles and role behaviour should not cause surprise. Another, related, conclusion is also possible: to someone who only knows you superficially, slight changes in your behaviour will be hardly noticeable.

– Some kinds of behaviour are considered normal in one social role, but odd or abnormal in another. *Role behaviour*, after all, is bound up with a particular role. Take the sergeant in an army unit who addresses his troops harshly in a loud voice if something has gone wrong. The loud voice, tone and other behaviour would cause hilarity if a nurse were to try it out in a ward.

The difference is obvious in an extreme situation like the above. Situations, however, are not nearly always so clear-cut and slightly aggressive remarks, for instance, are more acceptable in some environments than in others. Differences may also occur if a patient comes from a different culture.

c. Role problems

Case study: Mrs Campbell

Mrs Campbell, aged sixty-four, is in the medical ward. She was admitted because of a serious metabolic disorder. Nurse Helen Smith is on good terms with the patient.

Because of various complications and the side effects of some medicines, Mrs Campbell's health has not yet improved much. One of her friends has urged her several times to try homeopathic medicines, but when she mentioned this to the consultant, he rejected the idea as 'nonsense' and 'unscientific'. Mrs Campbell has also discussed the matter with Helen Smith who, in fact, suggested that she spoke to the consultant about it. Helen had always been interested in homeopathy and was therefore a sympathetic person with whom to discuss the matter.

After the consultant had rejected the suggestion, and because there was still very little improvement, Mrs Campbell began taking the other medicines 'illegally'. She acquired them from her friend during visiting hours and, appealing to their good relationship, she also took Helen into her confidence.

Being made a party to the 'secret' placed Helen in a difficult position. On the one hand, the patient expected understanding and support from her in her nurse's role. This was made easier because Helen does not genuinely consider such support to be stricty inconsistent with her role. The consultant, on the other hand, will expect Helen to support his policy: he regards a nurse as the person who carries out his instructions.

In the example, conflicting expectations arose in respect of the same role, and Helen could not satisfy them both at the same time. If she were to give away the secret, as the consultant would expect her to do, she would no longer be a nurse in the eyes of the patient. If she were to say nothing, as the patient expected, the consultant would certainly regard her as a bad nurse.

The example provides an illustration of role strain, one of the two role problems that are dealt with in this chapter.

Role strain occurs if there are differences in expectations regarding a particular role and if such expectations are in conflict with each other.

There are various causes of role strain, and in the example these were the good relationship and the nurse's own interests. Religious consider-

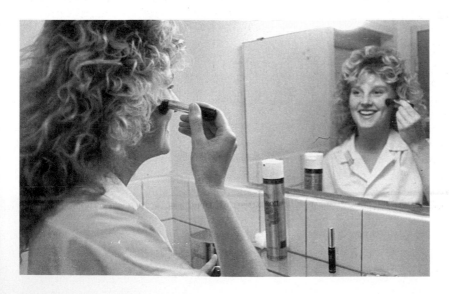

Figure 3.2.9
Too much make-up
may cause role strain

ations might also be a cause of such conflict, for example in cases relating to abortion.

Study activity
21. Compare your role as as a prospective independent adult and your role as your parents' child. To what extent might the two roles conflict with each other?

In the above task, there is not just one role about which there may be different expectations, but two. As was mentioned previously, everyone has a number of roles, and usually all goes well. Sometimes, however, the situation leads to conflict.

Role conflict occurs if someone's various roles conflict with one another.

There is an important difference between role strain and role conflict. In the case of role strain, there is one role and different expectations about it, but if there is a role conflict, more than one role is involved. The literature on the subject sometimes refers to role strain as an *internal role conflict*. The concept of role conflict dealt with in this chapter then becomes an *external role conflict*.

This kind of role conflict occurs quite frequently in hospital, if patients cannot relinquish their paternal, maternal or work roles. It then becomes difficult for them to combine their role as patients with their 'other' roles. The consequent role conflict may even lead to people discharging themselves or refusing to go into hospital.

It is important to distinguish between role strain and role conflict. In the case of role strain you will have to consider what your views are on a particular role. In the second case, in that of the role conflict, you may well have to decide not to perform a certain role, temporarily if need be.

Helpful behaviour
We help people several times a day, often in small ways such as handing someone something or holding a door open. Sometimes we need to do more, give blood for instance. In exceptional circumstances it might even be something extremely brave. To a greater or lesser extent, we are therefore concerned with the phenomenon of helping or the role of helper every day.

What induces us to help others? Do humans possess an innate inner goodness or do we only do such things in order to better ourselves? Unselfish help without benefiting from it is what the dictionary calls *altruism*. As we shall see, however, it is rare.

L. Berkowitz (1975) mentions two important norms that are crucial to answering the question of whether we help or not:
– the reciprocity norm;
– the social responsibility norm.

We mean by the *reciprocity norm*, (also called the economic motive), that we expect something in return for our help. This norm is based on the deeply rooted moral code that one has to reward someone for what one has been given. It is easiest to illustrate in terms of business transactions. Companies or shops selling goods also provide services along with their products. Such services or help are not provided because it comes naturally to a business. Their aim, obviously, is to make a profit and the reason for the service is that they hope to keep their customers. If a customer considers that he is well served by a company, it is more likely that he will give the same company his custom next time. Service, therefore, is provided in the expectation of reciprocity.

Reciprocity does not only play a part in the business world. If you hold a door open for someone, you expect thanks or a friendly smile. You also expect that the other person will do something for you next time. Helping like this is a means of placing someone under an obligation towards you. The 'price' of help may take various forms, e.g. tips, positive attention, a favour in return, or acquiring greater prestige.

Another reason for helping, according to the reciprocity norm, is the desire to avoid punishment. Another nurse, for instance, may ask you politely to fetch a cup of coffee for her.

For no particular reason, you refuse. The likelihood is that this does not only result in an angry look but also in a few negative remarks or thoughts about you as a person, 'You're not very helpful', 'You're selfish', or worse. That kind of incident makes it less likely that the other person will do something for you in the future.

We are therefore more likely to do something for someone else because of the reciprocity norm. If reciprocity is lacking, either in reality or according to our expectations, we are not inclined to do something for the other person. Someone known to be selfish will therefore be less inclined to receive help from other people. As will have been noted, while rewards or indeed punishments may be material, they are often in the nature of social rewards or punishments. In the *Social Exchange Theory,* Blau (1964) suggests that individuals attempt to maximise their satisfactions and minimise their dissatisfactions through *interaction* with others. In essence individuals, in their interactions with others, are bargaining for group or social benefits in a complex social exchange relationship.

The extent to which we know a person plays an important part in reciprocity. You would probably be willing to hold a door open for a stranger, but giving him or her money would usually be going too far. In the case of people you know, you are more willing, or feel more obliged, to help, but you also venture to expect greater favours in return.

According to the reciprocity norm (or social exchange theory), and depending on how well you know a particular person, you help because:
– you expect something attractive in return;
– unpleasant surprises are thereby avoided.

Apart from how well you know the person you are helping, there are two other factors that play a part in the reciprocity norm. They are: the extent to which the proffered help appears to be voluntary, and the other person's position in an organization or social group.

The first factor means that one feels more obliged to repay someone for his help if one believes that such help was wholly voluntary. If he or she had been acting on instructions, the reciprocity norm would hardly apply.

A person's position in an organization or social group also plays a part. It is true, in general, that the more responsibility one has in an organization, the more inclined one feels to do something in return, at least if the help was provided by a subordinate. This is less true in the opposite circumstances. An employee who receives some help from his employer will be more inclined to think that he has earned the help. Reciprocity therefore does not apply in this case; he has paid enough through his work.

The *social responsibility norm* was the second norm to be mentioned in this context. It tells us that we must help someone who clearly needs help. The social responsibility norm has a long history: remember the good Samaritan in the Bible story. The basic principle for this norm is not helping for its reciprocity, but the help that is needed. If, for example, another nurse asks you to fetch her a glass of water because she is feeling dizzy, you will undoubtedly do it. In that case, your prime motive will be your sense of responsibility rather than any idea of reciprocity.

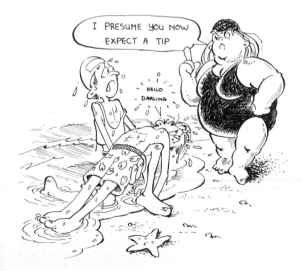

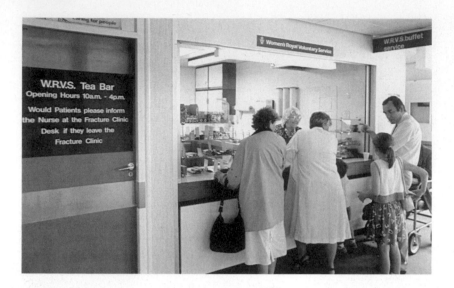

Figure 3.2.10
The social
responsibility norm

Although fear of punishment may sometimes play a part in this kind of situtation, it is not your main reason for helping. You would otherwise have to say that people punish themselves by having feelings of guilt if they do not offer to help.

Personal responsibility is a special form of social responsibility. A good example occurs if a teacher asks a class whether anyone would be prepared to help by playing a role, e.g. the role of a patient in hospital. If the question is put to the class as a whole, it often happens that everyone sits staring at the ceiling at first. At a given moment there are usually several people who begin to feel personally responsible and volunteer for the job. The teacher may also tell someone to do it. She then makes that student personally responsible for the job and it will be fairly difficult for the latter to refuse.

As we have seen, the reciprocity norm and the social responsibility norm play an important part in the problem of whether or not to help. The same obviously applies to the relationship between nurses and patients. How, for instance, should one regard the chocolates that many patients present to the ward when they are discharged? From the point of view of the reciprocity norm, this may be seen as payment for help received.

Matters are more complicated in the case of the social responsibility norm. Take, for example, a patient who tells you in confidence about her unhappy experiences. It is likely that you will subsequently devote extra attention to the patient. The example of Mrs Campbell on page 231 showed you that this may also put you in an awkward position. Feeling personally responsible is therefore not necessarily by definition a positive reaction.

Since helping has a lot to do with our norms, there may also be conflicting norms. There is, for example, the saying, 'Mind your own business', which stresses the norm of not interfering with other people's business.

Take, for example, a matrimonial row at the home of your neighbours. At what stage should you call for help or go to see them? When you hear them shouting at each other? Or when you hear china being hurled at the wall? Or when you hear them assaulting each other? Somewhere along the way, the norm 'mind your own business' will no longer apply. That, however, does not always mean that you will actually do something about it.

There are dramatic examples of help not being offered for fear of involvement. Some kind of instruction or mandate appears to be required for offering help. Your own sense of responsibility may give you that instruction, or it may be provided by someone else.

Fear of the consequences may be a reason for not helping, but help may even fail to materialize when obviously unpleasant consequences do not seem likely. A special example of this is known as the spectator phenomenon. You read about it in the newspaper sometimes, for instance when somebody has fallen into the water and none of the spectators lends a hand or fetches help. A well-known example in the US is that of Catherine Genovese, who was murdered in between several blocks of flats without the murderer being restrained. None of the large number of people who had heard the screaming took any action to help her.

The above example has been thoroughly researched along with several others. These studies have highlighted the conditions that decide when and how quickly spectators take action:

- The situation must be recognized as a dangerous one. Whatever is seen or heard must therefore not be attributed to something else or regarded as innocuous.
- There must be a sense of personal responsibility. This may occur when the number of spectators is small, but it also applies when someone designates certain people to perform certain tasks.
- Action is taken more rapidly if no-one in authority is present. The presence of, say, a single policeman will give the spectators the sense of having been relieved of their responsibilities. It is worth realizing that if you are present in your nurse's uniform when there is an accident, this will also apply: people will look to you and feel less responsible;
- The final condition is that another spectator must not be responsible for the situation. If someone is clearly to blame, he or she is also expected to resolve the situation that has arisen.

It is certainly true that the mere presence of others can have an influence on how individuals behave. Latane (1978) describes a *Social Impact Theory* which states that the actual presence of others exerts an arousing influence on individuals and influences how they behave. However, this depends on the magnitude of impact (e.g. the number of people and strength of feeling) and the extent to which the individual is the target of group impact. Where impact is *diffused* across a group i.e. where there are multiple sources of impact and where the *strength* of impact or urge to act is not high, an individual may not feel compelled to act. In an interesting and well-known study of crowd behaviour, Latane and Darley (1970) found that at the scene of accidents individuals tended not to help, apparently assuming that others would do so. Zajonc (1980) also suggests a principle of *compresence* in such situations. This recognizes that while the mere presence of others has an arousing effect which causes anxiety e.g. stage-fright in some, others in fact react differently and play to the audience. Thus, in crowd situations some people may react by inactivity, some may be frightened, especially when they are the target of crowd attention, while others may adopt naturally to a centre-of-attention role. Clearly social impact and compresence are powerful social influences.

4. Power and leadership

The concept of roles was considered in detail in the previous section. Within a group, the various roles bear a certain relation to one another, and the concept of power plays an important part in this.

Case study: Tom Baker

Sister Young has had years of experience as a nurse and she has been ward sister in the Neurological Department for the past fifteen years. She is known to be kindly, but strict on occasion. If one of her nurses is having problems with his or her private life or work, she usually makes allowances for this when drawing up the duty roster.

Tom Baker is a student nurse in Sister Young's ward and is faced with a problem. He would like to have the day off on Wednesday week as there is to be a trade fair that he would like to visit. One of his colleagues is willing to take over the day shift to which he had already been assigned. Swapping duties, however, is not on as far as Sister Young is concerned, and certainly not without her prior consent. She knows from experience that swapping duties easily becomes a habit as a result of which she loses control of the situation.

When Tom went to ask Sister Young whether he might swap duties with another nurse, his request was refused. Sister Young was, in fact, rather annoyed that Tom had already asked someone to take over his shift. He was therefore unable to visit the fair.

Study activity
22. Describe the emotions that the above kind of situation arouses in you and consider what basis there is for Sister Young's power.

In the example, Tom wants to do something but can only do it with Sister Young's consent. Apparently, she has the power to control at least part of Tom's conduct. All of us are faced with the concept of power every day of our lives. Sometimes someone has authority over you, and on other occasions you take decisions for someone else.

Differences in power occur in all the groups that you find yourself in every day. Power is sometimes open and visible, as in the case of Sister Young. At other times it is more covert, for instance when someone has power because he can manipulate social situations.

If, like Tom, you are prevented from doing something, you will normally take an unfavourable view of power. Power, however, can also be viewed in a favourable sense if you manage to arrange something that would not be possible without it.

Study activity
23. Check whether you take a favourable or an unfavourable view of power. Give reasons for your answer.

There are several angles from which to view a concept such as power:
– power as a negative concept;
– power as a pleasure-giving element;
– service-rendering power;
– power as a sociological concept.

Your evaluation and definition of the concept will vary according to your line of approach. A useful definition based on the sociological point of view is as follows:
Power is the ability to control the behaviour of others so that it accords with the intentions of the person with power and irrespective of the agreement of the person without power.

There is a major difference between this definition and definitions based on other approaches. Here there is no evaluation of the concept; it is of no importance whether power is evaluated positively or negatively. A second important difference compared with other definitions is the fact that the emphasis is on power relationships.

It is helpful to pause briefly to consider a concept that is sometimes confused with power, namely *authority*. Authority is not the same as power, although there are many similarities. A person with authority is also able to control the behaviour of someone else so that it accords with his or her own aims. The major difference concerns the consent of the person whose behaviour is prescribed. In the case of power, consent is unimportant but, in the case of authority, there is a measure of acceptance, either tacit or otherwise.

Combining the two concepts gives an extra dimension to an unequal relationship. If someone has power and authority, he not only lays down what the other person is to do or not to do, but he is also appreciated for it. If a person has power but no authority, such appreciation is lacking.

There are three kinds of authority:
– *Rational authority*. Faith in order and rules plays a major part in this. Since you consider the existence of rules to be important, you

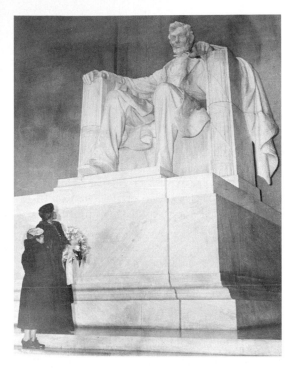

Figure 3.2.11
Power and authority
can coincide

'The power of the strongest'. In the first case i.e. that of Sister Young, power is based on someone's position, whereas in the second case physical strength forms the basis of power.

Power can be based on many things and the following are just some of them:
- power of sanctions;
- legitimate power;
- expert power;
- power of the word;
- power of numbers;
- reference power.

Before reading about the various kinds of power you should realize that they are not mutually exclusive. Combinations occur in which a person's power is based on more than one principle.

The power of sanctions means the power to reward and punish. The concept of sanctions was dealt with in Chapter 1 when the subject of social control was being considered.

The power of sanctions usually occurs in combination with *legitimate power*. This is the power that goes with formal positions; boards of management, heads of departments, teachers, policemen, etc. all have legitimate power. The examples also show that although power of sanctions often forms part of legitimate power, the opposite is not always true. The head of a department, for instance, may need the consent of the board before punishing or rewarding someone.

Expert power is the power derived from one's knowledge of facts. The saying, 'Knowledge brings power' is directly concerned with this form of power.

There are sellers of goods or services who, because of their excellent sales talk, are almost capable of forcing people to buy things. The form of power related to that is *the power of the word*. You also come across it in discussions in which the outcome is decided by the debating skills of the participants, sometimes because of, but at other times in spite of, the arguments.

bestow authority on the person who is upholding the rules.
- *Traditional authority*. This is a deeply rooted traditional faith in the authority of certain other people, e.g. the Queen, lawyers, doctors, teachers, etc.
- *Charismatic authority*. This means bestowing authority on someone with special gifts. It is difficult to indicate exactly why some people have charisma, this special gift. Possible examples are: Gandhi, John F. Kennedy and Martin Luther King.

Study activity
24. Give three examples of people who have power over you. Consider whether they also have authority and on what such authority is based.

a. Forms of power

There are various reasons why someone has a particular power. One example of power was mentioned in the example of Sister Young above, but you might also consider the phrase

Many people have experienced the sense of impotence that you feel if you are unable to express yourself in public. You can sometimes win discussions with words, but they also give you the power to reassure, console or, if you wish, anger someone.

The power of numbers again brings to mind phrases or sayings such as, 'United we stand, divided we fall'. This kind of power also plays an important part in politics and trade unions. It does not, however, mean that the power of numbers on a smaller scale is unimportant. Consider the experiment by Asch (1952) that has become a classic example.

In this study, groups of six to eight students (usually about seven) were presented with simple perceptual problems. The seven students involved in each trial in the experiment were told that they were taking part in research on judging visual relationships. During each assessment, the students were shown four lines consisting of one standard line and three with varying lengths. On each occasion, the simple task was to decide which of the last three lines was the same length as the standard line. Each student had to express his opinion aloud. One of the students, however, was unaware of the fact that the others knew all about the purpose of the experiment and that he was the only one involved in it.

As agreed, the other students gave incorrect answers on a number of occasions. They all pointed out the same incorrect line. The object of the experiment was to find out how the uninformed student would react. On most occasions the student gave the same wrong answer as the others, even though, as he later admitted, he sometimes knew that his answer was wrong. These astonishing findings have become known as the "Asch effect".

The student in the example apparently did not dare to express a different opinion. It seems to be difficult to put forward a dissenting opinion in a group. Other experiments have shown that the size of the group and the extent to which you are supported by one or more of the others is important. The experiment proved to be a good

example of the power of numbers. This kind of power can evidently ensure that we do not simply tell other people about what we see or feel, especially if we think our views may be unpopular minority views.

Study activity
25. – Everyone in the ward is concerned about a patient who is very sad. You think she is putting it on.
    – Hardly anyone is taking the behaviour of a certain patient seriously. You, however, are concerned about him.
    State whether you would make your opinion known to the others in each of the two cases. Also give your reasons.

Reference power is the last of the six kinds of power mentioned above. It is the power that one derives from factors in one's immediate environment. Take the kind of advertisement that appeared in a newspaper once:
'Widow of a senior civil servant would like to meet a man of similar status'.

The widow in the advertisement evidently derives her power and the status that goes with it from her deceased husband. A pop star might have a similar function in that behaving or looking like such a person could convey a sense of power. The idea behind reference power is that something of another person's power rubs off on the person who is in some way closely connected with him or her.

If you know that one of your colleagues is very friendly with the ward sister, it may be that you will attribute more power to that colleague, even though there is no genuine reason for doing so. Reference power can also be derived from a group. If you put on naval uniform, this may give you a sense of power that you derive from the navy.

Study activity
26. Argue the case that a nurse's uniform also provides reference power. In formulating your argument consider the advantages and disadvantages of some psychiatric units where nurses do not wear uniform.

Power gives people a certain *status*. Such status or prestige is made plain in various ways. In the case of reference power that is even essential, since you have to state or show how your power is derived, e.g. in the case of the widow or in that of the person in the navy.

Symbols often serve the purpose of showing that one has power, whether it be reference power or one of the other kinds. The mayoral chain of office, the managing director's expensive car, the stripes on the sleeve of a policeman may all be regarded as status symbols.

It would be wrong, however, to think that one must have a lot of power to be able to use status symbols. Belonging to a group – remember the power of numbers – is frequently another reason for making use of status symbols. The motoring organization's badge, the local café's T-shirt and somebody's ID card are also status symbols.

Study activity
27. List at least five status symbols to be found in a hospital.

b. Leadership

After the concepts of power and status, we must now consider the concept of a leader. You can, if you wish, find a large number of synonyms for the term *leader*, e.g. head, director, commander, chief, etc. They each possess a certain amount of power and use it in their endeavours to provide leadership for a group. The aims of the group form the basis for this.

Case study: Mia Bloomer

At the weekend Mia Bloomer was the senior staff nurse on duty in the children's ward. That meant that she, the person who had been qualified longest, had to make sure that everything in the ward was running smoothly. She had allocated the various tasks first thing in the morning and prepared the medicine trolley herself. Joseph Wilson's first job was to check the drips. He noticed that Peter, a little boy aged four who had not been in the ward for long, was looking very pale. Joseph's impression was that the small patient was not reacting quite correctly either. He went in search of Mia to discuss whether it would be necessary to inform the paediatrician on duty. Mia, however, first wanted to see for herself, and decided to wait for a while. This annoyed Joseph considerably. He, too, had been qualified as a children's nurse for some time and was confident of his own judgment. He had always found it hard to put up with the way in which Mia behaved when she was in charge. He thought she took too many decisions herself and did not allow enough discussion.

Study activity
28. How would you describe the style of leadership adopted in the story? Would you opt for the same kind of behaviour as that exhibited by Mia? Give reasons for your answer!

In the example, Mia is the boss, the leader. Not only does she decide on what is to be done, but also how she will share her responsibilties with the others. She can do that in a strict fashion, without much in the way of discussions, but she may also leave all the decisions to other people. The way in which leadership is exercised may vary considerably from one situation to another. The difference in style has two important causes:
– the aims of the group;
– the personality of the leader.

In the first case, we sometimes refer to *functional leadership*. The leader adapts his style to the aims of the group. This means that, depending on the situation, he will discuss matters more on some occasions than on others.
The leader's personality is also of importance to the style. Depending on his personality, values and skills, he will choose a style with which he thinks he is most likely to achieve his aims. Charismatic leadership occupies a special position in this. We looked at what it meant when we were considering the concept of authority.

Depending on the above causes, it is usual to identify three types of leader. You need to realize that there may be mixed types, particularly in the case of functional leadership. The three types of leader are:
– the autocratic leader;
– the democratic leader;
– the laissez-faire leader.

Autocratic means ruling alone. The *autocratic leader* is therefore someone who takes decisions alone. The other members of the group contribute little or nothing to such decisions. There are situations in which autocratic leadership is almost a condition for the satisfactory performance of a task, for instance when an emergency case is brought into Casualty. Lengthy consultations and discussions until everyone agrees may cost the patient's life. In that kind of situation it is important for one person to be in charge and assign the various tasks.

It is not quite so simple to justify this type of leader when less urgent cases are concerned. The needs and possibly the tolerance of the members of the group are one of the factors to be considered in such instances. Depending on that, the leader either will or will not be appreciated. In the latter instance, there may be a lack of motivation, which may have a negative effect on group functioning.

Study activity
29. Mention three situations in which you would opt for autocratic leadership. Mention three others in which you would not do so. Give reasons for your answers.

The second kind of leader is the *democratic* one, the kind of leader who allows plenty of opportunity for discussion. In the example at the beginning of the subsection, this is what Joseph would

have chosen in view of his opinions. Many democratic leaders regard themselves as co-ordinators rather than leaders. In the most extreme cases, decisions are only taken when the entire group is in favour of them. Motivation in that kind of group is usually good, although the time required for consultation is often long, particularly if there is personal friction between members.

A democratic leader is usually considered to be one who allows adequate time for consultation. The leader will take the ultimate decision, even if not everyone agrees with it at the time.

Study activity
30. Give three examples of situations in which you would opt for a democratic leader. Give reasons for your answer.

The *laissez-faire* leader was the third one to be mentioned. This term does not really refer to leadership in the strict sense, rather to the lack of it. Laissez faire is French for let things go. The appointed leader of a group does not act as such, which does not mean that there is no leader at all.
Informal leaders often make the decisions, which may be because they dominate discussions, produce better arguments, have a certain charisma or the most expert knowledge.

Study activity
31. Try and think of a situation in which you would opt for a laissez-faire leader.

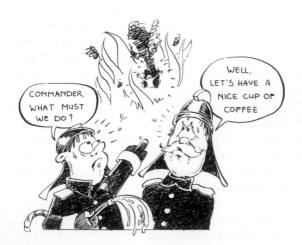

Finally, it is important to refer again to the concept of functional leadership, since it can incorporate any of the three forms mentioned above. Depending on the situation and the needs of the other members of the group, the style of leadership may change. To return to the Casualty Department example: if an emergency case is brought in, the task requires an autocratic leader. Transferring another member of staff to the same department might, within certain limits, be done more democratically. A social evening with the department staff might be an opportunity for the official leader to choose a more laissez-faire style.

5. Co-operation

The concept of co-operation forms the basis of the present section, which begins with a consideration of groups with a clear task function. A hospital ward team may be regarded as a prime example of a group with a task function.

There is a connection between this section and Module 5 of this book. The emphasis in the present module is on the theory of co-operation, whereas Module 5 stresses the skills required for co-operation.

Case study: Joan Girvan

Charge Nurse Burgess is retiring next year. He has had a long career but now feels that he has had enough.
He is gradually cutting down on work so that he will not have to switch suddenly from a busy life to one without any fixed duties. He usually lets other people perform certain jobs such as preparing duty rosters.

Joan Girvan has been his deputy for two years. She is hoping to succeed Mr. Burgess but it is by no means certain that she will. There are nurses in other wards who have been at the hospital for years and have as much right to promotion as she has.

In the corridors, speculation is rife. Most people would not be too happy if Joan Girvan were to become the new ward sister. For the sake of convenience, her opponents may be divided into two camps. One of them thinks that although Joan Girvan has the required ability, it would be better if she were to be put in charge of another ward. A prophet, after all, is rarely honoured in his own country.

The other camp opposes her because people do not like her personality. They think that she is already behaving as though she were in charge and are afraid that matters will be worse once she is promoted. In any event, the consequence of all these discussions is that the atmosphere and therefore co-operation in the ward are not very good just now.

Good co-operation is an extremely difficult process, and we rarely see it taking place in perfect harmony. In the course of your career you are likely to find on various occasions that co-operation within a group is not working too well for short or long periods. Open or concealed personal conflicts, lack of clarity about tasks and role-switches as described above may be the cause of this.

Working in a group with poor co-operation is disheartening. The quality of the job that needs doing is adversely affected. The obvious thing to do would be to identify the cause of the co-operation problems and then find a solution to them. In practice, however, it is rarely easy to pinpoint a simple cause. Sometimes it is not even simple to acknowledge that there is any co-operation problem at all.

If a group wishes to work together in the best possible manner, four general conditions need to be met, i.e.:
- clarity about the method of co-operation: the organization needs to be clear and everyone should know the rules governing the required conduct towards one another;
- clarity about the common aims: the task to be performed by the group must be known to all those taking part in it;
- everyone should be aware of his or her possible contribution and limitations;
- each person should also be aware of the possible contributions by other people.

In a well-run ward, these conditions have been met. It is sometimes said that the organization is in balance. Everyone knows what he or she has to do, what the others are contributing and how to respond to one another. It is important to protect that balance. If one or more of the basic conditions have not been met, in a ward for instance, it is said that the organization is out of balance. In the example of Joan Girvan, a situation like that threatens to occur. Her possible contribution, both now and in the future, has become less clear.

Study activity
32. Reference was made above to a number of

Figure 3.2.12
The task-orientated
process

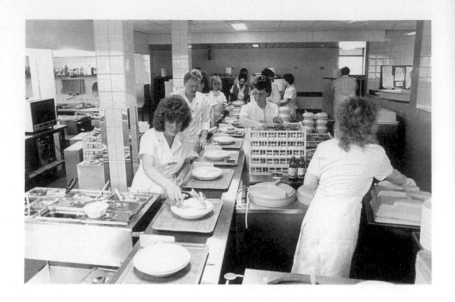

basic conditions which must be met to allow for good co-operation. Even if the conditions have been met, things may still go wrong sometimes. Mention a few possible causes.

a.   The co-operation process

Something has already been said about organizations being in balance. This may have created the false impression that such a balance is stable. When considering group dynamics (page 224), we found that a group experiences a certain development. This means that each new phase in a group, each new development, requires a fresh balance.

Co-operation is a process bound up with the developments in a group. There are in fact two processes, inseparably linked:

The task-oriented process. This is centred on reaching and/or carrying out a common objective. Your work as a member of a hospital ward team is an example of behaviour appropriate to a task-orientated process.

The group-oriented process. This is centred on the people that are working together and social relationships in the group. The group may perform a task together (figure 3.2.13) but this is not the normal function of the group.

Talking about co-operation or asking a colleague how things are going are examples of behaviour appropriate to a group-oriented process.

The general conditions referred to on page 241 apply to both processes and precede, as it were, a satisfactory task-oriented or a satisfactory group-oriented process.

Study activity
33. List at least five activities appropriate to a task-oriented process and five activities appropriate to a group-oriented process. Base your lists on a hospital ward.

In most cases, everyone in a well-run organization knows his or her own contribution to it and also those of other people. This applies to both the task-oriented process and the group-oriented process. Playing a positive role in a task-oriented process or in a group-oriented process is therefore counted as a *functional role.* *Dysfunctional roles* may also occur in an organization. They are roles which run counter to the constructive activity of a group.

Case Study: Mick Black
Mick Black works in the same ward as Mr. Burgess and Joan Girvan. He has been qualified

243

for two years and is very ambitious. He privately thinks of himself as Mr Burgess' successor. He is unlikely, however, to say so in public, because he feels that he would antagonize Joan Girvan. Although most of his colleagues quite like him, he rather overestimates the support he expects from the others. He does, however, show his ambition, though not always clearly, for instance by complaining about Joan Girvan to other people.

Mick Black has a dysfunctional role in this example. It applies to both the task-oriented and the group-oriented process.
Dysfunctional roles can usually be traced back to two underlying causes, i.e.:
– dissatisfaction within a group;
– personal ambitions and/or disappointments which are worked off in a group.

Both causes play a part in the example. The lack of certainty about the succession causes dissatisfaction and thus clears the way for the second cause. Had the matter of succession been settled, Mick Black would probably have displayed his ambitions less openly in his own ward.

If a group is out of balance, tension is aroused as a result. It is important to trace the reasons for this. Possible questions are:
Have the organization's conditions been met?
What is the significance of possible dysfunctional roles?

Depending on the answers to these questions, appropriate action may be taken. Asking the above questions and taking appropriate action are quite often postponed in many groups. Fear of open conflict is frequently the reason for this, but its consequence is that due to the lack of clarity, dissatisfaction and tension last longer. A new and possibly different balance is not achieved. This finally brings us to two propositions, as follows:
– tensions occur from time to time in every group or organization;
– such tensions, provided they are properly handled, may ensure that a fresh balance is achieved.

b. Co-operation between groups

Attention has so far been focused on co-operation within groups. Our society, however, consists of a large number of interconnected groups. Sometimes groups hardly know one another, or do not know one another at all, whereas there are

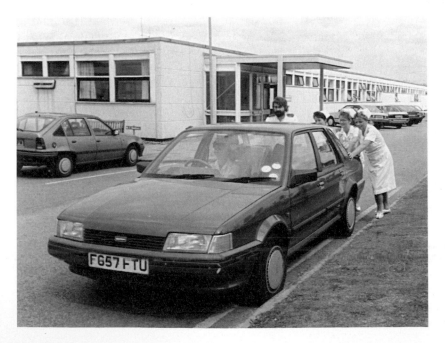

Figure 3.2.13
The group-oriented process

others which are in contact every day. There are groups which pursue the same aims, and others which are poles apart.

The society in which we live is a kind of super-group, in which all groups are united. Considered from this angle, 'society' means an organized network of interconnected groups.

The groups that make up society rarely have the same norms and values. Partly because of that, their image of mankind is not always the same either. As a result of such differences, we think in terms of a pluriform society, in which the concept of pluriformity refers to the different and sometimes diametrically opposite views of various groups.

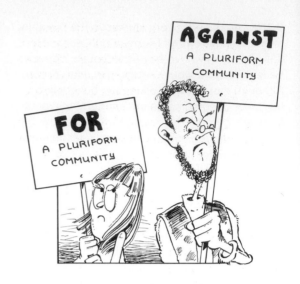

Study activity

34. a. Give at least three examples of two groups with different views on the same topic.

b. Do the same as in a., but now with reference to groups within your own class or student group.

The pluriformity of society has certain consequences for co-operation and therefore for problem solving. In our culture, i.e. a society with more or less common norms and values, the ways in which such problems are to be solved are fixed. This is expressed in rules of behaviour partly laid down in laws. By means of such laws, our culture decides how groups co-operate with one another and how they solve such problems as may arise.

You might take a topic like abortion as an example. Many groups feel concerned about it. There are occasional heated arguments between advocates and opponents. Such discussions as well as protest actions and the lobbying of politicians are some of the ways in which problems may be solved within our culture. The ultimate aim is for these accepted differences to be converted into some degree of consensus which is expressed as guidelines or legislation.

This method of solving conflicts is of course related to culture and as such is bound by time

and place. The way in which we deal with differences between groups these days is not the same as it was a hundred years ago. Culture is also bound by place. The ways in which groups deal with one another differ from one community to another. Every society bases the rules for the way in which people and groups deal with one another on its cultural background.

c. Co-operation between groups in a hospital

In the health service and also in a hospital, various groups co-operate with one another. Looked at in this way, a hospital is a kind of pluriform mini-society. The ultimate aims may well be the same for everyone, but the course to be followed and incidental aims sometimes give rise to problems in the area of co-operation.

Case study: cost cutting

A fierce conflict is threatening in a medium-sized hospital. There is a budget deficit. Although it was expected, no action has yet been taken. Certain cost cutting measures, however, cannot be postponed any longer. The medical specialists take the view that economies must not lead to a loss of quality.

The purchase of new equipment cannot therefore be postponed. They also consider, as does the nursing staff, that it would be impossible to do all the work with fewer people. The nurses feel that they have economized enough in recent years. The maintenance, administrative and catering departments are afraid that, because of the position taken by the others, their sections will bear the brunt of the economies. Consequently, they never miss an opportunity for producing arguments to demonstrate that there are no economies that they can make.

The example shows that different interests may make themselves felt within an organization in spite of common aims. Each group will obviously feel that its contribution must remain unaffected. Arguments that are partly factual, partly emotional, cause groups to oppose one another or else to co-operate with one another. The hospital's culture will determine how the problems are solved. You might ask the following questions in this context. Which consultative bodies are tackling the problem? Is it just the management, the board and the medical staff, or are others involved as well? Depending on the power structure, the style of leadership usually adopted is another important factor.

Opposing views, however, are rarely as clear-cut as they were in this example. Groups may be opposed to one another even when less practical matters are concerned. What, for instance, should one think of the arguments between the *holistic* and *reductive* approach to man. In the former approach, the human being is considered as a whole: a patient is not regarded simply as someone who is ill, but as a human being with a large number of needs, desires, fears, etc. This overall view is not taken in the reductive approach: only part of the patient, i.e. the complaint, is important.

The debate between the two views has consequences for co-operation and policy. Some hospitals, for example, include extensive psycho-social care in their services, whereas others pay far less attention to that aspect and take a reductionist approach concerning themselves only with the disease – its diagnosis, treatment and care. In the former instance the holistic approach is sometimes described as a *social* or *psycho-social* or *humanistic model* of care. In the latter reductive approach the term *medical model* of care is often used.

Study activity
35. Think of a few differences between groups or opinions in hospitals.

6. Summary

The title of this chapter is 'People in their Environment'. In the present context, this means specifically the group. Everyone is a member of a large number of groups. The more or less firm contacts that we have with them make up our social network. Social networks are different for everyone.

Groups differ in a number of ways. There are four aspects: creation, function, significance and organization.
The concepts of group dynamics and group cohesion were considered at the end of the section on groups. Group dynamics is the development that takes place in a group. A new group functions differently from, for example, a group whose members know each other better. One of the differences is the amount of involvement or group cohesion, which refers to the extent to which members wish to be members of the group to which they belong.

After the group and all its aspects, an important function within the group was dealt with, i.e. social role. How such social roles are created and the way in which they are learnt was also considered. The fact that one performs more than one role at a time and that roles are often complementary, is characteristic of the concept of roles. That is also true of the fact that roles are frequently more stable than individuals and that some behaviour is considered normal for one role and not for another.

At the end of the section, some mention was made of role problems. We made a distinction between role strain and role conflict. In the case of role strain there is a single role which has to meet different and opposing requirements. In the case of role conflicts, two roles are in conflict with each other.

Some attention was also devoted to the various aspects of power and leadership.

The final part of this chapter dealt with the subject of co-operation. The first topic was co-operation within a group: clarity about the organization, aims, one's own and other people's contributions are basic conditions. These conditions apply to the inextricably linked processes that always occur in a group, namely the task-oriented process and the group-oriented process. All members of the group perform a role in these processes. If it is a positive role, then it is called a functional role. It is also possible to have a dysfunctional role, which may be a sign of dissatisfaction within the organization, or else it may be based on personal motives.

Health and sickness as social concepts

3

1. Introduction

Health and sickness seem simple enough as concepts. They are words which are used so frequently in everyday language that we often do not even think about their meaning. We learn, and may have experienced, that the concept of sickness is inextricably linked to physical functions. The trouble caused by sickness is experienced in the form of pain or other forms of discomfort. Irrespective of whether the cause is physical, psychological or social, when considering the concepts of health and sickness we think first of all of our bodies.

It is remarkable, however, how differently people cope with the same psychological, physical or social complaints. Serious headaches, for instance, will make some people think they are ill, but not others. This fact makes it important to wonder whether the concept of sickness is really so firmly bound up with our bodies. We are accustomed to looking at sickness and health through somatic 'spectacles'.

This chapter approaches the matter differently, from a social angle. This does not mean that we consider only the social causes that may result in sickness. In addition, the concepts of health and sickness themselves are also looked at through social 'spectacles'. The social inconvenience, or sometimes even the social advantage, is seen as an important determination as to whether or not a person is defined as being well or sick.

The principal aspects of this topic, of great importance to nurses, will be considered:
– the concepts of health and sickness;
– social processes as bases for diseases;
– the consensus theory;
– the conflict theory;
– the interactionist theory.

Learning outcomes

After studying this chapter the student should be able to:
– give a definition of the concepts of health and sickness in which social processes play a part as well;
– discuss health and sickness in terms of somatogenesis, psychogenesis and sociogenesis;

- mention a number of social processes which, in addition to favourable aspects, may also have unfavourable or pathogenic influences on health;
- explain what is meant by clinical and social iatrogenesis;
- describe the consensus theory view on order in society;
- describe how the concepts of sickness and health are explained from the point of view of the consensus theory;
- explain order in society in accordance with the conflict theory;
- explain the concepts of sickness and health care in terms of the conflict theory;
- explain how order in society is achieved according to the interactionist theory;
- describe the concepts of sickness and health care according to the interactionist theory.

2. The concepts of health and sickness

Case study: Jean Barlow

Jean Barlow works as a nurse in a medical ward. She is away sick quite often, so that other nurses have to take over her duties. This causes occasional problems, certainly during evening and night shifts. Ken Lee is Jean's opposite. He is never ill and prides himself on the fact. Because of Jean's frequent absences, people tend to complain about her, usually behind her back. Ken, in particular, has expressed his doubts about Jean's complaints on more than one occasion.

If you looked at the number of days of sick leave, you would think that Jean is less healthy than Ken. She considers herself unfit for work more frequently than he does.

Supposing, however, that the workload in the ward is quite heavy. Jean's colleagues, on average, have more days off work than people in other wards, always excepting Ken of course. Armed with this information, you may still think that Jean is less healthy than Ken. It is likely, however, that you will take a less serious view of Jean's ill health. In fact the workload in the ward, as well as people's physical condition, also plays an important role in this situation. This ward has very heavy workloads and the higher incidence of staff sick-leave *may* be related to this fact.

Supposing, furthermore, that Ken was brought up in a family where being sick was scarcely

acceptable, where the general idea was, 'Don't fuss, carry on', except, of course, if he was very seriously ill. You may therefore assume that Ken would do almost anything rather than give in to his own major or minor complaints, fatigue or discomfort.

Study activity

1. **a.** How would you regard the difference in health between Ken and Jean in the light of this new information?
   b. To what extent do you consider that Ken's views on sickness will affect his work as a nurse?

Three factors which play a part in the concept of health have been mentioned above, i.e.:
- physical or somatic factors;
- social factors: the workload in the ward;
- psychological factors, e.g. Ken's attitude.

Health, and therefore also sickness, may be defined in terms of these factors. This may be done in two ways.

Firstly, we can take one of the factors and decide whether a person is sick or in good health on the basis of that factor. This principle is called the *reductive* approach. It occurs most frequently if the physical factor only is considered, but it is also possible if only the psychological or social factors are taken into account.

Secondly, it is possible to consider all three factors together to define the terms healthy and sick, the *holistic* approach. That is the approach

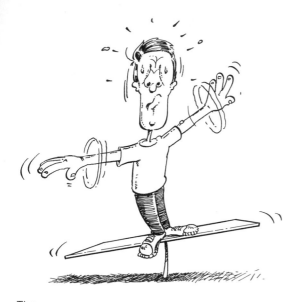

The
sociopsychosomatic
balance

adopted in this module, except where it is expressly stated that this is not the case. The following definition of health will therefore be applied:

Good health may be regarded as a balance between social, psychological and somatic functioning.

In much of the literature on the subject these concepts are explained by linking the concept of health to the sociopsychosomatic balance. From the point of view of the definition, sickness is regarded as a disturbance of that balance. It is important to realize not only that there are three factors in the above definition, but also that they are interrelated. The term balance expresses this. Changes in one area therefore have consequences in the other areas. If there is no adjustment, or no proper adjustment, sickness ensues.

Study activity

2. Mr Arnold is in hospital with a slight myocardial infarction. Try to think of a physical, a social and a psychological cause. Explain, from the point of view of the balance model why the causes that are found do not always lead to a myocardial infarction.

The interaction between psychological, social and somatic functioning is highly important and leads to three conclusions:

- Interaction indicates, for example, that somatic complaints may arise from somatic, psychological or social functioning. Serious headaches may thus have a psychological or social cause as well as a somatic one; they may be associated with problems at work or people's difficulty in coping with emotions.
- Another possibility is compensation. This means that poor functioning in one area may be wholly or partly made good by functioning in another area: a lot of stress at work (social) is not so much of a problem for someone who has learnt to cope with tension (psychological), in comparison with someone who has not learnt to do so.
- The interaction between the three factors provides an explanation for the differences shown by people in their reactions to comparable situations: one person reports sick because of a headache, another does not. Some people can still function properly when depressed, others cannot.

There are three concepts connected with the above, i.e. *somatogenesis, psychogenesis* and *sociogenesis.*

Sociogenesis means that a situation or condition (e.g. an illness), whether or not it is a primarily

Figure 3.3.1
People are reduced more
and more as a result
of further specialization

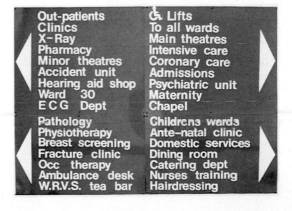

Figure 3.3.2
Health care is becomir
more complicated

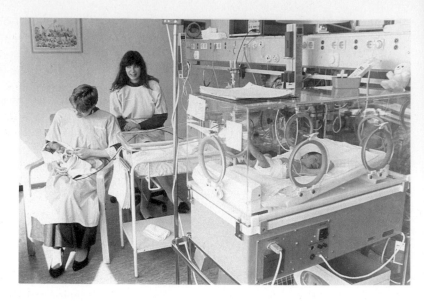

social, psychological or physical condition, has a social cause (socio = social; genesis = origin).

Study activity
  3. Give your own definitions of psychogenesis and somatogenesis.

This module is based on social psychology and sociology. The explanations and theories in the following sections should be seen above all as a sociological approach to the concept of sickness. In view of the definition of health adopted above, the somatogenetic and psychogenetic approaches are not, however, neglected.

There is a further important conclusion in addition to those already mentioned. First consider the following proposition:
  – *Sickness and pain lose their possible significance when they are regarded merely as inconvenient factors which should be eliminated as quickly as possible.*

This proposition emphasizes the important fact that the complaint, the sickness, may perform the function of a signal. In Jean's and Ken's ward, at the beginning of this section, there was a lot of absenteeism because of illness. This may have signalled that the work in that particular ward was too hard. Merely treating the complaints or illnesses does not remove their cause. Myocardial infarctions, backaches, stomach

trouble etc. may, for example, be signals of problems that are not somatic. If the complaint alone is treated, the cause will remain. It is not inconceivable that the signal will assume a more serious form next time. The same complaint may return, or there may be a different complaint, in which case we speak of a *symptom shift*. The signal function is dealt with in further detail in the next section.

3. Social processes as bases for sickness

In general, our society tries to care for its members as well as possible. In numerous areas, measures have been taken to provide the *social processes* that are important to the community, and we are concerned with them from the cradle to the grave. Some of the measures are taken by the government, e.g. education and social security. Others are in the hands of private organizations such as firms of undertakers or solicitors, but in such cases there are often government regulations and checks.

At the same time, many of such provisions also have a negative aspect. Although many provisions have advantages, they also constitute a threat in other areas. A number of important contemporary examples are mentioned below.
  – *Natural environment*
    Industry produces goods that benefit us all to

a greater or lesser extent. The production processes, however, also cause air, water and soil pollution. An important example is the global influence of CFCs from refridgerators and aerosol cans on the earth's ozone layer

- *Working conditions*
Because of the way in which we are organized, problems arise that are related to the work climate. You might think in terms of dangerous work, excessively long hours, too much or too little responsibility, dull and monotonous work, etc.

- *Living conditions*
Some parts of the country are overpopulated; noise pollution and the number of road accidents are therefore increasing.

- *Living and eating habits*
We are always in a hurry and therefore our food needs to be prepared quickly and conveniently. This hurried, stressful way of life and dependence on fast foods may cause threats to health. This is sometimes called prosperity or cultural sickness.

Study activity

4. Give at least five concrete examples of processes that may constitute a threat to our health in some way or other. A suggestion: make use of this week's newspapers.

Of particular interest here is the extent to which socially constructed living conditions, in total and in interaction, influence the health of a whole society and individuals within it. It is only within the last quarter of a century or so that medicine has started to recognize that disease may not be the result of a single agent such as a virus, but a consequence of many factors, including environmental factors such as poverty, overcrowding, poor housing etc. Hinkle (1964) has described this perspective as a 'human ecology' approach to medicine.

A major contribution in this area was the controversial Black Report published in Britain (DHSS, 1980). This report entitled 'Inequalities in Health' illustrated that the main determinants of the Nation's health were not the quality of Health Service provisions at all, but issues of *social* inequality, i.e. housing, poverty, unemployment and social class-related cultural attributes (eating habits, tobacco and alcohol consumption, etc.). This indicated that simple National Health Service strategies were, in effect, treating the symptoms (sickness and ill health) rather than the underlying social disease (poverty, housing, ignorance, etc.). The premise arising from Black was that the provision of what was, in effect, an *Ill Health* Service was inadequate; what was needed was a *Health Promotion* Service and a radical inprovement in social conditions. The social policy and public expenditure implications would have been significant.

Some critics have suggested that the British government of the day was extremely concerned about these implications and deliberately 'swept the Black Report under the carpet'. It is certainly true that only a limited number of copies of the report were made available initially. Indeed two of the Report's research working group published an account in a commercial paperback version in an attempt to make the Black Report findings more readily available (see Townsend and Davidson, 1982).

Study activity

5. Consider your own town or neighbourhood. If you have time, as you walk around observe: the housing; the people – how they are dressed; the amount of smoking and drinking which goes on; the extent of unemployment. Write in about 500 words a brief description of the locality and any implications for the health of the community.

An interesting aspect of environmental influences on health is the sheer rate of advancement and change in society today. This was brought to international attention by the American sociologist Alvin Toffler in his now classic publication entitled 'Future Shock' (Toffler, 1976). He described in vivid terms the accelerative thrust of change in modern life – in terms of science, medicine, technology and culture. The term 'future shock' was used to describe the shattering stress and disorientation which is caused by too much change in too short a time. Toffler analysed in some detail the detrimental influence of *rapid change* or *future shock* on health. This argument has been supported by research. In America, Holmes and Rahe (1967) were able to demonstrate the detrimental influence of life changes on health and illustrated how various kinds of life changes strike people with different force. Brown and Birley (1968) in England found similar correlations between significant life changes and mental ill health.

Social processes are a threat to health in many respects, even if they were originally favourable. Steps are taken whenever feasible to limit these negative aspects as much as possible. There are installations to purify water and furnaces to destroy chemical waste. There are laws dealing with working conditions and an inspectorate to check up on whether they are being obeyed. Radio and television devote more and more attention to health guidance.

In addition to the above examples, there is also a reverse of the health care coin. Take the following example.

'The following side effects may occur: serious liver damage, sometimes with fatal consequences. Allergic reactions, mainly exanthema, nettle rash, malignant neutropenia (after long use) and a reduction in the number of platelets may also occur'.

The above description of side effects belongs to

paracetamol, a well-known cure for headache, toothache, influenza and fever. It is used in many of the well-known patent medicines on sale at any chemist's shop without prescription. Many people take this kind of medicine regularly and run the above risks. They are not very great, of course, otherwise the medicine would have been taken off the market long ago; it is certainly not the intention to denounce it here.

In fact, nearly all medicines have side effects. What we are concerned with here is the negative aspect of medicine. Apparently we, as a society, accept a certain risk to health simply to preserve that selfsame health.

The threat to health of health care itself is called *clinical iatrogenesis*. Clinical iatrogenesis does not only mean the side effects of medicines, but also mistakes made during treatment.

In addition to clinical iagrogenesis, there is another way in which health care may have a negative effect

Case study: KUP Limited

The KUP company in Birmingham makes parts for various domestic appliances. There is a great demand for them, and employees have to work very hard. Shopfloor workers are chivvied by supervisors keeping close checks on their output.

There is also a sophisticated reward system for achieving certain production targets. As a result, production has increased more than tenfold in recent years. The consequence is that there are really too many people and machines in too small an area. Moving to other premises is not being considered since it would be very expensive and a lot of money has been invested in new machinery in recent years.

At least half the current staff are temporary workers, usually recruited from agencies. Absenteeism among permanent staff is very high. The number of complaints is even greater than the number of people off sick. Visits to GPs and the use of household remedies is increasing alarmingly.

Figure 3.3.3
Medicines are there to cure us,
but there is always a risk of side effects

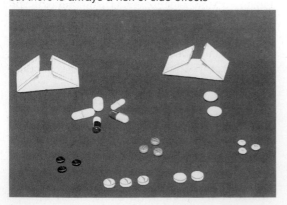

So what does Mr Bowman do if he works for this company and has a headache? He takes a pill and then goes off to work as usual. It is logical, since he would otherwise lose his extra pay for not achieving the targeted output, and taking sick leave would, in that way, prove expensive.

If the remedy does not help and the symptoms continue at home as well, he will probably visit his family doctor in the end. The latter will give him a prescription. If the symptoms continue, Mr Bowman will eventually be referred to a consultant. A similar tale could be told about Mrs Peterson, Ms Horton, Miss Newbury, etc. They all take patent medicines at first, then go to their family doctors and are finally referred to a consultant.

The question arising from this tale is how soon – if ever – 'treatment' will be given to the company rather than to the patient. The likelihood is not very great, particularly if the patent medicines or the doctor's prescription are effective for a while.

The health authorities often assure us that the patient comes first, and that is how health care is organized. The danger, however, is that the search for the cause will not extend beyond the patient. Even if the patient's background is taken into consideration, it is often impossible to do anything about it. This unhealthy aspect of health care is called *social iatrogenesis* – the situation whereby social factors or processes lead to ill health and sickness.

The underlying social inequalities and negative influences of poor housing, unemployment, faulty living habits, etc. referred to earlier in this chapter when the Black Report was discussed illustrate how concealed social factors may influence health. In other words this means that because the health service's practices and organization are designed to treat only the patients, there is a risk that health care conceals genuine problems.

Another interesting facet of the social iatrogenesis issue is the way in which society conjures up or constructs ill health classifications to explain and manage what are essentially social issues or problems. The argument here is not that social factors cause illness, but that often illness does not exist at all. It is, in fact, a myth concocted by society or its agents to control social problems. One of the most well known exponents of this type of argument is the American psychiatrist Thomas Szasz. In his now famous treatise on 'The Manufacture of Madness' (Szasz, 1971) he compares 20th century psychiatry with 17th century witchcraft. Society in the middle ages dealt with social behaviour it did not understand and viewed to be dysfunctional as witchcraft – those accused were tried and punished, often executed. In the 20th century, similar people are labelled as mentally ill by friends, disenchanted family or the community at large and incarcerated in mental institutions. Szasz was among the first to draw attention to the situation in the USSR during the post-war years, where those who dissented politically were confined to mental institutions and subjected to extreme treatments such as electric shock therapy.

On a wider plane, it has been suggested that today we are increasingly willing to recognise illness in ourselves. Ivan Illich (1977) an influential thinker in this area has claimed that we are increasingly prone to this because we have handed over responsibility for health to the medical profession. This, he argues, has led to a degree of medicalisation of social life. Doctors who have a vested interest in the medicine or ill health industry, lay claim to professional wisdom in dealing with many problems of a social or personal nature. It is in their vested interests to attach medical labels to these problems; suddenly these problems become illnesses. Homosexuality becomes sexual deviation or disorder, sleeplessness becomes insomnia, stress becomes neurosis and if we are a little fed up we run the risk of being labelled as suffering from depression.

The extent to which we succumb is, of course, to some degree, dependant on individual outlooks, as illustrated in the case of Jean Barlow and Ken Lee described above. However, often our family or close friends may attempt to deal with the difficulties we present to them by *labelling* us as ill and succeed in this despite resistance on our part. This labelling process is returned to again in the discussion on interaction theory below.

Study activities

6. Describe the conditions in which nurses have to work. If need be, interview colleagues who have been in the profession for some time.

7. Give an example of clinical iatrogenesis and one of social iatrogenesis; explain how, in each case, your examples may lead to ill-health.

4. Theoretical perspectives in sociology

We must now proceed to consider how sociological theory can give us insights into health and illness. It is important to recognize, however, that sociology does not adhere to a single perspective, shared by all social scientists in this field. Just like psychology, discussed in earlier chapters, it includes a number of perspectives. In-deed, some of these perspectives are vastly different from, and even incompatible with, each other!

It is not possible to refer in detail to these various perspectives here. However, it is possible, without losing accuracy through summarising, to group them into three broad sociological approaches or perspectives.

The first two sociological theories in essence belong to the same tradition. They concern themselves with how society as a whole or large social groups, nations or communities are structured and how they function. Although this *macro-sociology* approach has its origins in the work of the founding fathers of sociology – such as Comte (see Module 3 Chapter 1) – its broad title 'Structural–Functionalism' derives from United States sociology in the post-World War Two years. The seminal works in the first of these theoretical stances were those of Talcott Parsons (1951) and Robert Merton (1968). Both concerned themselves with issues of how society as a whole is structured, how it functions in terms of how its composite parts relate to each other in maintaining the overall social system and social order. In essence the concern is with how social consensus, which is 'functional' is maintained and how lack of consensus, which is 'dysfunctional' arises. It is, thus, essentially a *social order* or *consensus* theory.

The second theoretical stance within the macro-sociology or 'structural' tradition is also concerned with social structures and social order. However, here the similarity ends. Theorists in this perspective are concerned with structural – conflict rather than structural – functional issues. They see society as often being split in terms of the advantaged and the disadvantaged. Inequalities in terms of e.g. wealth or power, the dependence of the poor on the rich and the dominance and coercion of some social groups by others are the issues addressed in this perspective. Society is thus viewed in terms of *conflict* rather than *consensus* and some theorists in this tradition advocate values of egalitarianism and conflict reduction through major social change or revolution. Social order here is viewed as being dysfunctional rather than functional. Social order in fact involves socially constructed systems which maintain the status quo and protect those in power. The perspective finds its origins in the French revolution which influenced Karl Marx, the most famous theorist in this area (see, for example, Marx, selected writings in Bottomore and Rubel (1965) and Marx and Engels (1968)). It is essentially a *social conflict* theory.

The third sociological perspective differs significantly from the first two described above. One significant difference is that of scale. It is by definition a *micro-sociology* in that it is concerned with social interactions, social processes and how individuals experience their social worlds. Because it is concerned with understanding experiences, the terms *interpretive sociology* and *phenomenology* are sometimes used; because it is also concerned with interactions, it is also often termed *interactionist sociology* (the terms interaction theory and interactionism also being used). The concern here is with small groups and individual experiences. It is also concerned with how others with whom we interact influence our behaviour and how we act out social roles. George Herbert Mead (1934), to whom you were first introduced in Chapter 2 of this module, is one of the main influences in this perspective. Indeed, if you now scan Chapter 2 again, you will note the similarities between the micro-sociology introduced here and the social psychology perspective which is dominant in Chapter 2. Both disciplines share much in common and there is considerable overlap in subject matter and terminology. Indeed, the difference is difficult to discern and mainly rests on the fact that social psychology addresses *how groups function* and how the group *influences* the individual while interactionist sociology is concerned with the *social processes themselves* and how individuals *experience* their social worlds. While terminology varies in this perspective the terms *'social action'* or *'interactionist'* theory are common and will be used here.

There are thus three broad theoretical perspectives in all, that is:

(i)   Consensus theory   (both being structur
(ii) Conflict theory   }   alist perspectives)
(iii) Interactionist theory   (being a social
                              action perspective)

We will now proceed to consider how these theoretical perspectives can inform our understanding of health, illness and care.

As mentioned in the introduction, we are considering three sociological theories. They are firstly general theories on the way we associate with one another in the community. The concept of sickness can also be viewed from that angle. In the following three sections the theoretical aspects will be considered first, then the concept of sickness, and finally the role of health care agencies.

It is important first to refer back to two matters. Firstly the comment that was made about the holistic definition of health. In the following sections we take a sociogenetic approach, which means that the concept of sickness is explained from the point of view of social functioning. But somatic and psychological functioning is not denied; nor is the fact that the cause of sickness may also lie in those two areas. A second point to be borne in mind is that the point of departure is not practical but theoretical. Theories try to explain a great deal in this way and are often very abstract and vague. There is often more than one explanation for concrete examples.

5. The consensus theory

The first sociological theory to be considered here is the *consensus theory*. As indicated above, this is a theory within that sociological tradition which is concerned with the structure of society as a whole and the function of social systems within society. You will recall that it was described as a structural – functionalist or social order theory.

Culture and socialization are key concepts in consensus theory. In the sense suggested here, culture consists of:

– *Knowledge*, i.e. ideas, beliefs, symbols (language) and values related to those ideas and beliefs shared by a society;
– *Social rules*, also known as institutions or norms, i.e. the *folkways* (weaker rules generally applied) and *mores* (stronger rules or customs insisted upon) which are held by that society, and some of which in modern societies – whether these be folkways or mores – are formulated into laws and become legal requirements;
– *Artifacts*, i.e. social or man-made objects – ranging from eating implements, to books, to means of transport, to buildings such as banks, churches, and colleges of nursing – within and with which the society functions and lives from day to day.

Still within this line of thought, socialization is the process by which new members of the society, whether they be new infants or those entering the society from outside, learn this culture.

There are two points worth keeping in mind here. The first of these relates to the view of socialization shared by the consensus theorists. You will recall that we previously addressed socialization in Chapter 1 of Module 3 from a social psychological perspective. There you were first introduced to the idea of norms as folkways and mores. Indeed, the above explanation of culture is taken from the work of Sumner (1906) who first popularized these terms. However, in Chapter 1 the social psychologists and micro-sociologists were concerned primarily with the overall processes of socialization. The consensus theorists are concerned primarily with how socialization and learning the society's norms maintain, protect and promulgate a society's values and social order. The second point applies also to the other theoretical perspectives which will be discussed later. This is to draw attention to the fact that the theory is an approach to giving meaning to our social world. While it is discussed as though it is the only valid source of understanding our social situation, it is important to remember that there are alternative and in some cases conflicting explanations.

a. Order in society

The term consensus means agreement, and that is the basis on which the consensus theory is constructed. According to this theory, society has a number of general values which are accepted by everyone. These occur alongside the differences within society which occur in many areas. These general values ensure that a certain amount of order is preserved within a society. If these values did not exist, various people or groups would scarcely be able to associate with one another, or could not do so at all. The likelihood of chaos and disorder in society would be very great.

One example is the fact that the authorities administer the law. We accept that if we are involved in a serious conflict, the courts will give a verdict on the matter. We usually accept such a verdict.

Study activity

8. Check whether you can indicate a number of norms and values which you think are accepted by large sections of the community.

The existence of different norms is not denied by this theory, but interest is focused on what people have in common. In the context of this section, one general value is especially important, i.e. the value concerning work. The idea that we must work, or make a productive contribution, is accepted by most people.

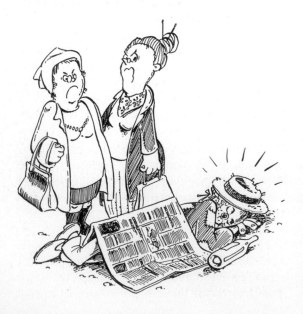

Working in any manner is regarded as normal behaviour, and not working is therefore considered to be a departure from the existing values. Such deviance, however, is accepted in a number of circumstances, e.g. when someone is studying: it is generally accepted that a person is relieved of a duty to work for the duration of a course of studies. It may also happen that someone is looking for work: if a person's willingness to work is evident from job applications, the fact that he or she is not currently working is accepted. That kind of person is therefore not treated as being 'deviant'. In other words: if someone does not come up to people's main expectations (in this case in respect of working), he or she will certainly have to satisfy certain conditions. Studying and looking for work have been mentioned already, but sickness is another frequently occurring circumstance which is accepted as overriding the requirement to work. If people are ill, they are relieved of their duty to work.

If you think in terms of roles, you are expected to assume the role of a working person. If you do not, this will only be accepted if one of a number of other roles is assumed, e.g. the student role, the role of a person looking for work, or the role of a patient .

Before going on to the next subsection, we must first take another look at order in society. The question of how such order is achieved will be asked in the case of the consensus theory and also the conflict and interactionist theories. The three theories give different answers to the question. It would therefore be useful to make a special note of this question alongside the possible answers to it.

Why is there a certain order in society?
The answer according to the consensus theory would be, *'Because, in the final analysis, the members of society share a number of identical values'.*

b. Sickness according to the consensus theory

Case study: Mr Bolger

Mr Bolger is head of the Maintenance Department of a medium-sized hospital. He is a rather boisterous person who works hard and has many friends in the hospital. Most of his colleagues find it easy to get on with him. He is fond of a joke, but not at the expense of other people.

Last week he suddenly felt a stab of pain in his back while he was at work, and after that he kept on having back aches. He continued to come to work for the first few days; his reluctance to stay at home was quite true to character. He was obliged, however, to pass on several jobs to other people. He was also less cheerful than usual. Various people had already advised him a few times to go home. Only when the staff medical officer diagnosed a slight hernia did Mr Bolger give in and report sick.

Several of his colleagues visited him at his home and met a Mr Bolger who was quite different from the one they knew. Instead of being cheerful, he was was rather gloomy and, though they did not like to admit it, almost querulous. He was allowing people to wait on him even when he could have done something himself.

Being sick may be seen as assuming a role. The role is assumed because a different role cannot be performed. In the above example Mr Bolger thus exchanged his role as a hospital worker for the patient's role. Different demands are made of each role and, in this particular example, the two different roles lead to different behaviour. This brings us to a very important point if we are looking at the concept of sickness according to the consensus theory. The emphasis, in fact, is on the behaviour and not on the complaint. It is usually assumed that you are sick, or assuming the sick role, if you have some kind of a complaint. According to the consensus theory, you assume *the sick role,* along with the appropriate behaviour, if you can no longer function normally.

As explained by Talcott Parsons (1966) in his now famous essay entitled 'On Becoming a Patient', once an individual is defined as being sick he has the *rights* and *obligations* of the 'sick role'. That is, the right to be exempted from normal social role responsibilities, the right to be taken care of, the obligation to want to get better and the obligation to seek expert help. The consensus theory provides the following definition for sickness:

– Sickness, according to the consensus theory, is a reaction to a disturbance of the normal functions of the total human individual; this refers to the condition of the organism as a biological system as well as to its personal and social adjustment.

Assuming a sick role, according to this definition, is therefore no longer linked automatically to a physical complaint, which may or may not play a part. Research carried out in 1971 by Wadsworth, Butterfield and Blaney may serve as an illustration (diagram 3.3.1). The researchers asked 2,153 people whether they had had any physical complaints during the past fortnight. Only 104 (4.9%) said they had had none at all. The most frequent complaints were:

– shortness of breath
– tiredness;
– rheumatic complaints;
– digestive complaints;
– skin complaints.

Complaint of group	Visited a doctor *	Away from work *	Bed rest *	Asked non-medical advice *	Medically prescribed medication *	Non-medically prescribed medication *
Respiratory	4.1	3.0	1.0	0.6	13.0	21.1
Tiredness, worries, etc.	3.7	1.7	0.8	0.3	11.1	19.0
Rheumatic	5.1	1.6	1.0	0.1	16.4	29.8
Digestive	4.2	1.5	1.4	1.4	13.6	36.1
Skin complaints	5.0	2.2	1.2	0.8	17.7	50.4

* During the past 14 days

Diagram 3.3.1
The treatment of the five commonest groups of symptoms expressed as a percentage of all the symptoms in the group

Source: Wadsworth et. al. (1971)

Of the total group 19% had not taken any action. The rest had either been to their family doctors, taken patent medicines, stayed in bed or combined several of these courses of action.

Your first reaction may be that the above 19% probably had less serious complaints. This research, however, showed that the seriousness of the complaint did not provide an adequate explanation for assuming the sick role.

This makes it important to take another look at the concept of a sick role. We first establish what rights and duties are associated with this role. Then we find out whether there are factors which indicate whether an individual is more, or less, inclined to assume a sick role.

Study activity
9. Before reading the following paragraphs, try to express what you mean by a sick role.

If being ill is linked to behaviour, as in the consensus theory, it is possible to speak of assuming a role. There has been a substantial amount of research regarding the behaviour that goes with this role. One thing that became evident was that the duration of the illness was an important factor. The following are a few of the rights and duties about which there is general agreement.

– People are relieved of their normal daily duties.
– People are relieved of responsibility for the sickness. This means that care is transferred to someone else.
– The patient is expected to regard his condition as undesirable. Everyone sighs on occasion, 'If only I could be slightly ill for a week', just 'slightly' ill, so that it is possible to be away from the bustle of everyday life for a little while, without feeling really ill. If you are genuinely sick, it is more difficult to say to other people that you are glad to be relieved of your everyday responsibilities for a little while.

– The patient must seek expert help. This applies even more if the illness lasts for some time. If you stay at home for some time when you are ill, there will be increasing pressure from those around you, including your employer, to call in a doctor. In the case of a very short illness, you are sometimes left to judge for yourself.

The various characteristics, or rights and duties, are not the same in all instances. It has been mentioned already that the duration of the illness may play a part, and so may the apparent seriousness and visibility of the complaint. If your legs are in plaster, the sick role is accepted by you yourself and those around without any hesitation. Nervous exhaustion is harder to accept.

Study activity
10. The Mr Bolger mentioned at the beginning of the subsection is suffering from back trouble. Indicate a few domestic chores which one would not normally take on in those circumstances.

Apart from the duration of the sickness, it is also possible to find out whether there are other factors which lead to the assumption of a sick role.
Research has identified the following factors (in order of importance):
– overcoming financial or social obstacles. This means that people assume a sick role more readily if it costs less. The 'cost' may be expressed in terms of money but also in terms of the amount of effort that is required;
– the seriousness of the complaint and people's upbringing;
– gender;
– education and age.

The factor mentioned first may be either financial or social. If your income depends on the amount of work you produce, you will be less inclined to assume a sick role. Your relationship with your family doctor might provide an example of social effort. If that relationship is not very good, it will require more effort to visit him and therefore more effort to assume a sick role.

The seriousness of the complaint is an obvious factor and it is surprising that it did not come first. Upbringing plays a more complex part. The research showed that people with a more traditional approach to illness were more inclined to adopt a sick role. Traditional is used here in the sense that health and sickness are viewed as something over which you yourself have no control.
If you consider yourself responsible for your own body, you will be less inclined to assume a sick role.

The research also showed that gender played an important part. Women, on the whole, are more inclined to assume a sick role than men. The level of education was also significant. The higher it was, the less inclined people were to assume the sick role.

Study activity
11. Try to explain why gender and the level of education appear to play a part in the assumption of a sick role.

Age was mentioned last of all. In general, willingness to assume a sick role increases with age.

To recapitulate, we may say that according to the consensus theory being ill means assuming a sick role. The sick role is assumed because it is impossible to meet the requirements of a different role which rests on a basic value. The basic value relates to work.

The seriousness of the symptoms affects the assumption of the sick role but is not the most important factor, and certainly not the only one. Finally, certain rights and duties are associated with the sick role.

c. The role of health care

In view of the above, we may say that, according to the consensus theory, society makes certain demands on its members. Such demands are based on generally accepted norms and values. Release from those obligations is allowed on certain conditions only. Assuming the sick role is one of the possibilities.

We may wonder, in this context, what kind of position health care occupies in all this. The consensus theory regards health care mainly as a control mechanism. This implies that those who provide health care have a duty to help (or indeed to coerce) anyone who has assumed the sick role to abandon it as soon as possible, and also to check whether a person has rightly assumed the sick role. You are therefore not genuinely sick unless the doctor agrees that you are.

It is important to realize that these comments apply to the entire area of health care. It is not only the consultant who decides whether or not you may assume or retain the sick role, but general practitioners and nurses also contribute to that decision. Imagine a patient who tells you, a nurse, about some physical symptoms. Whether you pass on what he has told you will depend on your assessment. Such an assessment of the symptoms may have some connection with the reason why the patient was admitted to hospital and in this case you will probably pass on the information. If, however, you think the patient is a person who complains a lot and who may just be making a fuss, it is not very likely that you will pass on his grumbles. In this way you decide whether you will allow the complaints to become part of the patient's sick role.

Study activity
12. How do you think health guidance is regarded from the point of view of the consensus theory?

6. The conflict theory

The second sociological theory to be considered is the *conflict theory*. This, too, is an abstract theory. Much of what is said about it will be familiar to anyone who has studied communist ideology. It may seem rather other-worldly to those who have not done so. The somewhat extreme terminology generally seems strange to our culture and also now outdated in the face of the rapid collapse of the communist system of government throughout most of the world.

While consensus theory emphasises social order and maintenance of the social status quo, conflict theory points – sometimes rather uncomfortably – at inequalities in society, structures of advantage and disadvantage and relationships of domination and subordination.

There are different perpectives within the conflict theory.

The most well known is, of course, Marxist theory. Marx and Engels (1968) argued that society is stratified into classes according to the distribution of capital or the means of production. There are the owners of capital who arc a small, powerful group (Marxists describe them as *'the bourgeoisie'*) and a more numerous mass who do not possess capital and whose only contribution is labour (Marxists describe these as *'the prolitariat'*). It may be suggested that workers, having control over the labour they supply, have significant power. However, it must be remembered that it is difficult if not impossible for workers to withold labour, as they must eat and survive at the end of the day. Students may remember the example of the British coal miners strike in the 1980s, when lack of money and other influences such as political and legal pressures and confrontation with the police led to eventual failure. In modern day life it is common to classify in terms of social status (e.g. upper, middle and lower or working class) or occupational status (e.g. in the UK we identify five social classes from 1, the professions through to 5, unskilled occupations).

Before proceeding to consider conflict theory in relation to social order, sickness and health care, there are two additional points which should be noted. Firstly, Marxist theory is often more than a sociological theory. It is also a political ideology, a justification for revolution and resolution of inequality and conflict as in the case of communism referred to above. As was indicated at Section 4 of this chapter it was, after all, a theory arising from the influences of the French revolution. However, this is not always the case and many Marxist sociologists see this theory as a means of understanding society and *not* as a plan for social action.

Secondly, Marxist theory and conflict theory are not synonymous. Marxist theory is just one theoretical approach within the conflict perpective. For example, Max Weber (1948) – see

Gerth and Mills (1948) – a prolific sociologist, who also wrote in the social action perpective (see page 264) considered sources of inequality other than capital. He suggested other social influences such as *caste* – where people are divided into strata on the basis of status differences based on religious, social or racial barriers. The prime, though not the only example, is society in the Indian sub-continent. A second example is the perspective of some structural-functionalist sociologists, such as Davis and Moore (1945) who saw society as being divided in terms of merit, prestige and esteem. According to this approach inequality has a positive social function. That is, some more able people – a meritocracy or elite minority – are destined to be the ruling minority, and this is a general pattern in all societies Such ideas orginate from writings such as those of the Italian, Mosca (1939), who in his work 'The Ruling Class' suggested that the tendency for a small influential group to rule is a constant tendency in all cultures. The influence wielded may be in relation to military valour, religious standing, political ability, or whatever is adjudged important in a particular society at a particular time. The tendency for minority elitist rule is a constant. Mosca's writings in the period leading up to and including the 1930s has often been identified as a theoretical rationale adopted by fascism in Germany and Italy. Mosca himself did not, however, identify himself with such movements.

Study activity

13. The common example of Indian society as a caste system is given above. But consider the racial divides in South Africa and the religious divides in Northern Ireland. Do you think class, or caste, or a mixture of the two best describes the social disharmony in these societies? Do some background reading in the sociological literature on caste and class to inform your judgement.

a. Order in society

Study activity

14. The term conflict is an important concept in this theory. What do you think of when you hear this word? Has it a positive or a negative value? Give reasons for your answer.

The term conflict has a negative sound to many people. It usually makes one think of quarrels or worse. The supporters of the confict theory view the matter differently: to them, conflict equals change. It is the creative force out of which renewal and improvements in society may arise. To the supporters of the conflict theory, the concept of conflict thus has a positive sound: conflict is desirable. Another concept that plays a central role in the conflict theory is the concept of power. The difference in power is the source from which the conflicts arise.

If you think of the concept of conflict, it is understandable that the conflict theory is all about change rather than stability. The theory consequently has its problems when it comes to the subject of order in society, in the sense that order does not really exist and is furthermore undesirable. That is, society is viewed as not really being in a state of order. In fact the majority of its members are being oppressed by actual or potential social constraints. Society is *really* in a state of conflict and ideally a state of social conflict (perhaps even revolution) to overcome this oppression may be necessary. Various authors have written about the view of society that goes with the conflict theory. Consider, for example, Marx's Communist Manifesto (Marx and Engels, 1968).

In the conflict situation, the concept of alienation is linked to the production process. The domination of workers by those with most power alienates the oppressed from the work that they are doing. People are not given an opportunity to join in discussions and deliberations concerning the whole process, so that satisfaction about the work produced by them is lacking. A worker in a car factory therefore cannot say, 'I made that car', and feel pleased about that. The part that one contributes to the whole production process is too small to give one a sense of satisfaction about one's achievements.

Study activity

15. You have been dealing with a patient from

admission to discharge and did most of the nursing. Can you regard yourself as the person responsible for his or her recovery? Give reasons for your answer, drawing from the literature on *primary nursing*.

Because of people's alienation from the work that they do, they ultimately become alienated from themselves, according to the conflict theory. It is therefore not merely a matter of dissatisfaction, their sense of self-respect diminishes as well. It is important to remember that this *felt* disadvantage is usually accompanied by real, material disadvantage. It will be recalled that a basic tenet in the social class theme is that wealth is unequally distributed in society. Thus, people do not only feel disadvantaged, they actually are disadvantaged in that they may have less money, poor housing, inadequate clothing and diet, etc. In a large-scale study in the UK, Townsend (1979) estimated that over half the population in Britain may experience relative deprivation or poverty at some stage in their lives. By this he meant that people felt (and were) disadvantaged in relation to norms or accepted standards (for example, having meat at least once per week or adequate heating in the winter). The problem is, that there is much disagreement about poverty. For example, politicians motivated by a consensus theory approach suggest that social scientists such as Townsend are unrealistic and are just scare-mongering.

Study activity
16. The next time you are in the coffee bar or pub with your friends put the following premise to them. Poverty is not just about having so little money for food that you are starving. Being unable to afford to send Christmas cards is poverty. If the discussion lags, stimulate debate with statements as:
    – If the unemployed stopped smoking and drinking they would have enough money for food, or
    – lack of money for home heating in winter is an exaggeration – if the unemployed and eldery wrapped up warmer and took exercise they would not need so much heating fuel.

Listen to your friend's views and compare them with your own and those of Townsend (ibid).

To return to order in society: in spite of the theory's problems on the subject of order, the following is an attempt to provide an answer, so that it will be easier to compare the various theories.
Why is there a certain order in society?
The answer according to the conflict theory would be, '*In fact there is no order. There is an apparent order in the more or less open conflicts between opposing interests*'.

b. Sickness according to the conflict theory

The conflict theory is concerned with differences in power. It is usual to talk about the exploiters and the oppressed. The exploiters have most power and dominate the oppressed by coercion.

The distinction between the two groups is important, since the conflict theory therefore has two sickness theories instead of one. One of them is based on the exploiters, and the other on the oppressed.

Like all contrasts in the conflict theory, the two sickness concepts are in conflict with each other. The sickness concept based on the oppressed will be dealt with in this subsection, and the sickness concept based on the exploiters in the subsection on health care. The classification is linked to the fact that the conflict theory regards health care as the tool of people with most power.

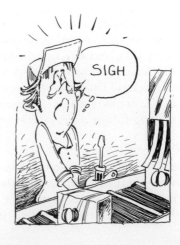

Study activity

17. Take another look at the case of the company in Birmingham in Section 3.

    Explain the illnesses of Mr Bowman and his colleagues in terms of the conflict theory.

As indicated above, conflict theory is concerned with differences in power. One power differential, and that central to Marxist conflict theory, is based on the unequal distribution of capital or wealth. The implications of being poor – as are the lower paid, the unemployed and many of the elderly population – in regard to health and sickness must not be overlooked here. You will recall the brief discussion of the Black Report at Section 3 above. This highlighted how poverty and its travelling companions – poor housing, lack of adequate diet, overcrowding, poor sanitation, ignorance, etc. – were important determinants of health and disease. It is still the case in Britain that infant mortality (i.e. infant death rates), general mortality and morbidity (i.e. incidence of diseases) are higher in the lower classes as defined by occupational status. The conflict theory would thus claim that the unequal distribution of wealth and the consensus status quo which maintains this adds to the litany of disadvantages of the working classes or proletariat. To these disadvantages (i.e. poverty, ignorance etc.) is added the disadvantages of ill health and shorter life-span.

c. The role of health care

We now come to the second sickness concept according to the conflict theory, i.e. the concept of sickness in terms of the exploiters. When an employee becomes ill it will be evident that medicines, surgery and other treatments may improve the patient's health. However the main object is to return the patient to the production process as quickly as possible, so that the exploiters can benefit again from the employee's labour.

In this way, health care becomes an important control mechanism, an idea that we also came across when considering the consensus theory. There is, however, a major difference. According to the consensus theory, being ill is an accepted role. It is in the interest of society as well as the patient to preserve this role. In the conflict theory, the role is viewed by the exploiters as being dysfunctional and a burden on society.

The comments above relate primarily to the exploiters' reaction to ill health and sickness. However, the issue of prevention of ill health and health promotion is also an important consideration. Public health and prevention of ill health has traditionally been an initiative originating in the upper classes and directed toward the welfare of the lower classes. A consensus theory view would see this as an altruistic, welfare-orientated motive. However, conflict theorists would take a different view. Public health actions such as sanitation reforms in the 19th century to stamp out cholera and immunisation against tuberculosis in the 20th century may have been motivated as much by fear as by humanitarianism. There was the risk of these diseases breaking out of the slums and into the homes of the rich if action was not taken. And there was a need, as indicated above, to protect for capitalism the labour so vital to the production of wealth. Thus, to the motive of maintaining a healthy and profitable work force, can be added a second motive, i.e. protecting the rich themselves from diseases spreading from the poor.

Study activity

18. It has been suggested that one form of inequality in society relates to ignorance about health matters. According to conflict theory, if this holds true, working class people would not eat a healthy diet, would indulge in more smoking and alcohol and would make less use of preventative measures such as cervical screening. According to consensus theory, maintenance of social order through welfare means that there is more health education and facilities provided for people to maintain good health. Which of the theories holds true in your town or locality? List your points of evidence in support of each theory and discuss them with your fellow students.

7. Interactionist theory

The third sociological theory to be considered is interactionist theory. As opposed to consensus theory, interactionist theory is not based on generally accepted fundamental values. Indeed, it is not primarily concerned with such issues. Its prime interest is in social interaction and in particular in the reciprocal influences of the social actions of individuals on each other. According to this perspective each situation is unique and dependant on the definition of the situation by the actors involved in it.

As will be recalled from Section 4, this is in essence a social action theory. In this context Max Weber (1978) one of the originators of this theoretical perpective, suggested that social happenings or actions are given subjective meaning by those who act out these happenings. Mead (1934), whose work was also referred to in Section 4, stressed that our understanding of the social world around us and thus how we ourselves behave within it is taken from others with whom we interact. This is particularly the case with 'relevant others' i.e. people who are highly important to the individual. Mead's now-famous term *'taking the role of the other'* was used to draw attention to how our roles are not static, rule bound 'givens', as suggested by the consensus theorists but dynamic and unique phenomena constructed out of social actions. In simple terms, this is all about seeing yourself as you are seen by others and acting accordingly, in effect, behaving as you think you are expected to behave, or being influenced by others.

As individuals interact with others, they take in, develop and share with them symbols or conventional meanings of the social world. Some interactionist sociologists are primarily concerned with this shared meaning and are known as *symbolic interactionists*. They are concerned with knowledge and how it is developed and constructed (i.e. reified) by the social group (see, for example, Goffman, 1968 and Blumer, 1969).

Study activity

19. Consider the nurses in the wards in your hospital. Do they all act out their roles the same in every ward or does the role of, say, the staff nurse vary from ward to ward? If the roles do vary, try to ascertain the extent to which this is a function of social interactions. In particular try to identify relevant others who may be influential on how the staff nurse role is acted out in each setting.

Here again, it is important not to forget that we are concerned with a theory. The consequence is that the examples are sometimes open to more than one interpretation. Furthermore, just as in the case of the consensus theory, the theory is described as if it had a monopoly on the truth. This, of course, is not usually the case.

a. Order in society

Interactionist theory is not based on common values and norms. According to the interactionist theory, human society is based on human interaction.

In Chapter 1, of this module, the concept of *interaction* was defined as people's influence upon one another.
According to interactionist theory, this kind of reciprocal influence forms the basis of human thought and action.

Figure 3.3.4
A ward round

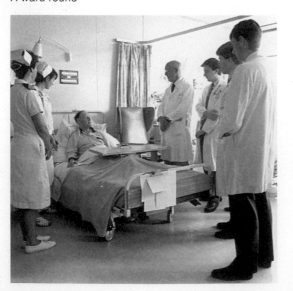

Interaction is also viewed as a process, in which how we act in any situation is determined by our interpretations of each other's expectations and behaviour.

For example, if I hold up my right hand, that is objectively observable behaviour. But the person facing me will react according to his interpretation of such behaviour. He might regard the raised hand as a greeting or as the beginning of a blow, and his own behaviour will be based on that interpretation.

Apart from interaction and its allied concepts, interactionist theory has another basic concept, i.e. *the self*. This self – and in everyday speech this comes closest to the idea of self-image – is the interpretation of oneself. In interactionist theory, this may be defined in the following way:
– Everyone has an image of himself or herself, the self. This is formed above all by the image which you think other people have of you. Therefore the self is formed mainly by others.

Study activity
20. Mention a number of people, from your own environment or far beyond it (e.g. famous personalities) who in some way or other influence you, or have influenced you.

An interesting demonstration of the formation of the self is taken from an experiment by E.R. Guthrie (1938).

A small group of students at an American university agreed on the following course of action for research purposes. They would treat a certain girl, who was usually thought to be shy and awkward, as though she were popular. They made sure that she was invited to all kinds of campus events, and that she was always surrounded by admirers. Before a year had passed, she had developed a more relaxed manner, and was quite convinced herself that she was popular. Even when the experiment ended and the students should have stopped their agreed approach, her attitude remained, as did her social popularity. The students taking part, and others as well, had accepted her as popular and continued to treat her as such. What her future at the university would have been without the experiment is hard to say. She would probably have scaled down any social ambitions and developed interests that were more in keeping with her awkwardness.

The description of human interaction and the self show that behaviour patterns are not fixed. It is clear that behaviour which has been displayed once, does not continue to exist by itself; its continuation depends on confirmation by other people. Behaviour patterns, but also norms and values, are constantly in motion; they change or continue depending on the environment.

Finally, there is a third concept which plays an important part in interactionist theory, i.e. *joint actions*. They concern the behaviour *patterns* of groups of people. To give an example: members of a class of students develop a certain type of behaviour towards one another, in public as well as in private. Teachers will therefore experience the group quite differently from the way they do other groups, and they will adapt their own

Figure 3.3.5
The self-image is formed
in contacts with
other people

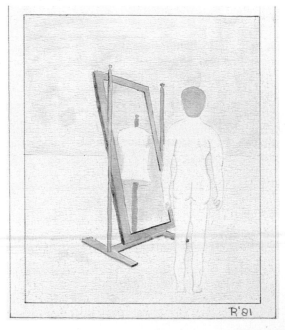

behaviour to it. Joint actions are formed by the accumulation of the interactions between the individuals in the group. Society as a whole is also a group. The way in which society as a whole behaves towards groups in society is also a joint action .

With the aid of the above concepts we can take a look at the key question asked in the case of each theory:
Why is there a certain order in society?
The answer according to the interactionis theory would be, *'Coexistence is possible because, by acting creatively, people to some extent adjust their behaviour to one another. A certain order and regularity in action patterns is thus created (joint actions). Such order, however, is a constructive and certainly not a self-evident order; behaviour patterns must be maintained and may, in principle, be replaced by other behaviour patterns'.*

b. Sickness according to the interactionist theory

Case study: sickness behaviour
For years I have occasionally suffered from sinusitis. I am prescribed antibiotics and it usually clears up in a week. Sinusitis produces various symptoms. One of them is a slight pain when the side of the nasal bone is pressed. This action and the reaction of pain is used by many general practitioners in their diagnosis, but I have never been troubled by that kind of sensitive spot. When I had to visit a different doctor, for some reason he first wanted to take X-rays. That had never been done before and I thought it was rather unnecessary. The doctor, however, was insistent and I was refused antibiotics until the X-rays had been taken.

Next time, and again there happened to be a different doctor, more X-rays were required. Since then I have adopted a different approach. Whenever I have sinusitis and the doctor presses my nose, I groan softly but audibly. No more X-rays have been taken since then and I get my antibiotics immediately.

This anecdote reaches the crux of sickness and

sickness behaviour as viewed by interactionist theory:

If certain symptoms occur, people start behaving in a particular way because it is called sickness (not because it is sickness). People as it were create sickness behaviour because they behave in a certain manner.

Study activity
21. What kind of sickness behaviour would you expect from:
    - a man of fifty-five troubled by serious headaches ;
    - a woman of thirty-five with cancer;
    - an elderly person with a fractured hip?

According to interactionist theory, sickness behaviour is a subjective concept. The objective element, the symptoms, is not, however, denied. A broken leg is a broken leg, even according to interactionist theory. The behaviour of someone with a broken leg, however, is subjective. In practice it is rarely possible to make a clear distinction between the objective complaint and the subjective behaviour.

As will be recalled in Section 5 on consensus theory, the sick role has a clear status and has explicitly laid-down rules of behaviour. You may find it helpful to refer back to Parsons' (1966) presentations of the two sets of rights and two sets of obligations essential to this role (see page 258). The interactionists take an entirely different point of view. They see the sick role as developing out of interactions between patients and carers, and patients and patients. One illustrative example is Goffman's (1968) celebrated study of asylums. He demonstrated how patients and staff negotiated living patterns in mental institutions and how an almost secret underlife existed, whereby, seemingly mute mental patients interacted with other patients to gain daily living advantages. A second example is Julius Roth's (1971) equally celebrated study of the sick role as a bargaining process. He found that while at first it may appear that patients are passive and co-operative (in line with the sick role in consensus theory) there is in fact a lot of interaction which goes on between, for example,

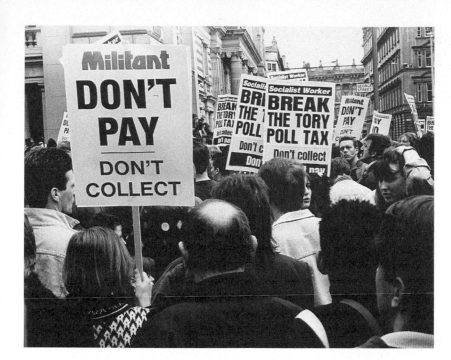

Figure 3.3.6
A joint action

patients and nurses, patients and patients, and patients and visitors. Roth found patients actively attempted to control and manipulate their situations by negotiating extra medication from nurses, bargaining for food outside of their prescribed diet from other patients or visitors and faking or exaggerating symptoms to gain preferential treatment.

It is clear from this that nurses cannot assume that their patients adhere to a static co-operative role and clearly laid down behaviours. A deeper understanding of how the patient feels and sees his position is essential in the nurse/patient relationship. In Mead's terminology, discussed above, this means the nurse being able to 'take the role of the other' – in this case the 'other' being the patient. In our professional vocabulary we describe this as having 'empathy'. It is only by having this insight into the patient that we can interact effectively with him.

c. The role of health care

Health care agencies feature twice in the creation of sickness or sick behaviour. Firstly, the individual members such as nurses and doctors contribute to the creation of sick behaviour through interaction with the patient. Secondly, the health care 'community' as a whole plays a part in the form of joint actions. There are generally agreed and accepted expectations concerning behaviour in the case of various complaints.

Study activity

22. Look at the descriptions of behaviour in the previous study task and compare them with the descriptions of other students in your class. Establish whether there are similarities relating to the expected behaviour. Remember that to the extent that you all share cognitions or views about sick behaviour, you will all probably share ways of behaving (i.e. joint actions) toward patients exhibiting such 'complaints'.

Interaction has been described as mutual influence, which means that sickness behaviour is not created by health care workers alone. Patients (as a group) also make sure, through their joint actions, that their generally agreed expectations of how doctors, nurses etc. should

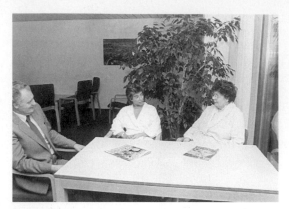

Figure 3.3.7
Who is the patient and
who are the visitors?

behave are conveyed to (and thus influence the behaviour of) these health care workers. The anecdote in the previous subsection provides a single-case illustration: the person learnt to groan at the right moment when he was being examined. The doctors' view that this was an essential symptom and indicative of sinusitis meant that the patient's goal i.e. to be diagnosed as having sinusitis, was achieved.

Diagram 3.3.2 shows the results of research carried out in USA (Bakwin, 1945). 1000 New York children aged eleven were examined. The first column shows that 611 of the children had already had their tonsils removed. The remaining 389 were examined by a group of doctors who were ignorant of the research. They decided in the case of 174 children that their tonsils should be removed. The remaining 215 were examined by a fresh group of doctors. Column three shows that 99 of those children were diagnosed as requiring tonsillectomy. Even in the third examination of the remaining children, the same advice was given in a number of instances. In the end there were only 63 children left in whose cases the doctors had not recommended surgery. The research was then terminated. The reason was that no further group of New York doctors could be found. Otherwise it is likely some of those 63 children would have been advised to have a tonsillectomy.

The research shows that the line between the objective complaint and the subjective behaviour is not always clear-cut. As appears from examinations 2 and 3, the tonsils of a great many children were considered unhealthy even though they has been declared healthy in the

Diagram 3.3.2
Theoretical
survival rate
of tonsils after
three medical
examinations

Source:
H. Bakwin (1945)

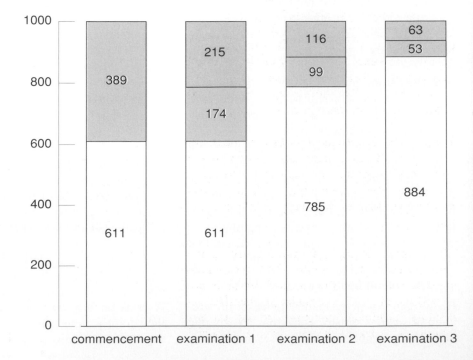

first examination. The research shows that subjective interpretation plays an important part in diagnostics.

These subjective opinions make it possible for the interaction between doctor and patient to play a part. The examination then constitutes confirmation that the interaction between, for example, doctor and patient may create sickness or sickness behaviour. As for the research programme, it should be borne in mind that it took place in 1945 and medical diagnosis has greatly improved since then! In spite of improvements, however, the 'clinical impression', or subjective judgment, continues to play an important part in diagnosis.

Study activity
23. Imagine that you are ill, not seriously, but you are unable to work. Your GP says it is all right for you to go out of doors. How likely is it that you will go and sit out in the sunshine in front of the hospital or nursing college?
    Give reasons for your answer.

8. Summary

In the above sections, the concept of sickness has been considered from the point of view of the social environment. Social factors form part of the concept of health. Health is linked to the balance between somatic, psychological and social factors. This is called the sociopsychosomatic balance. This holistic approach regards sickness as an interference in that balance.

The balance between the three factors and therefore their influence upon one another has a number of important consequences. The question arises why some people are ill and others carry on working even if their complaint is the same.

The purpose of the definition according the equilibrium model is to look a little beyond the somatic complaint. The somatic illness is not denied but placed in a broader perspective, especially a sociogenetic one in the present module. This means that the focus is on social

factors and that their effect on the psyche and somatics is considered.

The first topics to be considered from this angle were various social processes which might have an adverse effect on health. As a rule they are intended primarily as positive contributions to society, but they may also have adverse consequences in the areas of environment, working conditions, and social climate.

Theories provide a second basis for the sociogenetic point of view. Three sociological theories were discussed, i.e. consensus theory, conflict theory and interactionist theory. All three are theories which try to explain order or meaning in society.

4

Community, family and health

1. Introduction

In the previous chapter we considered sickness and health as social concepts and addressed these issues from the point of view of major theoretical perspectives in sociology. You will also recall that in Chapter 1 we considered socialization and how individuals learn the 'culture' of their society and the norms or expected patterns of behaviours within that society.

It is important to remember that our day-to-day social behaviour, and the norms of social conduct we adhere to, occur within particular social frames or social structures. Sociology was, after all, described in Chapter 1 as a discipline concerned with the study of human society (i.e. people together, rather than the individual case) and of human social behaviour (i.e. behaviour between individuals, or at least behaviour which takes cognizance of, or is influenced by, others).

This begs a fundamental question. That is: how *do* people exist 'together' in society? In the previous chapters of this module, we discussed some ways in which people can be grouped 'together'. There is of course the all-embracing but rather unclear concept of 'a society'. Even this term is not blessed with unambiguity. Most sociologists use it to describe the totality of people in a major geographical area, such as a nation-state or country. But when we hear people use terms like West Indian society, or Boston society, or high society, we know that the term is rather vague. We in fact can only be sure of what someone means if we note the context within which the word is being used. Other social groupings defined with a little more precision were those of class and caste.

All of the above social groupings exist at a macro-social level i.e. they are ways of considering how people in a country or society as a whole are classified or grouped together. Because they are large scale (as in the idea of society) or relate to the classification of society into major categories (as in the ideas of class and caste) people do not always identify with them. For example, few people are conscious on a daily basis of the fact that they belong to a particular social class or caste. They tend to identify more with smaller-scale social groupings, such as their family, friends, work-place group or neighbourhood. In this chapter we will consider some of these smaller groupings and how they may be important for health and health care.

Learning outcomes

After studying this chapter the student should be able to:
- recognize the nebulous nature of community and family as sociological concepts;
- make definitive statements about community;
- describe different types of community, including:
  - rural, urban and surburban communities;
  - gemeinschaft and gesellschaft communities;
  - mechanical and organic communities;
- define the term 'family' and describe different family structures;
- recognize alternatives to the traditional family in society;
- explain the function of the family with regard to children, adults and the elderly;
- discuss the position of elderly people in the community;
- analyse the implications of modern community and family structures for health and health care.

2. The concept of community in society

The problem with *community* is that there is no general agreement about what it actually is. There is some general agreement on the matter of scale or size. Robert Nisbet (1967) suggests that 'society' refers to the 'large-scale' impersonal social groupings of people in the modern age while 'community' is the smaller-scale grouping of people mostly in localities in which there are social bonds of sharing, emotional cohesion and fullness. He suggests that the modern trend is away from community toward society. Others, for example Chaplin (1968), see community as something at a different level to society; community consists of a group in close proximity and organized into a social structure. Using this line of thinking, a society is composed mainly of a collection of communities, which in turn are made up mainly of family units and others – people living alone, communes, religious orders etc.

Another different conceptualization of community sees it not in term of locality (though this may be involved) but in terms of social relationships or sentiment (Azarya, 1985). Chaplin (1968), referred to above, recognizes this alternative definition of community as 'a group of people, not necessarily in proximity, who share common interests and goals, for example, 'the community of scholars''. This type of definition suggests that in community there is a shared consciousness of belonging.

It is therefore possible to attempt a catch-all definitive statement including both of the ideas presented above, by defining community as:
- *a group of people in a locality who share a sense of belonging and living together in that locality to greater or lesser extent, and/or*
- *(a group of people) who share common interests and goals in relation to a particular facet of social life.*

We must beware of complacency in adopting such a definition and assuming that it will please everyone. As far back as 1955 Hillery identified 94 different definitions of community (Hillery, 1955) and in most years since then there have been other sociological writers foolhardy enough to attempt to crack this nut!

Example
By far the most popular television soap-opera in Britain today are those set in particular localities. Most of you will be aware of (and may regularly follow) programmes such as Eastenders, Coronation Street, Emmerdale and Brookside or their popular Australian counterparts, Neighbours and Home and Away. These depict neighbourhoods or localities. The people in them

spend a lot of their time together – they visit each other's homes, may go to the local cafe for lunch and often meet in a local pub at lunchtime or the evening. You may have noted some differences. In Emmerdale they are farming folk – they live and work in the locality. It is a little different with Brookside. Here there is no corner pub and most people work away from the locality. They tend to live as separate family groups and interact mainly when there is conflict between residents of Brookside Close or when they unite against a common enemy such as property developers.

Study activity

1. Do you think locality communities such as those in the soap operas exist in reality? Take your own locality (or your parents' locality, if you are living in student accomodation) and write a 500 word description of it. Pay attention to such issues as:
   – whether a locality with boundaries can even be identified;
   – the extent to which people relate and share their lives;
   – whether it resembles an inner city neighbourhood like Eastenders, a suburban neighbourhood like Brookside or a rural setting like Emmerdale.
   Discuss your write-up with fellow students. If possible divide into small groups of 5-6,

ensure that everyone has a copy of everyone else's write up, and discuss and compare. Use a poster to list key words descriptive of communities as these arise in your discussion.

When you were doing the latter activity, you may have noted a subtle difference between a new suburban community such as Brookside and older, more stable communities such as in Coronation Street or Eastenders. In the latter communities most people know each other and indeed often spend a lot of time in each other's company. In newer suburban neighbourhoods it is not uncommon for people not to know even their next-door neighbours. The population in surburban neighbourhoods is often quite transient as well. Often as you walk or drive through them you will see a forest of Estate Agents 'For Sale' signs.

In older rural or inner-city communities such movements in and out are not so common. Sometimes, of course, inner city communities are fragmented by economic patterns and/or redevelopment programmes and mass movements out and in occur. This occurred in cities such as London and Glasgow in the late 1950s and 1960s when whole communities were fragmented, with families being re-housed in new

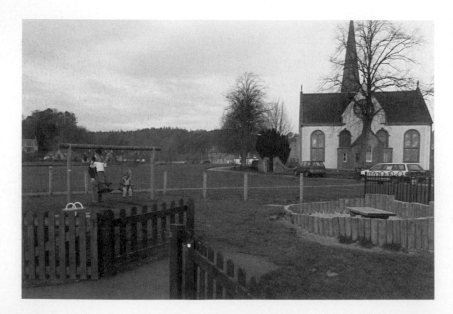

Figure 3.4.1
The rural community:
a green and
pleasant land

towns or out-of-town housing estates. As they moved out, immigrants and transient tenants moved into the inner-city areas to take their place. But of course, the old communities in these areas had died forever. Those who still remain and those who move in are unwilling to invest in the locality or even in the improvement of their homes because of uncertainty about what central or local government intend to do about the locality. This phenomenon, described by Hill (1976) as 'planners' blight', results in a gradual deterioration in what was previously a vital, living community.

3. Size of community

It is more difficult to think of community in terms of size if the criterion of locality is excluded from the definition of community. Using Chaplin's (op. cit.) second definition presented above, the example of a community of scholars could stretch beyond even the boundaries of a country. However, most people set aside this definitional subtlcty and think of community in terms of a geographical locality. It is then possible to give some consideration to size.

Warren (1973) is helpful here in promoting a view which essentially sees the community as being a microcosm of the wider society. According to Warren the community must include not just a sense of belonging and shared familiarity among members, but the performance of basic social functions. These include: provision of basic economic needs, socialization, social control, social participation and mutual support. The community does not have to be like the total society in that *all* these functions are *fully met* in some way. But there does have to be some activity in each of these spheres. This is of course not really very precise. However, at least we know that, to meet such conditions, a community must be larger than a family living in a single house and fairly limited to a neighbourhood. In the example presented above, in densely populated areas this may be a single street – as in Coronation Street, or the Albert Square of Eastenders – or an area covering several square miles – as in the sparsely populated rural Emmerdale.

This increasing acceptance of community as something which exists in a locality or neighbourhood is illustrated in the context of social policy. Thus, when in Britain a Community Development Project was introduced in the late 1960s by the Home Office to combat 'social' problems – neighbourhoods, especially those with concentrated social problems, were the assumed unit for targeted action (Marris, 1985). But as nurses we must also be aware of a less precise use of the term community, which is

Figure 3.4.2
Inner city decline

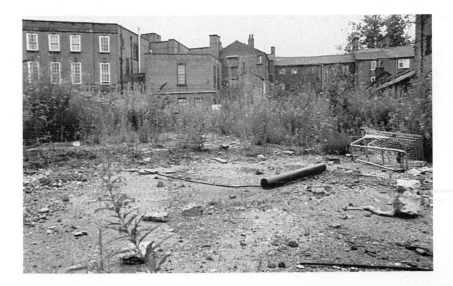

returned to in greater detail below. This is the use of 'community' as meaning the opposite of institutional living. In this sense patients or clients are divided into those who are in-patients or residents of institutions – particularly in the sense of large mental institutions originally isolated from urban areas – and those who live outside these, who are said to live 'in the community'. In this context the term 'community care' implies care of patients/clients outside hospital – in their own homes or other smaller residential settings.

4. Types of community

The two sociologists most notable for their work in this area are the German, Ferdinand Tonnies and the Frenchman, Emile Durkheim. Their ideas on community bear similarities, but there are marked and fundamental differences.

Tonnies (1955) suggested that society has two fundamental forms of social life. One of these he entitled *Gemeinschaft* (which translated means 'community'); the other he entitled *Gesellschaft* (which translated means 'association'). He suggested that the trend in modern life was a move away from community and toward association. In gemeinschaft, relationships are direct, intimate, enduring and all embracing. The community is a territorial entity. People live, work, marry, have families, are cared for when old, die and are buried in such communities. Kinship ties are strong. In the extreme form they are self-sufficient social entities in their own right. Conversely, gesellschaft is characterized by a lack of intimate and enduring relationships. People are associated in certain ways eg. by contractual arrangements (the milk delivery man brings the milk each day, the doctor and nurse tend the sick when required). However, there is no sense of attachment to place and the individual members seldom spend most of their day to day life in the neighbourhood of their homes – usually going to school, work or recreation elsewhere.

The approach taken by Durkheim (1974) is rather similar. Durkheim described a move from *mechanical solidarity* in pre-industrial society to *organic solidarity* in modern industrialized society.

In mechanical solidarity small, locality-based homogeneous groupings exist as self-contained communities. Each 'community' is like all others and each to a large extent is self-sufficient. Because each functions independently as a unit in its own right, the *mechanical* metaphor is descriptive – the communities are like so many clockwork timepieces, ticking away in isolation from each other. This is very similar to the gemeinschaft community described by Tonnies.

In organic solidarity, the emphasis is on interdependence and a division in relation to social functions. Family life, education, work and often leisure are all separated. In the context of work, there is a division of labour. Some are involved in producing goods, others in providing services such as caring for the sick and educating the young etc. The typical family group is a small nuclear family (husband, wife and children) living in an urban setting. The wife looks after the home. The husband may be a mechanic servicing other people's cars. Other 'workers' deliver his milk, educate his children and treat him and his family when illness strikes. The contractual social relationships and network of interdependencies are similar to the interdependence of organs within the human body. The *organic* metaphor is thus meaningful in this context. Organic solidarity has some similarity to Tonnies' concept of Gesellschaft.

The fundamental difference between Tonnies', and Durkheim's viewpoints is in the value attributed to these social trends. Tonnies viewed this in negative terms, deploring the dehumanizing nature of association or gesellschaft. Nisbet (1967) describes this as *alienation,* a situation in which the individual is seen as being estranged, *anomic* (i.e. deprived of social identity, standards for behaving and sense of belonging) and rootless when cut off from the ties of community and moral purpose. It is widely held that such states of *alienation* and *anomie* can lead, in vulnerable individuals, to feelings of desolation, depression and suicide.

Durkheim, however, was of the view that a move towards organic solidarity was desirable. He was well aware of the dysfunctional effects of alienation and anomie. Indeed it was Durkheim who originally introduced the concept of anomie in his famous study of suicide (Durkheim, 1952). Nevertheless, he firmly believed that organic solidarity gave society order and cohesion. He also felt that as the contractual obligations between people were limited and specific, members of society would be more liberated than in mechanical solidarity. For example, the doctor's obligation to his clients is to provide treatment. When he has done this, his time is his own – as with the miner at the end of his shift or the teacher at end of term. People would no longer be tied to intense social relationships and responsibilities for twenty-four hours a day, and social functions would be performed more efficiently by those specially trained in such functions.

There are perhaps two additional points to note about the study of community. The first relates to the positions taken by Durkheim and Tonnies. While both sociologists wrote in the late 19th and early 20th centuries, their views about community are still live debates and they are strongly disputed and discussed among sociologists today. You should therefore take time to consider their conceptual frameworks.

The second point relates to the assumption arising from these ideas that the transition from gemeinschaft or mechanical solidarity to gesellschaft or organic solidarity is a transition from traditional to modern or from rural to urban. While this may generally be the case, sociologists have found that society is not in reality so predictable and that in fact variety appears in all sorts of ways. Consider the example of the soap-operas in Section 2 again. Most rural communities are in fact just like Emmerdale and gemeinschaft-like in their social structures and processes. Similarly most urban settings are like Brookside and gesellschaft-like in their social presentation. But what about Eastenders? This is a presentation of the people living in the heart of London, yet the close kinship ties, sense of identity, extent to which people live and work in the immediate area and share in most of their social lives is decidedly gemeinschaft-like. The extent to which people in recent years have set up communes or moved into Kibbutzim (small Israeli communities within which members live and work together), suggests that many may be rejecting the modern gesellschaft model of social living.

Example

A typical scene in modern society. A fast food hamburger restaurant in North London. On a particular evening there are a number of people in the restaurant. Beverley is a member of the staff. She is a student on holiday-work and stays in a hostel in South London. She walks up and down clearing tables, mopping the floor, stacking trays etc. Tom and Molly Smith, who live in the neighbourhood, are at a table with their daughters, Judy (6 years old) and Natalie (who is celebrating her 12th birthday). At another table are Joey Porter and his girlfriend, June Sandford. They are passing the time with a coffee until it is time for June's bus home to Harlow in Essex. At yet another table is Jonathan Randall a young stockbroker, dressed in dark business suit and working with an electronic organizer. A young man, Alec Butterworth enters the restaurant and sits at the table next to Jonathan. He came to London last year hoping to obtain work, but has been unlucky. He gradually ran out of money and he now sleeps rough, surviving by begging and stealing from market stalls. He is drunk from cheap wine and has come into the restaurant to get warm. It is extremely cold outside. He has no money to buy food. He is dirty and smelly, and mutters incessantly in a strange accent which is almost unintelligible to the others. This occasionally escalates into loud shouting and swear-words directed at the other customers. However, everyone studiously ignores Alec, except little Judy who stares at him in amazement until Molly whispers something to her, when she looks away and sits quietly though appearing uncomfortable. As Alec gets more boisterous Jonathan gets up and leaves. At this stage Beverley speaks to the manager who comes out and looks down at Alec. A few minutes later, two policemen arrive and escort Alec out.

Study activity

2. Would you say this situation is taking place in a community characterized by mechanical or organic solidarity? Explain your views in terms of:
   - the extent to which close social ties exist;
   - the level of interdependence, in terms of how performing certain functions are seen as the responsibility of certain individuals;
   - the existence or otherwise of alienation and anomie.

5. The family

It is generally accepted that the family is a social unit in which the members reside together and are directly related by marriage (i.e. a legal, or religious, or custom-based contract to live as man and wife) and blood (i.e. the off-spring of a married couple). This is of course the most fundamental of family units. For this reason the term *nuclear family* is usually used.

The nuclear family is the most common form of family in modern Western society. You will recall that at Section 2 above it was noted that some people view society as being made up of communities (locality or neighbourhood groups) which in turn are formed by families or other sub-community units e.g. people living alone, single-parent families etc. This draws attention to the fact that living in a family in the community is not the only option. Indeed even those who do subscribe to the idea of a heterosexual, monogamous (i.e. one man, one woman) relationship, do not always subscribe to the need for a formal legal or religious-legal marriage bond. More and more young people are cohabiting as an alternative or as a prelude to marriage; more young women are electing to have children but no permanent male partner; people increasingly appear to be seeing mar-

riage as a less permanent contract, with divorce rates rising and serial marriage being common. In the UK over one-third of partners at marriage ceremonies have been married previously.

Society today is also more accepting of alternative life styles. Many people choose to live in communes; the example of the Israeli Kibbutz referred to at Section 4 above is a well-known example. There are also, at least in more liberated Western societies, more homosexual relationships being established in terms of residental living patterns i.e. male couples and female couples living together.

6. Family types

The family type described above i.e. the nuclear family, is just one option. Family as a social concept is as nebulous as that of community and can mean different things to different people. Even if the ideas of kinship and shared residence are taken as joint definitive statements, there are variations in family types. Generally speaking, it is possible to classify these in terms of extension beyond the minimal or basic nuclear unit. In this sense, family may be extended horizontally or vertically.

a. Horizontal extension

Here the extension relates primarily to marriage or mating patterns. Where there is more than one husband and/or wife, the term *polygamy* is used. This is usually related in some way to economic circumstances, and includes:

Polygyny: Here a husband has more than one wife. This meets the need for children to ensure a continued lineage and/or to provide labour. It is common in agricultural economies, particularly in some African cultures such as the Yoruba of Nigeria.

Diagram 3.4.1
The nuclear family

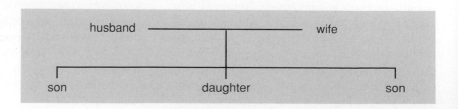

Polyandry: Here a wife has more than one husband. This is again often a response to an agricultural economy. For example, in some Himalayan cultures, with poor agricultural land, brothers share the same wife, primarily because they cannot afford one each.

b. Vertical extension

Here the extension relates primarily to the wider kinship goup. It is the most common form of extension found in Western society, and indeed many take the term 'extended family' to relate specifically to this type. In essence, if it can be stated that a nuclear family normally has one 'generation', i.e. offspring of the husband and wife. A vertically extended family consists of two or more generations. That is, grandparents (the parents's of one or other of the husband and wife), the husband and wife and their offspring. The family may of course extend back to include great-grandparents or forward to include the marriage of offspring and their subsequent offspring.

It is commonly said that vertically extended families were common in the past but were replaced by nuclear families in the industrial era. Such small nuclear families were taken to be ideal in industrialized societies. The wife kept the home, the husband worked. They had offspring to ensure a future supply of labour. They socialized the offspring into the norms of social behaviour necessary to ensure that they would be useful members of industrial society. The family group was small and mobile, capable of moving in response to the demand for labour. Many functions such as education of the young and health care became specialized functions provided more efficiently by others, thus freeing the family to perform as an effective social unit. Even if the main breadwinner became ill, a social security system supported the family until a cure-orientated health service prepared him to return to work as soon as possible. The work motive was viewed as sacred. It was necessary to work, to contribute to production in society and to accumulate wealth and provide for the family.

Weber (1952) described this as 'the Protestant Ethic', as the austere work motive in European reformationist protestantism was aligned to 'the spirit of captalism' (and indeed may have been its precursor).

Referring back to our consideration of community, a picture evolves of gemeinschaft or mechanical solidarity and extended families in the past and gesellschaft or organic solidarity and nuclear families today. However, as in in the case of community, the situation is a little complicated in reality. For example, Laslett and Wall (1972) in a famous and influential study of families in Europe over the past three centuries found that the extented family was as unusual in the past as it is today, with most households, going back as far as the sixteenth century, consisting of small nuclear groups. However, if the criterion of residence is removed, and family is

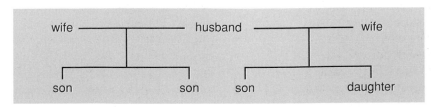

Diagram 3.4.2
Horizontal extension:
polygyny

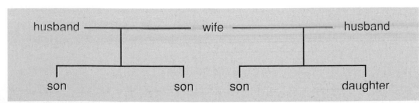

Diagram 3.4.3
Horizontal extension:
polyandry

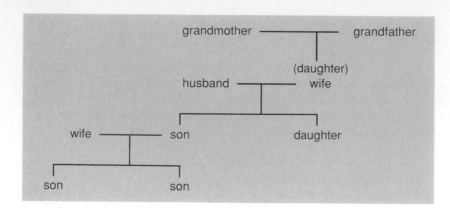

Diagram 3.4.4
The vertically
extended family

defined as a close kinship group, it is found that there is often an extensive close-knit kinship network. This is well documented in the work of Young and Willmot (1962) and Townsend (1957), who described close-knit and supportive extended family circles in inner city London.

It should be noted, however, that writing more than a decade later Young and Willmot had formed slightly differing views. In their important work entitled The Symmetrical Family (Young and Willmot, 1973) they suggest three distinct stages in the development of the British family. In Stage 1, the pre-industrial stage, the family was stable and based on production. By virtue of his control over production the father was master of the household. Stage 2 (from 1750 to 1900) was characterized by the disruption caused by industrialization as the industrial revolution took hold. Home and work place were separated; fathers, mothers and even children laboured outside the home and relationships were less intense. Stage 3, beginning around 1900 and continuing today is characterized by what Young and Willmot describe as 'the symmetrical family'. This family is a more stable unit, with greater equality between men and women and less role segregation on the basis of sex. Life is very much centred on the nuclear family home and there is less involvement in extended family networks. In effect, Young and Willmott argue for the productive unit nature of the modern nuclear family, but stress the more symmetrical, liberal nature of the family group. This has not been supported by

other studies. For example, Hartmann (1981) reports that there is not in effect an equalization of work in the household; men still do less and spend much less time in the home than their wives. (See also The family, pages 217-218.)

7. Functions and the family

Despite difficulties in definition and classification, the family is a constant social unit in almost all societies, so much so, that some claim family groupings are an essential aspect of human behaviour. This of course begs the question of why 'family' is so popular world-wide. It obviously serves a number of useful human and social functions. If you scan the earlier sections of this chapter you will be able to identify a number of these. For example, family functions already identified include:

(i)   providing a socially accepted context for sexual relations (in our society monogamy or single-partner relationships are the norm);

(ii)   ensuring a stable social structure for reproduction;

(iii) primary socialization of the young into the culture (i.e. language, knowledge, norms etc);

(iv)   acting as a stable base for the means of production – whether this is in the form of extended families in rural, agricultural settings or nuclear families in industrialized society;

(v)   caring for the young and – in some instances – the sick, disabled and elderly.

Study activities

3. Scan the earlier sections of this chapter and the references provided in relation to the sections on the family. Using your reading, attempt to extend the above list of family functions. Share your work with fellow students, so that you all end up with a comprehensive written list of functions of the family, upon which you all agree.

4. Much of the literature on families referred to in the above sections relates to family within the social structure and the functions family performs within society. You have probably recognized the dominant perspective here – it is the social order or consensus theory approach described in Chapter 3. However, what do you think conflict theorists might have to say about the family? Might a Marxist, for example, be of the opinion that the nuclear family is an alienating social constraint which serves capital but disadvantages workers and their families (the proletariat) in some ways? Go to the library and do a literature search, using key words such as:

conflict - family

Marxism - family

capitalism - family

socialism - family

Do a brief analysis of approximately 500 words on the conflict theory perspective on family.

Discuss your write-up with your personal tutor or fellow students.

8. The elderly in the community

In line with common usage in the UK, elderly people tend to be defined here as those who are 65 years or older (i.e. the official age when men are entitled to a state retirement pension). There are almost 8 million people in the age-range in the UK. Although it is anticipated that the total will remain static over the coming years, by the year 2000 the proportion of the 75 years and over age group will have increased by 45 percent (OPCS, 1979). In the oldest group of elderly people, those aged 85 years and over, an increase of at least 37 percent is anticipated. It has

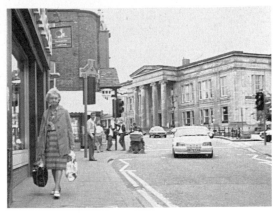

Figure 3.4.3
Surviving alone.
Happy or lonely?

been estimated that over two-thirds of those in this age-group will suffer some degree of disability and one-fifth will be severely disabled or bed-fast (i.e. confined to bed) (Carstairs, 1981). In a recent report by the Audit Commission (HMSO, 1986), it was reported that approximately one million of those aged 65 or older were receiving care of some sort. It is obvious therefore that the elderly are a sizable proportion of the UK population and that they make a disproportionate demand on health and personal social services provisions.

Given that the elderly are so numerous and so vulnerable, their status in society assumes particular importance. Some sociologists, e.g. Levin and Levin (1980) have suggested that in general elderly people are not held in high regard and indeed are largely devalued within society. They describe a pattern of 'ageism' whereby our culture is largely youth-orientated and whereby elderly people are viewed as being inferior, held in low esteem and even discriminated against. This is accompanied by prejudices (i.e. unsubstantiated negative attitudes), characterized by seeing elderly people in terms of stereoptypes, as being slow, forgetful, conservative, set in their ways, frail, cantankerous, feeble-minded etc. These views are said to be accompanied by a tendency to exclude elderly people from many aspects of social life.

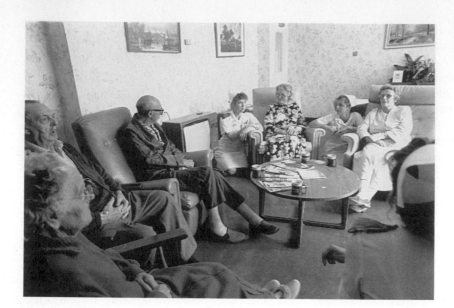

Figure 3.4.4
How will old people
live in the future?

The attitudes of the elderly themselves to their position in society is a matter of controversy. There are essentially two sociological stances which address this issue and they are in direct opposition to each other.

One of these is the so-called *Disengagement Theory,* proposed by Cumming and Henry (1961). On the basis of research on elderly people in the American mid-west, they suggested that the elderly person prepares for the ultimate disengagement of death by a mutual and accepted disengagement from society. In simple terms, the individual wishes to withdraw from society, the society wishes him to withdraw, so he does so gradually with minimum disruption to the social order. This in essence involves a relinquishing of social roles, a reduction in social activity and the severing of affecive ties with other members of society.

The other theoretical stance, which is in direct opposition to the disengagement theory, is referred to as the *Activity Theory.* As expressed by one of its original proponents, Havighurst (1963), the activity theory assumes that the natural course of old age is to remain active and to replace previous centres of activity e.g. work, political activities, etc. with new forms of active behaviour to compensate for such losses. Ac-

cording to Blau (1973) high morale and life satisfaction are correlated with social integration. The argument here is that disengagement from social networks is not the natural course in old age. Indeed it is argued that disengagement is both undesirable and unhealthy.

The problems here are two-fold. Firstly, if traditional neighbourhoods are in decline and if the modern family structure is the inwardly-centred symmetrical family, it will become increasingly difficult for elderly people to maintain ties with old friends and younger relatives. And secondly, if ageism *is* an increasing trend in society, there is the possibility that rather than being nurtured and supported by younger people in their neighbourhood, elderly people will be shunned and rejected.

Study activity

5. Think back over the last month. Have you visited or been visited by an elderly friend or relative in that time. Ask five friends the same question. Then ask them to quickly say five words which come into their minds when they think of old people. Divide the 25 words you collected into positive, negative and neutral words. Compare notes and discuss with your fellow-students who have also undertaken this exercise.

In a recent study Willmott (1986) found evidence to support the suggestion that traditional neighbourhoods are in decline. He also found that fewer elderly people than in the past live with or near younger relatives and that local extended families are now rare. While there is evidence to suggest that younger adults frequently visit their elderly relatives (according to Willmott, on average three times per week) and that friends and neighbours do provide support, the future social and demographic trends are not favourable. With the trend towards dispersed communities, symmetrical families, fewer young people and more frail elderly people, it is likely that health and social care of the elderly will be the major concern of those who plan, manage and provide health and social services as we move into the 21st century.

9. Family, community and health care

It is impossible to give a full consideration to health care in modern society without taking into consideration the family *and* the community. Both have implications for health promotion, aetiology of disease, and management of the sick, disabled and elderly.

a. Health promotion

When you progress in your nursing career you will understandably come across some tragic cases, situations for instance where young women with cervical cancer were unaware of the importance of cervical screening, situations where patients are overweight and have coronary heart disease, or who smoke and have developed lung cancer. You will feel that this is all a great pity; you will constantly ask yourself why this could not have been avoided.

Often the origins of these problems can be traced back to community environments and family life styles. Some would suggest that with young people who live and grow up in an Edinburgh housing scheme, or in Harlem or South Bronx in New York, it is almost a miracle that they do not become involved in drug abuse. Similarly, in a family where – perhaps because of poverty and social background – there is a habit of taking a high carbohydrate, high fat diet

and heavy smoking, it is again not surprising that coronary heart disease is common. For example, Northern Ireland, the most economically depressed region in the UK, also has the highest incidence of coronary heart disease.

The socializing influence of parents on their children is of particular importance in the context of promoting healthy life styles. Children often model their behaviour on that of their parents. It is of course true that when children leave the home they are influenced by secondary socialization processes in school and with their peers and they do not necessarily mindlessly adopt parents' lifestyles and values. Indeed, it is normal for older children and adolescents to strive for independence by resisting their parents. However, the promotion of healthy life styles in the family will reinforce the health education provided by the school and by community health services. Similarly, a strong basis in knowledge pertinent to health risks provided within the family – and an openness in discussing issues such as alcohol, drug abuse and sexual relations – will help young people to resist health-threatening influences from peers and other sources within the wider community.

b. Aetiology

Community and family aspects can be identified here, in line with the sociogenesis hypothesis discussed in Chapter 3 of this module. It has long been recognized that in deprived communities, particularly in inner city areas, there are various risk situations. Some of these relate to crime, poverty and unemployment. But some also relate to health and the interrelationships between material deprivation and health were well documented in the Black Report (DHSS, 1980) and by Townsend (1979) – both of which were discussed in Chapter 3 of this module. Where people live in overcrowded, substandard, damp, cold housing schemes; where there is unemployment and poverty; where local health care provisions are inadequate; in such circumstances respiratory disorders, accidents, gastro-intestinal infections and the failure of young children to thrive mentally and physically are rife.

Aetiological influences are not of course confined to deprived communities and the less well-off. The greater affluence of middle and upper class families, with busy parents whose socialite life style leaves little time for their own children, has its own risks. There is the absence of supervision and support, and the greater availability of money for young people to get involved in drug and alcohol abuse.

It must also be recognized that families, usually considered as nurturing environments, can in reality be very dangerous places to be. Family relationships are often very intense and can place individual members – particularly the less powerful offspring – under unendurable stress. Indeed such stress may drive a young person to alcohol abuse or even overt mental disorder. The Scottish psychiatrist Ronald Laing illustrated how oppressive family relationships, and the young person's attempts to reject these, can lead to his/her behaviour being labelled as schizophrenia (a psychotic mental illness) (see, for example, Laing, 1965 and Laing and Esterson, 1970).

One particularly interesting phenomenon here is the so-called '*double-bind hypothesis*'. This refers to the situation in which a hostile parent reacts apparently positively to the child at one level and negatively on another level. The child receives ambiguous messages e.g. 'Do this in this way' but then, immediately, 'You should not have done this.' In effect, the child can do nothing right and is torn apart by stress. This pattern of parental behaviour has been associated with the onset of schizophrenia in young people. Indeed double-binding is so common a pattern in some mothers of schizophrenics that the term *schizophrenogenic mother* has been used.

Example
A community psychiatric nurse is called to an emergency in a family home on the local army base at 9.00 am in the morning. When he arrives, the sitting room is wrecked - smashed television set, broken china, tables and chairs overturned. The mother is crying hysterically. A young man (the son), dressed in black leathers, with shoulder length hair and wearing an earring is hovering in a corner. He is 18 or 19 years old. He has dilated pupils, is breathing heavily and appears to be slightly drunk. He has a cut eye, bleeding nose and is holding a hammer. He has been out at an all-night party. The father immediately accosts the nurse. He is a 50-year old man, with short back-and-sides haircut and is dressed in an army Sergeant-Major's uniform. He is shouting aggressively: 'We are not prepared to put up with this nonsense any longer. If he can't be in by 10 at night he can **** off out of here. We'll have no drinking and whoring in this house! He needs treatment. Cart him off to the loony bin. I'll sign the forms all right!'

Study activity
6. What do you think may be the basic problem here? Might this young man be mentally deranged? Is his all-night partying abnormal, or is his father's reaction to it abnormal? If possible, try to remember similar highly charged situations in your own or any other family you are familiar with. Discuss these types of situations with your fellow-students using the following agenda:
 – Do parents understand their children?
 – Do children understand their parents?
 – What should the community psychiatric nurse in the above example do?

c. Health care
Both family and community also have implications for health care. Indeed, after considering the above example, you may feel that in many instances we should be treating sick families rather than sick individuals – as suggested by Laing and Esterson (op. cit.). Even when an illness such as asthma or leukaemia appears to primarily effect the individual, the traumatic effects on the family should not be under estimated. Indeed you will find that, when you obtain experience in clinical areas such as radiotherapy or coronary care wards, the most progressive practitioners will include in their care programmes the provision of information, reassurance, counselling and support for the spouse and family of the victim.
A particular area of concern here is the increasing emphasis on community care. This is yet

another term about which there is ambiguity, and which will tax you throughout your course. Bayley (1973) summarizes the problem well when he distinguishes between 'care *in* the community' and 'care *by* the community'. The former refers to care of the patient *in* the community by professional workers such as GP's, District Nurses, Health Visitors, Community Psychiatric Nurses etc. The latter relates to the voluntary care of the patient *by* non-professionals in the community, that is, care by family, friends and voluntary workers – often known as 'informal carers'.

The aspiration of care *by* the community may be problematic if the nature of the community approximates gesellschaft or organic solidarity (see Section 2 above) and if the nuclear, symmetrical family (see Section 6 above) is the norm. Can a family with young children, with husband and wife working, really support a sick member or a frail elderly relative? Critics of the recent trend towards community care claim that in particular long stay mental illness patients and individuals with learning difficulties have been discharged into a community which is not capable of supporting them. Families can be put under considerable pressure by having to care for disabled children or frail elderly people. Where close-knit communities no longer exist and there are not extended family networks the capacity for families to support relatives, or indeed the capacity of discharged long-stay patients to survive alone in the community, may be limited. In such circumstances the availability of comprehensive community-based health and personal social services is of vital importance.

In the United Kingdom, government has now recognised the need to review community support services. It is now proposed that, under new *care management* structures, each patient or client will have a *case manager* (e.g. nurse, doctor or social worker) who will be responsible for and coordinate community-based services. In the particular context of nursing, the new *Patient's Charter* advocates that when a person is admitted to hospital, he/she will have a *named*

nurse, who is the *primary nurse* responsible for his/her care during the period of stay in hospital.

Study activities

7. Do a literature search of critiques of 'community care' in your College library. Write a brief summary (2 pages, 1000 words) of criticisms and relate this to sociological theories of community and family.

8. Review recent literature and write descriptions of each of the following:
   – care management;
   – case manager;
   – primary nursing;
   – named nurse.

10. Summary

This chapter addressed the related concepts of community and family. You will have found that these apparently simple and straightforward concepts are infinitely more complex when you start to give them detailed attention. What will also hopefully have become clear to you is that these are vitally important unit ideas or concepts in sociology. They are particularly important for nurses and other health workers. Not only does illness occur in the context of family and community, but these structures are important influences in the prevention, cause and treatment and care of the sick, disabled and elderly.

Finally, you may find it useful to supplement the reading and study tasks in this chapter by consulting another sociology text which addresses these issues. A particularly useful reference is Berger and Berger (1979) whose book, 'Sociology: A Biographical Approach' includes helpful chapters on family and community.

Final test Module 3

Instructions

- This section comprises 70 yes/no questions.
- Each proposition, claim, statement, etc. may be *true* or *false,* either *yes* or *no.* There is no middle way: you must make a choice.
- Your assessment of whether items are true or false should be based on your reading of the book.
- The questions are arranged in order relating to subject or chapters.
- Check that all questions have been answered.
- Finally, mark the test yourself. You will find the answers at the end of the book.

1. Relationships differ, particularly with regard to their purpose, but not with regard to their form.
2. The psychological situation is included in the environmental factors.
3. Norms are opinions on what is right or wrong.
4. Norms and values are tied to specific societies, cultures and periods.
5. The imposition not to indulge in incestuous behaviour is one example of social mores.
6. Formal norms are also rules of behaviour.
7. Universal norms apply, for instance, to everyone within a particular culture.
8. An example of a special norm is wanting, or not wanting, to eat vegetarian food.
9. All laws of the land are by definition folkways.
10. Social control is an effective mechanism for maintaining central values and checking their observance.

11. The key to the socialization process lies in children's education.
12. Primary socialization takes place at school level.
13. Socialization is effected by means of a great variety of interactions.
14. Two learning processes play a part in socialization, i.e. conforming and identifying.
15. Attitude is the way in which an individual thinks about a social fact, appraises it and behaves in regard to that fact.
16. A social role refers to the position that someone occupies within a group.

Items 17 and 18 are the factors which affect children's socialization process:
17. Biological heritage.
18 Attitude.

19. An example of an internal attribution is a woman who attributes her irritation to premenstrual tension.
20. Three criteria for an internal or an external attribution are consensus, congruity and consistency.
21. In the fundamental attribution error, there is a tendency, in the assessment of someone else's negative behaviour, to underestimate the external attributions and overestimate the internal attributions.
22. The dissonance theory describes the process of changing attributions in those situations in which the original attribution is incompatible with the behaviour that has been displayed.
23. A group can exist only if it is in some way perceptible.

24. Groups can be created spontaneously.
25. Dictated groups frequently consist of people against whom there is discrimination.
26. Secondary socialization is one of the family's most important tasks.
27. As a result of changing economic circumstances, the family formerly had far more opportunities for exchanging emotions – what is known as the emotional family.

Items 28 and 29 are group-bonding aspects:
28. Security function.
29. Task function.

30 It is a characteristic of members of a secondary group that they are also members of several primary groups.
31. Formal groups may also be created spontaneously.
32. In informal groups there are usually no clear arrangements about internal relations.
33. Lack of structure is another characteristic of informal groups.
34. An informal group is also an open group.
35. Patients in the coffee shop constitute a formal group.
36. Group cohesion refers to the extent to which group members wish to remain members of the group to which they belong.

Items 37 to 41 are factors which determine group cohesion:
37. Dissonances manipulated by individuals.
38. Involvement with one another.
39. Tolerance of dissenting opinions.
40. Regular achievement of group aims.
41. Differences in power and status between members of the group.

42. Conforming plays the principal part in learning roles.
43. Internalization is the same as identification.
44. Roles are usually complementary.
45. Role strain occurs when the internal and external attributions relating to a particular role are in conflict with one another.
46. Helpful behaviour is encouraged by reciprocity and social responsibility values.
47. Power and autocratic leadership are the same.

48. The leadership of nursing sisters is a good example of charismatic authority.
49. Nurses in our society have little power of sanctions.
50. Reference power is derived from factors in people's (immediate) environment.
51. Nursing sisters usually exercize laissez-faire leadership.
52. Dysfunctional roles have a particularly negative effect on the task-oriented process within a group.
53. A hospital may be regarded as a small pluriform society.
54. The reductive approach to sickness and health means that, on average, nurses need devote less time to a patient.
55. Sociogenesis is the influence of personal functioning on the psychological and physical balance of human beings.
56. It is evident that social processes may affect sickness and health.
57. According to the consensus theory, sickness is a reaction to the disturbance of the normal functioning of the total individual.
58. According to the consensus theory, sickness is linked to a physical complaint.
59. In the consensus theory, being sick is linked to assuming a role.
60. Overcoming obstacles (financial or social) is one of the factors that determine the assumption of the sick role.
61. According to the consensus theory, society makes certain demands on its members based on generally accepted norms and values.
62. The concept of power is a central feature of the conflict theory.
63. Contrary to the consensus theory, the interaction theory does not stem from sociology.
64. Joint actions are the common views of people regarding the 'self'.
65. According to the interaction theory, sickness cannot be objectified.
66. According to the interaction theory, health care also results in sickness.
67. Gesellschaft describes a small neighbourhood community in which all members are intimately acquainted.
68. According to disengagement theory society wants elderly people to withdraw from

socially active roles, but elderly people themselves do not want to do this.
69. Polyandry describes a family structure in which the wife has more than one husband.
70. When a parent conveys conflicting messages to a child, this is known as double-bind.

References

Allport, G.W. (1975), The historical background of modern psychology. In Berkowitz, L. (Ed.), *A Survey of Social Psychology*, Illinois, Dryden Press.

Asch, S.E. (1952), *Social Psychology*. New York, Prentice-Hall.

Audit Commission (1986), *Making a Reality of Community Care*. London, HMSO.

Azarya, V. (1986), Community. In Kuper, A. and Kuper, J. (Eds), *The Social Science Encyclopedia*. London, Routledge and Kegan Paul.

Bakwin, H. (1945), Pseudodoxia pediatrica, *New England Journal of Medicine*, 231, 691-697

Bayley, M. (1973), *Mental handicap and Community Care*. London, Routledge and Kegan Paul.

Berger, P.L. and Berger, B. (1979), *Sociology: a biographical approach*. Harmondsworth, Penguin Books.

Berkowitz, L. (1975), *A Survey of Social Psychology*. Illinois, Dryden Press.

Blau, P.M. (1964), *Exchange and Power in Social Life*. New York, Wiley and Sons.

Blau, Z.S. (1973), *Old Age in a Changing Society*. New York, New Viewpoints.

Blumer, H. (1969), *Symbolic Interactionism: perspective and method*. Englewood Cliffs, New Jersey, Prentice Hall.

Bottomore, T.B. and Rubel, M. (Ed.) (1985), *Karl Marx: Selected Writings in Sociology and Social Philosophy*. Harmondsworth, Penguin Books.

Brown, G. and Birley, J.L.T. (1968), Schizophrenia relapse and life change histories. *Journal of Health and Social Behaviour*, 9, 3, 263.

Carstairs, V. (1981), Our elders. In Shegog, R.F.A. (Ed.) *Impending Crisis of Old Age - a Challenge to Ingenuity*. Oxford, Oxford University.

Chaplin, J.P. (1968), *Dictionary of Psychology*. New York, Dell.

Comte, A. (1983), *The Positive Philosophy of Auguste Comte*. London, Bell. (From original 1896 publication).

Cumming, E. and Henry, W.E. (1961), *Growing Old: the process of disengagement*. New York, Basic Books.

Davis, K. and Moore, W.E. (1945), Some principles of stratification. *American Sociological Review*, Vol. 10, 242-9.

Department of Health and Social Security (1980), *Inequalities in health: Report of a research working group (the Black Report)*. London, DHSS.

Durkheim, E. (1952), *Suicide*. London, Routledge and Kegan Paul.

Durkheim, E. (1974), *The Social Division of Labor in Society*. New York, Free Press.

Elkin, F. (1960), *The Child and Society*. New York, Random House.

Festinger, L. (1957), *A Theory of Cognitive Dissonance*. Illinois, Row Peterson.

Franzini, L.R., Litrownik, A.J. and Blanchard, F.H. (1978), Modelling of sex-typed behaviours: effects on boy and girls. *Developmental Psychology*, 14, 313-314.

Gerth, H. and Mills, C.W. (1948), *From Max Weber: Essays in Sociology*. London, Routledge and Kegan Paul.

Goffman, E. (1968), *Asylums*. London, Penguin.

Guthrie, E.R. (1938), *The Psychology of Human Conflict*. New York, Harper and Bros.

Hartmann, H. (1981), The family as the locus of class, gender and political struggle: the example of housework. *Signs*, Vol. 6, 366-394.

Havighurst, R.J. (1963), Succesful aging. In Williams, R., Tibbits, C. and Donahue, W. (Eds), *Processes of Aging*. New York, Atherton.

Heider, F. (1958), *The Psychology of Interpersonal Relations*, New York, Wiley.

Hill, M. (1976), *The State, Administration and Individual*. Glasgow, Fontana.

Hillery, G.A. Jr. (1955), Definitions of Community: areas of agreement. *Rural Sociology*, 1955, 20.

Hinkle, E. (1964), The doctor, his patient and the environment. *American Journal of Public Health*. Jan. 1964, p. 11.

Holmes, T.H. and Rahe, R.H. (1967), The social readjustment rating scale. *Journal of Psychosomatic Research*, Vol. II, 213-18.

Homans, G.C. (1950), *The Human Group*. New York, Hartcourt and Brace.

Illich, I. (1977), *Limits to Medicine*. Harmondsworth, Penguin.

Kelley, H.H. (1967), Attribution theory in social psychology. In D. Levine (Ed.), *Nebraska symposium on motivation*. Nebraska, University of Nebraska Press.

Laing, R.D. (1965), *The Divided Self*. Harmondsworth, Penguin Books.

Laing, R.D. and Esterson, A. (1970), *Sanity, Madness and the Family*. Harmondsworth, Pelican Books.

Laslett, P. and Wall, R. (Ed.) (1972), *Household and Family in Past Time*. Cambridge, Cambridge University Press.

Latane, B. and Darley, T.M. (1970). *The Unresponsive Bystander: why doesn't he help?* New York, Appleton.

Latane, B. (1981), *The Psychology of Social Impact*. Ohio, Chicago State University Press.

Levin, J. and Levin, W.C. (1980), *Ageism: prejudice and discrimination against the elderly*. Belmont, California, Wadsworth Pub. Company.

Marris, P. (1985), Community Development. In Kuper, A. and Kuper, J. (Eds), *The Social Science Encyclopedia*. London, Routledge and Kegan Paul.

Marx, K. and Engels, F. (1968), *Karl Marx and Frederick Engels: Selected Works*. Moscow, Progress Publishers.

Mazlow, A.H. (1970), *Motivation and Personality*. New York, Harper and Row.

Mead, G.H. (1934), *Mind, Self and Society*. Chicago, University of Chicago Press.

Merton, R. (1968), *Social Theory and Social Structure*. New York, The Free Press.

Moreno, J.L. (1953), *Who shall Survive? Foundations of Sociometry, Group Psychotherapy and Sociodrama*. New York, Beacon House Inc.

Mosca, G. (1939), *The Ruling Class*. New York, McGraw-Hill Book Co.

Nisbet, R.A. (1967), *The Sociological Tradition*. London, Heineman.

Office of Populations Census and Surveys (OPCS), (1979), *Population projections 1977-2017*. Series PP2, No 9. London, HMSO.

Parsons, T. (1951), *The Social System*, London, Routledge and Kegan Paul.

Parsons, T. (1966), On becoming a patient. In Folta, J.R. and Deck, E.S. (Ed.), *A Sociological Framework for Patient Care*. New York, John Wiley and Sons.

Ross, L. (1977), The intuitive psychologist and his shortcomings: distortions in the attribution process. In Berkowitz, L. (Ed.) *Advances in Experimental Social Psychology*, Vol. 10, Academic Press.

Roth, J. (1971), The treatment of tuberculosis as a bargaining process. In Rose, A. (Ed.), *Human Behaviour and Social Processes: an Interactionist Approach*. London, Routledge and Kegan Paul.

Sprott, W.J.H. (1958), *Human Groups*. London, Penguin.

Sumner, W.G. (1906), *Folkways*. New York, Ginn and Co.

Szasz, T. (1971), *The Manufacture of Madness*. London, Routledge and Kegan Paul.

Toffler, A. (1976), *Future Shock*. London, Pan Books.

Tomalin, N. and Hall, R. (1970). *The Strange Voyage of Donald Growhurst*. London, Hodder and Stoughton.

Tonnies, F. (1955), *Community and Association*. London, Routledge and Kegan Paul.

Townsend, P. (1957), *The Family Life of Old People*. London, Routledge and Kegan Paul.

Townsend, P. (1979), *Poverty in the United Kingdom: a survey of household resources and standards of living*. Harmondsworth, Penguin Books.

Townsend P. and Davidson, N. (Ed.), (1982), *Inequalities in Health: the Black Report*. Harmondsworth, Penguin.

Wadsworth, M.E.J., Butterfield, W.J.H. and Blaney, R. (1971), *Health and Sickness, the Choice of Treatment*. London, Tavistock Publications.

Warren, R. (1973), *The Community in America*. Chicago, Rand McNally.

Weber, M. (1952), *The Protestant Ethic and the Spirit of Capitalism*. London, Allen and Unwin.

Weber, M. (1978), *Economy and Society*. Berkeley, University of California Press.

Willmott, P. (1986), *Social Networks, Informal Care and Public Policy*. London, Policy Studies Institute.

Young, M. and Willmott, P. (1962), *Family and Kinship in East London*. Harmondsworth, Penguin.

Young, M. and Willmott, P. (1973), *The Symmetrical Family*. London, Routledge and Kegan Paul.

Zajonc, R.B. (1980), Compresence. In Paulus, P.B. (Ed.), *Handbook of Small Group Research*. New York, The Free Press.

Module 4

THE PSYCHOLOGY OF HEALTH

Introduction to Module 4

In this module we examine the areas of clinical psychology with the emphasis on skills rather than theory. Three main areas are considered, as follows:

the application of psychology in different clinical settings, i.e. in somatic, psychiatric and learning difficulties situations;

the use of measurement in psychology;

the concept of support of people in stressful situations.

Clinical psychology is therefore seen as being concerned with people who:
- as a result of a physical condition have developed an emotional problem;
- have functional complaints, i.e. complaints for which no physical reason can be found;
- have a poor relationship with the helper and as a result of this, the progress of the illness is influenced negatively;
- have a behaviour problem resultant from a psychiatric illness;
- have a learning difficulty which limits their ability to cope as full members of society.

In Chapter 1 the term *stress* is examined. Stress is not always a negative phenomenon. In the somatic-medical sector it is predominantly the negative results of stress that are seen (myocardial infarction, hyperventilation and suchlike). In our consideration of stress, we pay particular attention to Moss's model, especially in relation to adaptation tasks and to the process of coping, i.e. the ways in which people behave in threatening situations. The emphasis in Chapter 1 is on the description of illness as a stressor and on the converse, becoming ill as a result of the influence of stressors.

In Chapter 2 the area of psychology related to *mental illness* is considered in more detail. The concept of abnormal behaviour is identified as the response to mental illness, and the causes of such illness are explored from a biological, social and psychological perspective. The final section of this chapter introduces the areas of psychotherapy and considers the relevance of an understanding of the psychotherapeutic perspective within the nurse's role.

In Chapter 3 the area of psychology related to *learning difficulties* is explored. The concept of IQ is investigated and the relationship between mental age and ability is discussed. Consideration is given to the effects of learning difficulties on individuals, their acceptance into society, and on the effects on the family. The chapter concludes by looking at psychological processes in the care of people with learning difficulties, especially at the concepts of social role valorization and gentle teaching.

In Chapter 4 *tension complaints* and *functional complaints* are described. Tension complaints are all complaints which are connected with an excess of stress while functional complaints are characterized by difficuties for which no physical reason can be found. In this chapter the principles of conditioning are discussed, as is Moos's model of coping and the SORC diagram.

In Chapter 5 *psychological assessment* is examined in more detail. Important elements are the psychosocial history and questions about the trustworthiness, validity and standardization of the measuring instruments. These are questions which also have a direct practical significance on the way in which nurses observe and measure.

In Chapter 6 the *psychological treatment and support of the individual* is the main concern. In this chapter we expressly refer to the psychological treatment and support which is practised without being perceived as psychiatric treatment or the long-lasting psychological treatments which are referred to in Chapter 2.

In this module the role of the nurse is examined in the context of the treatment of the patient/client. The continuity of the care plays an important part in the support of patients/clients. The patient/client always has the right to support when the psychologist is not available. The knowledge necessary for the nurse in the treatment and support of patients/clients is described. The social skills which the nurse must have at her disposal with the aim of being able to support patients/clients are addressed in Module 5.

Somatic-medical psychology

1

1. Introduction

Medical psychology has an important significance for the professional training of the nurse. Every nurse is confronted with patients/clients who exhibit behavioural disturbances owing to illness, admission to hospital and so on.

In Section 2 medical psychology in general is described. Section 3 discusses stress. There is a good deal of confusion about the notion of stress. That is why consideration is also given to the following concepts:
– stressors;
– being ill as a stressor;
– coping skills.

In Section 4 of this chapter Moos's model is described, with the different factors which determine the outcome of a crisis.

Learning outcomes

After studying this chapter the student should be able to:
– describe and explain what medical psychology is;
– understand the following concepts:
  • stress
  • stressor
  • coping
  • illness gain
  • illness loss;
– describe and explain being ill as a stressor;
– describe, explain and apply Moos's model.

2. Medical psychology; exploring the field

In the somatic-medical field the clinical psychologist deals with behaviour which is within the range that society calls normal but which is considered by the person himself or by others as undesirable. For example: the patient feels down, is anxious, is afraid that he is sickening for a serious illness. Or: the patient's wife is worried about him because he is so unsettled. Or: the General Practitioner asks for an opinion about a patient's (un)fitness for work. The clinical psychologist can investigate such questions and investigate also whether it is possible to change the undesirable behaviour. If that is the case, he offers help in the matter.

One area of medical psychology can therefore be considered as the application of clinical psychology in the somatic-medical situation. Medical psychologists in this setting deal with undesirable behaviour that is linked with physical complaints. The undesirable behaviour is part of the illness itself, but the psychologist also deals with the reaction to the illness. The situations that he has to deal with are:

– people with a physical condition who have developed emotional problems. Examples of this are patients with a chronic illness (such as rheumatism), kidney dialysis patients, or cancer patients;

– people with a physical condition which is caused by stress and/or tension, for example: patients with cardio-vascular diseases;

– people with a functional condition, that is to say physical complaints for which no physical cause can be shown, such as patients with a tension headache;

– a poor relationship between helper and patient, which can have an influence on the course of the illness process.

3. Stress and stress reactions

In everyday life the term 'stress' has a variety of meanings. In this book we do not use the term stress as a designation for all kinds of threatening situations. These situations are the sources of stress and the term that is used to indicate a source of stress is *stressor*. In the hospital many stressors are to be found, such as the admission itself, being away from home, being alone in the strange white world with its own unfamiliar rules and customs. In addition there is the physical examination, the exhibition of your nakedness to strangers, the pain before and after the medical intervention, and the trauma associated with anaesthesia. The apparent contradictions in information about the course of the illness which are sometimes given to patients, are also stressors. For this type of stress, in the sense of a situation experienced by the patient as threatening and therefore as a source of stress, we shall always use the term stressor.

The term *stress* is used to indicate the reaction to a stressor. If we find ourselves in a situation which we experience as threatening, we react in different ways. We may react in a physiological manner: a rise in blood pressure, alterations in the frequency of respiration and in the tension level in the muscles. We may also react in a more mental manner and display anxiety, anger, irritation, disturbances in concentration and thinking, and tension. In addition our reaction to a threatening situation may affect our behaviour: aggression, panic, apathy, depression, being unable to carry out daily duties such as work, school or looking after the household, are all examples of this.

The second meaning which is accepted for the term stress refers to the interaction between the environment and the individual. The person feels that threatening demands coming from the environment are being made on him and he reacts to this as best he can. We talk of stress if the threat from the environment is too great, or if the adaptation to this threat is not adequate. We all know from our own experience that not everyone reacts in the same way to a particular situation. What is a worrying occurrence for one person may be of no concern for another.

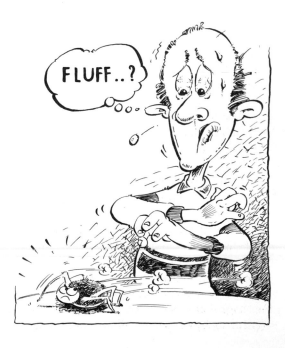

Another way of discussing stress is to consider it in terms of conflicts and life changes. By conflicts we mean those situations where two or more motives conflict, the satisfaction of one leading to the frustration of the other. We referred to these conflicts in Module 2 in terms of the stages of development: independence vs. dependence; intimacy vs. isolation; cooperation vs. competition; and the making of life choices. The effect of life events as a stress were investigated by Holmes and Rahe (1967). The Social Readjustment Rating Scale produced from this research scores 38 life events in terms of their stress effect. Studies have shown that 79% of persons whose stress score for a year on this scale was greater than 300 became ill in the following year. One factor of important note is that the scale consists of items that might be considered of a positive nature e.g. 'marriage' (score 50), as well as items that might be considered of a negative nature, e.g. 'personal injury or illness' (score 53) and 'fired from job' (score 47).

As indicated above not everybody responds to stress in the same way, and what is stressful for one person may have no effect on another. In fact a state of no activity, leading to boredom, may be the most stressful situation for some people. A more recently developed scale asks subjects to judge events as good or bad and to estimate the effect of these on their lives. People who reported a large number of events they regarded as bad were found to be more likely to suffer physical and emotional problems six months later than were people who reported similar numbers of events in total but fewer bad events. (Sarason, Johnson and Siegel, 1978).

Individual processes are important in the formation of a stress situation. Two concepts which play an important part in this are 'cognitive judgement' and 'coping'. By *cognitive judgement*, we mean the individuals process of judgement which determines why and to what extent a situation is judged to be threatening. We are continually dealing with this sort of classification. We constantly judge to what extent an event is of importance for ourselves, for our career, and for our physical and mental welfare. A cognitive judgement in fact involves the answering of three questions.

The first question asks, 'Is this event as it ought to be or not as it ought to be or indeed is this situation threatening for me or not?' If the answer is, 'Not as it should be: it is threatening', then the second question follows, 'What can I change about the event, so that the extent of threat emanating from it decreases?' The third question concerns the control of the effect of the measures taken, 'Is it in fact the case, that the extent of threat which the event contains within it is reduced now because of the measures I have taken?'

By *coping* we mean all possibilities, all capabilities, all manners of intervening which we have at our disposal to reduce or eliminate the threatening character of an event or situation.

Examples of coping techniques are facing up, combating, being a match for, managing all right. If you have successfully divested a threatening situation of its threatening characteristics by means of coping techniques, you have 'faced up to the situation', or – in everyday language – 'you have got through it OK'.

Coping therefore has to do with the methods people use to deal with threatening situations; it concerns getting control over such situations. But sometimes we cannot do anything about a situation in itself, as in the following case. Your boy friend ditches you for someone else, quite definitely, with no second chance. You don't just let matters rest, but it soon becomes clear that all your attempts to win him back are in vain. You can no longer change anything about this situation, but you can certainly do something to deal with your feelings of loneliness, hurt and grief. You can comfort yourself with thoughts such as: there are plenty more fish in the sea, or, that you are better off without him. Coping therefore not only concerns the actual changing of situations, it also concerns the changing of the experiencing of situations.

Study activity

1. **a.** Are defence mechanisms (see Module 1) coping skills?

   b. Describe what coping skills you use in stress.

One last remark before we go on to the next section. Stress is widely regarded as something which leads only to negative things; stress is therefore something which must always be avoided. This idea is incorrect. Stress can also entail a challenge. Having to complete a certain task before a certain date frequently results in an improved performance. Competition also motivates many a student to succeed. Stress therefore is not bad in itself although we in health care often see only the negative side of it. Finally a connection has been made between conditions such as myocardial infarction, skin rash, headache, nervousness, hyperventilation, and stress.

4. Being ill as a stressor

a. Introduction

In this section we discuss being ill as a stressor, that is the ways one can react to an illness. The converse, being ill on account of the influence of stressors will be dealt with in a subsequent section.

For patients, admission to a hospital can often be an uncertain, worrying and threatening situation especially if it is the first time that they have been admitted. On the one hand there exists the hope of a cure, whilst on the other hand this admission is often accompanied by anxiety about the unknown, anxiety about pain, about an operation or about an examination. In the hospital the patient is confronted with staff who are unknown to him. He is confronted with unfamiliar rules and procedures, and he must adapt to them. On admission the patient must accept the role of the sick person (see Module 3) and to some extent relinquish his role of, for example, being a father. Being well looked after will be for one patient a release, but for another a bitter confrontation with his own failure: 'A fully grown chap who, if he has to pass water, has to do it with the help of such a young girl.' Becoming angry is no use as it is always supposed to be for your own good. In short, illness and admission to hospital usually cause stress.

Being ill is, certainly in the first instance, a form of crisis. A crisis is a disturbance of equilibrium. If this is disturbed, the patient will try to restore the old equilibrium or to find a new, different equilibrium. One cannot, in the long run, remain in an extreme condition of disturbed equilibrium.

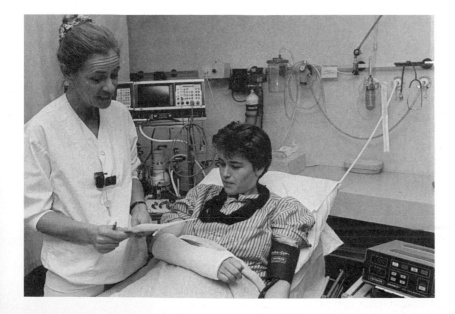

Figure 4.1.1
Confrontation with
unknown staff

A crisis is always limited in time. After a period of time a new equilibrium will occur. This new equilibrium may be a healthy adaptation to the new situation, but it may also be an unadapted reaction which in fact means a decline. We shall give an example. You could compare it with a tight-rope walker who balances high in the air on the rope: he is in equilibrium. If something suddenly happens, for example he is distracted by a noise and begins to sway back and forwards, the balance is then disturbed. This cannot continue for ever. At a certain moment he either recovers his balance on the rope or else he falls down. In both cases he reaches an 'equilibrium'. A fall is not a desired balance, but it is a sort of equilibrium, in the sense that the tight-rope walker is now no longer swaying back and forth.

Similarly, a patient can also appear to come out of the disturbed equilibrium of illness in a desired manner: he has applied adequate coping skills. He may also come out of it in an undesired manner. An example is the driver seriously injured in an accident. After his physical cure he appears to be so afraid of anything to do with cars that he cannot leave his house any more. This driver applied inadequate coping skills.

Rudolf Moos (1989) published a model (diagram 4.1.1), in which different factors are collated to determine the outcome of crises. With Moos's model it is possible to give a good description of the behaviour of sick people and to understand their reactions to illness.

The model takes as its starting point the fact that the reaction to being ill is dependent on a number of personal factors. We list these factors here and then we will examine them more carefully:
– cognitive judgement: this is the significance which the sick person ascribes to the illness and his expectation of being able to handle the illness;
– adapting to the illness: this means the carrying out of a number of tasks, e.g. the handling of pain;
– the availability of adequate coping skills: this means that if you have to adapt to illness and pain, can you actually do so?

These three personal reactions are further influenced by:
– personal background of the sick person: is this the person's first experience of illness or has he a history of such events being effectively coped with?;
– illness-linked factors: cancer is harder to cope with than a broken leg;
– environmental factors: is the patient lying in an overcrowded, overheated ward, or does he have a private room with colour television and a telephone?

Diagram 4.1.1
MOOS'S model

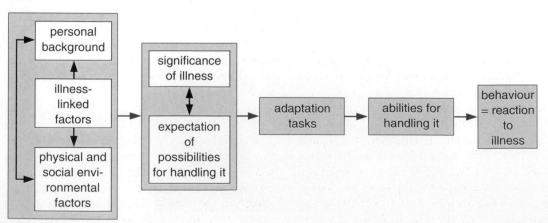

Study activity

2. Use Moos's model for a stress situation and analyze in what manner the different components of the model can be recognized.

b. Cognitive judgement of the illness

The concept of cognitive judgement is introduced in the previous section. It is defined here as: the individual judgement process that determines why and to what extent someone judges a situation as threatening. This concept has a central place in Moos's model, which starts from illness as a crisis situation. The significance that the individual attaches to the illness plays an important part in this. Illness can be considered by a patient as loss, as gain, or as something that has no definite significance for him.

Illness as loss can involve the loss of pleasure-giving events. Through the illness you can no longer participate in a party, an excursion or a holiday. Illness is also the loss of being able to fulfil certain tasks in daily life. A housewife can no longer do the housework, she can no longer look after the children; another person can no longer go to her work. Illness sometimes means loss of functional capabilities, certainly when the patient is bedridden and cannot look after himself, cannot get up and cannot walk, so that he is dependent on the help of others. Often this loss signifies loss of self-esteem and loss of self-respect. Sometimes illness also means loss of love and recognition of other people. In general, illness is loss of normality: the patient cannot do the things which every 'normal person' can do. Illness can sometimes even mean a threat to the person's life. The consideration of illness as a loss also includes negative feelings such as grief, sorrow, anxiety and anger.

Illness can sometimes also signify gain for a patient. Illness may be a relief from the stress of work. For someone who has worked for years under stress, it may be a relief when he is ill and does not, at any rate in the early stages, need to go to work. Illness may be an escape from family conflict: the sick person will be respected by the members of the family. Feelings of guilt can sometimes be reduced by illness. If someone is ill, he does not need to think of others, he can then think only of himself. Suffering in illness can for some people have a religious significance. They feel they are being put to the test and try to show that they can handle suffering. Illness can also offer people the opportunity to receive consideration, attention and friendliness from others. Without illness they would not have experienced this consideration and friendliness.

Study activity

3. Try by means of your own experience to give real life examples of the concepts illness gain and loss.

If the patient considers the illness as unimportant, he will attach little significance to symptoms or possible consequences.

The significance that the patient gives to the illness influences the amount of motivation which he needs to solve problems connected with the illness. Someone who considers the illness as a threat or a loss will experience his illness differently from someone for whom the illness offers gain or for whom the illness has no significance.

The patient's belief in his ability to do something about the illness often has to do with the significance which the illness has for him. His expectation influences the handling of the problems. If the expectation is low, and the patient thinks that he cannot do anything about it, the chance that he will try to do something about it is very small. If he expects that he really can do something about it, the chance is greater that he will also try.

In the above we have proceeded as if three reactions can be ascribed to illness: a negative one, a positive one and a neutral one. In fact this is an oversimplification. Illness can often mean a continuously changing mixture of reactions for each person.

c. Adaptation tasks

The significance which the patient gives to the illness determines the course of the crisis (or illness) to a great extent. But there are other factors that play a part. These are the adaptation tasks and the coping skills. The former postulates that: (this) illness means adapting to the experiencing of pain. The latter asks: 'Do you have at your disposal the capacity to effect this adaptation?'

According to Moos if the patient is set a number of tasks, he will be able to adapt to his illness. Before a new equilibrium occurs, the patient must carry out these adaptation tasks. In order to do this he must have at his disposal handling skills: he must also be capable of carrying out the adaptation tasks.

Seven tasks are described. The first three adaptation tasks relate specifically to illness. The last four relate to life's crises in general.
We shall first discuss the three adaptation tasks which are illness-linked.

The first adaptation task concerns the pain and the attendant limitations. It concerns the ability to live with the discomfort of an illness and with the symptoms of the illness or the injury itself. It concerns a whole series of symptoms such as pain, weakness, incontinence, lameness or a permanent change in external appearance. More than any other symptom, pain means loss of control for a patient; this may be the most im-

portant point of consideration of his suffering. In such a situation pain can become for him the means of communication.

The second adaptation task concerns getting used to the hospital environment and to treatment. Many things which are seen as self-evident for hospital staff are often for a patient new and unknown and therefore threatening. More medical apparatus is constantly deployed, so that patients also undergo more and more complicated surgical interventions and special treatments. All these factors are for the patient a source of tension. Unpleasant side effects of treatments also require adaptations of the patient. In this second adaptation task the importance of clear information and explanations to the patient is highlighted.

The third adaptation task is the development of a good relationship with professional helpers. From the point of view of the patient, this means that as many social skills as possible must be brought into play. A patient should ask himself if it is really sensible to ask many of the questions he wants to ask. He can for example ask himself if there is any point in getting angry with

Figure 4.1.2
Ever more medical
apparatus

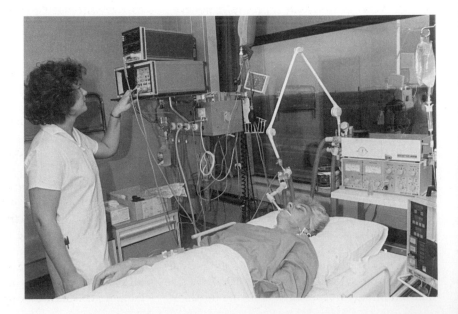

the doctor if the latter, in spite of his promise, has not come along; or if it is wise to ask for more painkillers than are strictly necessary? This requires a number of social skills from the patient, such as standing up for himself, expressing his own wishes, expressing dissatisfaction – all this at a time when he does not feel at his best. This third adaptation task is the mirror image of the task of the helper, who must build up a good relationship with the patient. The helper's task is discussed in Module 5.

Now come the four adaptation tasks which are connected with life's crises, but which now include illness.
The fourth adaptation task concerns the maintenance of a reasonably positive emotional state. That entails that you have to be capable of handling the confusing feelings which are caused by the illness. Illness, a physical crisis, evokes many negative feelings. There is anxiety and worry about the course of the illness as well as feelings of estrangement and isolation. An important aspect is that the patient should not lose courage, in spite of the difficult circumstances in which he finds himself.

The fifth task concerns the maintenance of a satisfactory self-image. In Module 1 we saw how great is the influence, positive or negative, of the self-concept on the functioning of the person. With a positive self-image, we feel competent to cope with adversity, that is: 'I am having a hard time now, but I can handle it'.
A constituent part of the self-concept is the body-image. Because the bodily functioning is altered in a negative respect, since the patient is ill, the body-image affects the self-image in its totality. The changes in body-image result in changes in the self-concept. This may assume the form of an identity crisis which makes it necessary to alter personal values and life style. In particular, victims of mutilating afflictions such as skin diseases, or leprosy; or of mutilating accidents, such as burns or traumatic amputations; are faced with the task of maintaining a satisfactory self-image. In spite of weakness, scars and/or the use of prostheses the person must maintain a reasonably positive self-image. Limitations on independence and the adapting

of life's aims and expectations also belong to this category. It is important that the person finds an equilibrium between the acceptance of help and the taking on of his own responsibility for his later life.

The sixth task concerns the maintenance of relationships with family members and colleagues. Someone who becomes ill must accept the role of illness. He must accept that he is a patient. Likewise he is confronted with the task of accepting that he can no longer properly fulfil the role of father, or boss of a department. In spite of his being ill, he still wants to remain 'father' or 'boss'. A new identity arises. Relations with household, family and colleagues may become disturbed through this and cause feelings of estrangement.

The seventh task concerns the uncertain future, such as having to face a future in which very significant losses may be suffered. It concerns the anxiety which is aroused by an uncertain prognosis. And if the prognosis is unfavourable, it involves questions such as: 'How much time is still left?' and 'Shall I die with dignity?'

These seven adaptation tasks all occur with every illness. The importance of each task differs from person to person. This depends on the type of illness, the individual's personality and on the circumstances in his life.

Study activity
   4. a. Describe in detail the seven adaptation tasks using three experiences from your own practice.
   b. Express the importance of Moos's model for the provision of patient care by the carer staff.

d. Coping skills

We have described the tasks which the patient faces. Whether he can fulfil these tasks properly depends on whether he has adequate coping skills at his disposal.

We shall describe the most important coping skills which are used in order to carry out the different tasks and face up to the problems. They can be used alone, one after the other or (as is mostly the case) in different combinations. That is, a certain skill or combination of skills may be appropriate to one situation, but is not necessarily appropriate to another.

The first group of skills concerns the denying of the illness or the minimizing of the seriousness of it. Feelings which upset someone can be tackled with the aid of this skill. One of the skills from this group is the ability to isolate the emotion, as a result of which it seems as if one is not emotionally affected in a certain situation: tiresome feelings are denied, anger is suppressed or ascribed to, or directed at another person, for example the doctor or the partner. In Module 1 this group of skills has already been described under the term 'defence mechanisms'.

Defence mechanisms are a special group of coping skills. Firstly it is characteristic of a defence mechanism that the person does not have it available to call upon at will. He can only apply it, he is (almost) unable *not* to apply it. For an explanation of this see Module 1. With the other coping skills the situation is different, since the person affected applies them willingly and knowingly. Secondly; a defence mechanism only brings about a change in the experiencing of a situation, it does not change the objective

Figure 4.1.3
No emotion?

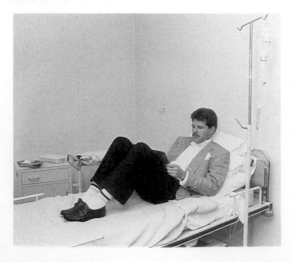

characteristics of a situation. Both of these are important aspects of defence mechanisms.

The second coping skill concerns the seeking of relevant information. The anxiety which arises through uncertainty and misapprehension can be reduced by relevant information. Patients feel that they can cope better if they obtain information which clarifies their situation. Good information, for example to explain medical intervention, may be important. In general, patients who have been properly informed beforehand about what is going to happen and what they can expect are less anxious after the intervention, need less pain medication and recover faster (Hayward, 1975). See also Chapter 6, Section 4.a, (Stress management).

The third coping skill concerns the seeking of reassurance and support from one's family, friends and helpers. Emotional support can be an important help in coping with illness.

People who conceal their feelings and so isolate themselves, lack this source of help. This coping skill does not only concern being able to accept this form of help. It also involves the ability to seek it out, as Moos has noted. It includes saying to a member of the family, 'I feel rotten, please just stay.'

The fourth coping skill concerns the learning of certain actions which have to do with the illness, for example, the diabetes patient who has to give himself the necessary insulin injections. The acquisition of the skill of carrying out for oneself a procedure which is important for the progress of the illness is of great importance. It gives the patient a feeling of competence, of pride, of his own responsibility. These actions serve as a confirmation of the fact that the patient can still *do* something and is still capable of useful action, at a time when there may be few opportunities for it.

The fifth coping skill concerns the setting of concrete, limited and attainable objectives. The patient must learn to divide a problem into small, attainable sub-objectives. This gives the patient a better chance of success. It makes no sense for a patient with a traumatic lower leg amputation to set himself the objective of running 100 metres next year in ten seconds. It is much more realistic if this patient, who knows that he can walk 50 metres with the aid of two sticks, sets himself the objective of walking 75 metres with two sticks in the following week. The capacity to split up apparently insurmountable problems into small, manageable parts is a key part of this coping skill.

The sixth coping skill is the practising of alternative outcomes. If a situation is very threatening, we cope with the anxious and uncertain aspects of it by looking at these from different angles. The following situation is an example. Mr. Jones never tires of telling nursing staff and visitors what Doctor Smith has been telling him about his illness. In this he frequently digresses. Through this disclosure the patient is preparing himself for what is going to happen. He is preparing himself for it by talking about it, and by thinking about it. In this he is confronting his options, and perhaps also seeking relevant information. In certain respects it is similar to the setting of attainable objectives; it is as if the patient breaks down his anxiety about what is to come bit by bit. It is important to realize that if a patient tells the story of his illness to the point of boredom, for the patient this is part of the treatment of the anxiety.

The seventh skill concerns the finding of a meaning in and a purpose for the (apparent) unreasonableness of illness and death. It is often easier to handle a serious illness if you know that your illness has a meaning. If you know that suffering can have a positive value, you then have a weapon with which you can keep your despair under control. Even if this value eludes you at the moment, you know for sure that it is not without meaning. For some people, belief in a God who is working out a purpose even with illness, is important.

The identification of seven coping skills is a more or less arbitrary number. Almost everything that anyone does can be a coping skill. Something is a coping skill if it serves to fulfil an adaptation task. A coping skill is effective if it helps to reduce unpleasant feelings, if it increases self-esteem, if it helps a person's relations with other people and if it improves the state of health.

Study activity

5. **a.** Describe the coping skills you use with illness. Discuss these with other students.
   b. Now compare these coping skills with other students. Is it possible or desirable to ascribe differences in the coping skills chosen to the personality structure? Give reasons for your answer.

Three important factors which play a part in determining the outcome of the illness as a crisis have now been discussed. These are cognitive judgement, adaptation tasks and coping skills. There are three other factors which also play a part: these are the personal background of the sick person, factors which are specifically linked to a particular illness, and the physical and social environmental conditions.

e. Personal background

This relates to factors such as age, intelligence, emotional development and a person's previous experience of dealing with illness. Age and intelligence, for example determine a person's chances of seeking and using information with the aim of reducing feelings of uncertainty and powerlessness. The time of life at which the illness occurs is often important; developing a heart condition, which has invalidity as a result, has a completely different significance for a person of eighteen compared with someone eighty years old. For a young woman the loss of a breast is probably more serious than for an older woman, although even in the latter case the trauma of mastectomy is great. Financial problems, as a consequence of illness, may also be a significant factor in the course of the crisis.

Personality factors, other than the style of cognitive judgement, also play a part. In general, people can be differentiated into three types: repressor, sensitizer and non-specific defender. A *sensitizer* fights against the illness, takes an active part in the therapy and gives a good deal of thought to details of the treatment. He admits to feelings of anxiety, aversion and fear and also expresses them. This is in contrast to a repressor.

A *repressor* tries to deny the illness and the negative feelings which go with it. He tries to reduce the threat of it by denying facts, rationalizing them or projecting them on to others; this is comparable with the defence mechanisms described in Module 1.

A *non-specific defender* is a combination of the sensitizer and the repressor. Sometimes he tries to deal with the illness by denying it, sometimes he fights against the illness. The extremes are reproduced on a continuum: at the one side stands the sensitizer, at the other side the repressor. Non-specific defenders come in the middle of the continuum.

Non-specific defender

Sensitizer ⟵⟶ Repressor

You will never encounter a pure repressor or a pure sensitizer in real life. Everyone applies more repressive or more sensitizing techniques according to the situation. See also Chapter 6, section 4.a (Stress management).

f. Illness-linked factors

The second group of factors which plays a role, besides cognitive judgement, adaptation tasks and coping skills, is the group of illness-linked factors. By illness-linked factors we mean the type of illness, the phase in which the illness is, the prognosis, the place where the body is damaged, the symptoms and so forth.

Sometimes an important organ is affected, for example the heart or the reproductive organs. Different organs and functions have a specific psychological significance which has little to do with biological factors. These parts of the body are especially important in the body-image that everyone has of himself. As we have already indicated the body-image is an important constituent of the self-image. A disturbance of the body-image, the self-concept, can go hand in hand with feelings of shame, dependence, contempt, reproach and the like. If the illness concerns the brain, for example in dementia or traumatic brain damage, the person is affected, literally at the core of his ability to adapt to the illness. Sometimes the brain can be so badly affected that the patient can no longer classify the physical possibilities of his behaviour.

g. Physical and social environmental factors

The third group of factors consists of the physical and social environmental factors. These too are factors which can influence the experience of illness. The unknown, often threatening environment of a hospital, with its profusion of apparatus and unknown sounds, can make patients anxious, just as the absence of familiar things can. The social support of family, helpers and other patients can be important. Interpersonal conflict can delay the recovery from an illness whilst social support and understanding can contribute to a better treatment of it.

Before we illustrate this in some worked out examples, it is important to emphasize one point. In a crisis (and getting through an illness is a crisis) people are more sensitive to influences from outside than in periods of relative calm. Intervention of third parties, however small, can play an important part in the promotion of adapted, effective behaviour. Furthermore the reverse can also happen. It is therefore important that the caring staff, and the other professional staff in health care, are fully aware of the importance of social support to the patient and his family.

h. The application of Moos's model

Two concrete examples, of the application of Moos's, model are given below.

Example 1

Preparation for an operation

Preparation for an operation has been shown to be important for the recovery after it.

From literature a number of coping skills and characteristics are known which play a part in this (e.g. Hayward, 1975; Boore, 1978).
- Anxiety plays a part as follows. Patients who as a whole are *not anxious* and patients who are *very anxious* before an operation com-

plain more of pain, and more often, and they need a longer recovery period than patients who are *moderately anxious.*

– Information contributes as follows. Better progress after the operation occurs if patients are informed beforehand about the operation itself and what they can expect after it. This information must cover three aspects: 1. the procedure which they will undergo, therefore the events that will occur; 2. the sensations that the patient will experience, what he will feel, see, smell and so forth; 3. a number of actions, things that a patient can do for himself to influence the course of the operation favourably, such as breathing and relaxation exercises. These three aspects concern both the pre- and the post-operative period.

– As far as personality factors are concerned, the following should be noted. As we have already noted, patients can be classified as repressors or sensitizers. It appears that repressors experience their behaviour as if it is caused by factors outside themselves, on which they exert no influence. They are inclined to deny problems and to think about them as little as possible. Sensitizers on the other hand have the impression that they are able to determine their own behaviour. They try actively to improve aspects of the situation. Research has shown that it is better for repressors to be unable to get information about the course of the operation, since they become more anxious as a result, so that after the operation they do not make such a good recovery. It is best to give them *general* information, and to give it relatively late. With sensitizers precise, detailed information which is given well beforehand has a positive effect on recovery after the operation.

– It is not only important that patients get information beforehand, it is also important who gives this information and how this happens. The information has more influence if the informant is trustworthy for the patient and if she has a good relationship with the patient. For one patient the surgeon will be the right person, since the patient feels she is the most expert. For another the right person will be the patient-carer, since he has the most contact with her and trusts her.

– Finally, the structure in which the information is presented is important. It should be presented in manageable units, not all at once.

In Moos's model these factors must be placed within the personal background:
– the options for treatment: is the patient a repressor or a sensitizer?;
– the environmental factors, that is to say, the person who is most suited to give the information;
– the coping skills, that is the seeking of information and reduction of anxiety.

Example 2

Mastectomy

A mastectomy is for women a very far-reaching event. Different factors play a role in the treatment of it, such as anxiety about return of cancer, anxiety about death, loss of femininity, feeling misshapen and so forth.
Within Moos's model the following factors can be recognized.
– Personal background: the age of the woman plays a part, as also do intelligence and level of education. Acquaintance with other women who have undergone the same operation can be important as a source of information.
– Illness-linked factors: the location of the amputation, the breast, plays a large part in its significance. Pain can cause problems later.
– Environmental factors: the reaction of the partner; will he still accept his wife after the operation, does he still find her attractive, does he react with aversion or is he worried, does he try to understand what this intervention means for her?
– The significance of the illness: loss of femininity, a threat of death, powerlessness.
– The adaptation tasks: the most important are:
  • dealing with the feelings of anxiety, depression, anger, powerlessness and inferiority;
  • acceptance of the loss of a breast;
  • building up of a positive self-image;
  • the uncertainty that cancer may return;

– The coping skills: help in the treatment may consist of the opportunity to talk about it, to express negative emotions. Support from the partner plays an important role. Information can be offered about likely side effects, about the possibility of help in coping, about the possibility of a prosthesis. In the help it is important to go over what effective treatment skills the woman herself has available. These can be supported and possibly supplemented with other skills.

5. Summary

In this chapter we have briefly looked at the kind of settings where medical psychology can be applied. We have differentiated between *stressors* (situations which are the sources of stress) and *stress* itself (the reaction to stressors).

By means of Moos's model we have seen that the *significance* a person attaches to an illness is an important factor in determining the course of the crisis or illness. The central role of *cognitive judgement* in this process was emphasized. The seven *adaptation tasks* were examined, three relating specifically to illness and four in the context of life's crises in general.

The question as to whether the patient can fulfil these tasks effectively depends to a large extent on the *coping skills* he has at his disposal. Seven coping skills were identified though the point was made that any means which serve to accomplish the adaptation tasks could be classified thus.

Finally two clinical situations were described as examples of the application of Moos's model.

Psychiatric psychology

2

1. Introduction

Psychiatric psychology is that area of psychology which concentrates on mental illness. Those carers involved in the care of people with mental illness have much to gain from its study. Cormack (1983) stated that insufficient emphasis was given to the practice of therapy within the training of psychiatric nurses. Psychiatric nurses were identified as operating in a medico-custodial role and most did not see themselves extending beyond such a role. There have been many advances within the therapeutic roles that nurses may take since that time. Roles such as behaviour nurse therapist, community psychiatric nurse, and involvement in group and individual psychotherapy, are examples. The need to understand and explain behaviours within this field is vital if a therapeutic role is to be adopted. This chapter cannot be a comprehensive treatment of the field. Instead it aims to focus attention on some of the key issues within the field and identify the needs of the nurse within this area.

In Section 2 the concept of psychiatric psychology is introduced focusing on how patients' problems are understood. The concept of abnormal behaviour is identified as are the mental health classifications used. Section 3 concentrates on the causes of abnormal behaviour from a biological, social and psychological perspective. Section 4 introduces approaches available in psychotherapy. Specific consideration is given to the:
- behavioural-cognitive approach;
- psychoanalytical approach;
- psychosocial approach;
- eclectic approach.

Learning outcomes

After studying this chapter the student should be able to:
- describe and explain what psychiatric psychology is;
- understand the following concepts:
  - mental health
  - abnormal behaviour
  - maladaptive behaviour
  - psychotherapy

- prepared conditioning
- systematic desensitization
- modelling
- labelling
- transference
- counter-transference
- abreaction
- therapeutic community;

  – explain how inheritance studies can help identify the causes of abnormal behaviours;
  – describe how neural transmitters are involved in behaviour and how psychotropic drugs act to reduce abnormal behaviours;
  – analyze the difference in approach between a behavioural-cognitive therapy and a psychoanalytical therapy;
  – discuss why an understanding of psychoanalytical theory can assist a nurse in the work setting;

2. Understanding psychiatric patients' problems

Experiencing periods of anxiety, depression, anger and other emotions are a normal part of our efforts to deal with life events. When we become unable to cope with life events is the time when the help of a professional is required. In this section we consider the development of serious mental disorders, that is those which require help of a more specialist nature than can be provided within the informal care setting. These disorders result in abnormal behaviour, including the development of self-destructive lifestyles.

When identifying normal behaviour it is usual to identify those traits which the mentally healthy person possesses to a greater extent than the mentally ill person. The mentally healthy person can live a more fulfilling life than can the mentally ill person. He can sustain meaningful and emotional relationships, partake in social activity, pursue a job of work, and make a realistic judgement of his own ability, or at least not make unrealistic and exaggerated claims about his ability. Such descriptions of normal behaviour are obviously socially dependent. The definition of normality in society will vary somewhat from place to place and from time to time. The use of 'soft' drugs, which some now argue should be legalized, was once considered to be totally abnormal. The severe physical punishment meted out to children under the adage of 'spare the rod and spoil the child' was considered normal in previous generations but is not now the accepted wisdom.

Normal or abnormal?

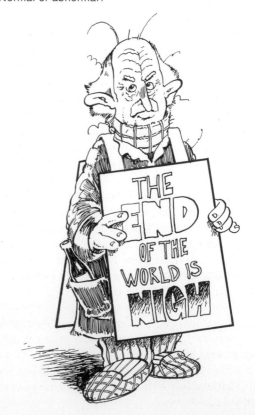

Abnormal behaviour can then be defined as that form of behaviour which does not conform to the cultural or social norms. It is behaviour which: deviates from the average of observed behaviours; deviates from the socially accepted norm; is maladaptive, i.e. it has an adverse effect on the individual or is harmful to others or causes personal distress. Each of the above criteria can be true in part, and in practice all four need considering when diagnosing abnormality. Abnormal behaviour is not a precise term; rather it lies upon a continuum from normal to abnormal. It can be difficult to identify the dividing line between 'normal' and 'abnormal' behaviour.

Case study: Jean Smith

Jean is 23 years old and has one son, James, aged 10 months. She lives with her husband in a flat on the third floor of a large block of flats. Since the birth of James, Jean has developed an elaborate cleaning routine to ensure that James does not catch an infection. She keeps James in the flat as much as possible, and has one room in the flat reserved for him. She cleans this room thoroughly every day, including washing of all ledges, handles and the radiator. Jean changes James's nappy 10 to 15 times a day, and all his clothes and nappies are soaked in disinfectant prior to being washed. Other examples of Jean's behaviour include bathing James before each meal and soaking all his feeding utensils in disinfectant before use. On the rare occasions that Jean takes James out, she wraps him up carefully and tries to avoid crowds. Jean finds it difficult to do the shopping, because she does not want to take James into a busy supermarket full of people who may infect him. Recently, as an extra protection, Jean has started to bath herself prior to feeding James, and she wants her husband to have a bath when he gets home from work before he plays with James. If Jean is prevented from following any of this behaviour she feels extremely anxious.

It must be noted in the above case study that Jean does not consider her behaviour to be abnormal. Instead she considers that she is doing a good job of looking after her baby. Jean's husband on the other hand considers that her behaviour is abnormal.

Study activities
1. Do you consider Jean's behaviour to be normal or abnormal? Give your reasons.

2. With other students (if possible), discuss how we might decide at what point Jean's behaviour would change from 'normal' to become 'abnormal'. Give your reasons.

Categorization of abnormal behaviour
To facilitate discussion of abnormal behaviour a classification schema is of value. The World Health Organization has defined a disease classification scheme which includes a section for mental illness. From these categories the following are identified within the area covering abnormal behaviour.
- Disorders first evident in infancy, childhood, or in adolescence; this includes any deviation from normal development plus others such as eating disorders (e.g. anorexia nervosa).
- Organic mental disorders; where symptoms are related directly to abnormality in brain functioning, perhaps due to degenerative disease (e.g. Alzheimer's disease), injury, or toxic substance (e.g. alcohol).
- Substance abuse; this covers all mind-altering substances.
- Schizophrenic disorders.
- Paranoid disorders; showing excessive suspicions, hostility and feelings of being persecuted.
- Affective disorders; where the person demonstrates abnormal mood states, e.g. extreme depression or elation, or maybe alternates between the two.
- Anxiety disorders; including those where anxiety is the main symptom (free floating anxiety), where situations have to be avoided to prevent anxiety (phobias), or where trying to resist performing rituals or thinking persistent thoughts leads to anxiety (obsessive-compulsive disorders).
- Somatoform disorders; where physical symptoms are present but no organic cause can be found and psychological factors seem to play a major part.
- Dissociative disorders; related to temporary alterations in consciousness, memory or

identity due to emotional problems (e.g. amnesia or multiple personality).

- Psychosexual disorders; covering problems of sexual identity, sexual performance, and sexual aim. N.B. Homosexuality is only considered a disorder if the person is not happy with their situation and wishes to change it.
- Conditions not attributable to a mental disorder; including marital problems, parent-child difficulties and child abuse, environmental issues such as housing and pollution, social issues such as isolation, loneliness, and incarceration.
- Personality disorders; covering long-standing maladaptive behaviour (e.g. antisocial personality disorder and narcissistic personality).

This section will not go into detail about any one of these disorders. The interested reader should refer to the texts identified in the reference section.

The reader may discern from the above that some of the 'conditions' we have identified are the classic 'mental illnesses' whilst others are not. Within this chapter no distinction will be made as to the severity of an 'illness' state; rather the requirments of understanding the concept of abnormal behaviour, regardless of cause, will be explored.

3. Causes of abnormal behaviour

When considering somatic illnesses a causative classification is readily apparent, e.g. infective, traumatic, degenerative, etc. A similar classification scheme can be advanced for psychiatric psychology. This causative classification considers the conditions under the headings of biological factors and social and psychological factors, which include consideration of psycho-analytic, behavioural, cognitive and phenomenological theories. We will take these categories in turn, giving examples from specific conditions to clarify the discussion.

a. Biological evidence

Toxic conditions such as high fever; various poisons such as lead or carbon monoxide; excessive use of alcohol or other drugs, and withdrawal from drugs or alcohol; disease of the kidney or liver; certain kinds of brain trauma; brain tumours; and degenerative changes of the brain: all these can all lead to delirium and dementia. These conditions which may be short-lived, lasting about one week in the case of some of the toxic causes, or long-lived and progressive in the case of the senile and pre-senile dementias, are known as the 'organic brain syndromes'.

Delirium varies greatly but sufferers generally have difficulty maintaining attention to environmental events or engaging in goal-directed behaviours. They are usually restless and over-alert with difficulty in sleeping, although reduced wakefulness may occur. They can also experience perceptual distortions which may progress to hallucinations, visual hallucinations being the most common.

Dementia on the other hand refers to a deterioration from the person's previous level of intellectual capacity. This deterioration is particularly evident in memory, abstract thinking and judgement. Senile and pre-senile dementia is a particularly sad condition where the sufferers progressively deteriorate in their ability to cope with their lives. Memory loss becomes so acute that recognition of family becomes confused or non-existent, personal presentation in terms of dress and language deteriorate, and the person loses the ability to initiate action.
The most common form of these conditions is Alzheimer's disease.

Other mental illness conditions for which no clear cause is identifiable, including the dissociative disorders (e.g. schizophrenic disorders), are considered to have a biological base. Although the cause of the presentation is less clear, heredity studies point to a genetic connection. Gottesman and Shields (1982) studied the probability of diagnosis of schizophrenia in relation to genetic similarity. They found that if one person was diagnosed as schizophrenic, the closer the genetic ties, the more likelihood there was of other related persons also being diagnosed. The linkage is not absolutely clear, which suggests that several genes are involved

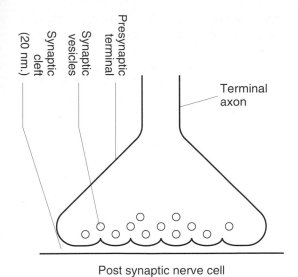

Synapse
Transmitter substances are released from the synaptic vesicles into the synaptic cleft.

Diagram 4.2.1
Chemical transmission of messages

rather than one dominant or recessive gene (Nicol and Gottesman, 1983).

Evidence from twin studies also show an inheritance probability for the conditions of anxiety (Torgersen, 1983) and depression, especially manic-depression.

Other evidence supporting a biological cause comes from studies of neural chemistry. The functioning of the nervous system is dependent on a series of neural transmitters and receptors. Neural transmitters are chemicals which are released from the pre-synaptic end of a nerve cell. Receptors are sites on nerve cells which can bind with a specific transmitter and stimulate the cell to act or not to act. Other chemicals produced have the effect of clearing the transmitter substances from the area of the cells so that a constant state of activity is not evidenced. Many chemicals have been identified as transmitter substances. Some of these substances have been shown to be involved in responses to pain, the general state of readiness of the body and to the emotional state of the individual.

Research into the schizophrenias has led to the conclusion that the presentation of the conditions is probably due to an imbalance in dopamine (a neural transmitter) usage although this is difficult to prove. Antipsychotic drugs used in the treatment of schizophrenia have been shown to reduce the useable level of dopamine in the brain. Creese, Burt and Snyder (1978) demonstrated that the therapeutic effectiveness of antipsychotic drugs paralleled their potency in blocking dopamine receptors. Further evidence comes from the effects of the use of amphetamines, a substance which increases the release of dopamine. Drug users who overdose on amphetamines exhibit psychotic behaviour which resembles schizophrenia. Further, when small doses of amphetamines were administered to schizophrenic patients it exacerbated the symptoms they were experiencing (Snyder, 1980). Whilst the evidence presented may seem positive proof of the connection between dopamine and schizophrenia the picture remains inconclusive. Not all patients respond to antipsychotic drugs. This suggests that there are other causes of this condition, or that schizophrenia is not a single condition but a group of disorders.

Neural transmitters have also been identified as involved in anxiety conditions, where the benzodiazepine receptors have been implicated, and in depression where the biogenic amines have been implicated. Research in these areas is leading to more effective drugs for the treatment of these conditions.

When considering the antisocial personality, research points not to one transmitter but to a generalized underactivity of the autonomic nervous system. For instance Hare (1970) identifies that people suffering from antisocial personality who are in prison do not learn to avoid shocks as easily as other prisoners and do not show as much autonomic nervous system activity as other prisoners.

b. Social evidence

Schizophrenia has been linked to lower social classes. The reason for this is not clearly understood, but the following hypotheses have been suggested. It is argued that one reason for the link with lower social classes is an unwillingness to label people from higher social classes as it would affect their career prospects. A further cause argued for this link to social class is that due to poor coping skills people who suffer from this condition do not complete their education, or if they do they have difficulty maintaining employment, so there is a downward drift to become part of the lower class – *the social drift hypothesis*. Finally it is argued that living under conditions of increased stress in areas of poverty, with poor housing and poor schooling, is sufficient to precipitate schizophrenic disorders, particularly in people genetically predisposed to this condition. Evidence to support these explanations, particularly the last two, comes from Brenner (1982), and Fried (1982).

c. Psychological factors

Family relationships and communication have also been identified as contributors to schizophrenia. Two types of family have been focused on, these being: those where there are sharply divided parents who fail to collaborate in mutual goals, each devaluing the other and competing for the child's affection; and those where there is a dominant parent who shows serious psychopathology that the other parent accepts as normal (Lidz, 1973). Observation of communications in schizophrenic families shows a tendency to be unable to focus attention and communicate a coherent message to their listener. Conversations tend to be disjointed and confused. Within these families there is also a tendency to deal with the child in a hostile and critical manner, i.e parents tend to criticize the child rather than his actions when he misbehaves, and tend to tell him how he should feel rather than listen to what he has to say. Goldstein (1985) claims that whilst both confused communication and negative parental attitudes appear to be individually involved in the development of schizophrenia, a combination of them both is more predictive than either in isolation. Whether these factors cause the condition or are an attempt by parents to cope with a child's disorganized behaviour is not yet known. What is demonstrable is that family disorganization and parental rejection are important in determining the severity of the illness and the prognosis for recovery (Roff and Knight, 1981).

When specific theories of psychology are examined, further causes are advanced.

Psychoanalytical – These theories based on Freud's work focus attention on the internal control of the individual (Freud, 1962). They argue that abnormal behaviour is related to the use of psychological defence mechanisms resulting in regression and behaviours linked to earlier developmental stages. Psychoanalytical theory argues that schizophrenia is a reflection of a weak ego which can no longer contain the ordinarily unconscious id. The combination of this weak ego and fixation at the oral stage of development leads to a regression to this earlier stage. This description is able to explain many features of the conditions, e.g. the failure to distinguish clearly between external reality and internal wishes. Such persons are also said to have withdrawn their libidinal attachments from other people and turned this energy inward, leading to detachment and autistic (the inability to differentiate between the I and the not I) preoccupation (Martin, 1981).

This use of internal and unconscious drives has also been used to explain the cause of anxiety and depression. Anxiety is seen as a repression of unacceptable or 'dangerous' impulses, i.e. those which can damage the self-esteem or relationships with other people if expressed. These impulses are usually sexual or aggressive in nature, and in situations where they are likely to be aroused the person experiences intense anxiety. This unconscious feeling of apprehension cannot be explained by the person due to its nature being within the mental defence process.

A similar explanation can be advanced for depression, except in this case it represents a reaction to loss. The current loss brings back memories of earlier loss of parental affection in childhood. Persons who are depressed also experience angry feelings towards the loss. Such people have learnt to repress these feelings as a protection against alienating those they depend on for support. Finally it is argued that the low self-esteem and feelings of worthlessness associated with depression stem from a childlike need for parental approval. A loss in later life, of a person, status, or whatever, causes the person to regress to an earlier and dependent state.

Behavioural – As one would expect, behavioural theories link abnormal behaviour to conditioning. Behavioural explanations tend to concentrate on those conditions for which a clear link can be seen. In this section we will concentrate on the causes of anxieties and depressions.

Anxiety is seen as being triggered by external events. Generalized anxiety is viewed as a response to an inability to cope with many everyday occurrences, whereas phobia is seen as an avoidance response learned from self-experience or vicariously. Whilst classical conditioning can provide theoretical explanations for phobias through the pairing of neutral stimuli with traumatic events, there are problems. Some neutral stimuli never seem to become linked in this way except in experimental situations, for example snakes and dogs do whilst kittens and lambs do not. Experiments into the ability of some stimuli to be more easily associated with fear (as measured by galvanic skin response) than others have led to the development of the concept of *prepared conditioning*. This is the idea that through evolutionary selection humans learned to fear certain stimuli such as heights, large animals, etc. whilst other stimuli such as guns have not been around long enough for natural selection to lead to this inherited ability to fear (Seligman and Rosenhan, 1984). Phobias are therefore considered as instances of 'prepared classical conditioning', as distinct from ordinary classical conditioning, and as such have the capacity to easily become conditioned to trauma.

Depression is seen as a lack of positive reinforcement, or a high rate of negative reinforcement. This reinforcement schedule leads to the inactivity of the depressed persons and their feelings of sadness. Persons who are prone to depression may lack the social skills to attract positive reinforcement or to cope with aversive events. Once a person is depressed his main source of reinforcement is sympathy and attention from family and friends, and this may actually reinforce the abnormal behaviour. It is difficult to maintain contact with someone who refuses to cheer up and so social contact is gradually removed, reducing any positive reinforcement even further and increasing social isolation and unhappiness. It is easy to see by this description how a vicious cycle of low reinforcement leading to further isolation can develop.

Cognitive – Theorists in this field tend to focus on how people think about situations.

Anxious people who suffer from generalized free-floating (everpresent) anxiety tend to be unrealistic in their appraisals of situations, especially where potential danger is remote. This overemphasis on the likelihood of danger, and on the degree of harm that can arise, leads to them being always on the lookout for danger, and interpreting innocent signs such as screeching of car brakes or sudden noises in the home as signs that the worst is about to occur. Because of this their autonomic nervous system is often in a state of heightened activity. Obsessions are seen as resulting from the difficulty experienced in getting rid of unwanted thoughts due to the general heightened level of anxiety. We all experience thoughts which are repetitive and sometimes abhorrent. The more anxiety-provoking the thought the less easy it is to get rid of. However, non-anxious people are able to get rid of these thoughts. Compulsive rituals in behaviour are seen as an attempt to neutralize these morbid thoughts by an action that ensures safety. The mother who has obsessive thoughts about harming her child may engage in compulsive rituals around the cleanliness of that child's environment.

Depression on the other hand can be seen as a general attitude of appraising events from a negative and self-critical point of view (Beck, 1976). Depressed people tend to expect to fail, and they blame themselves when things go wrong. They therefore magnify failures and minimize success in evaluating their performance. Another explanation of the cause of depression that has been advanced is that of 'learned helplessness' (Peterson and Seligman,

1984). This theory predicts that people who explain negative events in terms of:
- having internal rather than external causation, i.e. as an inability to control outcomes rather than having control of them;
- being stable rather than unstable, i.e. the feature is likely to persist;
- being global rather than specific on the global-specific continuum, i.e. as conclusive proof that they are totally helpless

will be more depressed than people who see the event as having an external cause; as being unstable, i.e. not a permanent feature of their behaviour; and as being specific to this situation.

Whilst such thought processes have been found in depressed patients who have been hospitalized, it appears that these thought processes do not persist once the depression has lifted (Fennel and Campbell, 1984).

Study activity

3. **a.** Is it possible to explain Jean's behaviour from a psychoanalytical point of view?
   b. Discuss this case study with other students and with qualified nurses to identify if it is possible to explain the behaviours from a biological and from a behavioural-cognitive perspective.

4. Techniques of therapy

Mental illness is subject to treatment and care in the form of drug therapy, physical therapy and psychotherapy. This text will only consider that range of therapies known as the psychotherapies. Excellent treatments of the other areas are available in numerous textbooks.

Within the psychotherapies the aim is either to change the abnormal behaviour directly, or enable people to reach an understanding about the causes of their behaviour so that they can change the behaviour themselves. The psychotherapies are therefore the attempts by one person to relieve another person's psychological distress (Frank, 1986), and can range over many varieties of individual and group therapies.

Within this text we shall group these areas together as the behavioural and cognitive, psycho-analytical, psychosocial and eclectic approaches.

a. Behavioural and cognitive approaches

This approach includes the behavioural and cognitive therapies. These therapies are concerned more with factors maintaining the symptoms and abnormal behaviours than with their causes. The basis of the behavioural technique is examined in greater detail in Chapter 4 of this module. What is important to remember here is that this technique is applied in specific ways for people suffering abnormal behaviour. Many cognitive and behavioural treatments are designed to increase the persons' ability to help themselves. Treatments may also encourage the patient to take an active part in planning and executing appropriate behaviours. The behavioural and cognitive therapies are most successful when dealing with:
- phobias;
- general anxiety;
- obsessions;
- depression;
- eating disorders;
- sexual disfunction;
- social inadequacy.

As the basis for this group of therapies is dealt with elsewhere in this book, we shall concentrate on describing briefly a few specific applications.

Behaviour therapies aim to reduce the occurrence of abnormal (unwanted) behaviour, or to increase the occurrence of wanted behaviour. Use is made of both classical, operant and social learning theories. The procedures are based on psychological experimentation and have limited and rather specific indications (Gelder, 1986). It is likely that nurses in the field of mental health will be involved in some or all of these therapies at some time during their career, although further training is necessary before the nurse can act as the leader in this field.

Systematic desensitization was first developed by Wolpe (1950) and is based on the model of classical conditioning. This system is seen as a form of extinction using the reinforcement of

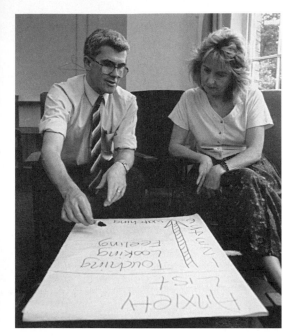

Figure 4.2.1
Developing a hierarchy of anxiety

relaxation. The assumption is that the person cannot be both relaxed and anxious at the same time. The technique can be effective using a hierarchy of imaginary stimuli (figure 2.4.1), or carried out using the real object (*in vivo* desensitization). When using this treatment the client is initially taught how to relax, and then practises relaxing while in the presence of, or imagining, lower levels of the anxiety-causing stimuli. Only when the client has mastered a lower level and feels confident at that level is the next level attempted. Ability to gain success is based on the expectation of a favourable outcome. The clients develop a sense of mastery leading to a change in their beliefs about themselves, from feelings of inability to cope with the anxiety-provoking stimulus to feelings of mastery of their own situation.

Covert sensitization aims to link undesired behaviour patterns with aversive stimuli. In this form of therapy, developed by Cautela (1967), both the behaviour and the aversive stimuli are imagined. Clients are taught to imagine the unwanted behaviour and then to imagine a very negative consequence. This approach has been used to reduce overeating and in helping people to stop smoking. The assumption is that the negative consequence will be conditioned with the unwanted behaviour and thus reduce its occurrence. This form of therapy can be explained in terms of both classical and operant conditioning.

Systematic reinforcement aims to increase the occurrence of wanted behaviour and extinguish the occurrence of unwanted behaviour. It is based on operant conditioning techniques (see Module 1, Chapter 2). Use of reinforcers and, less frequently, punishment, enable behaviours to be shaped. An illustration of this approach regarding a child who was inattentive in school is provided by Walker, Hedberg, Clement and Wright (1981). In this study, beans were used as currency that the child could trade for desired special privileges. Within the psychiatric hospital, attempts at the use of this system are based on the introduction of the 'token economy' (i.e. where desired behaviour is rewarded by tokens, e.g. plastic disks, which can be exchanged for desired goods, e.g. sweets, cigarettes, magazines). This system is of value in adapting the behaviour of regressed, chronic clients to induce socially appropriate behaviour. Use of this approach can not only bring about a change in the persons' behaviour, but also a change in their view of themselves. Social learning theory refutes the notion that there is no internal connection between stimulus and response (Bandura, 1969). This concept is taken up further in Chapter 4.

Modelling is a form of behaviour modification that uses the technique of observational learning. This technique, like systematic reinforcement, is based on the work of Bandura (1969). It has been shown to be an effective form of therapy in the treatment of phobias, and also in the field of social learning. Techniques used include 'symbolic modelling' where the subject can watch the desired behaviour on video, and 'participant modelling' where the subject models behaviour demonstrated by the therapist. Participant modelling, at least with regard to phobias for snakes, has been shown to be the most effective (Bandura, Adams and Beyer, 1976).

When modelling is used as a social skills training technique it usually incorporates role playing as a part of the process. The client observes the behaviour to be modelled, and then practises that behaviour in the relative safety of the role play situation prior to going live (figure 4.2.2). Within the role play situation the therapist provides feedback and positive reinforcement. Programmes of social skills training are developed for persons who possess low levels of social skills, have specific perceived deficiencies (e.g. interviewing skills), are lacking in assertiveness, or who have lost their skills through illness (e.g. schizophrenia).

Cognitive therapies attempt to both modify the behaviour and change unwanted beliefs. When discussing the causation of depression we identified Beck's cognitive theory. The aim of the cognitive therapists is to help the person identify the maladaptive nature of their beliefs and

Figure 4.2.2
Role playing:
safe to make mistakes

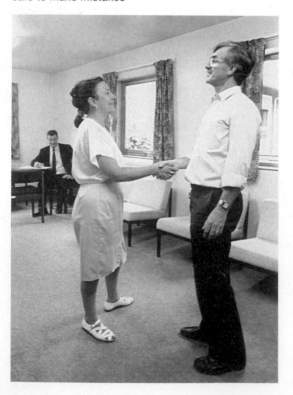

thought processes through carefully directed questioning. The person is taught through this therapy to use positive self-instruction in the place of his previous self-defeating thoughts. This form of therapy is usually combined with behaviour modification techniques such as systematic desensitization or modelling to enable the individual to achieve a change in his observed behaviour. As previously noted, a feeling of self-mastery is one of the strongest reinforcers (Bandura, 1984).

Behaviour modification can be an effective form of treatment in the changing of abnormal behaviour into socially acceptable behaviour. As we stated earlier, this form of treatment does not look at the underlying cause of the behaviour being modified, even when cognition is an accepted variable within the behaviour. Other modes of therapy do accept the underlying cause of the aberrant behaviour as the proper focus of therapy and these will be dealt with in the next section.

b. Psychoanalytical approaches

This area of therapy owes its orgin to Freud. Its focus is the underlying unconscious processes that are assumed to be causing the abnormal behaviour. In Module 1, Chapter 2, we examined the psychoanalytical approach to personality development. We further considered the mental defence mechanisms that enable a person to withstand attacks on his psyche. Within the field of psychoanalytical theory, abnormal behaviour is considered to be a symptom of unresolved conflict during the development of the person. Therapy therefore aims at the exposure of the causes of the behavioural difficulty (the unresolved conflicts), so enabling the person to deal with it more effectively. The classical approach to psychoanalysis, developed by Freud, has been modified in the light of current theories. These modifications place more emphasis on the social and cultural factors in the shaping of human behaviour. They also place greater emphasis on the ego instead of the unconscious sexual and aggressive drives. The psychoanalytical psychotherapies which have developed from these changes also demonstrate a modification in their methods; they are usually shorter and less intense than the classical approach.

Nurses require specialist training before becoming involved in the practice of psychotherapy. An understanding of psychoanalytical theory is important however in helping nurses appreciate the processes of behaviour within their sphere of influence.

Psychoanalytical approaches have been developed for many areas of therapy, including family therapy, child therapy and group therapy. In this section we concentrate on the adult individual psychoanalyses which are divided into two main forms: long-term psychoanalysis and brief focal psychoanalysis. Long-term psychoanalysis gives emphasis to both the intra-psychic and extra-psychic components of man. Its aim is the relief of symptoms and the modification of the basic personality (Crown, 1986). Brief focal psychoanalysis has the less grandiose aims of increasing self awareness and relieving the client of one or more 'focused' conflicts within a given time-frame.

The process of both the above forms of psychoanalyses is based on *free association*. This enables the client to make connections between unrelated events in an attempt to get to the root of the unresolved conflict. Prolonged silences and sudden changes of direction in the client's associations are taken as evidence of blocking by the unconscious of sensitive areas which the analyst should explore. The role of the analyst is to provide *interpretation* of the associations by calling attention to resistances evidenced through silences or changes in direction, and by helping clients draw associations. It is important that the analyst does not provide interpretations of what the client says, but instead hints at possible connections that the analyst may privately have reached by, for instance, pointing to areas for consideration that the client may consider trivial. During the process of psychoanalysis an important area of concern is *transference*. Here the therapist is made into the object of emotions relevant to the area of conflict by the client. By studying these emotional responses the therapist is able to help clients come to a better understanding of their emotional responses to others. *Counter-transference* also occurs during therapy. This is the transference of emotions felt by the therapist to the client. It is important that the therapist recognizes these

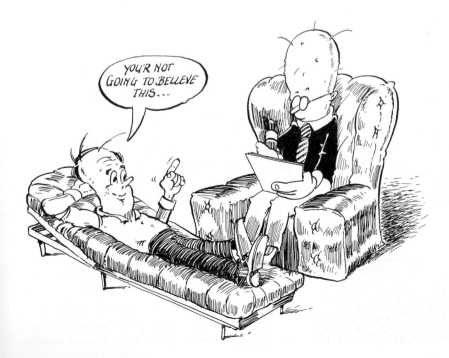

Individual psychotherapy: everything is of value

and does not let them influence the treatment programme.

Improvement by the client during psychotherapy is usually attributed to three experiences, these being: *Abreaction (catharsis),* which is the free expression of emotion which can occur in the relative safety of the therapeutic environment; the achievement of *insight* into the root cause of the conflict causing the behavioural abnormality; and the repeated *working through* of the conflict from many angles, thus enabling the client to face the original conflict without undue anxiety.

Transference and counter-transference are important concepts for the nurse to keep in mind when working with clients. It is probable that at some time the nurse will be the recipient of transference from a client. It is also probable that the nurse will experience counter-transference of her own unresolved conflicts towards clients. Working in the field of mental health is an emotionally demanding job, and the motivation for entering this area of work could have something to do with unresolved conflicts within the individual. The use of mental defence mechanisms is a normal part of everyday existence in helping us cope with the trauma of life. It is only when use of these mechanisms is prolonged and leads to maladaptive behaviour that they become the focus of treatment.

Use of defence mechanisms by clients is also a potential cause of conflict for nurses. One mechanism which we have not previously identified is that of *splitting*. Splitting is closely related to the mechanism of idealization and is a way of avoiding conflict by keeping two incompatible thought processes separate. If a person has both very intense good and bad feelings about others he can avoid conflict by projecting all the good feelings on one person and all the bad feelings on another. If a client behaves to one member (or group) of staff as if they possessed all the good qualities, and denigrates another member or group of staff, this can lead to disagreements and rivalries about the patient amongst the staff. It does not matter how emotionally mature members of staff are, nor how

good their understanding of mental defence mechanisms may be, it can be extremely difficult to tolerate being the recipient of negative transference. Some hospitals and day centres run group therapy sessions for their staff to help them cope with this form of tension and other emotional conflicts associated with work in this field. If these are available, it is important that the ground-rules for what can be raised and discussed are clear to prevent inappropriate disclosure and embarrassment.

One final point. Just because you are working within the field of mental health it does not mean that all the patient's feelings and statements about a nurse or group of nurses are the result of transference, neither are the feelings of the nurses necessarily counter-transference. We must always remember that what the client feels and says, just as what the nurse feels and says, may be an accurate reflection of their perception of the situation.

c. Psychosocial approaches

The psychosocial approaches to therapy accept to a larger extent the role of the environment in the determination of behaviour. These approaches therefore focus on the group interactions and other environmental issues which can influence the behaviour of people. Many of the forms of therapy within this area do not have a theoretical psychological underpinning, although some are based on psychological theory. The nurse will become involved within this group of approaches through group work within ward or day centre activities, where the group may serve many functions, and in centres operating under the concept of a therapeutic community. The therapies considered here are those based on humanistic theories and sociological theories either in isolation or in combination.

Groups operating on a humanistic approach aim to examine the here and now and not the past as would be the case with a psychoanalytically orientated group. Their purpose is to foster personal growth of the members through their interactions within the group and so enable them to live more fulfilling lives. Within these settings

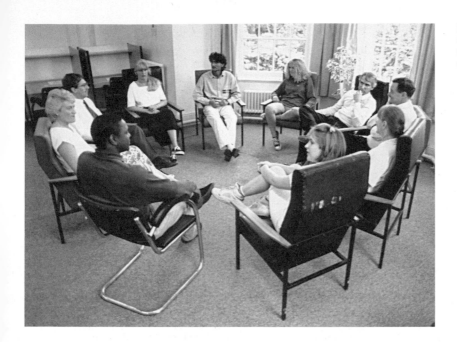

Figure 4.2.3
Security to disclose:
safer than in the
outside world

the therapist generally stays in the background allowing group members to exchange experiences, comment on one another's behaviour, and discuss their own problems as well as those of the other members. Whilst the members of the group may initially be defensive and uncomfortable about exposing their weaknesses, as they gain experience within the group they become more aware of the effect that their attitudes and behaviours have on other members (figure 4.2.3). Through their exchanges the members of the group become more able to identify and empathize with one another, and gain in self-esteem when able to help another member by offering understanding or meaningful interpretations. The ability of members of the group to explore attitudes and reactions with a variety of people enables learning to occur. Group members are able to acquire new social skills through modelling and by being given the opportunity to practise them within the group.

Therapeutic communities have the aim of affecting a change in behaviour by the very fact of living within that community. Some centres for disturbed adolescents, alcohol/drug abusers, and some wards are set up to run as therapeutic communities. These communities run on the principles of democratization, permissive-

ness, reality confrontation and communalism (Rapaport, 1950). *Democratization* refers to the degree of involvement of the members of the community within its management. Within therapeutic communities the demarcation between staff and client, and between professional groups in relation to what happens in the community, is broken down. This levelling of hierarchy is symbolized in part by the non-wearing of uniform by staff. Communities vary in their degree of democratization, but each community has its rules concerning who makes decisions about the day to day running of the community, admission to the community, and all other factors. It has been found that a strong background leadership is necessary for the continuance of a community, and when that leader departs, the community may flounder for a time until a new leader emerges. The *permissiveness* of the community is reflected in its greater degree of tolerance and acceptance of other people's behaviour than might be the case in other situations. This tolerance may be in terms of dress, such as the wearing of jewellery by nursing staff, or of the time that members get up in the morning. This greater freedom is counterbalanced by *reality confrontation*. This means that members of the community are continuously confronted by the effects of their behaviour on

Democracy can
be challenging

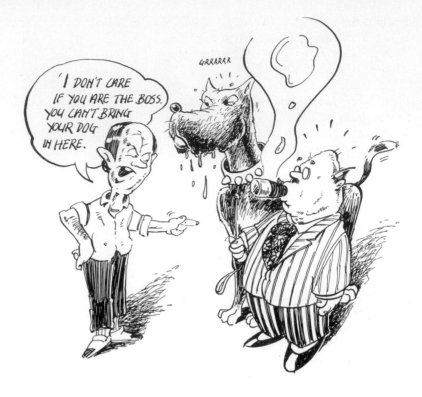

others. This confrontation may be by other members or by staff and shows itself in a greater openness between all concerning what they think of each other. This closeness within the community is the foundation of *communalism*. The staff may share the same dining facilities as other members, and the use of first names between all members is common. Communities such as these achieve their success through the confrontation of reality in a supportive environment. In effect the members of these communities cannot escape the consequences of their behaviour, but are able to try out new behaviours and learn their effects on others. The full gamut of feelings will be experienced within a community, but the facing up to these experiences and the working through of emotional responses assists people's understanding of themselves and their ability to cope with such situations outside the therapeutic community.

d. Eclectic approaches

As has been stated previously there is no 'right' or 'wrong' theory of psychology. Likewise there is no 'right' or 'wrong' therapy for an individual. Some therapies work better in some conditions than do others, and some therapists have more success with certain approaches to different conditions than do their peers. What is important is that the therapy used for the particular individual is acceptable to the client and works under the guidance of the therapist. It might be that a therapist faced with a person who exhibits strong obsessive compulsive behaviours with rituals initially uses a behaviourist approach to control the rituals and then moves to a psychoanalytical approach to gain understanding as to the cause of the behaviour.

Most psychotherapists do not stick to one particular method. Their primary orientation may be to a particular school, but they select from different techniques to suit the person being treated.

There are many other schools of therapy which we have not touched on here. These include such schools as Gestalt therapy, Transactional analysis and Hypnotherapy. The interested reader is referred to the reference section for specialist texts in the these areas.

Study activities

4. Which of the therapies identified might be of value in changing Jean's behaviour, and why?

5. Identify the focus that would be taken in treating Jean by:
   a. a behavioural-cognitive therapist;
   b. a psychoanalytical therapist.

5. Summary

Within this chapter we have identified that mental illness is not a unitary condition but a multitude of categories, all of which share in common the appearance of abnormal behaviour. An attempt was made to identify the causative features of these behaviours using biological, social and psychological explanations. Within the psychological explanations the psychoanalytical, behavioural and cognitive explanations were considered. It was found that these abnormal behaviours can be explained to some degree by each of these theories. The evidence from genetic relatedness tends to the view of a biological predisposition being inherited by the individual which is later activated by a psychological trigger. Within this framework the social factors act as an added source of stress which can lead to the activation of these psychological triggers. The 'truth' is not yet available, so we have to work on what is.

Regardless of the causes of mental illness and abnormal behaviours, treatment possibilities exist, and these were outlined. This chapter concentrated on the psychological treatment options, that is the psychotherapies, and viewed them from a behavioural-cognitive approach, a psychoanalytical approach and a psychosocial approach. We ended by identifying that most psychotherapists use an eclectic approach as one would expect from the availability of different schools within psychology.

3

Learning difficulties

1. Introduction

People with learning difficulties are those with an intelligence level within the lower 2 or 3 percent of the normal distribution of the population. Nurses and other carers in the field of learning difficulties are involved in assisting these people, who may need help to allow them to care for themselves or who are unable to care for themselves at all, to achieve the highest quality of life possible.

In Section 2 of this chapter we consider the definition of the term 'learning difficulty' and its causes. Section 3 looks at what it means to have a learning difficulty in terms of its effects on the individual in his development of self, and his ability to cope within society. This section also considers the effect on the family of having an intellectually retarded member. Section 4 considers the adaptation of the person with a learning difficulty into the community. The concept of social role valorization is examined, as are techniques used to train the person with learning difficulty, including behavioural techniques and gentle teaching.

Learning outcomes

After studying this chapter the student should be able to:
– describe and explain what learning difficulty is;
– understand the following concepts:
  • intelligence
  • Intelligence Quotient (IQ)
  • Mental Age
  • normalization
  • social role valorization
  • gentle teaching;
– explain how inheritance studies help identify the causes of learning difficulties;
– describe the relationship between mental age and chronological age, and discuss the presentation of mental age when less than chronological age;
– identify the effects of learning difficulties on the self-concept;
– discuss the issues relating to acceptance in society of the person with learning difficulties.

2. What is learning difficulty?

This first section considers what is meant by learning difficulty. In the past the term 'mental subnormality' was used and even today the term 'mental handicap' is used in legislation to describe people with learning difficulties. However, we prefer to use the more socially acceptable term 'learning difficulty' in this text. Following a definition of the term, the concepts of mental age and chronological age are further examined as is the quality of the thought processes. The section concludes with a look at the causes of learning difficulty.

Case study: Edward
Edward is 17 years old and has an IQ measured at 57. He has one brother, John, who is older than he is and a younger sister, Samantha. Edward went to a normal school but played truant on numerous occasions and was aggressive to other children at times. Besides the aggression at school, Edward showed disruptive behaviour at home, and has been to court twice for stealing. Recently his disruptive behaviour has increased. He shows aggression to his parents and is destructive of possessions in the home unless under constant supervision. His mother and father have always shown favouritism to Edward, but bringing up the children has been difficult. Neither Edward's mother nor father achieved much at school, both having been in remedial classes. Since leaving school Edward's father worked as a builder's labourer, but he has found difficulty finding work since the small firm he worked for went into liquidation. His mother works at home making soft toys for a local producer. Both his brother and sister have a below average IQ, John's being 75, and Samantha's being 67.

a. Definition of learning difficulty
Alfred Binet, a French psychologist who lived at the beginning of this century, is considered as the first designer of an intelligence test. Binet was given the job of designing a method with which children with learning difficulties could be 'tracked down' by the French government. Binet set out from the idea that a child who was a slow learner functioned as a normal child that was somewhat younger as far as age was concerned. Of a child that learned quickly he postulated something comparable: he functioned as a normal, but somewhat older child. Binet compiled, by age category, a number of tasks which a child of normal learning capacity of a particular age category could just solve within a certain time. For a child of normal learning capacity of a younger age category the tasks were too difficult. For a child of normal learning capacity of an older age group they were too easy. In this manner Binet was able to determine whether an individual child functioned in conformity with his (calender) age or diverged from it. Binet introduced two concepts: calendar age and developmental age. Calendar or chronological age is the age that is determined by the date of birth of the child. Development or mental age is connected with the level at which Binet's test is passed. Binet was in this way able to state whether a child functioned in conformity with, above or below his calendar age.

Study activity
1. Explain why the average calendar age is similar to the developmental age.

The German psychologist Wilhelm Stern devised the idea of dividing the development age by the calendar age. He multiplied the result of the fraction by 100 (in order to get rid of the decimal point from the fraction). The figure that resulted he called the intelligence quotient (IQ).

Thus: IQ = development age divided by calendar age, multiplied by 100.

An IQ higher than 100 means that the individual functions at a higher intellectual age than his contemporaries. An IQ lower than 100 means that the individual functions on a lower intellectual level than his contemporaries.

If a sufficiently large number of people are tested it is found that the distribution of scores at each age group inscribes a 'bell shaped curve' (a normal distribution, see diagram 4.3.1 on page 322). Learning difficulty is arbitrarily put at two standard deviations or lower below the mean. This means that an IQ of 70 or below indicates learning difficulty. Because 2 or 3 percent of the population fall into this group, this figure is

Diagram 4.3.1
Distribution of
intelligence scores

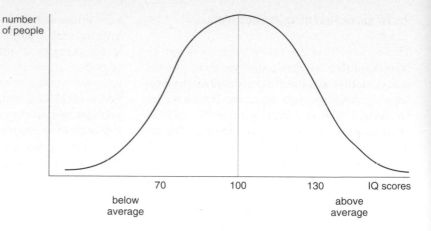

number
of people

70   100   130   IQ scores

below   above
average   average

Diagram 4.3.2
Mental development
of related to IQ
IQ of 100 = black line
IQ of 67 = red line

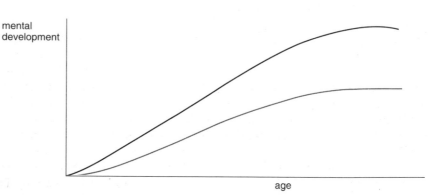

mental
development

age

Diagram 4.3.3
Graphs demonstrating
the 2% to 3% with
specific disorders

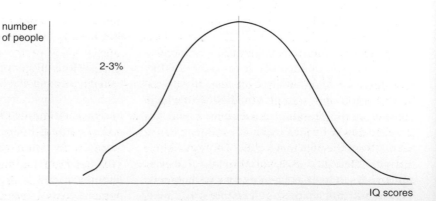

number
of people

2-3%

IQ scores

often quoted as the prevalence of learning difficulty.

The definition of learning difficulty might then be considered to relate solely to the intelligence of the person as measured by the IQ. This form of definition is not fully accurate however as there is great variation in the abilities we can identify between a person with an IQ of, say, 70 (two standard deviations below the average) and one with an IQ of, say, 60. Whilst it might be expected that the person with the lower of the two IQs is less able in all situations, this might not be the case. The degree of adaption to the needs of society can affect the person's ability to cope. A more meaningful definition of learning difficulty would be *'significantly subaverage general intellectual functioning existing concurrently with deficits in adaptive behavior, and manifested during the developmental period'* (Grossman, 1973). Using this as the base we can examine in more detail the nature of this deficit.

Intellectual functioning refers to general intelligence. In Module 2 we considered cognitive development without specifically considering intelligence. Intelligence usually refers to behaviours that reflect:
- learning ability, which encompasses both rate and depth;
- knowledge, which encompasses formal and informal learning;
- ability in coping with new situations.

Whilst deficits in all these areas are demonstrable in the person with a learning difficulty it is in the area of coping with new situations where their deficiency is most obviously shown. People with a learning difficulty are notoriously uneasy in new or unfamiliar situations.

The degree of learning difficulty may be defined in relation to the person's ability to profit from education, or in relation to a broader concept of overall ability. Educational ability can be identified as: educatable (50–75 IQ); trainable (25–49 IQ); and profound learning difficulty (below 25 IQ). A more descriptive categorization, but one which is less widely used, gives four levels of learning difficulty. As with other categorization systems the ranges are a guide only and are not meant to be definitive statements.

Mild comprising about 89 percent of the people with learning difficulties, with IQs in the range 55–69. These people are often not identified as having a learning difficulty until in their school years when they start to fall behind their peers. With persistence they can achieve an IQ of an 11 of 12 year old child by their late teens. As adults they can find work and become independent.

Moderate comprising about 6 percent of the people with learning difficulties, with IQs in the range 40–55. These people usually learn to talk during the preschool years but later and more slowly than children closer to the average IQ. They are also likely to show impairment in sensorimotor development such as poor coordination. Such children gain little from the normal academic activity at school, but can, with special training, gain in social and occupational skills. In adulthood they are unlikely to achieve total independence but can contribute to their own support if work is available in sheltered workshops.

Severe comprises about 3.5 percent of the people with learning difficulties, with IQs in the 25–39 range. People at this level show their deficiency in infancy or early childhood through poor motor development and minimal speech. Physical deformities are also a fairly common feature at this level of retardation. These people do not profit as much as those with moderate learning difficulty from training, but as they get older many can learn elementary health and grooming skills. As adults they may learn to perform certain routine tasks but generally require complete supervision and economic support.

Profound comprises the final 1.5 percent of the people with learning difficulties, with IQs in the range 0–24. Handicap in these people is extreme in both the intellectual and sensorimotor functions, and is apparent early in life. Some limited goals of habit training may be achieved in the older child, but usually they require total care throughout their lives. Many of these people also demonstrate severe physical handicap or deformities that further restrict their capacity to cope with the demands of the environment.

b. Mental age versus chronological age

As we stated earlier, IQ tests are standardized in relation to age. One often hears of people with learning difficulties who, although they have a chronological age of 9 years, have a mental age of 6 years. We need to consider what this means to the person in relation to his ability to function. Does a mental age of 6 years for a 9 year old boy mean that he is identical in cognitive functioning to a 6 year old boy? The answer to this must be an emphatic no. The meaning of the mental age is that the child achieves on average the same result as the mental age indicates. A normal 6 year old is likely to be inquisitive, and creative in solving puzzles. The child with learning difficulites is likely to be less inquisitive and less creative in solving puzzles than is his mental age contemporary. The child with learning difficulties is also more likely to be more dependent on external cues than is his mental age contemporary. He is more dependent on others pointing him in the direction to follow. On the other hand the child with learning difficulties may be more competent in some dextrous skills, and in social relationships, than is the average 6 year old. So the use of the term mental age implies that the abilities of the person being considered more closely resemble those of the average 6 year old: but not that they are the same.

The development of mental abilities, like the development of physical abilities, has a growth period. Depending on the test used to measure mental age this growth period ends between the late teens and early twenties. Mental development during this phase is dependent on the IQ. At its simplest, a child with an IQ of 67 (e.g. the boy with a mental age of 6 years and a chronological age of 9 years previously identified), is in effect achieving 67/100 of the average normal child. Such a child experiences only 67/100 of a year's development for each chronological

year, whereas the child with an IQ of 100 experiences a full year's development for each chronological year. The result of this is that the child with the lower IQ progressively gets further behind his age mates up to the point where mental development stops, from which point this difference remains fixed (see diagram 4.3.2 on page 322).

Study activity
2. Calculate the approximate mental age of Edward in the case study.

This concept of a mental development growth period should not be taken as indicating that learning stops at the point of cessation of mental growth. Learning continues throughout life as some of the older people reading this book will attest. The success of institutions such as the Open University in reintroducing retired people to education, who then progress to the award of a degree, illustrates well that learning does not cease when the mental development phase comes to an end. What does cease though is the development of our *learning ability cognitive structures*. The end of the mental development growth period marks the end of the growth of the equipment with which we learn.

The degree to which nature and nurture contribute in the development of the IQ was raised in Module 2 but is obviously of vital importance here. If through effective early developmental work the IQ can be raised by 10 points, it can have remarkable effects on the individual who is on the border of the normal versus learning difficulties divide.

Once the IQ is developed it is remarkably stable. There is little deterioration measurable throughout life. It is, however, observed that we find it more difficult to learn as we get older, and this might be true. The causes of this are however elusive, and it does not affect all people in the same way. Those whose job involves mainly or exclusively manual skills may not experience intellectual learning for long periods during their life, and so the ability to learn, like all skills, becomes rusty. For any skill to survive in peak performance it requires practice. People who are in jobs where mental ability is constantly required are able to maintain this practice with the mental skills and so do not lose the ability to learn.

Study activity
   3. a. List six difficulties that Edward with an IQ of 65 may have encountered at school which may have led to his repeated truancy;
   b. give reasons why his brother and sister might not have experienced the same difficulties.

c. Qualitative thought processes

It appears that learning difficulty is not only a quantitative deficit, but also a qualitative deficit. Definitions of learning difficulty related to IQ look to the quantitative elements of the difficulty. However, areas such as suggestibility, memory, and abstract thought also show effects.

People with a learning difficulty have long been considered to be *suggestible,* that is being more dependent on external cues for their actions than are people without a learning difficulty. The reason for this is probably that they learn a degree of helplessness through repeated experiences of failing at tasks with which they are presented. This *learned helplessness* not only presents them with more difficulties if the outside cues are misleading, but also stops them attempting tasks at which they may succeed (Weisz, 1979).

For learning to occur it is necessary to process information through the stages of memory as identified in Module 2. It appears that this *memory* process is slower in people with learning difficulties (Saccuzzo et al, 1979). Information from the environment which other people would assimilate may therefore be missed due to the load on the memory system of the person with learning difficulty. This will have the effect of reducing the overall quality of individual experiences.

Abstract thinking is also shown to be less able. The person with a learning difficulty has greater difficulty solving problems such as 'how are an elephant and mouse similar?' than do contem-

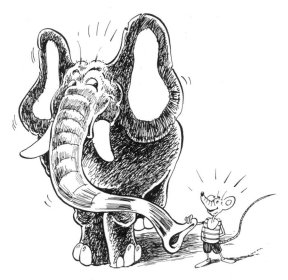

Can you see the similarities?

poraries without learning difficulties. As the differences between items grouped by similarity increases, the person with a learning difficulty seems to get stuck on the differences and is unable to break out of this difference mode even though the item group is known.

Finally, learning also tends to be context specific, and the person with a learning difficulty is less able to generalize learning across contexts apart from the one where learning took place.

d. Causes of learning difficulty

The causes of learning difficulty can be considered as belonging to two main categories i.e. those which are cultural-family related, and those due to specific organic causes. As with all abilities where there is a normal distribution within the population, there must be those people situated at the extremes. That is, for intelligence there must be those who are extremely gifted at the upper end of the distribution, and there must be those with a learning difficulties at the lower end of the distribution. In Module 2 we considered the findings of Bouchard and McGuie (1981) in relation to intelligence and inheritance. This work points to there being a genetic link acting within the area of learning difficulty. If one parent of a child has a low IQ there is a greater probability of the child also having a low IQ than if neither parent has a low IQ. Likewise if both parents have a low IQ the probability of the child being also in that category increases. *Cultural-family* related causation then refers to this group of people who occupy the lower portion of the normal distribution. It is estimated that about 75 percent of the people with learning difficulty belong to this group.

The remaining 25 percent belong to the group of *specific organic* causes. Within this latter group can be found some of the most severely retarded people. Zigler (1967) considers that the small bump found at the lower end of the distribution curve of intelligence (see diagram 4.3.3 on page 322) represents those people who would have had normal intelligence except for an organic defect. The classic conditions leading to learning difficulty can be found in this group. Examples of these conditions are:

Self-concept starts
with self-identity

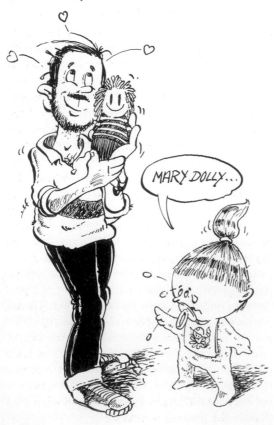

MARY DOLLY...

– Down's syndrome, a chromosomal abnormality;
– Phenylketonuria (PKU), inherited through a recessive gene;
– Tuberous scleroses (epiloma), inherited through a dominant gene.

Other conditions are also causative and the interested reader is referred to the references at the end of this module.

Regardless of the cause of the learning difficulty, the degree of retardation found may be greater than the cause ascribes. The reason(s) for this includes factors related to a *lack of experience and stimulation,* the nurture component. This may be either because the parents do not recognize the need for stimulation, do not have the capacity to introduce the stimulation necessary, or have reduced expectations of the child's ability and so do not want to 'pressure' the child.

Likewise if the child's teacher has a low expectation of achievements possible then the overall level of stimulation and experience offered may be less than for other children. A further reason is that as the child with a learning difficulty is less inquisitive than the normal child, self-initiated learning experiences, such as the learning play with rattles, wooden blocks, social experiences, etc., will be fewer than for other children, so reducing overall the level of stimulation and experience that the child with a learning difficulty receives.

Study activities

4. With other students if possible, list the types of activities that might help the child with a low IQ gain the most from his development.

5. Try to decide if the knowledge of the parents' IQ would be of advantage to teachers of a child with a low IQ.

3. Psychosocial effects of learning difficulty

a. Development of self-concept

In childhood we develop a concept of ourselves which we take forward into adult life. As we grow and develop, this concept of self is continuously being modified, a point emphasized in Module 2. Part of the development of the self-concept is related to interactions with others. As you have probably noticed, adults addressing a very young child often use the child's name instead of the general 'you', 'What is Mary doing?' rather than, 'What are you doing?' This use of the name would seem to help the child start to separate him/herself from others. It is the start of the concept of self. Linked to the traumas of potty training it aids in the establishment of the unique individual, a person, one who has a self-concept. As speech develops, young children often start by using their name instead of the impersonal 'I' when talking about themselves, e.g. 'Mary drink.' It is only later that the use of 'I' becomes standard.

It is possibly the case that for children with learning difficulties this development of the self-concept does not occur as quickly as it does for other children, and that the concept is weaker. It may be that this weakened self-concept is due in part to the child with learning difficulty being spoken to less, especially if the learning difficulty is marked. In such cases the child would show little recognition of being spoken to. It may also be due to parents and other adults having lower expectations than they have for other children, a part of the learned helplessness process we discussed earlier. Children with learning difficulties, albeit secondary school boys, were shown to use fewer constructs to describe themselves and others, and tended to combine many characteristics into one construct (Wooster, 1970); that may be one effect of this.

If these children combine many characteristics into single constructs, a process such as might be seen in the formal operations stage of cognitive activity (see Module 1, Chapter 2 for the work of Piaget, 1952), they will be more likely to be confused by people's actions. If the child with learning difficulties classes all children who are kind, as also not being bullies, as trustworthy, as doing what they are told etc. then it is easy to see where behavioural experience may not match the expectation from the construct used.

We have mentioned the concept of learned helplessness. A natural extension of this might be that children with learning difficulties would have low expectations about their abilities, resorting to a failure-avoiding scenario. This might not be the case however. Whilst it is true that children with a learning difficulty might not attempt things which they believe they will not succeed at, there is some evidence that they retain a high expectation of their abilities. One study found that school children with learning difficulties reported consistently higher expectations of their abilities in school subjects, games and popularity than did other children. This higher expectation persisted over the period when expectations of children without a learning difficulty were becoming more realistic (Ringness, 1961). The cause of this might be a reflection of the imputed expectations of parents and teachers, where it could be a symptom of the dependence on external cues, or it may simply be a reflection of the lack of cognitive ability.

b. Personality and behaviour

Major differences have been noted between the personality and behaviour of the person with learning difficulties and the 'normal'. When personality tests have been used to assess people with learning difficulties, differences in nearly all scales used have been identified. It has been noted that such children are less cheerful, less stable, less persevering, and more demanding than are other children (Wilcox and Smith, 1973). Related behaviour differences have also been noted, especially in relation to depression, inhibition, tension and aggression towards adults. These behavioural differences are seen more in older than in younger children. It may be that these behaviours are related to either disruption of the home environment or to mental illness. One bias identified in surveys on personality and behaviour has been that a greater percentage of the children with learning difficulties come from broken homes than do the control subjects. It is also relevant that estimates place the proportion of people with learning difficulties who also have a mental illness at between 30 and 50 percent which is much higher than in the general population.

c. Educational attainment

We identified probable causes of lower achievement than the measured IQ might imply when discussing mental age. The main element we discussed was lack of experience and stimulation. This is obviously a major cause of reduced attainment and one which has external as well as internal dimensions.

Absences from school will obviously affect the attainment of these children. The need to attend special clinics and to attend social training sessions will reduce the time at school. Behaviour disturbance may also lead to reduced school attendance.

Medication may also cause reduced attainment during the school period. It may be that the child is on drug treatment for behavioural disturbance or for, say, epilepsy. Drugs used in these circumstances reduce the level of activity of the person and so reduce the capacity to concentrate. The effect of this is that children may be less able to benefit from the learning experiences they are exposed to.

Lower expectations of teachers and/or parents can influence educational achievement. This has been discussed previously and so will not be expanded on here.

Perceptual difficulties may also be associated with learning difficulty. Perceptual difficulties related to visual perception, especially in relation to the recognition of vertical or horizontal lines, can create problems. These difficulties can lead to accidents and increased problems in coping with the environment.

Cognitive impairment is a factor in learning difficulties, as the term implies. Specific impairments which may be present include: reduced constructional ability, e.g. the child is less able to copy diagrams in matchsticks than are other children; reduced motor coordination, there is usually a reduced coordination ability in these children; motor impersistence, i.e. the child has a reduced ability to control action when instructed to e.g. keeping the eyes closed; sensory defects, affecting the auditory and visual senses are common; and speech and verbal development are reduced from the normal in these children.

d. Societal considerations

Society is not necessarily geared to accepting people with a learning difficulty. It has been said that the village societies of the past were more willing to accept those of reduced ability than is our present fast modern society. It might be true that a rural society, which functions at a slow pace, might find it easier to accept a person with learning difficulty. It could also be true that such a person might find it easier to cope in a society which changes only slowly, where there is more time to work out what is expected, and where there are fewer conflicting cues. The evidence available however does not strongly support this hypothesis.

With suitable support, i.e. support that is necessary and not overprotection, it is possible for the person with learning difficulty to live in society as a full member. Many people are currently moving out of the institutions developed for their protection and training into community accommodation.

Some of these people are getting married and managing their lives with minimal support. Others are settling into group homes or hostels and demonstrating self care skills well above those necessary within the institutions from which they have moved. Current practice is to maintain the person within the community as far as possible, and only admit them to institutional care if all else fails.

The ability of the individual to adapt to the society will depend on factors such as the individual's adjustment to society, and his potential employability.

Adjustment to society is related to issues such as independence, awareness of reality, the ability to maintain adequate interpersonal relationships, possession of a reasonable emotional maturity, and the ability to pursue appropriate goals.

Independence is an obvious issue when the per-

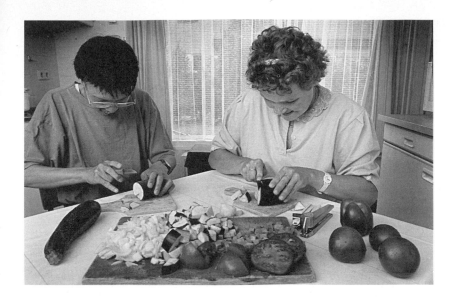

Figure 4.3.1
Developing
independence?

son has reduced ability to make decisions for himself. It may be that the person is not going to be able to become fully independent in all his actions. We must try to ensure, however, that the person is able to achieve the maximum independence possible commensurate with the degree of learning difficulty. We must be especially careful *not to expect too little* from the person. Risk- taking is a normal part of all lives and one that people with learning difficulties must not be deprived of. Just because the decision taken does not fit our perception of what is normal in a given situation does not mean that it is necessarily wrong. Not everybody will make the same decision as you, not even your friends on all occasions. We have to be be careful, however to ensure that sufficient measures are taken to assist the individual in such activities as managing money, managing the home, and being free of undue pressures (taking account of the greater suggestibility).

We have already indentified that the *awareness of reality* in relation to self-ability may not be accurate. There must be active attempts to enable the person to be realistic in his expectations of futures, including career options. It is not doing the affected person a service to raise his expectations above what can be achieved.

If the individual is to achieve independence and hold down a job there is a need to be able to enter into and maintain *adequate interpersonal relationships*. Social skills are a necessary part of everyday life. If the person displays inappropriate behaviours such as being aggressive or over-affectionate then others will quickly become alienated which can lead to an inability to maintain a job.

There must also be a demonstration of a *reasonable level of emotional maturity*. It is obvious that there is a great variation of emotional responsiveness within and between people. Too great a degree of emotional lability will however lead to others being less able to accommodate the person's behaviour. The person must finally have the *ability to pursue appropriate goals* if frequent changes in job or lodging are to be avoided.

Employment is an area of activity which affects the person's concept of himself, and his ability to achieve a degree of independence. Through employment the individual is able to earn the money which is the key to achieving a degree of independence. Depending on the degree of disability the person may be able to undertake open employment, niche employment, work in a sheltered workshop, or be employed in a special care unit. The closer the employment is to general employment the greater will be the income and the degree of independence that can be achieved.

Study activity
6. Review the list you made of difficulties

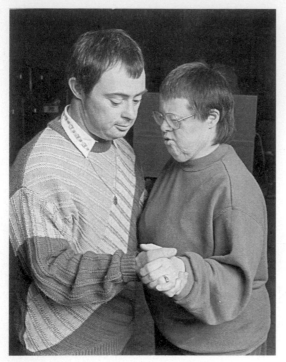

Figure 4.3.2
Distinctive characteristics
could lead to greater identity
with the specific group
than with the family

Edward may have encountered at school leading to his truancy.
a. Would you want to make any changes?
b. Justify your response.

e. Effects on the family

The degree to which parents accept or reject a child with learning difficulty will obviously affect the way the family operates. If the cause of retardation is due to a recognized diagnostic grouping such as Down's syndrome, the child may be seen as sharing more characteristics with others of that group than with his siblings. Such factors may lead to a weakening of the acceptance of that child as a full family member.

Most people who have a child with a learning difficulty raise him in the same way as other children, but taking account of the slower pace of development. It is however necessary for parents to make more decisions on behalf of the child with a learning difficulty. These decisions include issues such as the type of school and type of future that will be available. The need to make these decisions also tends to last for longer in the life of a child with learning difficulties. The parents may worry about what will happen to their child (who may be over the legal age) should they no longer be able to care for him due to their own inability or due to behavioural difficulties of the child. The issue of overprotection is obviously an additional factor here.

Certain challenges need to be faced by the family with regard to raising a child with a learning difficulty. These challenges are listed here as areas for thought, discussion, and further reading by the student:
– physical care of the child;
– fewer benefits of parenthood;
– discipline;
– going out with the child;
– going out without the child;
– care of the child if the mother is hospitalized;
– holidays;
– contact with other children;
– special housing needs;
– costs of raising the child;
– providing adequate stimulation;
– self feelings of inadequacy;
– child-parent relationships;
– effects of further children;
– effects of the child with learning difficulty on siblings.

The references listed at the end of this module provide suitable sources for introducing the student to these areas.

Study activity
7. Review the case study of Edward. Try to identify possible reasons for Edward's behaviour at home giving justifications for your answers. It will help if you discuss the subject with qualified nurses and the teacher.

4. Adjustment to society

When considering the adjustment of people with learning difficulties to society we must consider their support and training. Effective support and training is dependent in part on the professional staff in contact with the individual, and in part on the attitudes of society. The attitudes of society will in turn be influenced, as we identified earlier, by the behaviour of the person with learning difficulties. Two terms in common use today when considering the support and training of people with learning difficulties are: social role valorization; and gentle teaching. These two concepts will be examined in turn.

a. Social role valorization

Normalization is a principle advanced by Wolfensberger (1980) which represents an ideology; it is a system of shared values, attitudes and beliefs to advance the quality of life of people with learning difficulties. The concept of normalization includes the removal of all those features which might be termed institutional. Normalization is the 'regimen' geared to allowing freedom of choice, autonomy, risk taking; in fact being allowed all civil liberties and human rights to the maximum of the person's ability. In other words, the person is to be treated like everyone else in the community to the maximum of his or her ability; the person with learning difficulties is to be treated normally. One problem with this approach is found in areas of high unemployment. If unemployment in the community is high, and it is 'normal' for people to be unemployed, is this the normal existence that the person with a learning difficulty should be exposed to? Another factor is that freedom of choice may be interpreted over-liberally. Is it right that the person with learning difficulty should be allowed to withdraw from a regime of treatment without good reason? Surely the right to choose must be balanced by the responsibility that the choice brings. If people are allowed to start and stop agreed treatment regimes, at will and without cause, they are in effect being allowed to operate at the level of a child in a nursery and not at the level of an adult in society (Jackson, 1988).

Wolfensberger (1983) advocates the use of the term *social role valorization* instead of normalization due to the continuing misunderstanding and misapplication of the principle of normalization. Social role valorization has the goal of enhancing the social role of individuals or groups at risk of social devaluation. Wolfensberger believes that this can only be achieved through an improvement in these people's social image and social competence. Implicit in this is acceptance by professionals and society generally of the ideas behind this approach. If the person with learning difficulties is allowed to practise anarchy, then his acceptance into society is less likely. We have pointed out that current strategy within the UK is to care for people with learning difficulties in the community. This means admitting people into institutions only if no other care and support can be found, and returning people from institutions to community settings as an organizational priority (DHSS, 1981). Whilst the rationale for this policy has positive aspects (releasing people from large and negative institutions so relieving them of the process of institutionalization, Goffman, 1973), there is no empirical evidence that community based facilities are the best settings for the care of people with a learning difficulty (Zigler, Balla and Kossan, 1986).

b. Training

When considering training of the person with a learning difficulty we must examine behavioural techniques. These are considered in more detail in Chapter 2 of this module. The techniques presented there are the forms used in all settings. Systematic desensitization and covert sensitization work with the person with learning difficulties just as well as with other people. The need for social skills training has already been identified. Likewise therapeutic communities can be used for the development of skills in these situations. Obviously the methods need some modification to take account of the decreased cognitive skills of the person with learning difficulties. One specific technique used with people with learning difficulties is that of *backward chaining* which will be examined in more detail now.

Backward chaining presents the carer with the opportunity to increase the person's skill by using the techniques of operant conditioning in a social theory paradigm. This technique uses

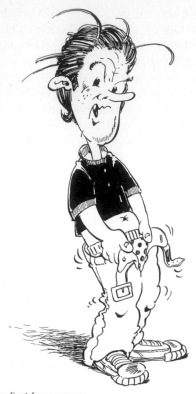

Last is first for success

the concept of cognitive intervention by gaining the benefits of success experience (Bandura, 1984). Instead of shaping the behaviour from the start, as was demonstrated by Skinner, the shaping occurs in a reverse order. The person is taught to perform the last act in a series which completes that activity. As an example let us look at putting on a pair of trousers, and assume no current ability. The putting on of the trousers is broken down by task analysis into a series of activities. To use this approach of backward chaining the carer would perform all the tasks except the last one. In this example the carer would put on the trousers and fasten the zip. The only activity left in the task will be the fastening of the waistband button. The person being trained is then taught to fasten the button. This process continues with physical, gestural and verbal prompting, etc. until the person fastens the button when required without prompting. Suitable reinforcers are used such as oral stimuli and praise to help shape this behaviour. Once the person is able to perform this stage of the procedure without prompting he has a clear state-

ment of success. The next step in the procedure is to require this person to perform the second last and the last stage. Again, prompting and suitable reinforcement are used to ensure success. This process is continued until the person is able to perform all steps in the task unaided, when required.

As can be imagined this can be a slow process. One of the most difficult aspects of caring in the field of learning difficulties is accepting the slow progress in all areas of activity. It is also probable that unless the behaviours being developed are reinforced at more frequent intervals than usual there will be decay of learning, and even extinction in a relatively short period of time.

Another area of special concern is that of coping with behaviour problems. We have pointed out that there is a tendency for behaviour problems to accompany learning difficulties, and these may relate to aggressive outburst and self injurious behaviour. We also pointed out that the integration into society of all people is in part related to displays of appropriate behaviour. If people with learning difficulties are to be able to live and work as members of society they must behave in a socially acceptable manner. Behaviour programmes have been developed to modify or change such inappropriate behaviours into socially acceptable patterns. Whilst other socially unacceptable behaviours may be witnessed and require modifications, this section will concentrate on that area of behaviour relating to aggression and self injury, the area referred to as challenging behaviour.

Many behavioural techniques have been developed to reduce the incidence of displays of *challenging behaviour*. These techniques have often related to extreme behavioural approaches using aversion therapy. Aversion is a technique of behaviour modification using punishment as the reinforcer to engender change. There are reports of cattle prods and ammonia sprays being used in a hospital in Western Ontario (Brandon, 1990). Whilst we in Britain do not use such methods we are reminded by Brandon (1990) of the extensive use of drugs, restraint mechanisms and time-out periods in this country to assist in the control of behaviour. Reacting against this use of punishment and aversive techniques, McGee (1987) developed the *gentle teaching* movement.

Gentle teaching is completely opposed to all forms of aversive techniques and to punishment being used with people with learning difficulties. This process of care identifies aggression and self-harm with expressions of anger. Seen in this light frequent expressions of anger can be viewed as a cry for help when something is wrong that the individual is unable to remedy. Help now focuses on identifying the causes of the anger and developing means of reducing it (Lally, 1988). Once this refocusing of the behaviour is undertaken then the way we go about correcting it changes. Gentle teaching is based on the following tenets:
- frequent and unconditional value-giving is central to interactional change;
- everyone has an inherent longing for affection and warmth;
- actions of carers focused on compliance and behavioural control need to be reduced and replaced with value-centred actions;
- dyadic (two way) change is critical (McGee, 1990).

Gentle teaching thus aims to create bonded relationships, within which change can occur. The development of such relationships can be evaluated by observing smiling, warm gazing, reaching out, increased participation, and sharing. The person with learning difficulties also learns to reciprocate and show valuing to the care giver.

Gentle teaching is based on a non-aversive behavioural strategy using an ignore-redirect-reward model (McGee et al, 1987). Supportive techniques used with this model are taken from the behaviourist school and include:
- task analysis;
- environmental management;
- the identification of precursors to target behaviour;
- fading assistance and the introduction of other care givers and peers into the relationship.

The need for all care giving interactions to begin with, centre on and lead to unconditional valuing is however the central tenet of the process (McGee, 1990).

Thus gentle teaching differs from behaviourist techniques in that these latter focus on conditional reinforcement, programmed learning and controlled responses. Whilst such techniques undoubtably work, McGee and his supporters believe that a recognition of the need of human interdependence can lead to a richer experience for clients and carers in this area where people can be so easily marginalized from society.

Study activities
   8. With other students and qualified nurses or teachers, devise a programme to reduce Edward's aggressive behaviour.

   9. Consider how Edward's family may be affected by his learning difficulty and behaviour, giving reasons.

5. Summary

In this chapter we have been considering the use of psychology when applied to an area of care where the recipients may not be able to fully appreciate what is happening. After considering what is meant by 'learning difficulties' and their causes, we examined the effects on the individual and his family. As part of this analysis we also looked at what it means to belong to society and why people with learning difficulty may not be accepted as easily as others.

The need of the person with learning difficulties to be accepted as a member of society was considered from the point of view of social role valorization. This was identified as more than giving the person choice. The need for a recognition of responsibility was also identified. It was pointed out that to allow the person with learning difficulties freedom of choice, without expecting that person to accept responsibility for that choice was in effect tantamount to treating him like a young child. Social role valorization is not a one way process. Whilst those in society who are fortunate to have a normal intelligence will need to initiate much of the policy and process to allow the person with learning difficulty to make choices and take risks, the need for reciprocal responsibilities must not be devalued.

We concluded the chapter by considering briefly the methods of training people with learning difficulties. The behavioural techniques were identified as the mainstay of training programmes, and the method of backward chaining was considered as a special adaptation of these techniques geared to achieve the best results in shaping socially acceptable behaviour. The difficulty of the person with challenging behaviour was finally considered, as was the rise of the gentle teaching movement as a reaction to aversive behaviourist techniques to reduce and eliminate aggressive and self-harming behaviours. The essential differences between behaviourism and gentle teaching were illustrated, although debate continues as to whether gentle teaching represents a unique method rather than an adaptation of non-aversive behavioural techniques.

Tension complaints and functional complaints

4

1. Introduction

This chapter begins with a consideration of the psychology of the body with particular focus on the concepts of 'body plan', 'body sense' and 'body idea'. In the rest of the chapter we concentrate on tension complaints and functional complaints. By tension complaints we mean those complaints which are linked with excessive stress. Functional complaints are those complaints for which no physical reason can be found.

After a general explanation of the SORC diagram, we study in more detail the relationship between stimulus and response in relation to tension and functional complaints. In this framework the concept 'classical conditioning' is discussed. We then explain the significance of the personality and of types of characteristic reactions.

Finally the relationship between behaviour and its consequences is explored. In this context we look at the occurrence and maintenance of low backache complaints and the role that 'operant conditioning' plays in this.

Learning outcomes
After the study of this chapter the student should be able to:
- explain the following concepts:
  - body plan;
  - body sense;
  - body idea;
- give a description of the SORC diagram;
- explain the difference between overt and covert behaviour;
- describe the concept 'classical conditioning';
- give an example of classical conditioning in daily life;
- give examples of the O category;
- explain the connection between psychosomatic conditions and the SORC diagram;
- explain the influence of consequent factors on the behaviour;
- describe the concept 'operant conditioning';
- explain the concept 'secondary illness gain' according to the SORC diagram;
- describe a tension complaint in an SORC diagram;
- describe a functional complaint in an SORC diagram.

2. The psychology of the body

The close relationship which exists between what you think of yourself, the self-concept, and what you think of your own body, the body-image, has already been mentioned in this book. We examined it indirectly in the discussion of the self-concept in Module 1. In Chapter 1 of this module, in the section 'Being ill as a stressor' the close connection was identified. In this chapter we list a number of concepts which are concerned with the mental experiencing of our body.

The body

The body as examined by a doctor is not the body that we mean when we speak about our own subjective body experience. The body, as studied in neurology for example, is an object, a thing. That thing has objective properties: weight, volume, temperature and the like. It has a certain construction: bones, muscles, blood vessels, nerve paths and the like. It has certain constituent parts: heart, lungs, liver, brain and so forth.

If the brain does not function properly, the body may no longer be able to think, feel or observe properly. In consultation with the neuropsychologist, the neurologist can consider the type of mental disturbance and thus determine what part of the brain is affected.The body as we discuss it in this chapter is the body that we both feel and experience. This body is someone; it coincides with the 'I'. In everyday life we are our body, we coincide with it. On the level of everyday functioning we do not say: 'My body is tired,' we say: 'I am tired.' If, after working hard, we feel hot and sweaty, we do not say: 'My body is sweaty, but I myself am fresh,' no, we say: 'I feel so sweaty, I'll go and have a wash.' The 'I' and the 'body' thus coincide.
A separation however can be applied. We can say: 'My leg hurts,' or 'My head is aching.' We can also do this with regard to our thoughts or feelings: 'My thoughts are so confused,' or 'He's really hurt my feelings.' However the metaphysical concept of mind and body, the question, 'Who are we really?' is, a philosophical problem, not a psychological one.

Body plan, body sense and body idea

When we speak about the body as a psychological subject, it is important to make a difference between three concepts: the body plan, the body sense and the body idea. These three concepts are now described in turn.
By *body plan* we mean 'the organized sum total of all sensory-motor structures which determines the automated behaviour of man'. It concerns the implicit idea that we have of our body as a spatial object. We know the spatial proportions of our body. For this reason we (seldom) run into walls, we go and sit on (and rarely beside) chairs, we scratch ourselves in places where we have an itch (and not beside them), we put a cup of coffee against the lower lip and not against the forehead and so on.

This body plan can, temporarily, be disturbed. With an excess of alcohol in the blood it can let you down. In adolescents who grow very fast, the development of the body plan does not always keep in step with the changing proportions. The adolescent then goes through a clumsy phase: he bumps against tables, knocks over cups and so forth. Pregnant women also experience this problem. In these cases however the disturbance of the body plan is a temporary one. The body plan can also become permanently disturbed so that the recognition of the body is not complete. In these situations the cause will usually be neurological, such as a stroke, where the effect has been that the brain is not functioning completely.

By *body sense* we mean 'the information which man can acquire through observation about the state of his body in space'. If we have to learn a particular body movement, for example at a dancing lesson, we probably learn first to move one foot and then to bring the other one to it. We are conscious of our movements, and we need to concentrate on the position of our body in relation to the movements. We then, in these terms, concentrate on our body sense. During recuperation from an illness, movements are relearnt through making use of body sense. The physiotherapist gives instructions about how movements must be carried out, and the patient then concentrates on carrying them out.

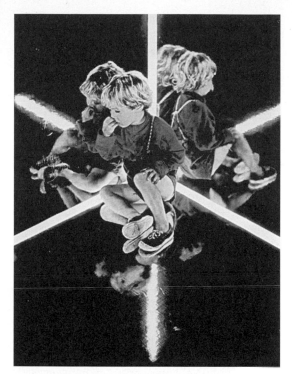

Figure 4.4.1a
Confused in the hall of mirrors:
concentrating on body sense

Figure 4.4.1b
On the moon:
new body sense, new body plan

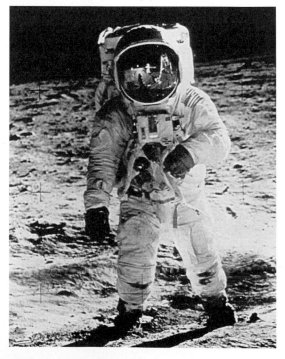

By *body idea* we mean 'the subjective judgement that man has of his own bodily state formed in relation to:
a. his own possibilities and the limits of his own ability;
b. the qualities or peculiarities of his own body and
c. the social interaction'.

The body idea is thus a judgement by ourselves about our bodily abilities and qualities. That judgement is partly dependent on the judgement that others have of our body.
The remark:
'You're lovely, no wonder people look at you' encourages in the recipient the idea 'I want to be seen.' And: 'How strong you are!' induces the notion 'I am strong.'

If someone realises that his body plan is disturbed, he will in the long term be conscious of the motor movements that he makes. That may then suggest that his body idea is 'bad': his value judgement about his body becomes negative. This value judgement (the body idea) is a constituent part of the self-concept. The *self-concept* is the totality of value judgements that we have of ourselves. In everyday functioning there is a close connection between the value judgement about the body and about ourselves. If our body is affected, we are ourselves affected.

Women who have been the victims of rape experience this. They identify that it is not just that something terrible has happened with the body, they themselves are also seriously affected in their integrity.

It must be clear to those who work in health care that, if they are occupied with the body of another, they need to approach the other person very closely. They enter into someone's intimacy. Being occupied with a body means being occupied with *someone*. It does not mean washing, cleaning or attending an object, a thing. You are occupied with the carrying out of actions which deeply affect someone else.

Study activity
   1. Put into words the consequences of the

concepts *body plan, body sense* and *body idea* for carers and patients in relation to:
- washing;
- giving an enema.

Although we have listed three seperate terms here that does not mean that everyone uses them. The *body plan* is often called in neurology the body scheme, or body schedule. The *body idea* is also referred to in different terms: subjective body experience, body picture, body concept, body feeling and body-to-body image.

The body idea is socio-culturally linked and is dependent on social and cultural attitudes. Certain body proportions are preferred to others. In Western society people do not like to be overweight. The idea that, 'My stomach is too fat' becomes, 'I am too fat,' which leads to 'I am not going to that party; people will look at me and laugh at me.' Being slim and athletic is much more in vogue and clothes are chosen to convey this impression of the body. One feels much better and more self-assured if one has the impression of being well dressed.

These self-assessments are of course culturally determined. In other cultures and in other times people have or had different attitudes to the body idea. Being overweight in some African cultures, for example, may be regarded as a sign of status or wealth, or think of the women in the pictures of Rubens where the preferences of the time were quite different from today.

Certain parts of the body are also more important than others for the total self-concept. Men have a preference for an angular appearance, with broad shoulders and narrow hips. These characteristics of their body give them the necessary security and self-esteem. Women have a preference for firm and well-proportioned breasts. The feeling that her breasts look good and attractive determines to some extent a woman's idea of looking attractive and of taking trouble with her appearance. Less well developed or badly proportioned breasts are camouflaged with full-fitting clothes and in this sense the 'breast idea' can be a negative component of the body idea.

3. Tension complaints and functional complaints: a closer examination

By *tension complaints* we understand the connection between the complaint and an excess of tension, or stress. This excess may relate to a single episode: witnessing a very serious traffic accident may cause such an excess of tension all at once. More often excess tension builds up over a long period. The most commonly found example of a tension complaint is the tension headache, a complaint that is largely determined by stress. We may take as another example a young woman who is physically exhausted by two pregnancies following quickly upon each other, with a lively toddler and an unweaned baby who needs a lot of care. Carers should not be surprised if such a woman complains of exhaustion and general malaise.

By *functional complaints* we mean complaints for which no physical cause can be shown. They may be termed as complaints where the cause is not understood. The patient complains about pain behind the left shoulder blade, though an extensive physical examination shows no irregularities. But the patient does have pain. He not only says that he has pain, he really does have it.

The misfortune of this sort of patient is that a physical cause is not shown. This pain can often be explained if we understand the pain as a form of learned behaviour. Learned pain, however, feels just as painful, and may be linked with the idea that the body is not fully fit, and also with the idea that the doctor has not made an exhaustive search for causes.

A close relationship exists between functional complaints and tension complaints. Stomach ulcers and myocardial infarction are examples of complaints where there is a clear underlying physical cause but where stress or tension is implicated in their development (see Chapter 1, Sections 3 and 4 of this module).

It must be noted here that not all doctors agree about the examples mentioned above. Some doctors believe that tension headache, stomach ulcers, myocardial infarction and other similar complaints are caused by strictly physical factors. They give as an explanation for these either that there was no thorough search or that knowledge in these areas is inadequate. Perhaps a misunderstanding plays a role here. The authors of this book adopt an integrated or holistic perspective taking as a starting point in illness and health the view that somatic *and* mental *and* social factors always play a part together. Sometimes somatic factors especially play a part, sometimes principally psycho-social ones (see Module 3). But it may also be the case that in strictly physical matters, such as a broken leg, psycho-social factors play a part, for example through the fact that the person affected becomes depressive because of it. The art of medicine, in addition to being the application of results of biological investigation, is also the application of the results of psychological and sociological investigation.

Study activity
2. **a.** Give at least three examples of tension complaints and of functional complaints.
b. Show why patients with functional complaints may not always be assessed as positively as patients with tension complaints.

One way of understanding and explaining tension complaints and functional complaints is discussed below. Through the use of the SORC diagram we can identify which behavioural factors precede the complaint and which follow it. Furthermore we can gain an insight into the personality structure of those with the complaints and what this has to do with the complaints themselves. After the discussion of the SORC diagram we consider the therapy plan.

4. The SORC diagram

Patients regularly come into hospital and to the family doctor with complaints for which no clear physical cause can be found. In many cases they are ascribed to stress at work or in the home (tension complaints), but it may also be the case that the doctor does not know what causes them and classifies them as having no identifiable cause (functional complaints). It may also be said that the patient's complaint is 'psychological'.

Whichever term is used, it tends to mean that the doctor cannot do much about it.

One way to understand these complaints is by considering them as a form of behaviour. By behaviour we mean: all human activities, such as moving, speaking, thinking, feeling and so forth. Some forms of behaviour are more easily observed than others, such as moving and speaking; this is called overt behaviour. Other behaviour, such as thinking and feeling, is only observable by the person himself; this is covert behaviour. Behaviour is the relationship of someone with the environment. Through his behaviour someone influences the environment and the environment in its turn influences his behaviour.

How does behaviour arise and how is it maintained? In order to give an answer to this question, we make use of a diagram from behaviour therapy. Behaviour therapy takes as its starting point the fact that nearly all behaviour is learned. It is a form of therapy which is based on the behavioural and the cognitive schools of psychology. One way of reproducing the relationship between behaviour and environment is by use of the SORC diagram. The letters S, O, R and C stand for *stimulus, organism, response* and *consequence*. The SORC diagram is given in diagram 4.4.1. Note the direction of the arrows.

Response
Response is positioned centrally in the diagram. It is influenced on the one hand by the stimulus via the organism and on the other hand by the consequences.

The response is the (complaint) behaviour. Every response has three components.
The first component is *overt behaviour*, which is visible or audible for other people. It consists of movements, facial expressions, words or sounds that someone utters. The second component is *covert behaviour*, i.e. thoughts, feelings and emotions which someone has about an event or about himself. The third component is *physiological reactions*, i.e. reactions of the body such as muscle tension, heart palpitations and increased blood pressure. The

Diagram 4.4.1
SORC diagram

$$S \to O \to R \leftarrow C$$

three components are not independent of each other, but mutually influence each other. This is represented in diagram 4.4.2.

We shall illustrate the mutual influencing of these three components with the following example. On getting up in the morning a man feels heart palpitations (physiological reaction). He thinks, 'I hope there's nothing wrong with my heart, I just hope I won't have a heart attack.' These thoughts (covert behaviour) lead to his going to the doctor to have his heart examined (overt behaviour).

Stimulus

Back to the SORC diagram. The first category in this diagram is the *stimulus*. A stimulus is a goad from the environment. It may be a matter of a simple goad, such as a prick from a needle. It may be a more complicated event, which consists of several stimuli. There is a relationship between the stimulus and the response. If a certain stimulus is present, the person reacts with a certain response: if you prick your finger with a needle, you will pull your finger back. However, not all people react in the same way. Another example of a stimulus is having an illness, for example flu. One person will react to it by going to bed. Another will generally try to

continue working. The flu stimulus does not always lead to the same response. We find an explanation for this among other things in the O factor: the characteristics of the *organism*.

Organism

In the SORC diagram the O stands between the S and the R. Every person is an individual with a certain life history. He has a personality of his own. He has experienced certain things and has learnt to react. These factors belong to the O category. In terms of the diagram: the response to the stimulus depends on the organism. Someone who has grown up in an environment in which a lot of thought is given to bodily complaints will pay great attention to his own body. He will notice changes in his body sooner than others and he will worry about them more. If this person gets flu, he will go to bed.

A certain manner of dealing with problems also belongs in the O category, for example trying to avoid problems as much as possible or asking for help from others. It will be clear that 'cognitive judgement' is a factor which also belongs to the O category. We met this factor in Chapter 1, Section 4.b, and also in the discussion of Moos's model (pages 296-300).

Consequences

The last category in the diagram is the C which stands for *consequences*. By consequences we mean the reactions from the environment to the behaviour. We make a distinction between two sorts of reactions: reinforcing and punishing. If a *reinforcing* consequence follows a certain form of behaviour, the chance is greater that that behaviour will recur. Examples of positive reinforcers are: money and the esteem of other people. Negative reinforcers also exist: something unpleasant does not happen. An example of a negative reinforcer: not having to perform a disagreeable chore. Punishing consequences

Diagram 4.4.2
Response composed
of three components

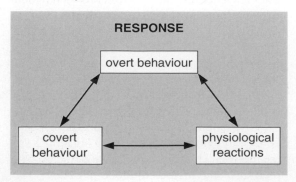

also exist. Punishing consequences have the effect of diminishing the likelihood that the behaviour will recur. Examples of punishing consequences are: being left on one's own and angry reactions from others. Consequences are not only present in the external world. One's own thoughts can also contain a rewarding (reinforcing) or punishing consequence of behaviour, e.g. the thought that you have done something excellently (reinforcing), or that you feel like an idiot (punishing).

Rewarding and punishing

Rewarding (reinforcing) has a much greater effect on making desired behaviour occur than does punishing. With punishing, the effect is that a certain undesired behaviour disappears. But as a disadvantage there is the fact that you do not know what new behaviour will replace it - possibly something even worse. Rewarding means that you know precisely what behaviour should occur more often. You can reward a patient who no longer needs to lie in bed, whenever he gets out of bed: the patient will as a result leave his bed more and more frequently. You can also punish him if he remains in bed unnecessarily by for example always finding fault with him. You then do not know what the reaction will be: does he stay in bed with the sheet over his head or does he become a peevish patient who sits in a chair only now and again? Be careful: the aim has to be an active, walking patient.

Study activity

3. Try to apply the principles of rewarding and punishing to the provision of care for patients with a deep anxiety about death, for example after an acute myocardial infarction.

a. The S - R relationship

If someone with hay fever gets pollen in his nose, his body reacts with a bout of sneezing, red and weeping eyes and an itch. If someone falls and breaks his arm, his arm then hurts. In neither of these examples has the person direct control over the response. Whether he likes it or not, the hay fever sufferer gets red eyes and a bout of sneezing when he gets pollen in his nose. How-

ever vehemently the person who has fallen may resist, he is going to feel pain in his arm when this is broken. The response, the bout of sneezing and the pain, is elicited by the stimuli, the pollen and the fracture. This is comparable with a reflex. If someone strikes the kneecap with a reflex hammer, the lower leg jerks.

At the beginning of this century the Russian physiologist Pavlov investigated the saliva secretion in dogs (see also Module 1, Chapter 2, Section 4). In due course Pavlov discovered a remarkable phenomenon: the dogs secreted saliva as soon as they heard the footsteps of the servant who came to bring the food. Pavlov investigated this phenomenon by letting a bell be heard before the food was offered. After the bell had been heard a number of times before the food was offered, saliva secretion took place on hearing the bell. In diagram 4.4.3 this sequence is reproduced.

This phenomenon is known as 'classical conditioning': if two stimuli occur a number of times together, one stimulus (the bell) can elicit the response (saliva secretion) which was first elicited by the other stimulus (the food).

Classical conditioning also occurs in people. If you are hungry and someone describes a magnificent meal, your mouth produces saliva; the saliva appears although no food is present. When someone with hay fever sees a photo of flowering grass, this can sometimes lead to a bout of sneezing. Children who have had an injection are often anxious at the sight of someone in a white coat.

Now what has this to do with tension complaints or complaints without an identified cause? In

Diagram 4.4.3
Classic conditioning

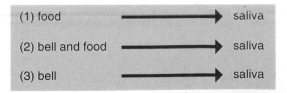

(1) food	⟶	saliva
(2) bell and food	⟶	saliva
(3) bell	⟶	saliva

these complaints a process of classical conditioning may also have occurred. This is explained by means of the case of Mr. Thomson.

Case study: Mr. Thomson
Mr. Thomson has a hard time working in a furniture factory. At his work conflicts often occur with his boss. Mr. Thomson bottles these problems up and does not talk about them.
He tries to make the best of his work. However, at his work he gets more and more trouble from stomach complaints. If he sees his boss, he gets a pain in his stomach. When Mr. Thomson goes to the family doctor, it turns out that he has a stomach ulcer.

Study activity
4. Translate the example from this case into similar experiences of your own in the course of practice.

In general the stomach reacts to conflicts with the secretion of stomach acid. Just as the broken arm and pain belong together, so also do conflict and the degree of acidity of the gastric juices. After a period of time, seeing the boss became a stimulus which could elicit this reaction. The connection between boss and degree of acidity is a conditioned one. The repeated secretion of stomach acid may finally lead to the development of a stomach ulcer.

In most tension complaints the relationship between S and R is very important. The complaints are elicited by certain stimuli, where the person does not know what to do about things. In this the thoughts that the person has about the situation play an important role. They are often thoughts like; 'I wish he wouldn't act so horribly again;' 'I shall immediately have trouble with my stomach again,' 'I can't do anything to solve this problem.' These are elements which belong to the O factor.

b. The S - O - R relationship
Earlier in this chapter it was indicated that the *organism* shares in determining what response follows a stimulus. Not every person always reacts in precisely the same manner in a given situation.

In the O category we have the life and learning history of a person. Every person learns in the course of his life to react in a certain manner to difficult situations. One reacts to a problem by withdrawing and brooding, another reacts by actively trying to find a solution. Yet another goes and asks for help from members of the family or friends. These ways of reacting also occur in dealing with an illness.

If a housewife gets a pain in her back while cleaning the house, there are different ways in

Diagram 4.4.4
SORC diagram
of a patient with
tension headache

S   stress-provoking situations,
        for example problems at work.

O   perfectionist;
        worry about failing;
        deficient social skills.

R   physiological:
        increase in muscle tension in the neck
        and head.

        covert behaviour:
        I hope I don't get headache again
        I feel the headache coming on
        I hope I don't have a tumour.

        overt behaviour:
        take medicines; rest;
        visit a doctor.

C   reinforcing (positive):
        time for hobbies.

        reinforcing (negative):
        avoidance of stress-provoking
        situations.

        punishing:
        problems with the environment;
        enslaved to medicines;
        less social contact.

which she can react. She might think that she really has been overdoing it and that she should stop working. She might react with; 'Dash it, the back again; but never mind, there is so much to be done' and carry on working as usual. A third possibility is that she is afraid that there is something wrong with her back and she goes to the doctor. Whichever of the three thoughts occurs to her depends on her life and learning history. In this her reaction may be affected by whether she has already had back complaints, what was the matter then and how her environment reacted to it.

The importance of the O category is principally in explaining people's behaviour, by accounting for their manner of dealing with difficult situations. This manner is relatively independent of the situation in which the patient finds himself, so taking account of it is of great importance. In the behavioural approach the illness behaviour is seen as simply the result of the situation in which the patient finds himself. The reverse also exists: the illness is the result of the personality structure of the patient. The O category is therefore very important since the individual differences between people can be explained by it.

c. Psychosomatics

The personality also belongs in the O category. The importance of the personality in the development of certain illnesses is emphasized in psychosomatic medicine. The so-called psychosomatic line of thinking has played a significant part in the development of medical psychology. For some, the term 'psychosomatics' is predicated as identical to 'medical psychology'. Everything that concerns the relationship between psychological and social factors on the one hand and physical factors on the other can be considered under this term.

Such a wide use of the term psychosomatics does not accord with recent developments. In this book this term is reserved for those situations where the personality factors are of importance for the occurrence and continued existence of illness.

In the 1950s three Dutch researchers, Groen, van der Horst and Bastiaans, formulated the specificity hypothesis. This proposes that a specific personality structure makes the individual receptive to the development of a certain somatically demonstrable complaint pattern. If for example you are characterized by suppressed aggression, anger and tension, you have a good chance of suffering from migraine. In the same way anxiety, passive and dependent behaviour are linked to asthma. This specificity hypothesis has had some influence on medical psychological thinking. The hypothesis has not turned out to be correct in all its applications, though neither has it been shown to be completely wrong.

Many illnesses are investigated from the standpoint of the specificity hypothesis. We shall mention two examples: coronary disease and rheumatoid arthritis.

Coronary disease

A well known example of the influence of the personality on illness is the type A personality in cardiac and vascular diseases. A type A personality works under continuing performance pressure, sets high standards for himself and sticks obstinately to them. It is someone who has a great need for recognition, who is continually active, very impatient and who lives under a constant time pressure.

From investigation it has become clear that type A people have a greater chance of suffering a myocardial infarction than people who have the opposite personality characteristics (i.e. type B personalities).

Rheumatoid arthritis

A second example concerns rheumatoid arthritis. If you examine a group of rheumatism patients, you find a number of mutual personality characteristics. But, for a proper understanding, two questions occur.

– Are these characteristics specific for rheumatism patients or:
– did the patients develop these characteristics as a result of rheumatism?

Research results show that the personality characteristics (in other words: the stable behaviour characteristics) are not specific for rheumatism patients; they are characteristic for those who suffer from a chronic somatic affection. The stable behaviour characteristics of the chronic somatic patient are gloomy outlook, dependence, and inhibition of expressions of feelings in general, especially feelings of anger and enmity. From some investigations it appears that these behaviour characteristics are the result of the affection and not the cause. As far as rheumatoid arthritis is concerned there is not yet much evidence that a personality structure exists which is characteristic of persons who afterwards develop rheumatism.

Study activity

5. Try to express the consequences of the specificity hypothesis for patients with (for example) epilepsy, cancer and rheumatism.

d. The R - C relationship

The fourth category in the SORC diagram is the *consequences*. People's behaviour is not only dependent on events which precede it, but also on the consequences that follow it. The relationship between the behaviour and the consequences can be explained with the aid of operant conditioning.
To understand it properly: R, the response, has a physiological aspect, a cognitive (or covert) aspect and an overt aspect.
All three of these aspects come under the control of the consequences.

The term 'operant' originates from the psychologist Skinner and derives from the verb 'to operate'. This means that the organism is active and carries out certain types of behaviour. This is in opposition to classical conditioning, in which the organism is passive and the response is elicited by the stimulus. If you peel an onion and rub near your eyes with your hand, your eyes will then water. If you do this many times on successive days, the sight of onions may then be enough for your eyes to water. If they do, you have no choice: it is a matter of classical conditioning. Compare this with an example of operant conditioning: if the telephone rings, you pick it up: there is no obligation for you to do so.

According to operant conditioning a behaviour which is followed by a positive reinforcer will occur more often in future. If a punishing consequence follows a response, the behaviour will occur less frequently in future. Whether a consequence is reinforcing or punishing is different for each person. There are a number of consequences which are reinforcing for most people. These can be divided into three groups:
- material consequences: money, sweets, presents, a dividend;
- the carrying out of a pleasure-giving activity or the avoidance of an unpleasant activity: watching television, lying in the sun; not having to work (if the work is unpleasant), not having to wash up;
- social consequences: attention of others, doing something with others, help, praise, a compliment.

Behaviour has consequences in both the short and in the long term. These are not always both reinforcing. Sometimes behaviour has a positive consequence in the short term and a punishing consequence in the long term. An example of this is smoking: in the short term it

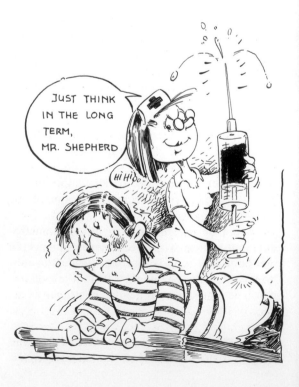

JUST THINK IN THE LONG TERM, MR. SHEPHERD

HI HI oo

leads to a pleasant feeling (removal of tension, belonging to a group); in the long term the 'punishment' is that the chance of lung cancer is greater.

Behaviour can also have a punishing consequence in the short term and a positive consequence in the long term. This is the case for example with being inoculated against a disease. In the short term the consequence is punishing: most people do not like having an injection. In the long term, however, it protects against catching the disease.

Consequences in the short term have a much greater effect on the occurrence and continuation of behaviour than consequences in the long term. This fact is evident in the case of someone trying to give up smoking. If the saying 'First impressions last the longest' is true in one way or another, it certainly is in the case of short and long term consequences. Why is giving up smoking so difficult? Because in the short term smoking gives relaxation, and only perhaps over forty years might it cause lung cancer. Another example: why does the patient keep on having pain in his back? Because the experience of pain in the short term provides sympathy and anxiety from the partner and only in the long term does it cause a sharp drop in income due to the inability to work. With functional complaints there is often evidence of reinforcing consequences in the short term and punishing consequences in the long term.

A much used term in this connection is 'secondary illness gain'. By this it is meant that an illness has positive consequences for a patient. This is not the same as simulating a complaint or malingering by the patient. If a patient simulates a complaint, he has no real complaints, but says that he does have them in order to obtain an advantage. The 'play' of consequences in the long and short term, however, goes on automatically and without the intention of the patient. If subsequent factors take over control of the behaviour, the patient feels precisely the same in his body as if a physical irregularity is present. He has also the same thoughts about the cause of it: 'There is something wrong with my body.' And he behaves in the same manner: he avoids certain activities and seeks help from the doctor.

Diagram 4.4.5
SORC diagram of a
female patient with low back pain

S   her husband is very busy and does not have much time and consideration for the patient; there is no medical explanation of the complaints.

O   she is very worried about her bodily functioning;
she needs the consideration of others;
she wants contact with other people;
she tries to avoid problems.

R   physiological:
increase in muscle tension in the back.

covert behaviour:
If I do anything, something will go wrong with my back;
If I have pain, my husband will get quite worried.

overt behaviour:
walking with crutches;
complaining of pain;
resting on the settee in the living room;
visit to the doctor.

C   positive:
the husband gets very worried, stays at home more, has consideration for her, helps with everything and organizes help with the housework.

punishing:
more isolation occurs from other people;
depression;
it is awful to be dependent on others;
the complaints become worse through not using the muscles.

Diagram 4.4.5 is an example of the SORC diagram worked out for a female patient with low back pain, for which no clear physical cause exists. In the maintenance of the complaint consequential factors play a big part.

e. The SORC diagram and Moos's model

The SORC diagram is comparable with Moos's model, which was discussed in Chapter 1. The differences between the two models are those of degree. Moos lays great emphasis on cognitive judgement. Cognitive judgement together with coping skills are the two central concepts in the understanding and explanation of illness behaviour.

In the SORC diagram great emphasis is laid on the influence of stressors (S - R) and consequences (R - C) in the understanding and explanation of behaviour.

With Moos's model we are better able to explain the reactions to being organically ill. Functional and tension complaints can be explained (and treated) better if we approach them from the SORC perspective.

Study activity
6. **a.** Apply the SORC diagram and Moos's model to the patient who is lying in hospital with unexplained attacks of giddiness.
   b. Show what differences exist between the SORC diagram and Moos's model.

5. Summary

In patient-care practice we are repeatedly confronted with stress and the complaints which have a connection with it. It is not always easy to identify tension complaints and treat them adequately. The patient also worries about functional complaints, since no physical causes for the complaints can be shown.

The concepts of body plan, body sense and body idea were considered as components of the totality of value judgements that we have of ourselves, the self-concept. The different aspects of the SORC diagram were described in relation to tension complaints and functional complaints.

The four constituent parts of the SORC diagram, stimulus, organism, response and consequences were described and the relationships and interaction between the parts were examined. Finally the SORC diagram was looked at in the context of Moos's model showing the differences in application between the two methods.

5

Psychological assessment

1. Introduction

This chapter examines the work of the clinical psychologist, with examples drawn from the area of somatic health care. The relation of psychology to psychiatry and learning difficulties was introduced in Chapters 2 and 3. We do not want to give the impression, however, that a strict separation can be made between the activities of clinical psychologists in mental health and those in somatic health care. Such a strict division does not exist. In mental health care the type of complaint is different from that in somatic health care. The former has to deal with a complaint like, 'I am so worried', while the complaint, 'I am so tired' comes into somatic health care. The methods which the clinical psychologist uses to carry out his work in each of these cases are usually rather similar.

In this chapter consideration is given to the necessity of measuring behaviour, as opposed to (chance) observation, on the basis of:
– reliability
– validity
– standardization
– measuring procedure.

Learning outcomes

After studying this chapter the student should be able to:
– show why the clinical psychologist deals with 'undesirable behaviour' and what dangers are linked with this labelling;
– reproduce the roles nursing staff, doctors and clinical psychologists play with the patient with a behaviour disturbance;
– describe the concept 'objectivization', and explain the manner in which the clinical psychologist can objectivize;
– describe the following concepts:
  • reliability
  • validity
  • standardization
  • measuring procedure
– explain the value of measuring instruments in psychology and nursing.

2. Undesirable behaviour

'Undesirable behaviour' is an ambiguous concept. 'Undesirable' can be taken to mean: deviant, strange, disturbed, unsuitable, criminal, abnormal, sick or even mad. Whichever meaning we take from this group, we should always remember that we are labelling the person who is asking for help.

Is the help seeker possessed by 'the devil', by 'demons'? Then she (*sic*) is a witch. She must be subjected to an exorcistic ritual, or even be drowned or burnt. With this idea we have transported ourselves back to the Middle Ages.

Is the help seeker 'crazy'? Then we can shut him up in a 'madhouse' and go and look at him from time to time, by way of an outing. This takes us back to the 19th century.

Is the help seeker a 'miscreant'? Then we must hand him over to Justice and it will remove him from society.

Is the help seeker a 'patient'? Then we must treat him in the medical circuit. The undesirable behaviour is then pathological and it is classified on the basis of symptoms, with a diagnosis as a result. Attempts to alter the undesirable behaviour are therapies. If therapies 'take', the patient is cured.

Is the help seeker a 'client'? Then we go through his problems with him. We give the client advice if the client wants that.

Theoretically the term 'undesirable' raises a wide range of problems. In clinical practice, however, and this book is practically orientated, it is hardly a problem. Clinical psychology deals among other things with back complaints, tension headache, spastic colon, suicide attempts, self-mutilation, anxiety, compulsion, depression and relationship problems.

We have already classified the problems with which the somatic medical psychologist has to deal, such as:
– people with a physical complaint who experience emotional problems as a result. Examples of this are patients with a chronic illness (such as rheumatism), kidney dialysis patients or cancer patients;
– people with a physical complaint which has to do with stress, or tension. An example is patients with cardio-vascular diseases;
– people with a functional complaint, that is to say physical complaints for which no physical cause can be shown. An example is patients with tension headache;
– problems in the relationship between helper and patient, which can influence the course of the illness process. An example is the problems which arise if a patient continually makes demands on the attention of nursing staff in a department.

Study activity
1. Describe from your own experience at least two examples of each of the above mentioned concepts.

3. The complaint as the angle of attack

Psychology is the study of human behaviour. The clinical psychologist is an expert on behaviour.

Figure 4.5.1
She behaves strangely and deviantly; she is a witch!

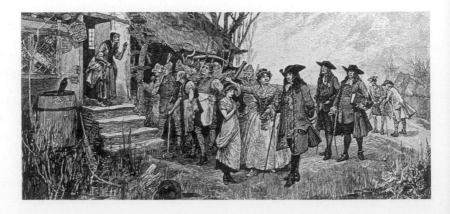

He knows about the way in which behaviour arises and how it is influenced. Nursing staff have not explicitly studied human behaviour to the same extent as psychologists have. Nursing staff (and doctors) are, however, experts with wide experience in the field of human behaviour. They deal daily with patients and in doing so they build up a wealth of experience about human behaviour in difficult (sickness and health) circumstances.

The clinical psychologist should appreciate this. He should listen attentively to the opinion of the nursing staff and the doctor treating the case, before making his own assessment. But the doctor and the nursing staff have called in the behaviour expert; the psychologist. This means that their own experience alone has failed to satisfactorily assess the behaviour of a patient. Nurses and doctor cannot deal with it on their own. The assessment that is requested of the clinical psychologist may therefore augment the assessment that is based on the experience of nurses and doctor, and should therefore add something to their assessment. Thus the clinical psychologist not only bases his judgement on the subjective assessment ('experience' is a subjective assessment!) of nursing staff and doctors: he also adds his own appraisal.

The clinical psychologist will try to objectivize the behaviour of the patient, as far as possible. By 'objectivize', we mean that the psychologist, making use of measuring procedures, will compare the behaviour of the patient with the behaviour of others. The question 'Is this behaviour disturbed?' is not answered with 'Yes, because I feel it to be disturbed', but with an objective judgement based on measuring procedures. Objectivizing means in the first place accurately charting the complaint.

Study activity
  2. Being able to measure 'disturbed' behaviour implies that a statistical norm for 'normality' is used. Define a 'statistical' norm, and name some advantages and disadvantages of this concept.

The clinical psychologist begins his study with the complaint. What is the complaint? Who has the complaint? What has he himself (the help seeker and his environment) done about the complaint? What have others (for example doctors) done about it? What has the effect of these actions been? Does the patient now have other, especially comparable, complaints? And what was it like before? The clinical psychologist tries to put the complaint in perspective: what are its characteristics, how has it arisen and what can be done about it?

He can for example do this by means of the two diagrams which are presented in Chapters 1 and 4 of this module. The complaint is the behaviour, the final reaction to being ill in Moos's model (page 296).

In the SORC diagram (page 340) the complaint coincides with the R of response. In each diagram the complaint is under the influence of various factors.

The task of the clinical psychologist is to trace the factors which influence the complaint in an individual patient. Consequently he will try to establish which factors have the most influence. The final aim of the investigation is:
  – to provide a description of the complaint from a medical psychological viewpoint;
  – to give a forecast of what is going to happen with the complaint in unchanged circumstances;
  – to state ways in which the patient and the helpers will best be able to deal with this complaint.

This means, if Moos's model is used, that the psychologist, after he has described the complaint, will try to assess the influence of the following factors on the complaint:
  – the personal background of the patient, such as intelligence, previous experience with illness and the methods of dealing with illness in the family;
  – the illness-linked factors, asking questions such as: Does the patient have a high temperature? What influence has medication had on his behaviour? Is the illness associated with pain?;
  – the environmental factors, i.e. the physical environment in which the patient finds him-

self; his social environment, especially the influence of conflicts with people from his immediate environment or the measure of support which he receives from these people;
- the significance of the illness for the patient and the expectation which he has in respect of his own possibilities of coping with it;
- the specific adaptation tasks which this illness sets for the patient;
- the patient's own coping skills: his chances of carrying out the adaptation tasks.

After the characteristics of the complaint itself are described the psychologist will study the following factors in terms of the SORC diagram:
- in what situation (S) the complaint occurs: what factors precede the occurrence of the complaint?
- what the characteristics of the person are (O): his personality, intelligence, previous experience with illness and method of dealing with illness;
- what consequences (C) has the complaint: how does the environment react to the complaint? Has the complaint direct positive consequences, such as for example consideration and help? Does the patient avoid negative events with his complaint?

Case study: David Jones

For about three months David Jones has been nursing in the Neurosurgery department. It is a department in which the sphere of work has a very stimulating effect on him. The expectations which David has of nursing are fulfilled in this department. He also plans to undertake specialist courses, and to apply himself completely to neurosurgical nursing.

But there is something which is bothering David. In one way or another, he has for some weeks been troubled by worries about death. This is not a passing emotion that you can as it were brush aside, but an all-pervading worry about death, in which his breath fails and his stomach contracts. To reassure himself, David has been checking in the mirror every morning for the past few days to see that his pupils are normal. He feels relief to note that his pupils are as normal as ever and

react well to light. At any rate still no brain tumour, he thinks. But he wonders how long it will be before he notices symptoms?

Study activities

3. a. Is it a question of undesirable behaviour in David Jones's case? Explain your answer.
b. Is David being responsible if he continues to work in the Neurosurgery department?

4. Try to objectivize David's behaviour with Moos's model and with the SORC diagram.

4. The psycho-social examination

If a patient is referred to the psychologist, the latter will try to find an answer to the question which was put to him by the referrer. This sounds straightforward and naturally the psychologist tries to give an answer to the question which has been put to him. But it not infrequently occurs that the referring doctor words the question very summarily: 'Complaint is beyond my comprehension; can the psychologist give a psychological explanation? If so, can he take over the treatment?'

With a question like that the psychologist must first clarify the question. He finds out from the nursing staff and the referring doctor about the background. He studies the medical and nursing records. Above all, he will make the question clearer in conversation with the patient and perhaps also with his partner. This is the *psycho-social interview* or *anamnesis*.

The aim of the conversation with the patient is to collect information about the patient's complaint and about his life situation. In order to achieve this aim, it is important that the patient feels that he can trust the psychologist. The patient must feel safe to tell a number of things about himself. The psychologist listens, is considerate, tries to get inside the patient's situation and accepts the patient as he is. We recognize the three conditions which Rogers formulated: empathy, honesty and unconditional positive acceptance (see page 57).

In essence, these three conditions entail that the patient is not subjected to an inquisition. The

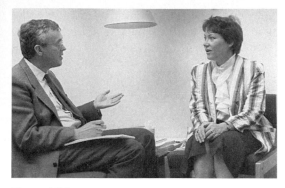

Figure 4.5.2
The recording of the
psycho-social background history

observations and questions of the psychologist are not intended to pillory the patient as an 'impostor' or as a 'poser'. The starting point is that the patient has a problem which is difficult to understand and difficult to solve. The psychologist ranges himself alongside the patient in order to help the patient solve this problem.

The psychologist asks questions, listens to the patient and observes the patient's behaviour during the conversation. The psychologist invites the patient to tell him his feelings and his ideas about the origin of the complaint. But the psychologist is even more interested in the patient's view about the why and wherefore of the continued existence of the complaint. Why did the therapies applied by the doctor not lead to a permanent desirable result?

The psychologist is trained in carrying out interview and in observation techniques. He must realize quite well however that, in spite of carrying out the examination in this style, the examination is still a subjective affair. If another psychologist carried out the conversation, he would perhaps pay attention to other things and go further into other subjects. Therefore his conversation data must not be the only source of information. The psychologist will also enquire, as said previously, into the views of the nursing staff and the referring doctor.

But even this is not enough. In order to ensure that the collection of psycho-social data is made as objectively as possible, use may be made of a psycho-social check list. By objective we mean that the information has been gained in spite of

the subjective influences of the psychologist. Thus the psychologist, where possible, makes use of psychological tests to obtain a more objective picture of the patient and his complaints. But tests are only one aid. Information from the tests, information originating from the psycho-social check list and information obtained from conversation with the patient together form the foundation on which the psychologist bases his opinion.

5. Reliability, validity and standardization

Measuring instruments, and measuring procedures more generally applied, must satisfy at least three conditions. We have mentioned the psychological test and the check list, and the interview with the patient, as measuring procedures. The three conditions which measuring procedures must satisfy are: reliability, validity and standardization of the recording.

Study activity
5. The recording of a nursing history is not standardized. Has the nursing history therefore become pointless? Give reasons for your answer.

Reliability means that if the measuring instrument is used by another psychologist, or if the information is recorded at another time (for example a week later), the measurement results are the same. The measuring instrument must thus not be dependent on the day on which it is used or on the person who uses it. The results must not depend on chance factors.

Thus it must be stated that the interview which the psychologist has with his patients does not provide completely reliable information. It is probable that another psychologist would put a number of other subjects on the agenda. It is also certain that the same psychologist would come to conclusions with a different emphasis depending on various factors such as whether he has slept well or badly. Furthermore this does not only apply for the psychologist: it is just as much the case for the junior doctor, the nursing staff and the consultant.

Validity means that the measuring instrument really measures what the designer of the measuring instrument says that it measures. An intelligence test must measure intelligence, and not perseverance or attitudes. A neurosis test must give the measurements of neurotic behaviour, not manual dexterity or intelligence.

If the psychologist carries out the interview taking into account Rogers's three conditions (empathy, honesty, unconditional positive acceptance), it is very probable that the conclusions will be valid. The conclusions then actually will concern the anxieties which the patient brought to the surface during the conversation.

A reliable test can also be valid but it does not have to be. It is quite possible to construct a test which is very reliable, but which obtains meaningless information, for example, a test for determination of the length of the nose. It is not known to us what psychological processes the length of the nose indicates. Such a test would thus be an invalid measure of aggresive tendency if that was its stated purpose. An unreliable test on the other hand is by definition invalid. A test for anxiety levels which can give different scores each time cannot really be measuring anxiety.

Standardization of recording requires that the individual recordings of the test are made in the same way. It also means that the scoring of the answers is done in the same way. Testers must try to keep the influence of matters not belonging to the measuring procedure on the test result as small as possible. You can indeed compare it with the carrying out of a test in a laboratory: the different experiments must be carried out in identical circumstances, so that the experiments' results are mutually comparable. Each test therefore has specific instructions about the way in which the test must be recorded and in which the answers must be scored. Tests are not taken in a noisy coffee shop, but in a quiet, well ventilated room. If the instruction in a test says: 'If the correct answer is not given inside 60 seconds, then stop and ask the following question', this is exactly what must happen. If you find the person being tested is struggling, you must not allow him 90 seconds'

time out of sympathy. It will be clear that complete standardization of the recording procedure cannot be achieved: the mood of the psychological assistant (who is recording the tests) changes; one day it is raining, another day the sun is shining; one person being tested is very anxious, another is quite uninterested in the examination; and so it goes on. That does not alter the fact that one must strive for as standardized a recording procedure as possible.

The reliability and validity of the test results depend to a high degree on the uniformity in the recording procedure of the test. But none of the measuring instruments which the psychologist has available is a hundred per cent reliable or valid, however standardized the course of the recording procedure is. This does not mean, however, that the tests are unusable.

Sometimes the psychologist does not require a very accurate answer to the questions asked, and a more general answer is sufficient. The psychologist then carries out an interview with the patient (and sometimes leaves it at that!). He may then record a test which is reasonably quick to record and relevant for the question, although he knows that the results of the test are of limited reliability or validity compared with a longer test. He knows that he could answer the question (much) more accurately, but makes do by adapting 'question' and 'answer' to the particular situation.

There are easily imaginable situations in which the psychologist must formulate his answer as precisely as possible and the tests which are available do not satisfy the high requirements set for reliability and validity. In practice the problem is solved by gaining information in different ways in connection with the aspect of behaviour concerned. For example, the question, 'To what extent is this patient depressive?' is then treated as follows. Firstly questions are asked in the intervieuw on the characteristic 'depression', and secondly different tests are recorded of which the makers state that 'depression' is one of the things measured in them. The degree of agreement between the results determines the reliability and validity of the answer to the question 'To what extent is this patient depressed?'

Furthermore the method of gaining information

in different ways is a sensible one. If the psychologist gets from the interview the impression that the patient is anxious, this impression is considerably more reliable if it is confirmed by, for example, the result of a questionnaire about anxiety.

6. The nurse and the assessment of behaviour

In the foregoing the impression is perhaps given that the psychologist is the only worker in health care who assesses the behaviour of patients and passes judgement on it. That is incorrect. The work of the nurse consists to a considerable extent in assessing behaviour. Before a nursing procedure is planned, carried out and assessed for a result, the nurse forms an impression of the state of the patient. This 'forming a judgement' is a form of assessment of behaviour. Assessment of behaviour for example takes place when the nurse takes the temperature of a patient or determines the amount of urine which is collected in a catheter bag, or notices that a post-operative patient starts eating again.

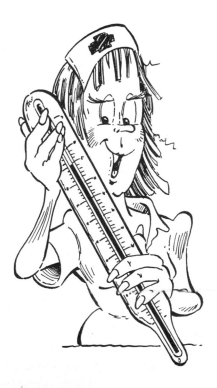

The majority of the assessments of patients by nurses fall into the category: direct observation. This means that the patient-carer uses her own faculties of observation (seeing, hearing, feeling and smelling) directly and immediately. We shall give a few examples: seeing a rose colour of the urine as an indicator of blood in the urine, feeling the heartbeat at the pulse (sometimes at different pressure points in order to trace differences), listening with the stethoscope in order to observe changes in the diastolic blood pressure during the recording of blood pressure, noticing a slight odour of faeces on coming into the room. Sometimes it is difficult to formulate clearly what the nurse observes. The observation may concern, for example, something like the 'degree of consciousness' and an indication of 'more or less than yesterday'. The nurse will make use of observation scales, such as the 'Glasgow Coma Scale' (GCS). By making use of this scale the assessor (usually a nurse) gives a score which can vary from 3 to 15. The score 3 indicates: brain dead, the score 15 entails: clear consciousness (Jones, 1979). In the assessment of both acute and chronic pain a pain assessment scale may be used. With this observation scale the nurse can, in 5 minutes, express the pain behaviour of an individual patient in measurement and figures (Bourbonnais, 1981). Just as is the case with the GCS, the value of the pain assessment scale comes from comparing the score of repeated measurements. From this comparison of the scores the state of the patient and the extent to which the treatment is successful can be seen.

The way in which an assessment is carried out helps to determine the outcome. This may be seen from the following example. It concerns the (routine) action of taking the temperature. Notice that taking the temperature is comparable with the measurement of the 'degree of consciousness' and the 'pain behaviour'. The significance of the assessment can be only seen from the comparison of the score with previous scores and/or with a known normal or average score.

A number of factors determine the figure which is given by the thermometer and which is re-

The Patient with an Altered Level of Consciousness

			Date						
			Time						
GLASGOW COMA SCALE	Eye Opening	4. Spontaneously							Eyes closed due to swelling = C
		3. To Speech							
		2. To Pain							
		1. None							
	Best Verbal	5. Oriented							Endotracheal tube or Tracheostomy = T
		4. Confused							
		3. Inappropriate							
		2. Incomprehensible							
		1. None							
	Best Motor	6. Obeys commands							Usually record best arm response
		5. Localizes to pain							
		4. Flexion / Withdrawal to pain							
		3. Abnormal flexion							
		2. Abnormal extension							
		1. None							
	Pupils	Right eye — Size							+ = Reacts − = No Reaction C = Eyes Closed
		Right eye — Reaction							
		Left eye — Size							
		Left eye — Reaction							
LIMB MOVEMENT	Arms	Normal power							Record Right (R) and Left (L) separately if there is a difference between the two sides
		Mild Weakness							
		Severe Weakness							
		Spastic Flexion							
		Extension							
		No Response							
	Legs	Normal Power							
		Mild Weakness							
		Severe Weakness							
		Extension							
		No Response							

Pupil Scale mm
1 •
2 •
3 ●
4 ●
5 ●
6 ●
7 ●
8 ●

Blood Pressure	210						42
Systolic = V	200						41
Diastolic = Λ	190						40
Blue = Lying	180						39
Red = Sitting	170						38
Standing	160						37
	150						36 °C
Pulse = •	140						35
(Red)	130						34
	120						33
	110						32
	100						31
	90						30
	80						Temperature = • (Blue)
	70						
	60						
	50						
	40						
Respirations = • (Blue)	30						30
	25						25
	20						20
	15						15
	10						10

Comments

Figure 4.5.3
Glasgow coma scale

ported by the nurse on the state of the patient. The first is obviously the temperature of the patient. But there are other factors that play a role. The place where the temperature is taken: mouth, axila or rectum. The extent of activity of the patient just before the taking of the temperature: lying on his bed or sweating after a vigorous treatment by a physiotherapist. The way in which the individual nurse deals with assessment problems: when the column of mercury stands between two marks, does she write down the value of the upper or the lower mark? Another assessment problem plays a part. The normal (skin) temperature is 36.9 degrees Celsius, that is to say the *average* normal temperature is 36.9 degrees. That means that there are healthy people whose stable body temperature falls outside the normal range. In the interpretation of a measured temperature it must be realized that the figure 36.9 is only an average. When a patient registers a temperature other than this, it need not follow that this individual has a temperature which is abnormal for him.

The conclusion that can be drawn from this example is that an agreement must be reached about the way in which the temperature is measured and assessed. In other words: the measuring procedure must, in the nursing situation, be standardized. Standardization is an important requirement which is also made for measuring procedures such as those carried out by the psychologist.

The second method of assessing the patient's state is by communication, specifically by talking with the patient. This has been previously mentioned. Talking with the patient can take many forms, from the 'Good morning' greeting when opening the curtains to the recording of an enquiry form. Module 5 pays particular attention to communication between nurse and patient.
Nurses do not only assess, in the framework of their profession, the behaviour of patients. They also carry out selection and assessment interviews. In carrying out this sort of conversation attention must also be paid to the requirements of reliability, validity and standardization.

a. Psychological tests

In this section we look more closely at the types of psychological tests. The word 'test' comes from the Latin word 'testatio' and means 'declaration' or 'evidence'. The test result is a piece of evidence, offering information about what can be concluded regarding the person examined. The intention is to make a statement which describes the patient examined, classifies his behaviour or predicts how this person will behave or develop in the future.

An example of a description might be: 'Patient looks normal for his age'. An example of a classification would be: 'The score of the neurosis scale falls into the category "very high", so the patient must be considered very neurotic'.
An example of a prediction would be: 'The level of intellectual functioning found is high, so passing the GCSE with success is considered very probable'. (See diagram 4.5.3, page 360.)

Statements of this sort can only be made if at least two test scores are compared with each other. The score of the patient examined is compared with that of other patients. Or two test scores of the same patient, but obtained at different times, are compared with each other. A test score only obtains significance in comparison with another test score. For example: a score in an intelligence test only has a meaning if this is compared with the average score of the total (British) population. Because we know how the scores of an intelligence test are distributed over the British population, this means that we can place the individual's score within that of the total British population. In the discussion of the intelligence test we shall come back to this point. Actually the psychologist reformulates the question 'What is wrong with the patient?' He rephrases this as: ' What is wrong with this patient in comparison with other individuals?' The psychologist understands the question as one about individual differences. It becomes: 'To what extent does this patient behave differently from others?' Tests are intended to measure individual differences.

Psychological tests are divided into two categories: tests for the level of performance and tests for the manner of behaviour. In tests for the level of performance it is a question of maximum performance, for example: how many sums can the person tested do successfully within one minute? Or: how many types of animals can he name within one minute?

In tests for the manner of behaviour it is a question of the usual manner of behaving of the person examined. It is a question of coming to know how he tends to do something, in what manner he usually reacts. For example: if he is unjustly accused of something, does he get angry or downcast or does he shrug his shoulders? Or: if she walks along a shopping street, is she interested in the displays of fashion goods or of books?

Tests for level of performance

We shall first look carefully at the tests for the level of performance. Two sorts of tests for level of performances are differentiated: requirement tests and aptitude tests.

With a requirement or achievement test we ask the question, 'What has been the result of a previous period of training or education?' A requirement test is aimed at going into whether the person examined masters a certain action or is able correctly to carry out or solve a particular task.

A well known example of a requirement test was the 11+ examination. This test was taken by children at age 11 or 12 years and determined whether they were admitted to a grammar school or to a secondary modern school. The type of school the child went to had long lasting effects on their future. The GCSE examination is also an example of a requirement test. The results of the examination indicate the performance of each child in relation to all other children sitting the examination. The results of this examination are also a good predictor of the child's progress after the age of 16 years.

You may hear cynical remarks about the value of GCSE examinations such as, 'You know Mark, don't you? Last week he got the results of the A level examinations and he passed all three at the first attempt. The results of his GCSEs were so poor he nearly wasn't able to stay on at school'. Or: 'Is there something wrong with Joan? Only last year she achieved good results in her GCSEs but now she is not able to keep up with her A Level studies'. These kind of remarks call into question the validity of the examination results.

The results of tests are never 100% reliable. On an individual level that can make a difference in terms of career options open to a school leaver when considering O or A levels. For this reason the judgement of teachers is often sought as supportive evidence for entry into post secondary school education. The more reliable the results of such tests are the less disappointment

Diagram 4.5.1
Subdivision of tests

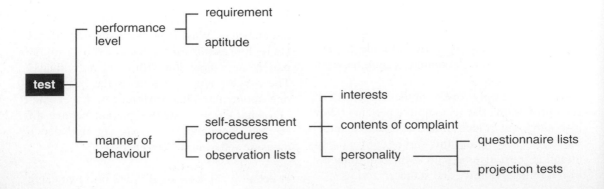

there is for individual people in terms of gaining post-school courses and having the ability to succeed in such courses.

Examinations for professions, including nursing, are also requirement tests. Demands such as reliability, validity and standardization must therefore be properly made on these examinations as well.

The second type of test for level of performance is the *aptitude test*. With an aptitude test we ask what performance someone must be considered capable of. The person examined does not have to demonstrate achievement now. It is a matter of predicting whether the person examined is capable, possibly after a learning period, of carrying out the task. Intelligence tests are well known examples of aptitude tests. Since intelligence tests are widely used, we shall go into these tests further. The concept of intelligence has been considered in Chapter 3, Section 2a.

At present the IQ is no longer determined by dividing development age by calendar age. There are other (difficult and less difficult) statistical techniques in use. The essence of these is reported below.

If one presents an intelligence test to a relatively large number of persons, chosen at random, it then turns out that the resultant IQs are distributed in a bell shape (diagram 4.5.2). This bell shaped curve is called the normal distribution. A well selected (that is: composed in a random manner) sample of the British population is a large group of such persons. If the sample is well (i.e. randomly) made, one can assume that the bell shape found also applies for the distribution of IQs over the British population in its entirety. This means that 50% of British people have an IQ lower than 100 and 50% an IQ higher than 100. Or, as can be seen from diagram 4.5.2, that about 16% of them have an IQ of 85 or lower. Since the normal distribution is symmetrical, this means that 16% also have an IQ of 115 or higher. We can also see from the diagram that 2.2% of the British population have an IQ of 130 or higher. And this means again that 13.8% have an IQ that lies between the limits of 115 and 130.

Study activity

6. **a.** Explain why the average intelligence quotient of the British population is 100.
b. Is the average intelligence quotient of the American population also 100? Why, or why not?

Tests for types of behaviour

We have examined tests for levels of performance. We now have a look at some of the tests for the assessment of behaviour. In this type of test, we have to elicit a person's *usual* manner or mode of behaviour. We have to try to find

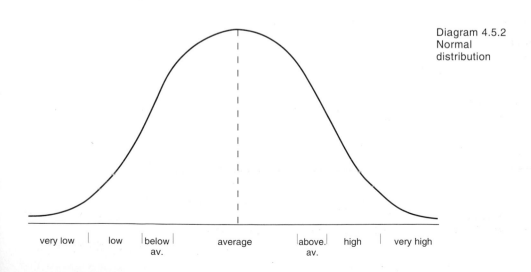

Diagram 4.5.2
Normal
distribution

| very low | low | below av. | average | above. av. | high | very high |

out how he will *tend* to do something, in what manner he usually reacts.

We also divide this group of tests into two sub-groups. This happens according to the manner in which the test data is collected: does the patient himself answer a number of questions about his own functioning or does someone else give a judgement about them? In other words: the tests assessing behaviour are divided into 'self-assessment procedures' and 'observation lists'. An example of an item which occurs in a self-assessment list is: 'I have had more than my share of all kinds of trouble.' An example of an item that occurs in an observation list is: 'Has a nap after a hot meal.'

Self-assessment procedures, in contrast to observation lists, are widely used in medical psychology.

Self-assessment procedures

We distinguish three types of self-assessment procedures. We distinguish self-assessment procedures with which information is gained according to whether they yield information on:
− interests;
− types of complaints;
− the personality.

Tests directed at *interests* are widely used in school and professional selection. These questions are often used by psychologists who work in rehabilitation centres. The psychologist will, for example, give advice based on the results of these tests on choice of occupation to the victim of a traffic accident who can no longer practise his profession. Making use of an interest questionnaire, the psychologist will advise the patient about the suitability of different careers. A *complaints* list is used if one wishes to enumerate the type of complaints which the patient has and has not got. To what extent does the patient complain of anxiety, pain or misery, or of vague physical complaints? The tester could obtain this information orally but making use of a complaints list has a number of advantages. In the first place it is systematic: all important complaint patterns are listed. Further the complaining can be given in measurement and number. The patient complains in the conversation about 'anxiety'. Making use of the complaints

list you know that the patient concerned belongs to the 4% of most anxious British people, because a normal distribution applies for anxiety too. Further, by recording the list for a second time after completion of the treatment, one can determine to what extent the treatment really has helped.

Study activity
   7. Try to think of other tests which could be of value carried out before and after treatment.

The third group from the category 'self-assessment procedures' concerns procedures aimed at the determination of *personality qualities*. Together with the intelligence tests the personality tests have for decades determined the 'public image' of test psychology.

A differentiation is made between two sorts of personality tests: the projective personality test and the personality questionnaire.

Projective tests address our imagination. A picture sheet of the Rorschach test, the best known or so-called 'inkspot test', is put before the patient with the question: 'What do you see in it? What does it make you think of?' The patient is encouraged to think associatively, helped in this by a number of blots of various shapes.

Another projective test, the Thematic Apperception Test (TAT) uses picture sheets on which an incident is depicted. The patient is asked to state what, in his opinion, is going on in the picture, how it happened and what will happen next. Here too the patient is thus enticed to give his own interpretation.

A third, widely used test in this framework is the so-called 'sentence completion test'. The patient must complete an unfinished sentence. Thus: 'My father ...', 'Women ...', 'The future ...', 'When I was at school ...'.

The underlying idea in projective techniques is a very obvious one. If you want to get to know someone, you give him 'meaningless' or incomplete material and you let him freely make associations with it. What he provides is not dependent on the material (that may be meaningless), but almost completely on the person who gives it the associations. The associations are thus certainly valid: they refer directly to the person making them. But the meaning of the associations raises a problem. The associations must also be able to be interpreted. In the interpretations the particular characteristics of the psychologist may be recognizable. That is not the intention. It is a question of the patient, not the psychologist.

In short, the reliability of the interpretation forms a serious problem for projective techniques.

Study activity

8. Why with projective techniques is the reliability in question rather than the validity?

The designers of *personality questionnaires* are of the opinion that they have solved this problem better than the designers of projective tests. A personality questionnaire is, in essence, a collection of questions with which the person gives his reactions in certain situations. Examples of some of these situations are: 'For every difficulty only one solution is the best', 'I sometimes get the feeling that I am a burden to others' and 'I like working quickly'. The answer that the person being questioned can give is limited to: 'correct', 'incorrect' and (in some lists) '?'. By precoding the answers in this manner the list can be scored easily and quickly.

In this a computer is often used to give a number of scores. The result of the scores determines the interpretation that must be given to the test. The scope that the psychologist has in interpreting the test scores is therefore considerably less than in projective techniques.

Most personality tests measure a number of qualities at the same time. One such test is the Minnesota Multiphasic Personality Inventory (MMPI) which has been developed to enable the diagnosis of particular psychiatric categories. The clusters of responses characterize the individual in terms of an index of vulnerability to a particular disorder. This test offers ten subscales which are: hypochondriasis, depression, hysteria, psychopathy, masculinity-femininity,

paranoia, psychaesthenia, schizophrenia, hypomania, and social introversion.

Whether the answer that the person gives to the question is true is (strangely enough) not so important. It is thus of no importance whether someone who answers the question 'I like working quickly' with 'correct' does in fact like to work quickly. What is of importance is: which of the three responses ('correct', 'incorrect' or '?') he gives to the stimulus 'I like working quickly.' This strange state of affairs will perhaps become clear with the following example. Assume that it turns out that as a rule very neurotic people answer the question 'Are you neurotic?' with 'incorrect.' Then in the testers' instructions it will be stated: reacting with 'incorrect' to the question 'Are you neurotic?' is indicative of a neurotic form of adjustment.

The MMPI is not quite as robust as an IQ test, so it does not give an average score for the population, but instead sufficient data has been collected to provide personality descriptions of people with different patterns of high and low scores on the various scales. Other personality inventories exist which score on different scales and for which an average score for the British population is known. One such test is the Maudsley Medical Questionnaire (MMQ) (Eysenck, 1958) which measures on the dimension of normal to neurotic. The results of such tests are however not indicative of a situation. As we said earlier for the MMPI, they provide an indication which a psychologist can use in reaching a diagnosis.

In the clinical situation it is necessary to compare the score from one patient with the average score from a population at large to enable an interpretation of the data to be made.

The group with which the individual score is compared is called the norm group. The score of the patient can then be compared with various norm groups: a random sample from the British population, a random sample from a group of psychiatric patients, a random sample from the practice of a number of family GPs and so forth.

A person's score on its own in a questionnaire has little meaning. The patient's score is therefore compared with the scores of what is called a norm group. This norm group can consist of a sample from the whole population. Use is often made of norm groups which consist of people who are in a similar situation to the patient. The raw scores of the norm group are divided into a number of categories. This can be done in various ways.

Two examples

The first example is from a (non-existent) test in which the division is into a number of classes. This test measures for example anxiety about injections. If a patient gets a score of 15, this means according to diagram 4.5.3 that in comparison with the norm group he is not very afraid of injections; in fact his score is low.

In the second (also non-existent) test the division is into decile scores (diagram 4.5.4). In decile scores the group is divided into ten equal groups, into each of which 10% of the people from the norm group fall. This test measures for example aggression. If a patient gets a score of 32, he comes into decile 9. This means that 80% of the people from the norm group get a lower score. This patient is therefore aggressive in comparison with the norm group.

Observation tests

The group of tests for types of behaviour consists of self-assessment tests and observation tests. In observation tests it is not a matter of an assessment, via introspection, which the person concerned gives about his own behaviour.

decile	score
10	37–
9	32–36
8	29–31
7	27–28
6	25–26
5	23–24
4	21–22
3	18–20
2	13–17
1	–12

Diagram 4.5.4
Division into decile score

Another person, the observer, reports on the behaviour of the person concerned, and in this he makes use of the observation method.

Observation tests occur in many forms: the journal that is handed over on changing duty is a form of observation test. The notes are then the scores, not very reliable perhaps, but mostly valid. Earlier in this section (page 353) a number of observations were mentioned: the recording of body temperature and the Glasgow Coma Scale.

As is the case with other tests, observation tests may also vary greatly in standardization. Whilst the already mentioned 'journal' is not a very standardized form, the Glasgow Coma Scale is highly standardized. In general it may be postulated that tests whose score is made via the observation method should achieve considerably better results than those whose score is based on self-assessment. By 'better' we mean more reliable and more valid. Observation methods are, however, much less usable. By 'usable' we mean that they are less easy to record. An observation list is filled in by a nurse, by a physiotherapist or someone in this sort of role. These people must make time available for observation tests and they must see the sense of them.

All in all, self-assessment tests are used much more than observation tests.

b. The neuropsychological examination

Neuropsychology is a subdivision of medical psychology. It deals with the cerebral organ-

Diagram 4.5.3
Division into classes

	Score
very high	40+
high	35–39
above average	30–34
average	23–29
below average	18–22
low	13–17
very low	0–12

ization of behaviour. This means that it is directed at the influence which the brain, as an organ, has on behaviour. In the neuropsychological examination the clinical psychologist focuses on defects of the brain itself. For example: when a person's brain is damaged in a traffic accident, how does this damage express itself in his use of language and so forth? Similarly, an assessment of the extent to which a person's behaviour is caused by dementia or other causes belongs in the field of neuropsychology.

In Section 6.a we divided tests into those which measure level of performance and those which measure ways of behaviour. In the investigation for defects in the brain no use is made of other sorts of tests apart from those already listed. In a neuropsychological examination the same tests we have mentioned can be used to measure the level of performance and the ways of behaving.

The difference is that in this kind of examination the kinds of question that are asked are different. Rather than questions which have to do with (presumed) disturbances which are of a neurological type, neuropsychological questions are mostly concerned with intelligence (a deterioration of intelligence), consciousness, speech, memory and so forth.

Case study: Mrs Banks

Mrs Banks is in bed at the Neurology department suffering from a herpes simplex virus. This virus seldom occurs in the brain, but if it does occur there various brain functions can be seriously disturbed. Thus the affected person is uninhibited, both verbally and in motor function. Mrs Banks curses the department roundly, sometimes pulls nursing staff by the hair and has to be strictly controlled. Although the cause is not strictly psychological, it is decided to place her in the psychiatric unit, in the hope that her behaviour can be more easily controlled there.

Figure 4.5.4
Example of becoming
demented: the patient is
in conversation with his reflection

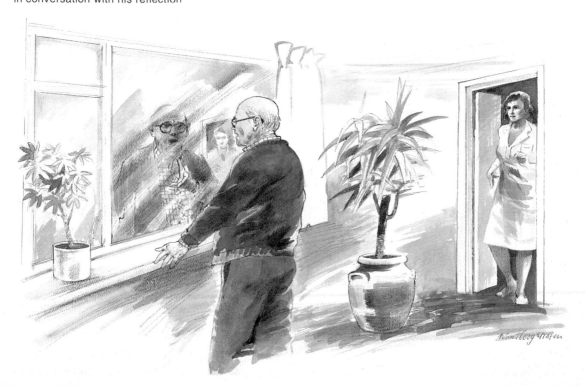

The cerebral organization of Mrs Banks's behaviour has become disturbed by a virus. She can be examined neuropsychologically in order to establish the type of behaviour disturbance. Is thinking disturbed? Is her observation still intact? and so forth. Assuming that with Mrs Banks the virus is properly under control or perhaps has completely run its course, that does not then mean that the behaviour disturbances will no longer occur. The virus may have permanently affected the brain in certain parts. Damaged muscles recover, a broken bone (often) heals completely, but as an organ, the brain's nerve tissue cannot recover from injuries. In this case the concept 'compensation' is of importance. This means that the parts of the brain are capable of taking over each other's functions. Thus a healthy part of the brain can take over from an affected part. We then speak of compensation.

Back to Mrs Banks. Her behaviour disturbances do not disappear when the virus has run its course. Compensation normally occurs only partly spontaneously, in the 'spontaneous recovery period', which on average lasts two months or so. This is termed plasticity of the nervous system. Some brain functions, however, cannot be compensated. Furthermore, compensation is dependent on the training that one undergoes. For that very reason the neuropsychological examination is of importance here. Training is dependent on learning capacity which in its turn is dependent on various mental functions, such as intelligence, memory, concentration and so forth. It is therefore important for the trainer to know which functions of the patient are affected and which can be properly addressed. With a neuropsychological examination one can thus make a statement about the state of affairs of the various psychological functions and the extent to which these are trainable in Mrs Banks's case.

Case study: Mr Thomas

Mr Thomas is 72. He has been admitted to hospital after a fall in which he broke a leg. During admission it becomes clear that now and again he is in a confused state when he does not really know where he is. In such periods he has also at times been known to look for his wife. She died ten years ago. His daughter says that this also happened now and again at home, but the frequency of these 'fits' now appears to be increasing. Mr Thomas is still living independently.

Is it a question of an incipient onset of dementia in Mr Thomas or is he sometimes confused because of, for example, anxiety about the hospital? The difference is of importance for the type of support Mr Thomas needs. This question is the start of a neuropsychological examination, which is used in order to bring about a differential diagnosis. A statement must be made about two different possibilities. Are the complaints the result of the influence of stressors i.e. the hospital as a strange environment, (see Moos's model), or is the brain no longer functioning optimally? In the latter case the complaints are 'organic' in origin, and it is a matter of deterioration of mental functions, that is to say of dementia. Suppose that the neuropsychological examination gives a diagnosis of dementia. In that case a subsequent line of questioning is important to find out how quickly this onset of increasing dementia is progressing. A statement about this can sometimes be made through comparing the test results obtained at two successive periods. Another possibility is the comparison of the test results with a reasonable estimate of the previous level of functioning. The latter is called the pre-morbid level. Thus you can to some extent estimate the pre-morbid intelligence level by taking into account someone's education and possibly his profession. Suppose that Mr Thomas, in his youth, completed an academic education and subsequently worked as a physicist. If the test examination now has as a result an IQ of 82, we can reasonably assume that the pre-morbid level of intelligence was considerably higher. As has already been said, it is important for the further support to know whether it is a matter of incipient dementia or not, and one should preferably know something also about the speed of the process. Whether Mr Thomas can go back to his independent home or remain in care are very important matters.

From the above two examples the impression could arise that only processes of increasing dementia and rare viruses are the subject of neuropsychological examination. This is not so. One can make use of this sort of examination in various fields of somatic health care. Think for example of the measurement of residual phenomena in a brain trauma after a traffic accident.

For the patient himself it is often of great importance to know where the boundary lies between actually no longer being able and his own lack of confidence. In one and the same example the extent to which the residual phenomena occur can be the determining factor for the (im)possibility of resumption of work. Another well known example presents itself with Korsakow's syndrome, an organic brain syndrome that can occur when someone consumes excessive alcohol for a long time. As with the previously mentioned herpes virus, it is necessary in this situation to get an insight into the extent to which mental functions are impaired. In addition it is also of importance to make an estimate of the trainability of these functions.

In the above examples various items are mentioned which can be the subject of a neuropsychological examination:
- the level of the different mental functions;
- the level of the 'residual' functions, in conjunction with their trainability;
- the rate of deterioration of the functions in conjunction with the assessment of self-reliance;
- differential diagnosis: is the deterioration due to a failing stress management or is there an organic cause?

A neuropsychological examination can sometimes also give an indication of the location of the brain injury. We mean by this the area of the brain where any neurological irregularity may be present. Certain mental functions are located in certain parts of the brain. Thus a disturbance in the area of speech, if this has to do with a brain injury, indicates damage in the left hemisphere. The Russian psychologist Luria has done a very great deal of research in this field. In the framework of this book, however, it would take too long to elaborate these location theories further.

Study activity
9. With the neuropsychological task, 'type', the person concerned must depress a button as often as possible in a certain time. Mr Stevens always carries out this task 'type' more slowly with the right hand than with the left hand. You do not expect that, as Mr Stevens is right-handed. If you assume that this difference between the performances of the left and the right hand has to do with a brain injury, in which hemisphere do you expect to locate this injury?

7. Summary

For the clinical psychologist the observation of behaviour forms is the basis for treatment.
The observations are carried out in order to be able to determine the diagnosis.
The psychologist aims to rid the observation of the chance factor, the incidental. Therefore psychologists use tests, examinations and other methods which can support them in objectivizing the behaviour of the client. Questionnaires and psychological tests are examples of such aids.
Obviously such measuring instruments must satisfy criteria in respect of:
- reliability;
- validity;
- standardization.

6 Psychological treatment and support

1. Introduction

This chapter will concentrate on those psychological treatments and the performing of support activities which will be found in all nursing settings. Several widely applied psychological treatment techniques are therefore mentioned, with special consideration being given to new treatment techniques which are attracting considerable attention.

The techniques covered here are those which are short term. Long term psychological treatments usually require the specialist support of a psychiatric department.

What must be understood by 'long-term' is a point of discussion. Some clinical psychologists feel that a treatment which lasts a year, with a treatment frequency of one session per day, is a short-term one. We take as a starting point that a treatment is called short if it does not last longer than a few months, with a frequency of one to two sessions per week being maintained. In many cases the duration of therapy may of course be much shorter than this. A section about support for the patient concludes this chapter.

Learning outcomes

After studying this chapter the student should be able to:
- express the differences between treatment and support and give two examples of each;
- explain what is meant by psychoeducation and name a few examples;
- describe the concept, execution and effects of the following treatments:
  - stress management
  - cognitive influencing
  - operant treatment
  - eclectic treatment
- express what is understood by support utilizing the following approaches:
  - the humanistic approach;
  - the cognitive-behavioural approach.

2. Psychological treatment and support

Study activity
  1. **a.** Try to describe when you as a nurse want to involve the psychologist in the therapy.
  b. In general terms, what criteria can you use for this?

We speak of *psychological treatment* when an attempt is made in a professional manner to alter undesirable behaviour. It has already been stated that by 'behaviour' we are to understand, besides motor activities, also experiences, emotions, thought processes and so forth. Thus the changing of negative feelings e.g. melancholy, anxiety also belongs to the package of psychological treatments. The clinical psychologist initiates treatment when the complaints are caused by mental or social factors or when these play an important part in the maintenance of the complaints. In the psychodiagnostic phase, which naturally precedes the treatment, it has become clear that such factors are significant.

We give *support* to the patient to help him handle the worries of a treatment, an illness, or the consequences of illness and treatment as well as possible. The patient learns to deal with his condition in a manner which does not view it as an insuperable obstacle. Support takes place with medical intervention (for example operations), with serious illnesses (for example cancer, AIDS), and with illnesses and medical treatments which have psychological or social consequences (for example amputations).The term *supportive therapy* is often used to describe such interventions.

The difference between psychological treatment (aim: cure) and support (aim: alleviation) is made clear by means of a number of examples.

Examples of treatment

– *Tension headache*
With the occurrence and maintenance of tension headache, the manner in which one deals with stressful situations plays an important part. The treatment is aimed at teaching patients to deal with stress in an alternative way to the development of headache. In the first instance the

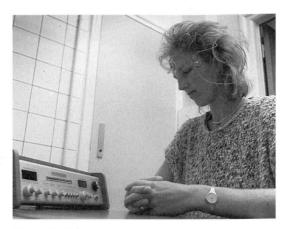

Figure 4.6.1
Learning to relax,
making use of the
bio-feedback technique

patient gets practice in relaxation. Secondly he learns to recognize the situations in which he becomes tense. Thirdly he learns to apply the acquired relaxation technique in tension-provoking situations. Sometimes relaxing in such a situation is not the best solution to the problem. In such cases the patient is taught another form of behaviour rather than the development of tension headache as a reaction to the stressor. This may be assertive behaviour, but also (more generally) the patient can be taught to behave in a more socially acceptable manner. In this way fewer situations will lead to tension and a reduction of the headache is the result.

– *Lower back pain*
Patients with lower back pain for which no physical cause exists are often caught in a vicious circle. Because of the pain these patients avoid all kinds of pain-causing situations, as a result of which they become more and more passive. Reduced activity leads to stiffness, and thus to more pain in movement. The result is that the patient will carry out still fewer activities: he will go and lie down more and more often, rest a great deal and use more painkillers. Because he is less active, he becomes more and more socially isolated and often the only contact with other people comes via the complaints of pain. People in this scenario react in two ways to pain: by worrying or by being aggressive. Neither reaction helps the patient, so it appears that in

both cases the pain increases. One way of treating these patients is to help them learn step by step, little by little, to become more active. It is also important that the family, the immediate environment, learns to handle the patient differently. We shall come back to this approach at length in Section 4.c.

– *Type A behaviour in cardio-vascular diseases*

Type A behaviour appears to be closely connected with an increased chance of cardio-vascular diseases. Patients with type A behaviour are continually active, feel attracted to competition and challenges, and their work is often their only source of satisfaction. The treatment of these people is directed at a change of life style and of reaction in worrying situations.

The patient learns to recognize worrying situations and learns to relax in these situations. He learns a calmer and more relaxed life style. This reduces the chance of cardio-vascular diseases.

Examples of support

– *Support for cancer patients*

The support is aimed at helping the patient and his family in dealing with the feelings that arise through the idea that one has a threatening disease. It concerns the handling of feelings of uncertainty about how the disease will develop. It concerns dealing with understandable feelings such as melancholy. But in the support you also have to deal with perhaps more open feelings such as anger. The family can also be involved in this kind of support process. This support is, besides the support of a fellow human being in need, also of great importance in another sense. It has a strong preventive effect on the development in the affected person of 'vague' complaint patterns which are not understood. The technique of this form of support is, in essence, effective listening to the patient. This means that you have time for the patient and his family, that you pay attention to his story, accept that the story if necessary is told ten times and that you do not find the story stupid or boring.

In Module 5 we study this technique comprehensively.

– *Support for patients with a chronic, somatic affection*

If we take as an example the support of a patient with multiple sclerosis, the following points are relevant.

1. The diagnosis. Often a long period of uncertainty elapses before the diagnosis is made. The fact that the diagnosis is made on the one hand means certainty, but on the other hand it gives rise to questions.
2. No longer 'being able to join in' with others while, especially in the initial stage, to the external world one is not ill.
3. The uncertainty about the future: how will the illness influence functioning? How quickly does the decline go?
4. Learning to accept increasing dependence on others, one's own aggression (with regard to the disease, the partner, the external world) and the changed body-image.

3. Psychoeducation

The critical reader may already have remarked that a sharp distinction between psychological treatment and support cannot be made. When is behaviour, which is essentially undesirable, altered? Why is support not treatment? Are the feelings about the condition more bearable, as a result of the support? Have these feelings in fact changed?

Between treatment on the one hand and support on the other there is a form of influencing the behaviour which is called 'psychoeducation'. Psychoeducation can be orientated to the individual, directed to the one patient. The explaining of the results of a psychodiagnostic test, to the patient is an example. The explanation of the results of such an examination influences the patient's thinking about and the experiencing of the affection. This affection was the reason for the psychological examination. It is sometimes incorrectly assumed that the discussion of the result of such an examination is a 'neutral' event for the patient. But if a patient (with for example chronic lower back pain) gets the result: 'Some psychosocial factors help to determine your experience of pain' (and if it is explained which factors these are and why they help to determine the experience of pain), the behaviour of the patient really is influenced.

Study activity
2. Give two more examples of psychoeducation.

Psychoeducation can also take place more generally. The provision of information about the affection can for example be understood as a form of psychoeducation. An example of the explanation programme is the back school. Back schools are information programmes intended for people with back pain. These back schools have best results in people who, in the psychosocial sense, are not too greatly handicapped by their pain.
By that it is meant that:
- they can meet their daily family obligations (they bear the usual responsibilities);
- they have a work cycle away from home; they perform a full day's work (perhaps with slightly longer periods of illness than non-back patients);
- the motor system in general is not disturbed;
- they complain of (sometimes violent) pain, for which the doctor has not been able to find a completely satisfactory explanation.

For a programme of instruction to warrant the term 'back school', it needs to offer the following types of activities:
- an explanation of the anatomical construction of the back, with the aim of being able to determine where the pain comes from;
- the learning of a number of exercises which strengthen the back muscles;
- the learning of postures in which one can carry out some frequently occurring daily tasks in a back-saving way (for example in housework);
- relaxation therapy, which is aimed at the effective learning of relaxation of the back muscles;
- explanation of 'What is pain?' and in this framework the discussion of the question 'How can it be the case that psychological

factors influence the experience of pain positively, but also negatively?'

In the last activity the course participants get the opportunity to discuss to what extent psychological factors have a negative influence on the experiencing of pain in themselves (and on what can be done about it). A programme like this may last for eight meetings of two and a half hours each. The results show that such back schools achieve the desired effect to a considerable extent.
For example:
- the somatic fixation (i.e. the obsessive idea that they are suffering from a serious physical condition) decreases;
- the depressed feelings decrease;
- the idea that one can do something to reduce the pain oneself becomes stronger;
- the seriousness of experiencing pain decreases;
- in more general terms, the negative influence of the pain on daily life decreases;
- the course participant seeks less support from his social environment (household, family) and the environment responds by acting less apprehensively.

Other examples of this sort of generally orientated, psychoeducative programmes are the sleep course and the headache course. Both courses are worth considering. Furthermore consideration can be given to meetings like those of the 'Weight Watchers'.

Study activity
3. Try to state whether a difference exists between explanation (to patients by nurses) and psychoeducation. Explain your answer.

4. Approaches to treatment

In this section four kinds of treatment for patients with physical complaints are discussed: stress management, cognitive treatment, operant treatment and an eclectic treatment. By an eclectic treatment we mean 'the application of different treatment techniques after each other without a clear theoretical connection existing between these techniques'.

a. Stress management

Stress management can be applied in all those situations where tension plays an important part with for instance headache, spastic colon, hyperventilation, attacks of anxiety and panic and when undergoing a (threatening) operation. With affections such as cancer, AIDS and suchlike illnesses it can also be useful for the patient to learn to deal differently with his tensions.

As the term 'stress management' implies, this treatment has to do with dealing with stressors and their resultant stress. A stressor is a stimulus or a situation which brings about stress. The strength of the stress response is partly determined by two cognitive processes: evaluation of the situation and evaluation of one's own possibilities of doing something positive about the situation. An example of the first process is the following.

Figure 4.6.2
A sleep course??

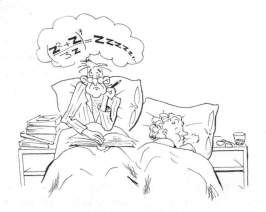

YOU CAN LEARN HOW TO SLEEP

SLEEPCOURSE

with information about f.i.:

> tv. braodcasting
> radio braodcasting
> the courseware
> audio-video cassettes

Two people are in an accident and both as a result have a broken legs. One thinks, 'This is a hopeless situation, I'll never manage to walk again.' He becomes depressed, has no longer any interest in, and therefore hardly cooperates with the treatment. The other thinks, 'I'll just show them, I'm going to surprise them all.' This person is optimistic and works hard to cooperate in his recovery.

The second process is the evaluation of one's own possibilities of doing something about the stress. Someone who thinks that he cannot do anything to change the stressor will withdraw, avoid the stressor and bottle up the tension. This tension can then lead to physical complaints.

In their clinical practice nurses have to deal with many stress-causing situations. We shall go more deeply into one of them: the preparation for surgical treatment.

That stress management in the preparation for operative interventions leads to good results was shown by Hayward (1975).

A group of patients in the pre-operative stage was told what they could expect of the post-operative situation. This group of patients was taught during the pre-operative phase how to relax and how they could best move with the surgical wound, by for example, going and lying down without making use of the stomach muscles if their operation was in the abdominal region. Further they were informed about the procedure of the operation, and also told what experiences (even unpleasant) could occur in this, such as the swallowing of a stomach tube. The patients were thus informed on a procedural and sensory level. The results showed that the 'informed' group of patients needed less pain medication post-operatively and were able to be discharged considerably earlier than a comparable group of patients who were not 'informed'.

From this it can be seen that 'telling a patient what he has to expect' is not just a correct 'bedside manner', but that it also has a demonstrably positive effect on post-operative progress.

The result of Hayward's investigation supported earlier work and is included as one of a large number of other investigations into this phenomenon. The present view on this matter is summarized by Suls and Wan (1989) as follows:

- the provision of information, *only* about the procedure of the intervention in question hardly influences post-operative progress;
- the same thing applies for information *only* about the feelings that will be experienced during the intervention;
- what is effective and clinically relevant is information about procedure *and* (unpleasant) feelings.

What therefore appears to be effective is the combination of procedural and sensory information.

Suls and Wan conclude that information about the procedure gives the patient a general idea of what is to be expected by him and that information about the (unpleasant) feelings enables the patient to contextualize and interpret these experiences as 'not threatening'.

By the giving of information, we certainly do not mean the relatively uninterested giving out of an explanatory pamphlet. Giving information means discussing with the patient with attention and with due consideration, the procedures and the experiences. The patient is thereby given the opportunity to put his questions freely and quite calmly.

This technique is also discussed in Module 5.

Study activity
  4. Design an information programme for the patient who has to undergo an abdominal resection, based on the principles described in the text.

Sometimes the reason for the fact that one patient has much more difficulty with post-operative progress than another is given as: 'Some people are worriers and some don't worry at all.' Translated into psychological terms, this means that the personality plays a recognizable part. In relation to this type of investigation, as far as personality is concerned, a differentiation is made between two sorts of personality: 'sensitizers' and 'repressors' (see also pages 301-2). By sensitizers we mean the patients who insist on hearing all that is going to happen. By repressors we mean the patients who say: 'Just don't tell me anything. I'll notice it soon enough when it happens.'

Repressors act just as if there were nothing wrong, they deny anxiety and make light of the operative intervention in hand. They deny anxiety.

The literature on this subject shows that to gain the best results the information provider, such as the doctor and the nurse, should relate to the personal style of the patient. With a sensitizer, carrying out an unpleasant, painful operation without previously providing information is asking for difficulties afterwards. The same applies for giving comprehensive information about the pending intervention, in advance, to the repressor. The repressor must only be told what is absolutely necessary beforehand; the sensitizer must be comprehensively informed beforehand. In clinical practice, however, an annoying 'complication' occurs: every patient is indeed a bit of a sensitizer and a bit of a repressor. It is important for the nurse to listen carefully to the patient and go into how he actually deals with stressors, before deciding how information is given.

Study activity
  5. Can one speak of repressors and sensitizers among students also? If so, what consequences would that have to have for support for students in the practical situation?

b. Cognitive treatment

A cognitive treatment is aimed at the thought content and at the style of thinking of the patient (see also page 42). By the thought content, we mean for example the depressed thoughts of someone who is sad, maybe thinking, 'I am worthless.' By style of thinking what is meant is that when this person is faced with anything at all, the style of thought which always comes to the fore is, 'Just look, I am worthless.' A more than usually cheerful woman can be depressed: her thought content is then depressed, but her style of thinking is not. With somatizing patients too a differentiation can be made between thought content and style of thinking. A somatizing patient with this negative style of thinking faced with a setback, literally feels the disappointment physically and the thought, 'Just look, my back, there really *is* something wrong with it' comes to the fore (style of thinking). Yet this patient can, from time to time, feel physically very good (thought content).

Many patients with tension or functional complaints (see also Chapter 4 of this module) are affected with a somatizing style of thinking. They are solemnly convinced of the fact that a physical cause for their complaints exists. The style of thinking, entailing that there is something fundamentally wrong with the body, is called 'illness conviction'. Such patients may be advised that no physical cause has been found for their complaints. Sometimes they may also be told that their complaints are psychological.

Study activity

6. Why, in this context, is the statement 'Your complaints are psychological' incorrect?

The positive conviction that one is physically ill can seriously stand in the way of a non-somatically directed treatment. This conviction will, if a psychological treatment is necessary, first have to be 'challenged'. A psychoeducative procedure can be the beginning of the treatment of the patient with the conviction that he is physically ill. He is given an explanation about how physical complaints arise and how it may be the case that these complaints remain in existence in spite of the fact that there is no longer any physical cause present. The person who is treating him explains that other factors also influence the complaints and that this does not mean that the complaints are not genuine. The patient may feel ill, miserable and exhausted, but what he is experiencing is not based on physical factors. The miserable feeling has not changed but the the explanation may lead to a different attitude. The SORC diagram can be used with this explanation.

Sometimes being given this information is sufficient for the patient to deal with his complaints

in another way, to be able to live with them. Sometimes the changing of the conviction that one is physically ill has in itself little effect on the complaints. It is a first attempt to set the patient on the track of a different kind of approach to his complaints.

In cases where the psychoeducative approach does not have the desired effect, it may be necessary to carry out a treatment directed at the thought content and the style of thinking. Together with the patient the person treating him analyzes precisely what the patient thinks about his complaints, what he (as it were) says to himself about them. Often these are negative thoughts, which only make him more ill, depressed or tense. During the treatment the patient learns to say in each phase different, more positive things to himself. These so-called self-instructions help him to remain calmer, become less tense and finally to have fewer complaints. This form of treatment was introduced in Chapter 4.

Case study: Mrs Peterson

Mrs Peterson has for years been troubled by headaches. She has a headache especially when her mother-in-law is staying with her. Together with the person treating her she writes down on paper the thoughts which successively go through her head. After that they consider together what she can say to herself instead of the unpleasant, self-destructive thoughts (see the diagram on page 372).

Mrs Peterson and her mother-in-law

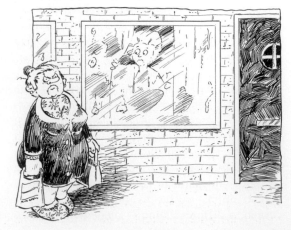

At first it will be strange for the patient consciously to think of something different in the different situations. 'I can't sit here like an idiot, come on!' or some-such retort is what the person treating him gets thrown back at her. Then the patient has to be re-convinced that the method *will* help, *if he sticks with it*. He will have to be told to correct his thinking in those terms. It is important that the patient gets a lot of practice in the application of positive self-instructions. The positive thoughts then overcome the negative ones. The positive thoughts then become a habit, and the positive effect is clear.

Study activity
  7. **a.** Work out an example of cognitive treatment with a patient who considers himself far too fat.
  b. Think of four other possible applications of cognitive treatment.

c.   Operant treatment

Operant treatment is suitable for chronic pain conditions where no physical explanation for this pain is found. Operant treatment is *not* suitable as the first option in the treatment of acute pain, although it may be used as an adjunct to other therapies.

This section deals with the operant treatment of chronic lower back pain. In the discussion of the back school it was stated that the back school is suitable for people who complain about back pain, but who are not or are hardly handicapped by this pain: they lead an almost normal life. They are troubled by their back, nothing more. Operant treatment is especially suitable for back pain patients who are handicapped because of their pain, sometimes very handicapped. These patients lie in bed, can only move in a wheelchair and so forth. The motor system is disturbed, sometimes seriously while there is no – or almost no – physical explanation.
Operant treatment was introduced in Chapter 4, Section 4 (systematic reinforcement), and has been refered to at other points in the text. In this section we go into this style of treatment in more detail: firstly, because this manner of treatment requires a style of nursing which does not conform to the usual one, and secondly because we

expect that this manner of treatment will be applied more and more for other 'unexplained' conditions also.

The operant style of treatment originates from the behavioural approach in psychology. Suffering pain, it should be repeated, is considered in the behavioural approach as a form of behaviour. Experiencing pain is that sort of behaviour from which an outsider, for example a doctor, deduces that pain is suffered.

The operant treatment of chronic pain was developed by Fordyce (1976). The treatment firstly concerns behaviour from which an observer deduces that it is caused by pain. Secondly it is aimed at behaviour that can be understood as learnt. This last aspect is essential though it should be noted that not every form of chronic pain which cannot be explained from a somatic standpoint can be treated in the operant manner.
During the psychodiagnostic phase attention is paid particularly to two aspects, since in the operant manner pain has, on the behavioural level, two striking characteristics. The first characteristic is called 'the avoidance aspect' and the second 'the learning moment'.

The avoidance aspect
The avoidance aspect itself has two characteristics. The first entails that the patient has learnt to avoid certain physical activities and/or certain physical postures. This learning process has taken place because the patient has the authentic experience that the activity avoided, if carried out, causes pain. The patient behaves passively and the gain which he intends to secure, on the basis of this behaviour, is being safeguarded from pain. The resultant picture is that of a passive, complaining patient, possibly with a compensatory physical posture.

A sad result of passivity and compensation is the 'disuse' syndrome with among other things the occurrence of 'secondary nociception'. By this we mean that the patient's sincere attempts to break through his passivity or to correct his physical posture provide experiences that are painful. The experiences strengthen in him the

1. The preparation for the visit

What Mrs Peterson usually thinks:
- she's coming immediately on a visit
- I've done far too little in the house
- she won't find the house tidy
- she always sees something that is not right

Positive thoughts:
- my mother-in law is coming immediately
- let me just see what I can do
- I shall stay calm, I shall relax
- let's drink a cup of coffee together as friends
- I can see how things are going

2. The confrontation

What Mrs Peterson usually thinks:
- she is sitting looking all round – she will immediately make a critical remark
- I have certainly not done a good job
- I shall immediately get a headache again

Positive thoughts:
- try to stay relaxed
- give her a cup of coffee and ask how she is
- tell her she looks good
- think of the relaxation exercises: relax

3. Dealing with stress at critical moments (mother- in-law makes a remark about the dirty windows)

What Mrs Peterson usually thinks:
- just look, I never do this right
- she thinks I am not good enough for her son
- I should have washed the windows too

Positive thoughts:
- relax, don't let this upset you
- you don't need to do everything the way she wants it
- say in a normal tone of voice that you were too busy

4. The evaluation afterwards

What Mrs Peterson usually thinks:
- why does she always do that?
- I have a headache again
- if I don't have a headache it was a better-than-usual visit

Positive thoughts:
- I've done that well
- I stayed calm I didn't get worked up
- I can be very proud of this

idea that he has to limit himself to a passive life style.

The second characteristic of the avoidance aspect entails that the patient has obtained the experience that having pain also gives an 'advantage' in the psychosocial sense. For example: a sub-assertive, socially phobic housewife thinks that because of pain, being at home gives protection from the stifling, violent feelings of anxiety which she experiences in the street and in the supermarket. She feels pain and has the impression that the pain is the reason why she cannot go into the street any longer. The woman does not see through the fact that the pain remains present because the experience of pain is rewarded by the falling away of the anxiety which she feels when she is in the street. The mixing up of cause and effect is something at which we humans are very adept. It requires the eye of an experienced clinically observant outsider to give cause and effect their correct place in this behaviour sequence. It is only rarely that we can recognize such patterns in our own behaviour.

The learning moment
The second striking aspect is what is called the 'learning moment'. We speak of a learning moment if during the experience of pain an *external*, confirming (i.e. learning) factor occurs. The episode of pain begins for example from a somatic standpoint in an understandable manner; a traffic accident, a fall or whatever. Subsequently an external, confirming factor occurs, for example, a husband who shows himself very sorry for his wife, a type of behaviour which she (the patient) has not previously known from him. She has never before experienced the attentive care he now gives her. Pain thus provides her with a form of advantage, a sort of gain.

The avoidance aspect and the learning moment both provide an advantage to be gained from pain behaviour. The difference between them is that in the latter, an additional external factor makes the pain into an advanatage whereas the avoidance aspect is a conscious evasion of actions and situations within the somatic setting itself. The situation can escalate: the family doctor who despairs of ever curing the pain, unsuccessful operations after which the pain still persists, periods of pain of ten to twenty years and so forth. In this situation too the case is that the patient and her partner do not see through this behaviour pattern.

Two principles of learning theory
The treatment of chronic pain of this type is based on two principles of learning theory. The first is called 'extinction', and the second 'shaping'.

Extinction
By 'extinction' we mean that the pain behaviour is deprived of its effects. Pain behaviour as a type of behaviour is placed in a behavioural vacuum. It no longer has the usual effect on the environment. Pain behaviour no longer has the effect of relief of anxiety, consideration, the administration of medication or anything else. It only provides negation.

This apparently unmerciful method is very effective in making complaint behaviour decrease, and even stop.

Those who apply this method for the first time must be prepared for a specific characteristic of extinction. Ignored behaviour has the tendency in the first instance to occur to an increased extent, and only after that to decrease in frequency (see also page 39). The period of increased extent of pain behaviour lasts about two to three days. It is to be expected that after that the frequency of the behaviour to be extinguished will quickly decline.

Shaping
The second principle is 'shaping' (see also page 38). This entails that the patient is taught desirable behaviour (for example a form of activity) step by step, bit by bit. You do not give a completely immobilized patient the task of walking five hundred metres. Instead of that you say: 'To-day you will walk ten metres, tomorrow fifteen, the day after tomorrow twenty and so forth.'
In this way you prevent the patient, owing to the phenomenon of secondary nociception, from 'snapping' after seventy-five metres. This would confirm the patient in the idea that he has pain because of physical irregularities. It confirms the idea that he is now being treated in a completely incorrect manner. Raising the level of the activity step by step improves the condition of the patient slowly but unmistakably, with the result that the patient, for example after a week, can indeed walk five hundred metres. The realization that he can do much more than he himself suspected is a terrific boost for the patient.
An essential factor in this procedure is that the patient carries out the task exactly as instructed.

He must not do more than he is told, nor must he do less. Rest (reward) follows when the task is carried out. Therapeutic skill is necessary in order to correctly choose the degree of increase in the activity.

As an illustration of an operant treatment we shall discuss the results of the treatment of a forty-nine year old married woman who has had pain in the back for seven years. The pain made her a complete invalid. In somatic-medical parlance she has been 'treated to the limit'. From a medical standpoint the pain was and still is unexplained. From a learning theory point of view this is not the case. This lady was admitted to a general hospital for six weeks into a 're-habilitation bed'. Measurement was carried out before and after, and by a further follow-up measurement three months after discharge. We shall go into the progress of the treatment, by means of three important forms of activity. Two of them are in the field of physiotherapy: basic physiotherapy exercises and walking. The third form of activity is in the field of ergo-therapy.

First the two physiotherapy measures.

On admission the patient was capable of performing the basic exercises five times a day. After five times she had to stop owing to pain. Walking was completely impossible. We prescribed that the lady should have the activities increased gradually. After six weeks she performed the basic exercises twenty times a day, and she walked a thousand metres a day. In the follow-up, three months after discharge, the increase in activities was seen to have continued, although at a slower tempo.

The ergotherapy activity was concerned with working in the kitchen. On admission the lady kept it up for five minutes. Working in the kitchen was very important for her: cooking for the family has always been her hobby. She can now practise this hobby again. This gives her back a good deal of the joy of living. In the follow-up it was seen that she could now manage fifty minutes, and considering the family situation a longer time was not necessary.

Such operant treatment can take place if a number of conditions are satisfied. The treatment should take place clinically, or at least there is a strong preference for this. The influence of the patient's environment on the pain behaviour must be disconnected for some time. This can only happen in the clinic with staff who see the sense of such a therapeutic method and have the courage to persevere with it.

Study activity
  8. a. Explain why the person who is treating the patient needs to have courage to persevere with this approach.
  b. Would you as a nurse be suitable for carrying out an operant treatment?
  c. What qualities must those who treat the patients in this framework generally satisfy?

The treatment must also be carried out on a contract basis. This means that the patient is informed about the therapeutic measures including those of negation of the pain behaviour and that he declares himself in agreement with them. In this way those who are treating him point to the contract if the patient, despite the agreement, complains about pain. The treatment only succeeds if it takes place within a multi-disciplinary framework. That means that doctor, clinical psychologist, physiotherapist, ergotherapist and the nurse carry out the treatment together as a team from one standpoint.

This treatment has as its objective to break through the (learned) motor-disturbed, handicapped behaviour. If that is successful, it still does not mean that the patient is 'cured'. If the female patient in our example can walk a thousand metres and can prepare the meals again the treatment is still not completed. The pain may have been given the chance to become chronic owing to street phobia or lack of social skills or a disturbed partner relationship and so forth. That means that subsequently these aspects must be treated. The patient (and his partner) is highly motivated to do this after a successful treatment of the disturbed motor system. With the onset of the treatment the thought content and the style of thinking are likewise altered. 'I have a physical condition which only the doctor can remedy' has become 'The people who treated me had the right idea, now for the street phobia too.'

A question often asked is: do the patients who are treated in this manner still feel pain after the treatment? This question is difficult to answer. Some patients say at the end of the treatment, if they are asked this question: 'The pain doesn't bother me so much now' or 'I now know what I can do if I get such dreadful pain again' or 'I don't just give up any longer.' More often you also hear the answer: 'If I don't think about the pain and if I'm not reminded of it, I don't think I actually have the pain.'

Study activity

9. Explain the answers just mentioned from patients who have undergone an operant treatment. In your answer make use of the learning theory concepts.

d. Eclectic treatment

An eclectic treatment is characterized by two qualities: it is symptom orientated and short-term.

The treatment is directed at the symptom. Here the psychologist selects from the various possibilities the techniques which he thinks will have a positive effect in the present case. What counts is the practical effect of the technique applied. In an eclectically carried out treatment the helper, if it turns out that the selected technique does not 'work', will break this off and try another technique. This means that an eclectically orientated helper may use divergent treatment techniques in one treatment.

A second characteristic is that the treatment is short-term. The patient's supporter along with the patient looks for a technique which brings the patient relief. The application of the technique is subsequently taught to the patient. Now the patient is himself responsible for the keeping his symptoms in check. If an appropriate technique cannot be found, the treatment is then concluded. This too is agreed at the beginning of the treatment.

In the selection of suitable patients for treatment the eclectic support is pragmatic. Eclectic treatment can be directed both at the individual and also at a married couple or a family.

The first aim of the supporter is to raise expectations and give hope. The reasoning on which this aim is based is the following. Most patients do not go to a helper when the problems begin. They first try to deal with the problem themselves. If that is not successful, they try to solve the problems with the aid of people in their immediate environment for example in the family or the household. It is only when they themselves do not know any longer what they can do that they seek professional help. The expectations are then often low or just the opposite in that the patient either has little hope for a cure or expects a wonder cure through which the problems will disappear 'at a stroke'.

The therapist first checks which solutions the patient himself has already tried and what the result of them was. He can then present options for the solution of the problem which have not yet been used, and with which the patient perhaps does have relief. The treatment is tailored to the specific problems and the circumstances of the patient.

The techniques which are used are varied. These techniques are used in varying sequence according to the degree to which they 'work'. Two important groups of techniques are relaxation techniques and cognitive techniques. These two techniques are frequently applied by eclectically orientated treaters. We can also briefly note two therapeutic techniques which have not been previously mentioned: hypnosis and the paradoxical approach.

Hypnosis

Most people are familiar with hypnosis from shows in which volunteers perform funny tasks which they are given to perform by a hypnotist. The impression is thereby incorrectly given that hypnosis is a form of entertainment. Hypnosis is in fact a respectable, sometimes very effective, therapeutic technique.

As a form of therapy, hypnosis is used in order to achieve a state of deep relaxation in which consciousness is narrowed down and the patient concentrates intensely. In this state use is made of the imagination in order to help the patient to get inside a situation, to remember certain events better or to change certain symptoms.

For example: a patient with headache is given the task of concentrating the attention completely on the sensation of a headache. Tension headache usually feels like a tight band round the head. During hypnosis the patient is asked to imagine that there really is a band round his head. The therapist then gives the patient the task of making the band somewhat looser in his imagination.

Paradoxical approach
In this technique the patient is given a task which is opposite to what the therapeutic process aims at, i.e. the symptom is prescribed. For example, a patient with a twitch is given the task of intentionally twitching as often as possible. If the patient regularly pulls his face into a grimace, he is given the task of carrying out this movement again and again. It turns out that the patient thereby gets a feeling of control over the twitch by the very fact that he can do it at will. Furthermore fatigue occurs in the muscles, as a result of which the twitch will gradually occur less often.

Another example: a patient who is afraid of fainting is given the task of trying to faint. It turns out that if he tries this very hard, he in fact finds that he cannot faint and his anxiety decreases. These paradoxical tasks lead to a decrease in the symptom.

The eclectic approach is a pragmatic one. As a result it is assured of a certain sympathy in practically orientated somatic health care. However, there is a serious difficulty connected with this approach. Little (or no) attention is paid to the psychodiagnostic phase. The symptom is the central element, not the 'why and wherefore' of it. The root causes of the complaint are not considered in any great detail.

Study activity
10. a. Give the advantages and disadvantages of a symptom-orientated treatment.
b. List some cases from your own practical experience in which hypnosis and para-

doxical techniques could have been a correct treatment.
Explain your answer.

5. Support

The term 'support' was introduced in Section 2. We speak of psychological support if the patient is given support in handling the burdens of a treatment, an illness, or the consequences of treatment or illness. Support takes place with medical interventions, for example with operations, but also with serious illnesses, such as AIDS and cancer. In general what applies is that the support takes place if it turns out that the patient cannot manage the psychological pressure which the illness exerts on him: if the 'bearing load' exceeds the 'bearing strength'.

When we think of the term 'support' we mostly think of supporting patients with a serious affection. We then think of the effective, supporting help of people in psychological distress. These people have arrived at a state of distress through the idea that they have a serious (sometimes incurable) illness.

The boundary between treatment and support cannot always be drawn sharply. In Section 4 we discussed 'stress management' as a treatment technique. As an example we gave the preparation of a patient for an operative treatment. Such a form of stress management can also be described as a form of support.

It is not so simple to formulate briefly and concisely the meaning of what support is. In this text we refer to support as the 'general position' of the helper: it is a question of the manner in which one is present with the patient, of being available and expressing an essential solidarity with the other person.

Study activity
11. What position must the nurse adopt during support for the patients?

In this section we shall consider two styles of support. Firstly we shall discuss a style of support which originates from the humanistic approach. The second style is based on cognitive-behavioural starting points.

a. Support from a humanistic standpoint

It is sometimes said that the ability to give support is either something you can do or something you can't. We do not subscribe to that idea. 'Support' is the application of a number of actions and as such it can be learnt. The social skills which can be a help in the carrying out of these actions are described in Module 5. Of course the same thing applies for support techniques as for other techniques: you master one technique better than another. The 'special thing' about support is that it is often associated with (strong) emotions. These emotions may also be evident on the part of the carer as well as the patient. As such, support is a form of action which you cannot just provide without thought.

Supporting people in existential distress requires a high degree of concentration in the helper. This can really only be provided if she actually feels essentially involved with the patient who needs support. The supporter has to ensure, just as is the case in a Rogerian treatment, that the relationship which she builds up with the patient satisfies the following characteristics: honesty, acceptance and empathy (see page 57).

Honesty means that the supporter is herself, that she does not keep up a facade but is open. With this she awakens trust. The supporter tells the patient what she feels, even if it concerns negative feelings.

Acceptance means that the supporter reflects a deep and genuine care for the patient. She accepts the patient as he is, with all his 'peculiarities'.

Empathy entails that the supporter is capable of observing the feelings and experiences of the patient and their significance for the patient. This means active listening to and sharing the feelings of the patient.

If the carer uses social skills which only *suggest* empathy, honesty and acceptance, and therefore which are without essential involvement with the patient, it is unlikely that the support contact will succeed. The skills must be used from a standpoint of being authentically moved by the distress of the patient. Through these techniques you can convert your emotion into a form of effective provision of help. Menges (1982) speaks of this aspect of support as 'the general position of the helper' and says 'it is a question of the manner in which one is present with the patient, of being available, of bringing to expression an essential solidarity with the other person'.

If the aim is to support the patient in his anxiety or sorrow, one must arrange the situation for this purpose. This means: take the time and create calm (in yourself too), and then concentrate on it. This is easily said, but not so simply done. Some feelings, certainly if these have an anxiety-provoking content, are expressed by the patient more or less in passing, for example during washing. Reacting to these passing remarks is not so simple. A (correct) first reaction may be one made in passing. For many a patient, even a seriously ill one, such a passing expression of support suffices. The alert observation of the increase in the allusions that a patient makes also falls under the heading of

Figure 4.6.3
Support: honest, accepting, empathic

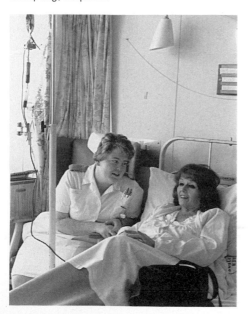

support. One can then consider, possibly after discussion with colleagues, building up a specific contact directed at support.

Study activity

12. Explain, making use of Moos's model, why a single uplifting remark is enough for one patient, while another needs psychotherapy support.

Dealing with psychological distress appears to have a phased character. That means, it looks as if there is a more or less fixed order of sequence in the feelings which the patient experiences.
A well-known division is that of Elizabeth Kübler-Ross (1970), (diagram 4.6.1), who has wide experience in the support of dying patients. She describes the acceptance of approaching death as a period which consists of five phases: denial and isolation, anger, negotiation, gloom and acceptance.

Denial and isolation

The first phase is that of denial and isolation. Normally the first reaction of the patient (and his environment) is, 'That can't be so', when he is told that he is incurably ill. Denial is the first reaction, and some patients use this defence mechanism in the whole process of illness. As Moos states in his model, denial has an important function. This function is 'psychological survival', and preventing 'psychological disintegration' owing to the serious threat which the message contains. Some patients keep on using this defence mechanism until the moment of death: they thus keep on denying that there is anything seriously wrong with them.
Most patients apply 'isolation'. They then 'forget' from time to time the illness and the seriousness of it. This means that they are capable of coping, sometimes very adequately.

Anger

The second phase is characterized by anger, fury, resentment. The patient asks himself aggressively why *he* has to be smitten by this incurable affection. He says for example: 'I didn't smoke, I drank no alcohol, I only ate health foods, and I get cancer! And what about my neighbour? She is older, smokes forty cigarettes

a day, eats anything she chooses and is as fit as a fiddle.'
Or the AIDS patient: 'Okay, I had various partners, but I make love safely, always with a condom. Why do *I* get this?' The jealous resentment which is fostered in this phase does not always come out 'adapted' like that. The fury can be seen in an uncoordinated manner, throwing things, pulling out infusions and so forth. Seen from the patient's position, the anger, which is apparently senseless, does have a justification.

Negotiation

The third phase is called negotiation. In the literature you also come across this phase under the term 'bargaining'. It is as if patients are making agreements about the further course of the disease. Sometimes it is God with whom they try to make a bargain. The idea that one is oneself to blame for the illness is often experienced in this phase. They then try to redeem this supposed guilt by undertaking a specific behaviour such as visiting Lourdes. The person may also make statements like; 'My daughter is getting married in two months, I want to be able to go to the wedding,' or, 'In eight months we will have been married for 25 years; if I can live until after that then I can die happy.'

The negotiation phase is a very treacherous one. The mechanism 'negotiation' destroys the 'moment of choice' that the patient has: 'Chemotherapy, shall I try that?', 'The doctor does not guarantee a single positive effect from that new medicine and I become very queasy with it; shall

Diagram 4.6.1
Five phases described by E. Kübler-Ross

| phase 1: denial and isolation |
| phase 2: anger |
| phase 3: negotiation |
| phase 4: gloom |
| phase 5: acceptance |

I just leave it alone?' Most patients undergo chemotherapy, take the new medicines. Why? Perhaps only because of the negotiation mechanism, 'They won't be able to accuse me of not having done everything to effect a cure.' Just continuing to go through with actions which in themselves have no sense can also occur in this phase. Opponents of the so-called Moerman diet interpret the consumption of the (mostly not very tasty) Moerman preparations from this viewpoint: 'I am doing everything possible, please, let it help.' The same applies for the sometimes unscientific and uncritical consultation of the alternative circuit: 'Then I have at least tried that.' That is not to pass comment on the effectiveness of the alternative therapies that are on offer. It is simply that the reason the patient has for attempting such therapies in this stage of grief may be more to do with the process of negotiation than with a belief in their efficacy.

The negotiation mechanism possibly also comes to the fore with chronically ill patients. The sufferer from chronic kidney disease who in spite of several serious complications continues with dialysis, despite the suffering: 'They won't be able to accuse me of not having done everything for my cure' may be another expression of negotiation.

Gloom

The fourth phase is gloom. The patient no longer believes in his recovery, he lacks the energy to become angry, denial and isolation no longer succeed. The end of life approaches unmistakably, and the patient has no other answer left apart from severe depression. Sometimes this depression can be so massive that one can no longer accept it as a non-pathological reaction. The depression is a manner of preparing for the loss of all that is dear to oneself.

Acceptance

The fifth phase is called acceptance. Sometimes this phase is indeed called a 'happy' time: a time of 'fullness', of the idea of 'having lived, a good life'. The patient becomes resigned to his lot, the gloomy and mutinous feelings are over. He has now taken his leave, and he awaits, in a certain sense calmly, the end.

It is a mistake to suppose that every dying person proceeds through this process in this manner. The sequence of these five phases is described by Kübler-Ross as one which in her experience is very prevalent. But many patients die without following this course. A patient who you think has reached the stage of acceptance may the next day speak in a very embittered way. Embitterment belongs back in the 'anger phase'. Some patients remain 'suspended' for quite a long time in one phase and pass quickly over another one. You should not expect therefore, each patient to follow this sequence through the five phases. It is however possible to recognize these phases in the behaviour of many patients, and a knowledge of them helps in our understanding of the process the patient is going through. It is much easier to provide understanding for a cursing, unmannerly patient if you can indicate his behaviour as 'the aggressive phase'. You understand a patient who does not want to know anything about his illness much better if you consider that there is such a thing as 'a denying phase', and that such behaviour has 'sense': the sense concerns the maintenance of an emotional equilibrium. We again refer to Moos's model.

A question which is of interest in the support of seriously ill patients is that of 'the truth'. In other words: when should the patient hear what is wrong with him? When should he know what the prognosis is? Does the patient have to know what is wrong with him? The answer would seem to be yes and no! The patient has the right to know what is wrong with him: this is a standpoint of medical ethics. This does not mean that every patient *must* be kept informed of his situation. There are always exceptions. There are situations imaginable in which one must confront the denying patient with the nature of his condition and there are situations where information should be given slowly. Each person must be considered as an individual and the pacing of the information given geared to their ability to cope. If the patient, once he has been given the information, enters the stage of negotiation then we should not decry this behaviour. One realizes that the patient, by negotiating, is able to maintain his psychological equilibrium.

Study activity

13. Try by means of a case from your own practice to show the value of the phase division according to Kübler-Ross.

b. Support from a cognitive-behavioural standpoint

Reasoning from the cognitive-behavioural standpoint, Fishman and Loscalzo (1987) developed a support protocol. These authors work with the famous Memorial Sloan-Kettering Cancer Center. This protocol is discussed below.

We should remind you at this point that 'cognitive-behavioural' means that one is working on the relationships between on the one hand the O (cognitive styles), the S (the factors preceding the pain), the C (the factors following the pain), and on the other hand the R (the patient's behaviour). They therefore think from the standpoint of the so-called SORC diagram.

In the introduction to the section about support from a humanistic standpoint (page 377), we spoke about the relationship between techniques and authentic emotion. From the cognitive-behavioural standpoint it becomes even easier to confuse the application of techniques with a cold lack of emotion. It should be emphasized that precisely through adequate application of techniques it is possible to convert emotion into an effective provision of help. What Menges (1982) calls 'the general position' of the helper also applies in the application of Fisher and Loscalzo's protocol. The relationship which the supporter offers is characterized by acceptance, understanding and respect.

A support protocol

The first aim of the helper in such an intervention is to establish in the patient the idea that he himself is capable of doing something about his condition. He can himself change something about his situation. Not much can be changed about the illness as a *somatic* factor with the application of psychological techniques. But patient and supporter can effectively work on the *suffering* aspect of the illness. The cognitive-behavioural interventions advocated are structured. That means that the agenda for each meeting of patient and supporter is clear. Agree-ments are made between supporter and patient about the goals to be aimed at. What they want to achieve is formulated in terms of the everyday problems. Furthermore the supportive actions are carried out in a standardized form. Various techniques can be applied in such an approach.

In the first instance a number of them are directed at the relationship between S and R. This means that work is carried out on muscle tension, on autonomous hyperarousal, on mental confusion. It is assumed, on good grounds, that the suffering factor is strengthened by muscle tension, autonomous hyperarousal and mental confusion.

This first group of techniques is completely centred around provoking the relaxation response. Well known techniques in this group are bio-feedback and progressive relaxation and its variants. Hypnotic relaxation technique also belongs in this category. It is assumed that hypnosis is a good relaxation technique. Further the patient can, by means of hypnosis, learn to transfer his attention from the suffering to other, pleasurable things. Hypnosis has an important disadvantage in that the term hypnosis evokes a lack of veracity. A number of patients therefore refuse to be helped with a hypnotic technique.

The second group of techniques belongs to the arena of systematic desensitization. which was discussed in Chapter 2, Section 4. In this setting the application of this process involves identifying clearly the situations which cause the patient to feel especially miserable and confused. Once the stimuli have been identified as precisely as possible, the patient is taught to relax in situations which gradually become more and more like the original misery provoking stimulus. After a few support sessions the patient is usually capable of undergoing relaxation in situations which to a large extent originally caused him misery. This style of support is especially effective if the patient, owing to his illness, has to undergo strictly necessary but unpleasant treatment, for example chemotherapy. For many cancer patients chemotherapy is an unpleasant experience. With 'systematic desensitization' the patient can influence his reactions to it positively.

Study activity

14. Try to show what advantages for the patient who is being treated with chemotherapy can be obtained by the application of sytematic desensitization.

In the second instance one can work on the relationship between the R and the social consequences. In the SORC diagram this means working on the operant connection between R and C. The application of this style of treatment has been successful with chronic benign pain (that is, roughly speaking, pain without somatic substratum). In the treatment of pain in cancer it is not much used.

The underlying idea in the application of the operant technique is that the patient is suffering more than is strictly necessary. One has the impression that reactions from the environment (strongly) influence the suffering factor. These reactions from the environment, although authentically supportive and intended as supporting, have the undesired effect that the patient suffers more than is strictly necessary. As an example of such an approach we shall mention a case described by Redd and Vazquez (1981). They were treating, in the operant manner, a patient who cried for a very long time owing to the realization that he had cancer. By the term 'for a very long time' we mean several weeks almost without interruption. This form of crying could not be cut out with the usual methods. By 'usual methods' we mean the techniques derived from the humanistic approach. The patient's crying prevented the somatic treatment to a great extent. Redd and Vazquez prescribed a nursing regime in which the patient got social attention whenever he was not crying. He was left alone if he did cry. Of course he did receive the attention which he needed for his somatic condition. The prescribed nursing regime was very effective. Within fourteen days the crying, or at any rate the degree of crying which was disturbing for the treatment, disappeared from the patient's behaviour repertoire.

The patient, who before the treatment began was informed about the style of it and had given his consent, was unwilling to speak about the result. To his own relief he could now speak with others about other things. His style of communicating with others was previously limited to crying. Other communication patterns had not been available to him.

In the third instance, so-called 'cognitive coping' is reinforced. It is directed at the changing of aspects of the O factor. It could be described as the learning of other thought contents about cancer or about the illness that one has. If such an intervention is going to succeed, the patient must assume active control over his attention function. The patient must therefore be capable of directing his attention to a previously agreed subject. For example: to a burning pain sensation he must be able to give the meaning of, 'I am burning myself on the stove, I shall now turn the stove off.' Or another example: a painful sensation in the legs becomes, 'I am a famous footballer, the match depends on me, they are trying to kick me out of it, they are not going to keep me down.' These examples sound trivial but it means a terrific relief for the patient if he notices that these, call them 'tricks' if you like, can be applied by himself and that the effect in fact is that the suffering aspect of the pain is then suppressed.

Study activities

15. Is the approach as described in Section 5.b an eclectic one?

16. Can the support protocol of the Memorial Sloan-Kettering Cancer Center be understood as a stress management programme?

6. Summary

In this chapter the psychological treatment and support of the patient is the central feature. It makes clear the extra value that the psychologist can give in the treatment and support of patients. Therefore a strong plea is made also for a multidisciplinary approach, in which nurses, doctors, physiotherapists, psychologists and others can each provide a relevant contribution from his own background.

Combating pain and coping with mourning are excellent examples from which the vital contribution of psychological support becomes clear. But however that may be, support and treatment do not stop when the psychologist goes away. In this too the nurse is 'the factor' that must guarantee continuity.

Final test Module 4

Instructions

- This section comprises 100 yes/no questions.
- Each proposition, claim, statement, etc. may be *true* or *false,* either *yes* or *no*. There is no middle way: you must make a choice.
- Your assessment of whether items are true or false should be based on your reading of the book.
- The questions are arranged in order relating to subject or chapters.
- Check that all questions have been answered.
- Finally, mark the test yourself. You will find the answers at the end of the book.

1. Clinical psychology is the application of medical psychology in a medical setting.
2. People with functional complaints are not treated by the clinical psychologist.
3. The cognitive evaluation of stress is individually determined.
4. Cognitive evaluation of stress has to do with facing up to stress.
5. Coping has to do with the ways that people deal with a threatening situation.
6. Illness and admission to a hospital are stressors.
7. Moos's model describes the factors which determine whether coping skills are adequate or not.
8. Moos's model sets out from illness as a crisis in the course of human life.
9. In Moos's model cognitive evaluation occupies a central place.
10. The concept 'illness gain' is according to Moos a determining factor in whether adequate coping skills are present or not.

11. Coping skills must emphatically be differentiated from adaptation tasks.
12. An example of an adaptation task is the necessity to develop a good relationship with the professional helpers.
13. An example of a coping skill is the maintenance of a satisfactory self-image.
14. An example of a coping skill is the seeking for relevant information.
15. An example of an adaptation task is the injection of insulin by the patient with diabetes.
16. An example of a coping skill is the setting of concrete, limited and attainable goals.
17. A treatment skill is used to carry out an adaptation task
18. A person classed as a 'repressor' is likely to try to deny having an illness.
19. A person classed as a 'sensitizer' is likely to try to ignore an illness.
20. A 'non-specific defender' has qualities of both a sensitizer and a repressor.
21. In crises people are more sensitive to influences from outside than in a period of relative calm.
22. There is a clearly defined difference between normal and abnormal behaviour.
23. All abnormal behaviour can be identified as mental illness.
24. The cause of anxiety can be explained in biological, psychoanalytic, behavioural and cognitive terms.
25. Behaviour therapy concentrates only on the observable behaviour and not on the causes of that behaviour.
26. Splitting is a mental defence mechanism.
27. Abreaction, insight, and working through are stages in psychotherapy.

28. Group therapy concentrates on the here and now.
29. Therapeutic communities work because of their strict regimes.
30. Psychiatric psychology is concerned with abnormal behaviour.
31. People can develop phobias to guns as easily as to rats.
32. Counter-transference is the projection of feelings by a therapist onto a client.
33. Dopamine has been shown to be involved in the schizophrenic conditions.
34. Learning difficulty relates only to the level of an individual's IQ.
35. Mental Age is equal to chronological age divided by IQ score.
36. Inheritance studies show no link between parental IQ and the IQ of their children.
37. Self-concept is weaker in people with learning difficulty than others.
38. Social role valorization is concerned with ensuring that the person with learning difficulty can get a job.
39. Gentle teaching is a system developed from behaviour therapy.
40. A method of training used with people with learning difficulty is backward chaining.
41. The quality of thought is affected in people with learning difficulty.
42. Learning difficulty relates to a significantly subaverage intellectual ability linked with a subaverage adaptive ability.
43. People with learning difficulty are no more likely to have a demonstrable mental illness than are the rest of the population.
44. Gentle teaching is based on a non-aversive behavioural strategy.
45. In neurology the body is studied as an object.
46. The body plan is the organized total of all sensory-motor structures that determines the automated behaviour of the person.
47. With an excess of alcohol the body plan will let you down.
48. Body sense is the subjective judgement that the person forms for himself of his own physical appearance.
49. By body idea we mean the information that the person can acquire for himself about the state of his body in space.

50. The body plan is also termed the body scheme in neurology.
51. The 'breast idea' is a part of the body idea.
52. Tension complaints are complaints without a physical substratum.
53. There is often a close relationship between tension complaints and functional complaints.
54. The stimulus is the central element in the so-called SORC diagram.
55. Every response is composed of three components.
56. A stimulus is a goad from the environment.
57. A thought can also have the role of a stimulus.
58. The personality is one of the factors which, according to the SORC diagram, are included in the O category.
59. The S-R relationship is the central feature in classic conditioning.
60. The R-C relationship is the central feature in operant conditioning.
61. The specificity hypothesis assumes a connection between a specific personality structure and a specific physical suffering.
62. That type-A personalities are more often affected by a heart disease than other personalities is in accordance with the specificity hypothesis.
63. The watering of your eyes when you think of the onions which you still have to peel is a connection that is learnt via the principles of classical conditioning.
64. Short-term consequences have less effect on the arising and continuance of behaviour than long-term consequences.
65. A dog's reaction to the auditory stimulus 'over' by swimming over the river is learnt via the principles of operant conditioning.
66. The SORC diagram is comparable with Moos's model.
67. Theoretically the term 'undesirable behaviour' provides no problems.
68. Objectivizing indicates especially the accurate charting of the complaint.
69. The task of the clinical psychologist is the tracking down of psychosocial factors which influence an individual patient's complaint.
70. A measuring procedure is called reliable if it 'measures what it is supposed to measure'.

71. Standardization entails that the individual recordings of the test run similarly.
72. None of the instruments available to a psychologist is 100% reliable.
73. Nurses predominantly use indirect observation.
74. A psychological statement which is based on a test result is always based on the comparison of at least two test scores.
75. Tests for performance level are measures of the usual behaviour of an individual.
76. An example of an aptitude test is an intelligence test.
77. An oral examination mostly satisfies the reliability requirements.
78. An oral examination mostly does not satisfy the validity requirements.
79. A self-assessment procedure is an example of a test for a manner of behaviour.
80. A projective test is as a rule more reliable than a personality questionnaire.
81. In the clinical psychological examination, tests are divided into tests for the performance level and tests for the manner of behaviour.
82. By psychological treatment we understand the curing in a professional manner of undesirable behaviour.
83. We talk of psychological support when the patient is professionally supported in bearing the burdens of the treatment.
84. We talk of psychological support when the patient is professionally supported in handling the negative consequences of his illness.
85. The operant treatment of a patient with lower back pain is an example of a psychological intervention which is especially directed at support.
86. Psychoeducation is applied during psychological intervention with the patient with MS (multiple sclerosis).
87. Giving information to the patient is an example of psychoeducation.
88. Giving information to the patient in the pre- and post-operative phases can be considered as an example of stress management.
89. Giving information about the procedure as preparation for a surgical intervention is mostly sufficient in the framework of stress management.
90. 'Repressors' are patients who deny anxiety.
91. With cognitive therapy a differentiation is made between style of thinking and thought content.
92. 'Illness conviction' is a characteristic of patients with a somatizing style of thinking.
93. With 'illness conviction' psychoeducation has hardly any effect.
94. Self-instruction can be used with the patient with tension headache.
95. With the passively complaining patient with 'disuse' symptoms we can speak of the presence of the avoidance aspect.
96. Extinction is the step by step learning of desired behaviour.
97. Eclectic treatment is symptom orientated.
98. Paradoxical treatment is seen as an important part of operant treatment.
99. Support at death according to E. Kubler-Ross belongs within support from a humanist standpoint.
100. A part of the cognitive-behavioural treatment can consist of the group of techniques which is based on the provocation of the relaxation response.

References

Bandura, A. (1987). *Principles of Behaviour Modification*. New York, Holt, Rinehart and Winston.

Bandura, A. (1984). Recycling misconceptions of perceived self-efficacy. *Cognitive Therapy and Research*, 8: 231–55.

Bandura, A. Adams, N.E., Beyer J. (1976). Cognitive processes mediating behavioral change. *Journal of Personality and Social Psychology*, 35: 125–39.

Beck, A.T. (1976). *Cognitive Therapy and the Emotional Disorders*. New York, International Universities Press.

Boore, J.R.P. (1978). *Prescription for Recovery*. London, Whitefriars Press.

Bouchard, T.J., McGuie, M. (1981). Familial studies of intelligence: a review. *Science*, 212: 1055–59.

Bourbonnais, F. (1981). Pain assessment: development of a tool for the nurse and the patient. *Journal of Advanced Nursing*, 6: 277–282

Brandon, D. (January 1990). Gentle teaching. *Nursing Times*, 86 (2): 62–3, 10.

Brenner, M.H. (1982). Mental illness and the economy. In: Parron, D.L., Solomon, F., Jenkins, C.D. (eds.), *Behavior, Health Risks and Social Disadvantage*. Washington, D.C., National Academy Press.

Cautela, J.R. (1967). Covert sensitization. *Psychological Reports*, 20: 459–68.

Cormack, D.F.S. (1983). *Psychiatric Nursing Described*. Edinburgh, Churchill Livingstone.

Collister, B. (1988). *Psychiatric Nursing: Person to Person*. London, Edward Arnold.

Creese, I., Burt D.R., Snyder S.H. (1978). Biochemical actions of neuroleptic drugs. In: Iversen, S.D., Snyder S.H., (eds.), *Handbook of Psychopharmacology*, Vol. 10. New York, Plenum.

Crown, S. (1986). Individual long-term psychotherapy. In: Bloch, S., (ed.), *An Introduction to the Psychotherapies*. Oxford, Oxford University Press.

DHSS, (1981). *Care in the Community: A Consultative Document on Moving Resources for Care in England*. London, HMSO.

Eysenck, H.J. (1958). *Sense and Nonsense in Psychology*. Harmondsworth, Penguin Books.

Fennel, M.J.V., Campbell E.H. (1984). The cognitions questionnaire: Specific thinking errors in depression. *British Journal of Clinical Psychology*, 43: 522–4.

Fishmann, B., Loscalzo M. (1987). Cognitive-behavioural interventions in the management of cancer pain: principles and applications. *Medical Clinics of North America*, 71: 271–87.

Fordyce, W.E. (1976). *Behavioural Methods for Chronic Pain and Illness*. St Louis, C.V. Mosby.

Frank, J. (1986) What is psychotherapy. In: Bloch, S. (ed.), *An Introduction to the Psychotherapies*. Oxford, Oxford University Press.

Fried, M. (1982). Disadvantage, vulnerability and mental illness. In: Parron, D.L., Solomon F., Jenkins C.D., (eds.), *Behaviour, Health Risks and Social Disadvantage*. Washington, D.C., National Academy Press.

Freud, S. (1962). *Two Short Accounts of Psychoanalysis*. London, Penguin.

Gelder, M. (1986). Cognitive and behavioural therapies. In: Bloch, S. (ed.), *An Introduction to the Psychotherapies*. Oxford, Oxford University Press.

Goffman, E. (1987). *Asylums*. London, Penguin.

Goldstein, M.J. (April 1985). *The UCLA Family Project*. Paper presented at the High Risk Consortium Conference, San Francisco.

Goldstein, M.J., Baker, B.L., Jamison, K.R. (1986). *Abnormal Psychology: Experiences, Origins and Interventions* (2nd ed.). Boston, Little, Brown.

Gottesman, I.I., Shields, J. (1982) *Schizophrenia: The Epigenetic Puzzle*. New York, Cambridge University Press.

Groen, J., Horst, L. van der and Bastiaans, J. (1951). *Grondslagen der Psychosomatiek*. Haarlem, Bohn.

Grossman, F. (1973). *Brothers and Sisters of Retarded Children: An Exploratory Study*. Syracuse, New York, Syracuse University Press,

Hare, R.D. (1970). *Psychopathy: Theory and Research*. New York, Wiley.

Hayward, J. (1975). *Information. A Prescription Against Pain*. London, RCN.

Hogg, J., Sebba, J. (1986). *Profound Retardation and Multiple Impairment, Vol. 1. Development and Learning*. London, Croom Helm.

Hogg, J., Sebba, J. (1986). *Profound Retardation and Multiple Impairment, Vol. 2. Education and Therapy*. London, Croom Helm.

Holmes, T.H., Rahe, R.H. (1967). The social readjustment rating scale. *Journal of Psychosomatic Research*, 11: 213–18.

Jackson, R.N. (1988). Perils of 'pseudo-normalisation'. *Mental Handicap*, 16, 148–50.

Jones, C. (1979). Glasgow Coma Scale. *American Journal of Nursing*, 79: 1551–53.

Kübler-Ross, E. (1969). *On Death and Dying*. Suffolk, Tavistock.

Lally, J. (1988). When anger is a cry for help. *Community Living*, 2: 1.

Lidz, T. (1973). *The Origin and Treatment of Schizophrenic Disorders*. New York, Basic Books.

Lyttle, J. (1986). *Mental Disorder: Its Care and Treatment*. London, Baillere Tindall.

Martin, B. (1981). *Abnormal Psychology: Clinical and Scientific Perspectives* (2nd ed.). New York, Holt, Rinehart and Winston.

McGee, J. (1990). Gentle teaching: the basic tenet. *Nursing Times*, 86 (32): 68–72.

McGee, J., Menolascino, F.J., Hobbs, D.C., Menousek, P.E., *Gentle Teaching: A Non-aversive Approach to Helping Persons with Mental Retardation*. New York, Human Sciences Press.

Menges, L.J. (1982). *Begeleiding van patiënten met kanker, Ten geleide*. Alphen aan de Rijn, Stafleu.

Moos, R.H. (1986). *Coping with Life Crises*. New York, Plenum.

Moos, R.H. (ed.) (1989). *Coping with Physical Illness 2: New Perspectives*. New York, Plenum.

Nicol, S.E., Gottesman, I.I. (1983). Clues to the genetics and neurobiology of schizophrenia. *American Scientist*, 71:398–404.

Piaget, J. (1952). *The Origins of Intelligence in Children*. New York, International Universities Press.

Peplau, H.E. (1988). *Interpersonal Relations in Nursing: A Conceptual Frame of Reference for Psychodynamic Nursing*. MacMillan.

Peterson, C., Seligman, M.E.P. (1984). Causal explanations as a risk factor for depression: Theory and evidence. *Psychological Review*, 91: 347–74.

Rapaport, R.N. (1960). *Community as Doctor*. London, Tavistock.

Redd, W., Vazquez, A. (April 1981). Conditioned version in cancer patients. *Behaviour Therapist*.

Rigness, T.A. (1961). Self-concept of children of low, average and high intelligence. *American Journal of Mental Deficiency*, 65: 453–61.

Roff, J.D., Knight, R. (1981). Family characteristics, childhood symptoms, and adult outcome in schizophrenia. *Journal of Abnormal Psychology*, 90: 510–20.

Saccuzzo, D.P., Kerr, M., Marcus, A., Brown, R. (1979). Input capability and speed of processing in mental retardation. *Journal of Abnormal Psychology*, 88: 474–89.

Sarason, I.G., Johnson, J.H., Siegel, J.M. (1978). Assessing the impact of life changes: Development of the life experiences survey. *Journal of Consulting and Clinical Psychology*, 46: 932–46.

Seligman, M.E.P., Rosenhan, D.L. (1984). *Abnormal Psychology*. New York, Norton.

Sugden, D., (ed.) (1989). *Cognitive Approaches in Special Education*. The Farmer Press.

Suls, J., Wan, C.K. (1989). Effects on sensory and procedural information on coping with stressful medical procedures and pain: a meta-analysis. *Journal of Consulting and Clinical Psychology*, 57 (3): 372–88.

Snyder, S.H. (1990). *Biological Aspects of Mental Disorder*. New York, Oxford University Press.

Tiemersma, D. (1989). *Body Schema and Body Image*. Lisse, Swets & Zeitlinger.

Torgersen, S. (1983). Genetic factors in anxiety disorders. *Archives of General Psychiatry*, 40: 1085–89.

Walker, C.E., Hedberg, A., Clement, P.W., Wright, L. (1981). *Clinical Procedures for Behaviour Therapy*. Englewood Cliffs, N.J., Prentice Hall.

Weisz, J.R. (1979). Perceived control and learned helplessness among mentally retarded and non-retarded children: A developmental analysis. *Developmental Psychology*, 15: 311–19.

Wilcox, R., Smith, J.L. (1973). Some psychological-social correlates of mental retardation. *Perceptual and Motor Skills*, 36: 999–1006.

Wolfensberger, W. (1980). The definition of normalization. In: Flynn, R.J., Nitsch, K.E., (eds.), *Normalzation, Social Integration and Community Service*. Baltimore, University Park Press.

Wolfensberger, W. (1983). Social role valorization: A proposed new term for the principle of normalization. *Mental Retardation*, 21: 234–9.

Wooster, A.D. (1970). Formation of stable and discrete concepts of personality by normal and mentally retarded boys. *Journal of Mental Subnormality*, 16 (30): 24–28.

Wolpe, J. (1958). *Psychotherapy by Reciprocal Inhibition*. Stanford, California, Stanford University Press.

Yule, W., Carr, J. (1980). *Behaviour Modification for the Mentally Handicapped* (2nd ed.). Croom Helm.

Zigler, E. (1967). Familial mental retardation: A continuing dilemma. *Science*, 155: 292–8.

Zigler, E., Balla, D., Kossan, N. (1986). Effects on types of institutionalization on responsiveness to social reinforcement wariness and outerdirectedness among low MA residents. *American Journal of Mental Deficiency*, 91: 10–17.

Module 5

SOCIAL SKILLS

Introduction to Module 5

This module is concerned with communication. How you communicate as a nurse is very important. You have a great deal of influence over how the patient feels. You exercise this influence through everything you do, and one of the most important aspects of this is conversation. The essential thing about a good conversation is that it is two-way traffic. You react to the patient and the patient in turn reacts to you. You will appreciate that it is impossible to simply lay down regulations about the practice of conversation with patients. That isn't the way it works. The guidelines which we offer in this module are different. They are guidelines such as:
– ensuring that your conversation remains a genuine two-way traffic;
– ensuring that you do not jump to conclusions too quickly, but that you really *understand* what the patient is saying to you.

These are less definitive and therefore more complicated guidelines. They are guidelines with which we describe in particular the form of a conversation, not so much the content. Although the content of your conversations is important, this is considered more in other parts of your education.

A great deal of research has been carried out into social skills. All these studies together give a useful picture of what kind of communication is important in which situation. We shall describe for example the type of questions with which you obtain more information. We shall also describe how you can deal with a patient if you notice that he is very afraid. We cannot tell you what words to use. We describe what your 'attitude' should be, the style and approach which may be most appropriate to the situation.

1. The benefit of good communication

We have already indicated above that you affect how the patient feels through everything you do. This can be explained as follows:
– Good communication enables you to track down important information better.
– With good communication you follow the normal, widely usual rules of etiquette.
– With good communication you show the patient that you are doing your best to understand him. If sick people feel that they are understood, this promotes the healing process.
– Through good communication you can help the patient to make the best

possible effort towards his recovery. You can, for example, help to reduce unjustified anxiety.

This module, as the title suggests, is concerned with social skills. Obviously you are already socially skilled. You have been making things clear to others ever since you were born. It started by letting your parents know you were hungry by howling. You learned to talk in due course and since then you have been able to deal with other people well enough (read through Module 3, Chapeter 1 on socialization once more). You might get tongue-tied occasionally but in general you can cope when you are communicating with other people. So why should you be reading about social skills? Don't you know enough about this already? We suggest that although you may be perfectly capable of using your social skills in your normal everday life, there are common principles which can be understood and applied, and these principles have particular application in health care settings.

The result of social skills training will be that you have more choice. In particular situations you will be able to choose what to do. In situations where you used to be tongue-tied you will know better how to say something and you can pay better attention to what the patient wants to tell you or ask you. Your conversations will not be as interminable as they perhaps were and you will be aware of some of the difficulties which regularly occur in the course of conducting conversations. In fact you will be able to use social skills as a vitally important therapeutic tool. Indeed in nursing, which is essentially an interpersonal caring activity, interpersonal or social skills are possibly one of the most important nursing skills you will learn.

2. The purpose of social skills

Social skills serve the following purpose: they enable you to communicate with patients and colleagues and to work with them as effectively as possible. Two aspects are important in this objective:

1. *Communicating as well as possible.* This can mean many different things. What we mean here is 'in a way that promotes the attainment of a good end-result'. A good end-result means optimum patient care and the best possible co-operation. Patient care and co-operation become better as clarity on what is meant increases. We can speak of good communication only when all the parties to the conversation understand the same thing from the words used. You achieve this good communication by making a conversation reciprocal. All parties to conversations must have the opportunity to ask for clarification. A conversation must be two-way traffic. Only then can you avoid being misunderstood and incorrectly interpreted, only then does communication become clear.

2. *Distinction between one-to-one conversations (i.e. between two people) and group discussions.* We deal with these two kinds of social skills separately. In one-to-one conversations you use a number of skills such as listening, continued questioning and so on.

In group discussions you also use those skills, but they are not the only skills you need. You must also for example be able to summarize a discussion; you sometimes have to try to get people who have different opinions to agree: these are additional skills. You can assume that for group discussions different social skills are required compared with conversations between two people.

If you have good social skills, you can deal competently with other people (patients and colleagues) with regard to conducting conversations, attitude and approach. You can prevent lack of clarity in communication and if this occurs accidentally you can help to clear it up.

What you cannot do by social skills alone is to solve problems. You also need knowledge and understanding for this and these areas are described in the remainder of this book and in many other books. Only if you apply your knowledge in a socially skilled way can you help others in the optimum way.

You often need the social skills in your task of trying to influence the situation of the other person (generally the patient). This influencing must then lead to a situation which the patient considers to be better than the previous situation.

The result of training in social skills will also be that you work according to a particular method. What we mean by method is that you work:
– *consciously*, i.e. expressly: you have chosen this way;
– *systematically*, i.e. step by step, you work to a plan;
– *resolutely*, i.e. you do not digress, you do no more than is necessary to achieve your aim;
– *by a process*, i.e. you are mindful of your plan for achieving the ultimate aim.

We want you to learn in social skills training how to reconcile the wishes of the patient and your own wishes. This might sound odd. Perhaps you are not often told that you should serve your own interests as well as the meeting the patient's wishes. What we mean by this is that you can imagine patients asking you things which you consider inappropriate. For example, someone may ask you if you will move his pillow, even when he can do it just as well himself. It is easy enough to oblige; that way the patient is happy and you can get on with something else.

However, if you stand back and look at this scenario, you will probably think; 'If I carry on doing that for long, I will be promoting dependence in my patient. It is better to make it clear to the patient at the first opportunity that he must do the things that he can do himself.' We want you to learn to anticipate situations of this kind in social skills training. Only if you understand these situations can you choose what you want to (or have to) do. And you follow this course because it is *better* than something else. This is different from ordinary, everyday behaviour where we generally improvise. We do not tend to make the best possible choice by improvising.

3. Exercises

This module is arranged in a slightly different way from the previous modules. The chief difference is the exercises. The social skills which are presented are supported by exercises. You do not become more socially skilled by reading alone. You become more socially skilled only by practising these skills. The exercises in this module are necessary if you wish to learn the material and the chapters are explained and clarified through the exercises. In addition, the exercises are fun to do. They can open up a whole new world to you. If you learn to direct your attention towards how social interactions are conducted (and not simply what they are about), you may find that these interactions take on a new significance.

You might perhaps get the idea in the exercises that you are being put in an unnatural situation. What you do is commented on; you must not do this any more and you have to do that more often ...
Look at the exercises as opportunities to try things out. See what it is like to do things differently from the way you normally do them, not because it is necessarily better, but simply because you can see in an exercise situation how you like it and how the other person likes it. Eventually you can choose for yourself out of a number of possible forms of behaviour. It is advisable to be aware that you are always receiving feedback on your behaviour: for instance, people give you a disapproving look or break off the conversation and start talking to someone else. The advantage of giving systematic attention to your social skills in these exercises is that positive criticism is facilitated and the comments are finally expressed loud and clear. In this way it is easier to derive benefit from them.

4. Skills and attitude

It could be said that social skills consist of a number of techniques (summarizing, asking questions, explaining etc) and that it does not matter so much why you apply these techniques as long as you apply them correctly. People who think this say that you can go a long way with techniques alone, that the other person feels understood and invited to speak through the techniques alone.
Another line of argument says that it does not matter so much how you say something as the meaning behind it. If you are honest, you conduct your conversations well enough anyway, according to this line of argument. In the social skills component of this book we take an intermediate position. On the one hand we believe that a conversation will not run well if you merely apply techniques; on the other hand, honesty, conscientiousness and good intentions are very important, but often not enough.

You will also notice in the exercises in this book that we pay a great deal of attention to the basic skills, the techniques of communication. However, because these basic skills are not enough, other points for attention are also considered, such as: why do you find this more satisfying and enjoyable than that? These motives for why you act as you do (and not differently) are what we call your *attitude*. If you check earlier references to attitude in this text, you will recall that it was defined as a relatively permanent disposition to think, feel and behave toward an object, person or issue. We shall not indicate what attitudes you must consider important. We believe that you must be curious about your own attitudes, that you must attempt to get behind why you act as you do. Examples of such points for attention are: what do you think if someone calls you 'doctor'? What would you like to do then? What do you actually do? Does it matter who says it?

In this module we shall first deal with the skills which are important in the contact between nurse and patient. We shall then present the skills which are important for co-operating with others, such as nursing colleagues and other members of the health care team.

Communication

1

1. Introduction

Everyone communicates. Meaningful human existence is impossible without communication. Communication is obviously important in any situation which involves working with people. Nurses therefore cannot function professionally without communicating. Effective communication should take place between:
– nurse and patient;
– nurse and professional colleagues;
– nurse and staff from other disciplines;
– nurse and family, relations or friends of the patient.

You are not born with effective communication. It is a skill which can be learned. In this chapter the theory and skills of communication are discussed in the context of the relationship between nurse and patient.

Learning outcomes

After studying this chapter the student should be able to:
– define the term *communication*;
– describe and apply six features of communication;
– explain what role hopes and expectations can play during communication;
– explain how questions convey information;
– explain the terms *sickness gain* and *compliance*;
– describe eight problems or pitfalls which can arise during communication.

2. Aim of the relationship between nurse and patient

Both the nurse and the patient have a special role to play in this relationship. The patient wants something from you and you decide whether you wish to comply with his wishes.
This relationship obviously becomes more fruitful if you can count on the assistance of the patient.

There are two sides to the nurse–patient relationship.
Firstly correct care has to be given and secondly this must be done in a way in which you can count on the assistance of the patient, this is referred to as good motivation. If the patient feels that you sympathize with him, that you have compassion for him, he will assist more quickly than if you are unwilling to talk about feelings.

It often appears that 'pleasantness' and 'expertise' are two things that do not go together. People who are experts often appear to bother less about friendliness, whilst pleasant people often appear to be less expert.

This is not true however. Pleasantness and expertise have nothing to do with each other. You can easily be expert and pleasant at the same time, whilst there are also people who are unpleasant and inexpert at the same time.

It is generally a question of social skills. There are social skills by which you demonstrate that you are compassionate towards the patient, as well as social skills by which you provide evidence of your expertise.

These skills will be discussed later. Let us first look at some theory.

3. Communication

Case study - Elsie and James Archer

Six o'clock in the evening. James is sitting in the living-room with his feet up on the table. He pretends to be reading the newspaper. His wife Elsie is in the kitchen. The cooker extractor hood is whirring, she is cooking.

She thinks: he's just come home and he's sitting in the living-room. Why doesn't he help, and then we could both sit down together? She says, 'Are you comfortable?'

He thinks: I've just come home, I've had a hard day, why doesn't she come and sit down with me, so we can tell each other what sort of a day we've had, and then we can cook and eat together afterwards. He shouts to the kitchen, 'Will it take much longer?' The cooker hood continues to whir.

If you listen to these people without knowing their thoughts, it appears impossible to understand what they want to make clear to each other. Only if you know their underlying thoughts do you begin to understand what they mean. Meanings are often badly packed into words, so badly even that we are often no longer able to find the meaning through the words. We then simply react to what we *think* the other person means. It is quite likely that the woman in the example above thinks: if he carries on doing this, I shall walk out tomorrow, I'm fed up with being treated like his servant.

But if she were to say something like that to her husband, he would be flabbergasted. He would not understand where this reaction came from.

Figure 5.1.1
The communication gap

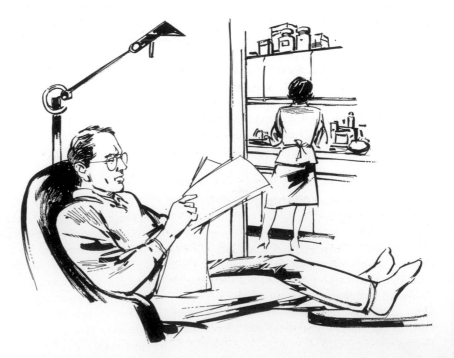

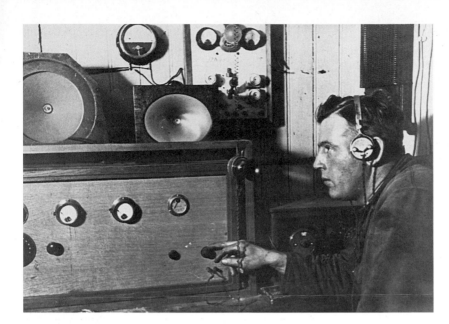

Figure 5.1.2
Communication
takes place between
transmitter and
receiver

Study activity
1. Give two examples in the relationship between patient and nurse in which communication can give rise to mutual misunderstandings, because meanings are unclear.

a. Definition of communication

The following definition is often given for communication:
Communication is the exchange of information between people. Important key words in this definition are *'exchange'* and *'information'*. Information is continuously being given and received (i.e. exchanged) during communication. You generally communicate with a specific purpose in mind: you intentionally make clear to the other person what you think about something or what, in your view, should be done.
Communication takes place between people. The case of the married couple illustrates that communication–or interaction (inter = between) –always takes place between people. If you listen to the conversation of someone who is making a telephone call, there is a great deal that is incomprehensible because you only hear half of the conversation. People always react to each other. We call this the *reciprocity of communication*. Because communication includes exchanges between people, it is by definition reciprocal. People respond in kind. If people respond inappropiately or with meaningless responses, communication is ineffective.

Study activity
2. The idea of reciprocity is important in communication. To make sure you understand the term, write a brief explanation. Make sure you include in your explanation important aspects such as mutuality, sharing, responding in kind, commonality. Illustrate your explanation with examples.

b. Features of communication

Communication roles

We have seen that communication always takes place between people, it is *interpersonal*. The roles played by those involved change constantly. One person relates something and the other person listens. We do not call the first person the narrator, because this would mean that only *his* words are important. However, there is more that is important: his facial expression, his body posture, his way of speaking and so on. We therefore call the person talking *the transmitter* and the other person, the one who is listening, is called *the receiver*. The transmitter and receiver usually alternate roles rapidly. We have already seen that you continuously react to each other in conversations. You tell your partner in the conversation something and he says something back: then you react again and so on.

Exercise 1. Communication roles

Aim: to be able to recognize that participants in a conversation between two people constantly change roles.

Number of persons: 3.

Materials: 3 chairs.

Time required: 15 minutes.

Procedure: two people sit opposite each other, the third acting as the observer. The task given to the two participants (**A** and **B**) is as follows: **A** tells **B** for 5 minutes how he has spent the past weekend. **A** must continue talking until the whole weekend has been described.

B listens and is not allowed to make any comments in response to **A**'s story; **B** must not react either verbally or non-verbally.

The observer monitors the roles described above. He pays close attention to **B**. As soon as he notices any reaction from **B**, he must interrupt **A**'s story. **B** must be 'whistled back' and **A** then continues.

In the subsequent discussion, the observer directs the conversation. He asks both partners in the conversation how they liked this way of holding a 'conversation'. Was it a conversation? What were **A**'s experiences? And what were **B**'s? Is it possible to remain strictly a 'transmitter' or 'receiver' in a conversation, without ever changing roles? If so, under what circumstances would that be possible?

Message

We call what is told a message. In ordinary language 'message' generally means a communication in words, but here it is understood to mean *everything* that is communicated to (one or more) others, whether this takes place by words, gestures, winking, saying nothing or walking away.

This definition has interesting implications. All your actions are statements. Even if you are just *present* in a roomful of people, you are conveying a message. If you are talking, your meaning will be clear, but even if you are merely sitting quietly reading a book, you are communicating. Your colleagues can see for example that you do not need their conversation and that you are engrossed in your book. If you, without realizing it, sigh, laugh or shed a tear, they can see from you that the book does not leave you unmoved. According to this definition of *message*, you never reveal nothing about yourself if you are in a room with other people. You cannot non-communicate even by staying silent. You convey information in the way you speak as well as in the actual content of the words. The tone, speed, volume, pitch and rhythm of speech and the inflections or emphasis placed on particular words all convey additional information and add new layers of meaning. This is known as *paralanguage* or *paralinguistics*. For example by emphasizing a word in a phrase, its meaning can be completely different. Thus:

'He could have WEPT'
tells us that he was very upset, while
'HE could have wept'
tells us that he alone was upset and not other people.

Exercise 2. Message

Aim: to be able to recognize that everything you do is communication.
Number of persons: 2 to 5.
Materials: none.
Time required: 15 minutes.
Procedure: person **A** stands or sits opposite the other person or persons. He is instructed not to say anything. The other person or persons must not ask person **A** anything and must not say anything to him. Continue this for at least one minute and no more than three minutes.
Each person then writes down what he saw or thought with regard to the behaviour of person **A**. Person **A** also writes down what he thought, felt and/or did during those minutes. In the subsequent discussion the descriptions are compared. Pay attention to agreed views or observations, however coincidental. The most important conclusion is that each person has probably had thoughts which in one way or another can be connected with what person **A** did. His slightest behaviour always gives rise to thoughts, feelings or actions.

Channels

We have seen that you need not necessarily make communication with words. You also reveal something about yourself in other ways. We call these various ways *channels*. The two channels which we have available to us are the *verbal* and *non-verbal* channels. By verbal channels we mean all messages which are conveyed in words. We are then talking about sentences and the choice of words in those sentences and nothing more than that. Everything that is not said in words is called the non-verbal channel. This means how a person looks, what gestures he makes and how he speaks, for example loudly, quietly, angrily, emotionally, smoothly, haltingly and so on. We will recall that earlier we described this as paralanguage. Non-verbal behaviour also means such things

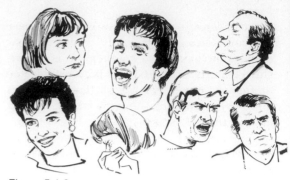

Figure 5.1.3
All behaviour is
communication

as eye contact, clothing, appearance, posture, proximity between individuals, and all the other non-speech ways in which people communicate something about themselves.

Exercise 3. Channels

Aim: to illustrate the distinction between verbal and non-verbal communication.

Number of persons: an even number between 2 and 20.

Materials: a sheet of drawing paper for each person, half of the sheets with a figure drawn by the tutor or a student. The figure is made up of various shapes (circles, triangles, rectangles, lines etc.) with a maximum of 10 items.

Time required: 1 hour.

Procedure: divide the group into pairs (person **A** and person **B**). Give person **A** the paper with the figure and person **B** the blank sheet. Person **A** sits back to back with person **B** and has to describe the figure to person **B** using verbal communication only. There should be no visual contact or non-verbal communication between the pairs.

Person **B** draws the figure on the blank piece of paper, trying to reproduce it from Person **A**'s description. When the drawing is completed the original and the copy are compared.

The subsequent discussion of this exercise is concerned with how necessary it is to have non-verbal behaviour in communication. Try to think of some situations when only one channel is available (blindfolded, telephone conversation etc.).

Levels

You can imagine how the question, 'I don't suppose you want any coffee?' will produce a reply from which you do not know for certain whether the other person does want coffee. Shy or cautious people react with, 'Well, no...' to this question, but someone who wants to assert himself answers, 'Yes please!'

A little sentence like this, awkward as it is, makes clear that as well as what is said in words, there is also often a resonance. By this we mean the words can have different or deeper meanings. In this example you could say that the resonance is, 'It doesn't suit me to give you coffee.' If you know the background, this becomes clearer. The fact that there is a resonance of information between the lines applies to everything we say. The words we choose ('He's thick', rather than, 'He's not very intelligent'), the way in which we speak (hesitantly or quickly and easily), and the gestures we make while speaking, all colour our communications. All these features help the other person to pick up our meaning. How something is said thus gives information on what is said.

We call what is said the content. If we assess what someone said, we look at communication on a *content level*. The way in which something is said is the *relational level*. The word 'relational' indicates a relationship. The relational level indicates something about the relationship between the speakers. In the example above, you can imagine the person who refuses the coffee not finding the other person to be very hospitable or pleasant.

Study activity

3. Give three examples in which the thing said at the content level has a different meaning at relational level.

In conversations it is possible to distinguish between the content and relational level. If someone says, 'Yes, I'll do that', with an expression of deep reluctance we can quickly perceive the relational message of displeasure on the part of the speaker. Although the content level ('I'll do that') may have a positive meaning, the relational message (the facial expression) indicates the speaker's reluctance to perform the action. Thus, we understand more than just the words that people use.

The way in which people put something in words is also perceived by us. If you watch closely how people communicate with each other, you will see that the relational level of their communications is quite visible. If the receiver yawns, the transmitter will take this as lack of interest. The transmitter will consequently also react, perhaps by talking louder, or by digressing. In any case the information he is giving will change at the relational level. If one person puts a grumpy tone in his voice, the other person will soon be inclined to react just as grumpily.

Study activity

4. Start a conversation with someone who does not know about this study activity. Look out of the window for 3 minutes, fiddle with your hands, rummage in your pockets and look at the other person as little as possible. Then enter more actively into the conversation – or what is left of it – looking at the other person with as much interest as possible. Nod, make sympathetic noises, and generally show your interest for a further three minute period. Observe how much the other person says in the first and second periods of 3 minutes.

Exercise 4. Levels

Aim: to be able to recognize a paradoxical task.

Number of persons: individually, where appropriate to be discussed in the group afterwards.

Materials: the message below.

Time required: 5 minutes with a subsequent discussion lasting 5 to 15 minutes.

Procedure: how must you react to the message below?

> ## DO NOT PAY ATTENTION TO THIS COMMUNICATION

What are the communications you can find in this message? Discuss your views with your fellow students.

Metacommunication

At the start of this chapter we gave an example of how communication works. The example concerned a married couple who tried to make something clear to each other but what became clear to the outsider was that neither of them grasped what the other was saying. Both of them attached meanings which the other person did not intend at all. They therefore reacted with a great deal of misunderstanding.

The nice thing about communication is that you can easily rectify mistakes if you follow a number of rules. For example, in the case of the married couple Elsie and James, it is not difficult to supply a commentary on the way in which the two of them communicate with each other. What if, for example, they said to each other, 'Can't you say that differently?' or 'You do sound angry!' or 'Why don't we sit down together and talk about this?'

This way of talking can be described as commentary on communication or communication on communication. You say something about the way in which the other person said something. We call this metacommunication. Metacommunication also covers such statements as: 'You looked rather sad when you were talking.' 'Every time you talk about your children, you cheer up' or 'Whenever I start talking about going home, you start talking about something else, why's that?'

With these forms of metacommunication a commentary is given on the course of the conversation. Because the course of the conversation is also known as the conversation *'process'*, these specific metacommunication remarks are known as process remarks.

Sometimes metacommunication can take the form of more subtle messages about the overt message a transmitter is sending. This may be in the form of non-verbal accompaniments to the overt verbal message. Or it may be in the way we say things, i.e. by the way we use paralinguistics, as discussed in the subsection on messages above. For example, a nurse may walk into the patient's room and say 'How are you doing today?' While she is saying this her voice may convey sincerity, she may establish eye-contact with the patient which conveys warmth and she will wait expectantly for a response. In doing all this she is communicating at the metacommunication level, that is, she is sending a message about her verbal question to the patient. She is saying, 'I care about you and I really do want to know how you are today.' However, if the nurse asks the question 'How are you doing today?' in a neutral and unconcerned voice, if she doesn't even look at the patient when she asks, but spends the time looking in a mirror, preening her hair and straightening her name badge, and then leaves without even waiting for an answer, she is conveying a completely different message. This nurse clearly does not really care about the patient and, perhaps without meaning to, she has conveyed this quite clearly to the patient. The message in these examples is clear. We usually convey to others information about our communication messages which communicates something about the messages themselves. In addition, we may not always be doing this intentionally; indeed we may be unaware of messages being transmitted by us on the metacommunication level.

Exercise 5. Metacommunication

Aim:	to be able to recognize in what way metacommunication can arise.
Number of persons:	2 to 20.
Materials:	none.
Time required:	5 minutes with a subsequent discussion lasting 20 minutes.
Procedure:	two people talk together. The task given to one person is: react normally to what the other person says. The task given to the other person is: react to your partner in the conversation solely with comments on the way in which she says something.
	In the subsequent discussion consider what course this conversation took. The person who must talk normally will herself start to make use of metacommunication within a very short time.

Direction

You can imagine that a conversation with a colleague will not run in completely the same way as a conversation with the head of department, although you are talking about the same thing. This is because something different is involved in the two conversations. The status of the two partners in the conversation is a factor. With a colleague you will perhaps feel more 'among ourselves' and at ease than with the head of the department.

In general two directions are distinguished which can appear in communication: horizontal and vertical communication.

Horizontal communication means communication between people with the same status or level of operating. In this form of communication the participants are equally important, in other words they have the same amount of decision-making authority; one of them does not have more power than the other. This communication is characterized by its two-way traffic. All the participants have just as much, or just as little, to say and all can join in making the decision.

Vertical communication means communication between people with differing status or power. One of them can give instructions or orders to the other, because she has more authority than the other one. The other person must do what she has been told. At most she can raise objections, but the one who does the saying decides. This communication is characterized by one-way traffic. One person says something to the other, and the other is not expected to say very much back.

Obviously two extremes have been described here. Most communication lies between these two extremes, and a mixed form generally occurs.

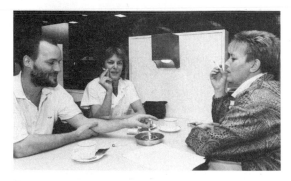

Figure 5.1.4a
Horizontal
communication

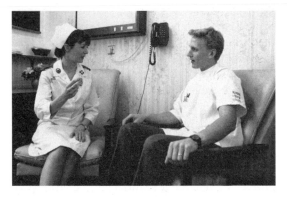

Figure 5.1.4b
Vertical
communication

Exercise 6. Direction

Aim: to be able to recognize that communication is affected by direction.

Number of persons: 2 players and observers

Materials: none.

Time required: role-playing, 2 × 5 minutes; subsequent discussion, 15 minutes.

Procedure: role-playing twice. The first time, it must be made clear to a colleague that his car is in the way, so that others cannot get past. The second time, this same message must be conveyed to the senior nurse.

The observer must pay attention to how the skills that have been described are applied.

The subsequent discussion is concerned with the differences in communication between these two role-plays.

4. Questions as communication

We are concerned here with information people convey by the questions they ask. That is, how questions tell us something about their wishes, concerns, hopes and expectations. The form of questions, and different types of questioning techniques, are discussed in the next chapter.

a. What does a question mean?

We have already suggested that when a patient asks you a question it is by no means certain whether he wants a reply precisely to that question. His question may very well be a try-out. It is possible that his question is a conversational gambit, to test out how pleasant or understanding the other person is. You may perhaps think that by reasoning in this way we are reading too much into what people say. But people often do act like that. Certain things are often not said for fear that the other person will find it odd, or will not understand it. A great deal of research has been done on communication between doctors and patients. One of the most striking findings was that patients in many cases did not get round to asking the questions they had intended to ask the doctor. They wanted information but did not ask for it. This was found to be one of the chief reasons why patients were dissatisfied with the conversations they had with their doctors.

A phenomenon which illustrates how people convey their information is what is called the door-knob phenomenon. In this scenario, people who go to the doctor with a particular symp-tom do not mention this symptom until they are about to leave. The patient instead discusses a trivial matter and only when the patient already has the door-knob in his hand in order to leave is what really matters mentioned. Many people like to circle around a difficult subject. It is as if they have to build up their confidence to discuss it.

Before people come into contact with health carers, a great deal has obviously happened to them. They do not start to think about what is wrong with them only when they are with the doctor or in the hospital. They have already thought about their symptoms, they have already weighed up whether it was worthwhile going to the doctor about them and whether the benefits (getting rid of the symptom) outweigh the drawbacks (going to the doctor, perhaps having to swallow medicines or having to adapt their lifestyle). Finally the balance swings in favour of going to the doctor, perhaps with considerations such as, 'This could be serious so it would be better for me to have it looked at early on.' The patient is unlikely to ask a doctor the question, 'Doctor, might I have cancer?' so directly. There are all kinds of reasons for not doing this, reasons which balance the need to obtain clarity on this point. The patient may think, 'What if the doctor says 'Yes'? What if he laughs at me, or gets annoyed with me for meddling in his specialist field.' Questions of this type are therefore more often gradually introduced. Other, minor questions are asked first which clear the way for obtaining an answer to the big, underlying question.

Exercise 7. Types of questions

Aim:	to be able to recognize that questions may have different meanings.
Number of persons:	individually, where appropriate to be discussed in the group afterwards.
Materials:	none.
Time required:	30 minutes.
Procedure:	write down three meanings which can attributed to the question: *'Nurse, how do you like my new wig?'* The question is asked by a patient who has lost her hair through radiotherapy.
	How can this type of question be defined?
	What do questions of this kind convey to you?
	How should you react?
	How would you react in reality?

b. Hopes and expectations

Other factors have a part to play in the types of questions people ask. We have already seen that a question need not be asked directly; it can also be asked in a roundabout way. In addition people often also have different things on their minds. If a patient has ideas about what might be wrong, he may also have ideas about what he can expect to happen. These latter fantasies can have the oddest, most illogical contents, but they do exist. On the one hand people have secret hopes about what will happen, such as, 'Perhaps there is a pill which will get rid of my symptoms' or 'I hope that I can go home in two days.' On the other hand, people have more worrying expectations such as, 'My neighbour was so ill from the anaesthetic; that'll probably happen to me too.'

Hopes and expectations need not be the same thing. Hopes are ideals, expectations have more to do with the (assessment of) reality. Both hopes and expectations can be expressed in the questions which people ask the nurse.

We have dealt in this section with the insights you can gain from the questions which patients ask you. We have not been concerned with the replies which you must give, since these obviously depend entirely on the questions. We hope, however, to have made clear, in this section and elsewhere, that the answers to questions from the patient also have to be accompanied by your (sometimes unspoken) question: 'Why are you asking that?'

Exercise 8. Hopes and expectations

Aim: to be able to recognize that hopes and expectations can be different.
Number of persons: individually.
Materials: none.
Time required: 5 minutes.
Procedure: imagine you have to ask for a day off during a very busy period.
What is your expectation for this conversation?
What is your hope for this conversation?
Which of these two has most to do with reality, the hope or the expectation?
What is the difference between the hope for such a conversation and the expectation for such a conversation?

Finally we wish to point out that when someone has a question this need not in itself mean that he will always accept the answer to this question. It may well happen that he only wants to hear a particular answer to his question.

Case study – Mrs Brown

Mrs Brown is a housewife. She has been admitted to hospital because her appendix was inflamed. She has been operated on and is recovering quickly. At home her husband and three children are doing something they never otherwise do: they are fending for themselves, cooking and washing up. Meanwhile, Mrs Brown asks Nurse Fransen, a nurse whom she has got to know well, when she will be able to go home. Nurse Fransen is surprised. Only yesterday she told Mrs Brown herself she would go home on Friday. Mrs Brown must remember that.

They talk, and during the conversation it becomes clear that Mrs Brown is dreading having to look after her family again; she is so happy with the care she has received in hospital. After she has heard this, Nurse Fransen understands better why Mrs Brown has blocked out the information about when she is allowed to go home.

Sickness gain

This phenomenon has to do with what we call sickness gain. This is the phenomenon according to which people sometimes derive benefit from being sick. You occasionally harbour the secret wish yourself to have 'flu. Along with the misery which it brings with it, being ill sometimes also produces something positive. Mrs Brown enjoyed the good care in hospital so much that she forgot (or rather, put out of her mind) what she had to go home to. It is not hard to imagine Mrs Brown suffering a complication around the time when her discharge from the hospital is approaching so that she has to stay in longer. You could say that she puts up with the misery of the complication in order to retain the 'gain' of the care. We do not wish to claim here that many people cause their own medical conditions in order to obtain attention or care, but it can sometimes be useful to try to look at the behaviour of patients in hospital in that way. It might help you to prepare patients like Mrs Brown for their approaching discharge.

When people go to the doctor, it is the result of a weighing-up process. The 'pros' and 'cons' are balanced and the 'pros' win, but sometimes only by 51 to 49 percent. So, the fact that a patient comes to the doctor does not mean that 'cons' are not still there! At most it means that the patient is considering committing himself to it. It also means that he is weighing up sickness gains against sickness losses and this may determine his *complaince* or co-orperation in treatment. This applies to people who have come to the doctor of their own volition; for people who are admitted as emergency cases, it is even less self-evident that you can count on their compliance.

It is not due to unwillingness that people find it difficult to adapt to a new situation. Reluctance to face an impending change, particularly when it relates to a new lifestyle, is a general human characteristic. You may perhaps have experienced what it is like to stop smoking. You realize then how firmly attached to habits you

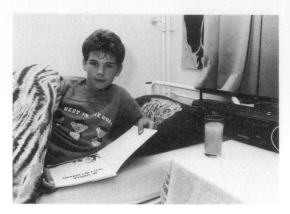

Figure 5.1.5
Sickness gain

can be. You notice that it is only now – when you are no longer allowed to – that you become aware of how often you lit a cigarette. Although you did it without thinking much about it, you discover that it is very difficult to stop this habit. That is how things often are in our lives. Without noticing it, we become accustomed to a particular habit and we also become attached to it. When we now get into a situation in which we have to give up this habit (for example because the doctor stipulates that we must), we find it difficult because there are many positive things which keep this behaviour going.

The positive consequences of a symptom or disease are thus called *the sickness gain:* what the patient gains through being ill. This sickness gain can be observed in all kinds of ways. But a patient may also dream up excuses for not co-operating or non-compliance if he feels losses outweigh gains, or he is antagonistic towards his carers.

Study activity

5. How would you describe these angry or uncooperative reactions of patients? In your answer refer to the literature you can search out on *sickness gain* and a phenomenon known as *compliance*.

Exercise 9. Sickness gain

Aim: to be able to recognize the concept of sickness gain.

Number of persons: 5 to 20.

Materials: none.

Time required: 30 minutes.

Procedure: group discussion. Everyone writes down four examples of how someone who is ill might derive benefit from this illness.

The group then discusses the following question: what is the difference between sickness gain and malingering?

5. Communication problems

As will by now have become clear, communication rarely runs flawlessly. Shortcomings in communication do not necessarily have dramatic consequences: things need not turn out disastrously in everyday life before we can speak of a communication problem. And, of course, we do not generally weigh up our words all that carefully in everyday language, and normally we have enough time and opportunity to identify and clear up misunderstandings.

During your work as a nurse, however, the situation is very different. It is of the greatest importance that communication runs as smoothly as possible and that the fewest possible misunderstandings occur. This chapter is concerned with how these misunderstandings arise.

We talk of communication problems when the intention of one person is misunderstood by the other person, when the message of *the transmitter* is not understood, or is understood in distorted form by *the receiver*. The path followed by a message from the transmitter to the receiver can be reproduced in a number of steps. Someone who wishes to make something clear to someone else must ensure that his meaning takes the following path:

1. He translates his meaning into words.
2. At the same time, or shortly afterwards, he speaks these words.
3. The words are heard by the other person.
4. The latter translates the words into a meaning.
5. The meanings attributed by both transmitter and receiver are identical.

Exercise 10. Communication problems

Aim: to be able to distinguish various communication problems.

Number of persons: individually, with subsequent group discussion.

Materials: exercises 1 to 9.

Time required: 20 minutes working individually with a subsequent discussion lasting 30 to 45 minutes.

Procedure: look at the previous nine exercises.

Point out for each exercise at which stage in the communication between a transmitter and a receiver the problem occurs.

Discuss in the group.

You will understand that a great many opportunities for misunderstandings exist. We shall now run through the five points in the path referred to above one by one.

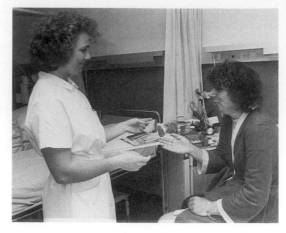

Figure 5.1.6
'Do you think that's clear to you now?'

a. The translation of a meaning into words

People often say, 'I cannot put that into words' or, 'I have no words to describe that.' These are expressions which indicate that our thoughts are sometimes difficult or impossible to capture in words. Some people are more articulate than others. But for some, less articulate people, this is the first problem area. If they have no words to describe their thoughts, how are they to transmit them? What sort of message will the receiver pick up?

Exercise 11. Communication problems: meaning in words

Aim: to be able to recognize communication problems which arise when you try to formulate words to describe a situation.

Number of persons: 5 to 20.
Materials: Figure 5.1.7.

Figure 5.1.7

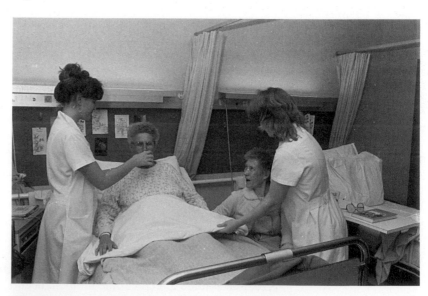

Time required: 30 minutes.
Procedure: write down for yourself what you see in this photograph. Then discuss with others in the group what they have written down.
Discuss the differences.

b. The words are spoken

If you as a native of London move house to Newcastle, you will regularly face this source of misunderstanding. Friendly people in animated discussion may lapse into a local idiom the significance or meaning of which completely escapes you. The same thing happens when a nurse in hospital says to a new patient that she is going to 'take his temp'. Words are often regarded as normal in medical circles which are completely unknown outside these circles. We call this technical jargon. Dialect, a different pronunciation, a different cultural background or just a speech impediment can produce misunderstandings or lack of clarity.

Exercise 12. Communication problems: the spoken words

Aim:	to be able to recognize communication problems associated with speaking.
Number of persons:	5 to 20.
Materials:	none.
Time required:	45 minutes.
Procedure:	each person tries to recall the last group discussion as well as possible. Agree with each other which discussion is meant.

Ask each student to summarize the discussion in writing. Then swap the summaries. Read out a number of summaries. Discuss the differences. Pay attention to descriptions of points of view, the reproduction of verifiable facts and interpretations.

c. The words which are heard by the other person

This process may also be obstructed in many ways. The words may not reach the receiver for one reason or another, for example, because an aeroplane is just passing overhead so that the message is drowned out. We use the technical term 'noise' for this type of obstruction. We also speak of noise when the television claims your attention, or when you are thinking about something else (so that you do not hear the words) while someone is speaking to you. Finally your words cannot reach the other person if he has a problem with his hearing.

Exercise 13. Communication problems: the words heard

Aim:	to be able to recognize communication problems associated with hearing or receiving words spoken by the transmitter.
Number of persons:	10 to 20.
Materials:	none.
Time required:	30 to 45 minutes.
Procedure:	ask two students to pay attention during a class. Ask the remainder of the class to be noisy. Then explain to the class what the difference is between perception and interpretation.

Ask each student to write down what they can recall of the explanation. Swap the reports. Discuss the differences. Pay attention to:
- the understanding that comes out of the descriptions;
  the number of details in the descriptions;
- the quantity of information reproduced.

d. The words are translated back into a meaning

When the words of the transmitter after over-coming the first three stumbling-blocks have finally managed to reach the receiver, the latter still has to translate them into a meaning before the message has really been conveyed. We noted in section **5.a** (the translation of a meaning into words) that thoughts or feelings cannot always be fully expressed in words.

A translation of these thoughts or feelings is always made. Logically the question is thus whether the 'back-translation' comes out with the same original meaning. The background, previous history and personality of the transmitter and receiver play a very important role in this translation and 'back-translation'. We use the term *reference framework* for this: i.e. the whole of the thoughts, emotions and attitudes with which each individual perceives the world. Since this can turn out very differently for different people, there is a great likelihood here of misunderstandings.

Question: Why are legal documents so wordy?

Exercise 14. Communication problems: the translated words

Aim: to be able to recognize communication problems associated with translating a message.

Number of persons: 5 to 10.

Materials: Figure 5.1.8.

Figure 5.1.8

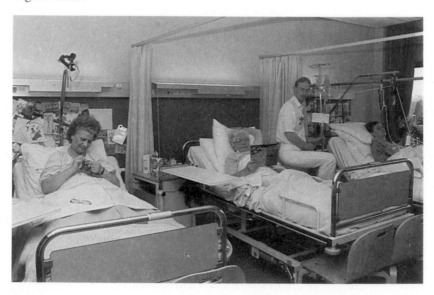

Time required: 30 minutes.

Procedure: each person makes a written description of what he sees in this photograph. Swap the descriptions. Discuss the differences. Pay attention to the difference between objective and subjective descriptions. Try to come to a unanimous description. What is left out? What was difficult?

e. The meanings are confirmed as being identical

The final stage in any successful communication is that of ensuring that the correct message got through. This usually involves *feedback*. That is, the receiver in turn feeds back what he understands he has received to the original transmitter for confirmation.

We do not normally feed back every single piece of information we receive for confirmation. This would seem odd and predestrian, unless of course the message is very important and we want to get it absolutely right. (*You are telling us that the Titanic is sinking. Please confirm that this is what you are really telling us.*) Normally, however, we simply check important facts or particularly difficult pieces of information with the transmitter just to ensure that we have got the fundamental meaning correct. This is in essence what you and your fellow students were doing when you tried to arrive at an unanimous description in Exercise 14 above.

f. Other communication problems

Alongside the misunderstandings which are concerned with the route which the message follows between the transmitter and receiver, there are also other causes of communication problems. However, these have more to do with how little one actually knows about communication in everyday life. They may involve errors of judgement about what to do or say in particular situations.

Exercise 15. Communication errors

Aim: to be able to recognize communication errors.

Number of persons: individually and to be discussed afterwards in the group.

Materials: the fragment of conversation below.

Time required: describing errors, 10 minutes; re-writing conversation without errors, 15 minutes; subsequent discussion, 45 minutes.

Procedure: part of a conversation between a nurse (**n**) and a patient (**p**) appears below. Both are at their wits' end. In this conversation a large number of pitfalls occur.
Write down what errors are made here.
Then re-write this conversation as it ought to have run, without communication errors.

n: What's this, Mr Vincent, smoking a cigar in the ward? You know you can't do that, put it out now.

p: Nurse, I am seventy-five years old, I have smoked all my life, I'm not going to give it up. I'm not going to spoil the few years I have left by suddenly stopping smoking.

n: But haven't you thought about the other patients? They are affected by the smoke from your cigar. That's no fun for them.

p: If it bothers them, they're big enough to tell me so themselves, but I've heard nothing from them. Why are you bothering about it?

n: Why am I bothering about it? There are rules in the hospital which everyone must obey, including you, Mr Vincent. One of the rules is no smoking in the ward. It would be a fine mess if everyone here started smoking. Yes, go ahead, don't let it worry you, they're just saying that for a laugh! Well that's not very nice of you. And now let's have that cigar.

p: Do you think I will allow myself to be treated like a kid? I could be your father, but if I was, you'd behave differently. Who do you think you are lecturing me like that? I am old and wise enough to look after myself, I don't need you or any part of this hospital for that matter, if you take my meaning.

n: Well if you're so clever, why don't you go home?

p: I'll do just that. I've been here long enough already.

First share the descriptions of the mistakes.
Then discuss how this conversation could have been brought to an end in a more constructive way.

Punctuation

Think back to that scene (page 396) with Mr and Mrs Archer at the beginning of this chapter. He was sitting with his feet on the table thinking how annoying it was that she was in the kitchen and did not come and sit with him. She, on the other hand, was annoyed that he was sitting back and was not helping her cook the meal. They exchanged rather cynical and sharp comments and did not come any closer to each other. He thought that she was to blame for the difficult atmosphere, while she felt that he was to blame. What these people did not realize (and it is something that everyone has difficulty with sometimes) was that people are continuously reacting to each other. Our dealings with each other can be described as a spiral. We are continuously working from previous history. So it is sometimes pointless to say who started it or who was to blame, because today's episode is based on some preceding episode, and so on: there is always something preceding the exchange.

People try to make sense of a conversation by *punctuating* its continuous flow (see for example Bateson and Jackson, 1964; McClintock, 1983). This involves pairing events which seem to have cause-effect connections. If effect, each punctuation consists of something like: *he said (cause), and then she said in response (effect)*. A total interaction sequence can be punctuated into units in this way, starting with an initial causative statement from one or other of the interactants. In conflict situations there is often dispute about which was the very first causative statement or *who started it all!* Attributing blame often assumes major proportions in arguments. Indeed the original dispute is often forgotten in a futile battle to settle this question of *who started it all* (see for example Bernal and Baker, 1979, for an excellent analysis of punctuation disputes).

Exercise 16. Punctuation

Aim: to be able to recognize punctuation problems.

Number of persons: individually with subsequent group discussion.

Materials: conversation below.

Time required: 10 minutes and a subsequent discussion lasting 30 minutes.

Procedure: read the following piece of interaction.

Write down who is to blame that this communication has gone wrong. That is, the first cause-effect punctuation.

Then share the descriptions.

Pay attention to the differences in the description.

10 o'clock in the morning.

she: I'm going to have a break now.

he: Of course, do that. I'll look after the patients; they don't have a break.

she: If you prefer me not to go, I'll stay.

he: I didn't say that. If you feel you have to have a break now, you must go.

she: If you react like that, I don't want to go any more.

he: And then I'll be blamed again for the fact that you can never take a break?

Paradoxical communication

We speak of paradoxical communication when there are apparent contradictions within the communication. These contradictions can appear in various ways. Someone says something that is in contradiction with itself. Can you for example believe someone who says, 'I am a liar'? How can you satisfy your mother when she complains, 'You always had to do what you wanted, and never did what we wanted'?

Paradoxes are highly complex forms of communication. It is difficult to recognise them at the moment they appear. A second reason why paradoxes obstruct communication is that it is so difficult to make comments on them.

Study activity

6. Think up a few examples of paradoxical communication for yourself.

Exercise 17. Paradoxical communication

Aim:	to be able to recognize paradoxical communication.
Number of persons:	individually with subsequent group discussion.
Materials:	the messages below.
Time required:	15 minutes with a subsequent discussion lasting 30 to 45 minutes.
Procedure:	Write down how you would react to the following message:

'We have always left you free to do what you wanted and never have you done anything for us!'

What messages can you recognize in the sentence above?

What do the messages say about each other?

How would you react if someone in the class rolled a cigarette, got out his lighter, looked round the class and said: 'Don't mind if I smoke, do you?'

How would you react if the teacher did this? Or the senior nurse during your performance appraisal? Or your father?

What are the differences between these four situations?

The subsequent discussion is concerned with paradoxical communication. The difficulty in making comments on this form of communication probably underlies the reactions to the four situations identified in this exercise.

Paradox

Disqualifications

A malicious way of admonishing someone is the use of what are known as *disqualifications*. Disqualifications are apparently honest comments which are made as sly digs to make it clear to the other person that he is doing or saying something wrong. The mean thing about disqualifications is that you can scarcely make comments on them because they happen so casually. They occur in many forms; we shall discuss a few of these.

Generalizations

If you are annoyed with someone who arrives late in the department and you talk in general terms to no-one in particular about people who come late, always being slovenly and how you cannot rely on them and so on, you are disqualifying through generalizations. You are making a sly dig at the person who was late, whilst you are purporting to talk about late-comers in general.

Asking questions which are intended as comments

'Do you really mean that?' 'Do you consider that normal?' 'Do you do that at home as well?' These are examples of questions by which you make your comment 'clear' between the lines.

Going into an unimportant detail

People sometimes try to take the force out of an argument by attacking a detail. The discussion then continues on the detail and the basic argument is lost from view. An example might be nit-picking about minor typographical errors in an important nursing policy document.

'Funny' or denigrating talk about a group

When you refer to a gathering of women as 'a hen party', or familiarly address patients as 'the old dears', you are denigrating the group.

Study activity

7. Think of some examples of these four types of disqualifications for yourself.

You can obviously also make comments if some of these disqualifications are applied to you but there is a good chance that your remarks will be laughed off. One of the most important characteristics of disqualifications is that they are given in such a way that they can be easily drawn into a particular context: 'I wasn't talking about you personally; it was just a joke!' It is thus difficult to pin the perpertator down; to prove in fact that he/she was talking about you. Indeed, if you accuse him/her, you are often yourself accused of being oversensitive or paranoid!

6. Summary

In this chapter attention has been devoted to the various aspects of communication.

It has become clear that communication always takes place between people. It was noted that effective communication was defined in terms of exchange of information and reciprocity. Five common features of interpersonal communication were described.

As well as a general introduction to the topic of communication, the following subjects have been described:

– questions as communication;
– hopes and expectations;
– sickness gain;
– compliance.

The chapter ended with a description of common communication problems.

Aspects of conducting conversations

2

1. Introduction

Before various types of conversations are discussed in Chapter 3, the building blocks used in conducting a conversation are presented in this chapter.
It is remarkable that we rarely think about how we conduct a conversation. In fact many communication problems occur because the transmitter and receiver have not communicated effectively.
This chapter therefore deals with some of the interpersonal skills which must form part of the behavioural repertoire of any nurse. As well as the various aspects of perception, attention is also given to the following topics:
– non-verbal concomitants of verbal interactions;
– paraphrasing;
– summarizing;
– reflecting feelings;
– speaking on behalf of yourself;
– assertive behaviour.

Learning outcomes

After studying this chapter the student should be able to:
– explain how people perceive actively and passively;
– define the halo effect;
– explain what is meant by the tough interview;
– recognize and use the following skills through role-play (during a conversation)
  • looking at someone;
  • nodding;
  • relaxed body posture;
  • following verbally;
  • identifying and asking closed, open and suggestive questions;
  • identifying and asking questions within and outside the reference framework of the partner in the conversation;
  • paraphrasing;
  • summarizing;
  • reflecting feelings;
  • speaking on behalf of self;
  • formulating criticism positively;

- making wishes concrete;
- applying metacommunication as communication;
- attuning use of language to the reference framework of the other person;
- using consistent, non-paradoxical communication;
- avoiding use of disqualifications;
- displaying assertive behaviour.

2. Perception

We have at least five senses available to us by which we obtain information about the world around us. Sight and hearing are the key senses in a consideration of conversation, and we shall restrict our treatment of perception in this chapter to these two.

Hearing and seeing can be looked at from the purely physiological point of view. It is important to get to know the anatomical structures of the eye and ear and also the neurological action of these organs. But we shall not dwell on that here. Alongside the physiological and neurological action of these organs, the psychological processing of perception is important. Whether you recognize what is perceived or not is important. Your emotions too decide whether you hear something or not. These psychological aspects of perception are presented here. To make clear what we are concerned with in this section, we use the terms 'observing' and 'listening' (instead of the sensory terms 'seeing' and 'hearing').

Halo effect

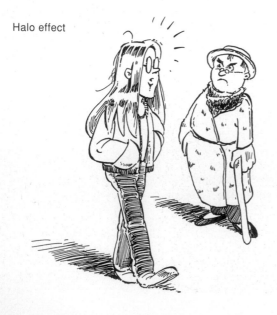

Halo effect

When we are dealing with comparative strangers, we tend to think that the other person is the same in all areas. If we consider the other person to be pleasant in a number of aspects (he is nice to his children and I can have a good chat with him about music), we tend to think that he is just as pleasant in all other aspects. It therefore appears unlikely to us that this person could be unpleasant.

The same thing occurs in dealing with people in whom we find disagreeable features. We tend to attribute an unpleasant personality to these people. We feel that nothing can be pleasant about this man or woman. This phenomenon is known as the *halo effect*.

When we react as described in the halo effect, we generalize enormously. We act as if the whole of someone is the way we perceive part of him to be. It will be clear that we are not responding to the whole of this person; we must try to perceive the other person as a personality with many different characteristics. Only then can we really offer much chance of help which is tailored to need.

When we are talking about perception, it is important to distinguish between actively obtaining information and passive perception. What we mean by this is as follows.

- Obtaining information actively means doing your best to get to know something. You can try to make something clear for example by asking the other person about it. You make an effort and take trouble to become informed. An example of this is that you watch an informative television programme with concentration, because it provides you with more information on a particular disease, information which you may well use in your work.
- Perceiving passively is concerned with things which strike you casually. They are

2 Aspects of conducting conversations

things from day-to-day living to which you do not pay much attention, but which nevertheless stay with you. You may for example think about the clothes worn by the presenter of the television programme referred to above. The things which you perceive passively have a great deal to do with yourself. They occur to you because you are in one way or another unconsciously paying attention to them.

Passive perception is a simple way of obtaining information; it takes place as it were automatically. If you pay attention to the conversations of experienced help-providers and compare them with your own conversations, you will probably notice that the experienced help-providers conduct their conversations easily. It appears that things occur to them automatically, whilst you have to have these things pointed out to you before you recognize them. In brief, it seems that they perceive far more passively than an inexperienced help-provider. People who conduct professional conversations all day have probably acquired a better eye for all the information other people give out. Do not be discouraged by this. As you devote more attention to perception, you automatically obtain a better idea of all the information that is transmitted. By listening

you automatically learn how to listen better, and by looking you automatically learn how to look better. By practising, you learn to perceive better, so that you need to take less and less trouble over it. You then gradually start to perceive more things 'automatically'. However, one word of caution in advance. It often happens that when we are developing new skills this increased sensitivity results in a decline in performance. We may even start to perform less effectively than we did before training commenced. This phenomenon, known as *the training dip*, is however temporary. With practice in the skill, smooth functioning develops and we start almost intuitively to perform at a higher level.

The tough interview
The word interview often makes us think about behaviour associated with reporters. In the 1960s what is referred to as the 'tough' interview appeared on television. Interviews of this type, following the example set by British and American reporters, was characterized by questioning in which the interviewee was confronted with a rejection of his policy or views. The interviewer held the person questioned (the interviewee) responsible and he (the interviewer) played the role of the prosecution. The underlying intention

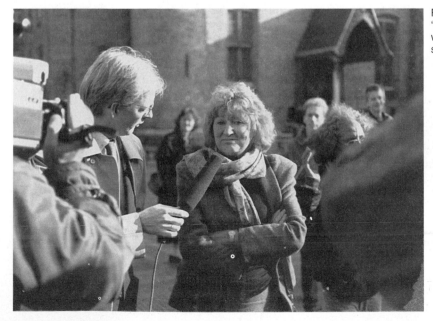

Figure 5.2.1
'Do you believe
what you are
saying yourself?'

was to entice the interviewee into making sensational statements, or ideally to make him angry. This style of interviewing has become effective as a procedure for getting sensational interviews into newspapers. The interviewee is certainly provoked and there is a great chance that he will open up.

However, the atmosphere of such an interview is very tense and there is clearly distrust in both directions. You will appreciate that this style of interviewing is not a proper way of getting at what patients have on their minds.

If you want to find out what the other person has on his mind, it is therefore important to make him feel free as much as possible to tell you what it is. You must try to achieve this by asking questions in a particular way. The person will feel free and start to open up only if you formulate your questions in such a way that he is convinced that you are seriously interested in what he wants to tell you.

How do you convey this sincerity to the person you are talking to? Imagine you are conducting a conversation with a patient who was admitted yesterday for observation. You do not know anything about her. She obviously does not know anything about you yet either, and for her that is only one of the uncertainties. She asks a great many other questions, 'What is going to happen? Will my husband cope at home without me?' and so on. We have seen in an earlier chapter that people who feel unsure cannot always overcome these uncertainties. They try to reduce uncertainty by their digressions: they start to behave more dependently than they are accustomed to in their ordinary life. They try, by paying close attention, asking many questions and looking for hidden meanings behind the answers, to find out more about what is unclear to them.

When you talk to this lady for the first time, you will probably not attach much importance to all these questions. You will probably see a woman who (perhaps rather grimly) is trying to keep up her spirits. She behaves like someone who is not afraid, like someone who can manage and who will not cause you any trouble.

Let us first look at how you can conduct a conversation with this lady, in such a way that she can get her worries off her chest.

The most important thing is to show her that you accept what she says. Make sure that you do not in any way disapprove of the questions she has to ask or the comments she has to make. In terms of learning theory you might say, 'I should reward the fact that she is telling me what she has on her mind.'

Acceptance or the opposite, condemnation, occurs very subtly. We have given some examples of communication problems in Chapter 1, Section 5. As you know, everything you say is considered to be very important by the patients, even if they do not indicate this directly. It becomes apparent for example from what you later hear indirectly, perhaps from the members of the patient's family. All the little comments made in passing, the way you look when you make them, all this is of great significance to patients who are worried.

People are very sensitive to attention. Attention forms one of the best rewards for human behaviour. Most people will therefore tell more if you give them attention.

You can indicate this attention through a number of basic skills which are easy to carry out:
- Look at the patient when you speak to him.
- Nod occasionally when the patient is talking.
- Make sure that you adopt a relaxed body posture.
- Make sure that you follow the patient verbally.

Before you close this book in indignation because you consider that this list does not do justice to the uniqueness and warmth of human interaction, you must bear in mind that these skills only work if you are sincere! We have argued earlier that we can help you to acquire a number of skills but that these in themselves are of no help if you have no interest in people. If you are not interested in others, you can at best keep a conversation going and convey correct information; this will never be capable of becoming a 'good conversation'.

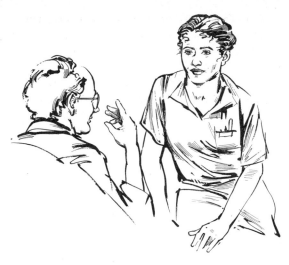

Figure 5.2.2
When you sit at someone's
bed relaxed, he will tell
you more than if you
stand over him

We have examined the basic skills associated with good and unprejudiced perception, because you must have these skills when you interact with patients. They are, in fact, the skills of active perception; that is, the skills of actively perceiving and in doing so letting the other person *know* you are actually perceiving, thus stimulating willing responses. We shall now proceed to address the important elements of active perception.

a. Looking at the patient (gaze)

The degree of eye contact has been studied at length. Very specific things about eye contact can be identified. It is known for example that a listener (receiver) looks at the other person for 25 to 50 per cent of the time that the other person is talking. This looking time is fairly evenly distributed over the whole talking time. The speaker (transmitter) looks at the other person for approximately half as long as he is looked at. In addition, the looking time of the speaker is differently distributed over the conversation compared with the looking time of the listener.

– At the start of the speaking time the transmitter looks at the receiver for a long time.
– Later on in the conversation he looks away more often, but always alternating with short glances in the direction of the receiver ('Is he still listening?' 'Is he still interested?')
– Towards the end of what he wishes to say, he looks at the receiver for a longer time again.

In this way we make clear to each other that it is now the other person's turn to say something. It is particularly through eye contact that we prevent ourselves from both talking at the same time. In addition, eye contact is an important way of gauging the attention the other person is paying to you. Just think what it is like to talk to someone who is constantly looking out of the window.

Study activity

1. If you have the opportunity to do so at college, record a conversation between two people on video. The topic of the conversation must be such that both partners in the conversation are only moderately interested. Ensure in addition that the receiver avoids eye contact with the transmitter. Pay attention to what happens.
Then do the same, with the same speakers, but this time the transmitter must speak about a topic which he finds very interesting. The receiver must try to do the same as in the previous conversation. Take note in this exercise of the difference between the behaviour of both partners in the conversations. Is there a difference in how the transmitter behaves between the first and second conversations? And the receiver, does he act differently? How would you explain the difference?

Figure 5.2.3
Eye contact

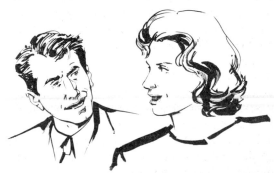

In an arbitrary conversation there are also limits to the duration of the glances or gazes. What are referred to as mutual glances last for a shorter time than individual glances. Individual glances, i.e. looking at the other person while he is not looking at you, generally do not last longer than seven seconds and mutual glances, i.e. both looking at each other, in a conversation last considerably less. The duration of mutual gaze is also influenced by intimacy. People who like each other have longer mutual gazes. In addition those involved can say fairly precisely when they are being looked at.

There is an innate interest in the shape of the eye and everything that looks like it. Children concentrate very early on in their life on the eyes of the mother. You can see quite well where he is looking from someone else's eyes, and the region around the eyes is exceptionally expressive.

Question: What exception would there be to the rule that people look the other person in the eyes when they are in conversation with each other?

Argyle (1972), a researcher who has written a great deal about eye contact, focuses attention on a number of aspects in which eyes are important:

- *Widening of pupils.* The diameter of the pupil can vary between 2 and 8 mm. In addition to the available light, excitement is a factor which affects the size of the pupil.
- *Blinking frequency.* People normally blink every 3 to 10 seconds. The humidity of the air is an influencing factor. The blinking frequency is also affected by emotional state.
- *Direction.* The look may for example be averted to the ground, when this is commonly explained as 'calmly taking everything in'; or to the ceiling, a sign of pondering.
- *Eye opening.* Wide-open eyes are a sign of surprise or shock. Downcast eyes generally convey the impression of being involved with a person who is shy or submissive.

Exercise 1. Basic skills: eye contact

Aim:	to be able to recognize amount and distribution of eye contact.
Number of persons:	2 role-players and 3 observers.
Materials:	paper for noting down observations and stop-watches or watches with second hands.
Time required:	role-play, 10 minutes; subsequent discussion, 30 to 45 minutes.
Procedure:	two students conduct a conversation on a topic which interests them both. The remainder of the group observe the eye contact of the two partners in the conversation. Get them to choose a good position for doing this. If the group is sufficiently large, appoint three observers: one observer notes how often and how long the speaker looks at the listener; a second observer notes how long and how often both partners in the conversation look at each other; the third notes how often and how long the listener looks at the speaker. Discuss and compare results in group discussion.

b. Nodding

Nodding is one of the most basic skills by which you can make it clear to another person that you are following his conversation. By nodding you encourage the other person, inviting him to continue talking. One of the difficulties in describing these forms of behaviour is that attention is artificially focused on these things. But this will make you more aware of these skills when you conduct a conversation. This applies to all the skills mentioned, but particularly to nodding. You already do that naturally during conversations and it may perhaps become more difficult once you are conscious of it. In this case just carry on nodding, as normally and spontaneously as possible, and be aware that in this way you are encouraging the other person to talk. But do not nod indiscriminately; only nod when you wish to encourage the speaker or acknowledge or agree with what he says.

Exercise 2. Basic skills: nodding

Aim: to experience that nodding is a normal, natural form of communicative behaviour; to become aware of communicative behaviour.

Number of persons: 2 role-players and a number of observers.

Materials: none.

Time required: role-play, 10 minutes; subsequent discussion, 10 minutes.

Procedure: two students conduct a conversation. The task given to one of them is to get to know as much as possible from the other person about a particular topic. The other group members are observers. The task of the listener is not to nod. The conversation must run totally naturally, except that the listener must not nod his head to show that he is following the speaker or that he agrees or disagrees with what is being said. If the listener does nod, the group must draw his attention to this.

Discuss afterwards to what extent nodding is a natural form of communication. This will be apparent from the exercise: it is almost impossible not to nod during a conversation.

The lesson of this exercise is that you do not need to make a special effort to nod during a conversation. With regard to this skill, you can usually keep to your normal way of doing things in order to achieve the best result.

c. Relaxed body posture

When someone stands up straight, chest out, shoulders back, hands on the hips and head back and looks at you in this way, you probably get the impression of being involved with a dominant person. Someone who has real power or status, on the other hand, more often adopts a very relaxed posture, for example by leaning back in his chair.

A positive attitude towards other people is expressed by bending towards them. If you sit by someone's bed relaxed, he will tell you more than if you remain standing. By sitting down you indicate that you are willing to give your time and attention to the patient. You show that you take the other person seriously and that you are curious as to what he has to say.

Figure 5.2.4
Relaxed posture

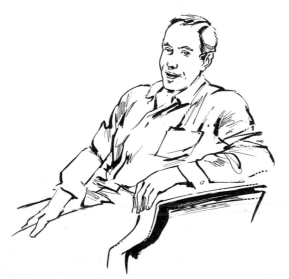

Exercise 3. Basic skills: relaxed body posture

Aim:	to be able to recognize that non-verbal and verbal behaviour should not be incongruent with each other.
Number of persons:	sets of three persons where appropriate; to be discussed afterwards in the group.
Materials:	none.
Time required:	role-play, 10 minutes; subsequent discussion, 15 minutes.
Procedure:	two students must argue with each other. Do not devote much time to choosing the topic, immerse yourself in the arguments for or against a particular opinion.

Possible topics are:

– equal distribution of income for nurses and (other) specialists;
– patients are capable of assuming responsibility for the progression of their treatment;
– you learn more in practice than at college;
– it is useful to devote a large proportion of training to social skills.

The third student in each trio is the observer.
The task given to the two players is: argue as much as you want, but stay slumped in your chairs.
The task given to the observer is: ensure that the two players do remain slumped in their chairs. As soon as one of the two starts to tense his body, the observer must intervene.
This task consists of two instructions which are mutually in conflict. You cannot argue and at the same time stay relaxed. One of the two instructions will be disregarded. You will see during this exercise that either nothing comes out of the argument or that the players do not stay sitting lazily. The latter is noticeable from moving feet (kicking movements), clenched fists, vigorous nodding of the head and so on.
Discuss the exercise afterwards.
Discuss the role that 'tension' plays in argument. Can this type of tension be utilized in a conversation? Why, and why not?

d. Following verbally

Here we come to the most difficult part of active perception in conducting conversations. Following verbally means formulating what you say so that you make the other person feel as free as possible to say what he wants to get off his chest. You are most likely to get an honest and frank answer if you do not put words in the other person's mouth. You can also make a great deal clear without words, for example by facial expression, but we shall deal with this elsewhere.

We shall be concerned here with the various formulations which you can give to your questions. You ask questions in order to find out more about something. You try to obtain an answer from the other person which contains information about the topic. There are various ways in which you can classify the different kinds of questions, for example:

– open and closed questions;
– questions within and outside the reference framework.

Open and closed questions

Open questions are questions by which you do not limit the possible replies. All answers are possible to an open question. Examples of open questions are; 'What do you like doing?' 'How do you feel about having this operation?' 'How do you like it in hospital?'

Closed questions, on the other hand, are questions to which you can only answer yes or no or with a brief, precise and usually factual answer. Examples of closed questions are; 'Do you want a cheese sandwich?' 'Is it a piercing pain?' 'I don't suppose you like being in hospital?' 'What time will your wife visit today?'

With closed questions you limit the other person's options for answering. You invite a brief, specific answer to the question you ask, but no more. The questioner has already decided what can be talked about by asking a closed question. Closed questions can also suggest a particular reply. We call this *suggestive questioning*.

Suggestive questions suggest an answer; 'You don't really want a drink, do you?' The 'answers' they elicit are of limited reliability.

If the other person wants to get something off his chest, the questioner must take particular care. We have seen that patients in a worrying situation such as during a hospital admission already have enough trouble finding things out. You do not help them by asking exclusively closed questions, and suggestive questions also work the wrong way.

An intermediate form which you must try to avoid is asking 'either...or' questions. There is no opportunity when asked the question 'Do you want coffee or tea?' to answer 'I do not want anything to drink'. Here again the patient has to go to extra trouble to make clear what he wants.

The most important rule in active perception is that when you ask questions you must try to formulate questions *openly* as far as possible.

Exercise 4. Following verbally: open and closed questions

Aim:	to be able to recognize open and closed questions.
Number of persons:	individually; and discussion in the group afterwards.
Materials:	list of questions below.
Time required:	10 minutes; subsequent discussion, 20 minutes.
Procedure:	listed below are 20 questions, of which some are 'open' and some 'closed'. Indicate for each question whether you think it is formulated as an open or closed question, and explain your opinion.

1. How is it going?
2. Do you want to do something for me?
3. Why did you do that?
4. What do you like reading in your spare time?
5. Do you think you could manage without alcohol?
6. Do you still live in London?
7. When can you help me?
8. Do you believe that yourself?
9. What are your favourite hobbies or pastimes?
10. How do you like my new shoes?
11. Do you think it's a good idea if I go on holiday on my own?
12. Don't you have to go to the eye specialist?
13. Do you by any chance know what time it is?
14. How did you get that idea into your head?
15. Who can that be from?
16. Did Avril say that?
17. Who wants to type this for me?
18. Is that everything you had on your mind?
19. What is your opinion about how this letter is worded?
20. It's a bit late, isn't it?

Exercise 5. Follow verbally: suggestive questions

Aim: to be able to recognize suggestive and neutral questions.

Number of persons: individually; and discuss afterwards in the group.

Materials: list of questions below.

Time required: 10 minutes; subsequent discussion, 20 minutes.

Procedure: the same 20 questions as in the previous exercise are listed below. Indicate for each question whether you consider this question to be suggestive or neutral. Indicate also why you think so.

1. How is it going?
2. Do you want to do something for me?
3. Why did you do that?
4. What do you like reading in your spare time?
5. Do you think you could manage without alcohol?
6. Do you still live in London?
7. When can you help me?
8. Do you believe that yourself?
9. What are your favourite hobbies or pastimes?
10. How do you like my new shoes?
11. Do you think it's a good idea if I go on holiday on my own?
12. Don't you have to go to the eye specialist?
13. Do you by any chance know what time it is?
14. How did you get that idea into your head?
15. Who can that be from?
16. Did Avril say that?
17. Who wants to type this for me?
18. Is that everything you had on your mind?
19. What is your opinion about how this letter is worded?
20. It's a bit late, isn't it?

Exercise 6. Following verbally: using open questions

Aims: to be able to use open questions.

Number of persons: individually; and discuss afterwards in group.

Materials: list of questions below.

Time required: 20 minutes; subsequent discussion, 30 minutes.

Procedure: 10 closed questions are listed below. Formulate them in such a way that they become open questions.

1. Did you have a nice holiday?
2. Is the pain in the left-hand side of your abdomen?
3. Did you have a nice sleep?
4. Do you think you are still getting better?
5. Do you also think it would be better to stop smoking?
6. That's not so bad, is it?
7. Do you understand?
8. You don't want any coffee?
9. Everything OK at home as well?
10. Are you very worried about that?

Exercise 7. Following verbally: using closed questions

Aim: to be able to use closed questions.

Number of persons: individually; and discuss afterwards in the group.

Materials: list of questions below.

Time required: 15 minutes; subsequent discussion, 20 minutes.

Procedure: 10 open questions are listed below. Formulate them in such a way that they become closed questions.

1. How do you find that?
2. What are you thinking about?
3. How could you imagine that?
4. Will you describe these headaches for me?
5. What sort of pain is that?
6. What do you feel like doing?
7. How has that come about?
8. How was your journey here?
9. What sort of drink do you prefer?
10. Will you tell me something about yourself?

Questions within and outside the reference framework

Continued questioning means trying to find out more about something by asking another question. Rule one in continued questioning is (see above) that it must be an open question; the same as has been argued for all questions applies here.

You can sub-divide questions of this type into two categories. You can continue asking about something else which *you* also want to know, for example because the other person has not thought about mentioning it. It is then a question which comes from the realm of your own thoughts, because you are curious.

A better term than realm of thoughts is *reference framework*, i.e. the whole of the thoughts, emotions and attitudes by which each individual perceives the world. This first type of 'continued questioning' derives from the reference framework of the questioner and not from the reference framework of the 'person questioned'. We therefore call this, 'continued questioning *outside* the reference framework' (of the patient).

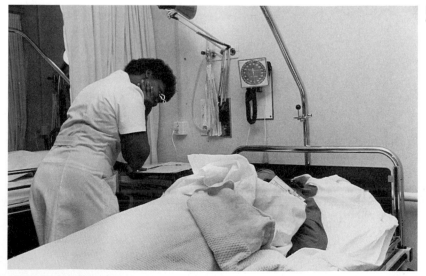

Figure 5.2.5
'How do you mean that?'

The other type naturally relates to questions for clarification of something that has already been touched on.

This is known as continued questioning *within* a reference framework.

The difference between within and outside the reference framework is a subtle one. If a patient for example says that his daughter plays the piano well, and you ask him how old his daughter is, that is a question outside the reference framework. It is a question which emanates from the realm of your thoughts, and is probably not something which the patient himself would have thought about.

The second important rule in continued questioning is that when you ask questions you should link your questions as far as possible to what the patient is telling you. A simple maxim is that you can continue asking questions on the adjectives used by the other person. 'Afraid', 'exciting', 'annoying', 'unpleasant', and so on are personal colourings which someone gives to his story. The word 'personal' says it all; these words personalize his story; they are not objective. You may know that someone is afraid of something, yet not know what it is that is frightening him, nor what he is thinking about and what he expects. It is therefore worthwhile continuing to ask questions about this.

Exercise 8. Following verbally: questions within and outside the reference framework

Aim: to be able to recognize questions within and outside the reference framework of the other person.

Number of persons: individually; and discuss afterwards in the group.

Materials: list of questions below.

Time required: 15 minutes; subsequent discussion, 30 minutes.

Procedure: a patient talks about his hobby. He is a very keen angler. He says that what he finds great about fishing is that you can sit undisturbed at the water's edge with your own thoughts.

Listed below are some questions which you could ask, prompted by the patient's story. Alongside each question an indication is given of whether this is within or outside the reference framework of the patient. Indicate why each question is within or outside the reference framework of the patient.

1. Have you been fishing for long? (outside patient's reference framework)
2. So it's the fact that nobody disturbs you, that's what you find great about fishing? (within patient's reference framework)
3. Does your wife go fishing with you sometimes? (outside patient's reference framework)
4. Do you fish for a particular type of fish? (outside patient's reference framework)
5. What do you mean, undisturbed...? (within patient's reference framework)
6. Can you tell me some more about that? (within patient's reference framework)
7. Are you often disturbed in other situations, then? (both within and outside patient's reference framework; indicate what is the good aspect of this question and what is the bad aspect)

3. Reproducing what has been perceived

It is not in itself sufficient for good contact with the patient for you to obtain information in the ways described above. It may not yet be clear to the patient that you understand what he means. It is necessary to actually show this to the patient, to reproduce it to him; only then does the other person know for certain that you understand him. It may perhaps appear an exaggeration to emphasize this so much, but it is regularly found that professional help-providers quite adequately nod, say 'ahem' and ask questions within the patient's reference framework but the patient still does not know what the other person has really understood from this. This is because the help-provider may have limited the conversation to one-way traffic. He asked suitable questions, but did not *show* that he was receiving his message. You can show the other person that you are receiving him in three ways: by paraphrasing, by summarizing and by reflecting feelings.

a. Paraphrasing

Paraphrasing means briefly stating the same thing spoken by the other person with the purpose of clarifying what that person said. The characteristic feature of a paraphrase is that it summarizes what immediately preceded it. It is no more than a brief re-statement of the last thing he said by the other person, using different words. Paraphrasing is not a matter of parroting; it is important to paraphrase at the right moment. This occurs when you sense that the other person only needs a small amount of encouragement or invitation to enlarge on what he is saying, or indeed to stop talking. You can often help him across the threshold in either direction by paraphrasing in a questioning tone.

Exercise 9. Reproducing: paraphrasing

Aim: to be able to use paraphrases.
Number of persons: individually; and discuss afterwards in the group.
Materials: list of statements below.
Time required: 15 minutes; subsequent discussion, 20 minutes.
Procedure: a number of statements by patients are listed below. Make a suitable paraphrase for each of these statements.
  - 'I am very afraid of it, nurse.'
  - 'Nurse, my husband has been coming to visit me less and less lately.'
  - 'I am so ashamed about it.'
  - 'I did laugh yesterday...!'
  - 'Do you think there's a funny smell here, or is it just me?'
  - '... and the food here is no good either...'
  - 'Oh, nurse, everything comes to an end...'
  - 'They are sitting behind me listening...'
  - 'Didn't you hear anything yesterday?'
  - 'They tell lies to you all the time here!'

b. Summarizing

Summarizing means giving a short reproduction of a longer part of the conversation. A summary reproduces the main points of what has been discussed. When you summarize, you thus necessarily limit what you include, you decide what the main points were in the other person's conversation. A summary should also always end with a question. You do not know for certain whether what you have learned from the other person is in fact the main thing which he wished to communicate. With your question, at the end of your summary, invite the other person to correct you if you are wrong, or to add something if you have been incomplete.

A summary generally has the following form: 'So if I understand you correctly, the doctor has not told you much about what he is going to do.

For that reason you do not know what will happen to you and want to know how long you have to stay here. Is that right?'
You thus give the other person the opportunity to confirm (or deny) that you have understood the message correctly. In this way the other person can easily make any additions that are necessary.

A summary is best if you also put it in your own words. If you do not do so, it tends to look like mere repetition, or parroting, imitating what has been said without understanding it.

A good summary:
– reproduces the main points of what has preceded it;
– is formulated in the summarizer's own words;
– ends with a question.

A summary has a stimulating effect, certainly if it ends with a question so that the other person is invited to carry on talking. The other person will also react to an incorrect summary. This does not mean that you must expressly attempt to make your summaries incorrect; it works better if you get it right!

Exercise 10. Summarizing

Aim: to be able to use summaries.
Number of persons: individually; and discuss afterwards in the group.
Materials: fragment of conversation below.
Time required: summarizing, 5 minutes; subsequent discussion, 15 minutes.
Procedure: part of a conversation between a nurse and a patient is given below. The patient is talking.
Write a summary of what is said.

'Yes, you know, I have not felt at my best recently, with this dizziness. And my wife has always said take that walking-stick with you, then at least you will have a bit of support. But when I took the thing with me a couple of times I had nothing but trouble from it. And I don't like walking with it, because that makes you disabled, I think. People look at you if you walk with a stick. No, I'd rather stay at home.'

Swap the summaries. Discuss them. Pay attention to the features of a good summary.

Do the same with the following piece of text:
'But now he's out of work and that takes some getting used to, you know. At first I thought: that's handy, he can do some jobs around the house and collect the children from school. But that's not the way it's gone at all. He just sits around. I don't like the man he's turning into ...'

c. Reflecting feelings

Reflecting feelings means reproducing particulary the emotional undertone. In a summary the emphasis is on the factual content of the conversation, whilst here we are concerned particularly with the emotional content. Generally the factual features of conversations are reproduced and not, or very inadequately, the emotional aspects. The good listener sees and hears these emotions constantly recurring in the conversation. But they are often not mentioned by the listener and the emotional undertone may dominate the whole conversation as a source of misunderstanding. This pitfall can be avoided by reflecting the feelings or emotions of the other person. This can take the following form: 'I have the impression you are getting angry about that as well, am I right?'
We often worry about 'stirring up a hornet's

nest'. This can also be given as a reason for not asking about feelings, but by not asking you are letting the other person down. If you decide not to examine these feelings, you make the other person's choice for him. You decide that feelings will not be talked about. On the other hand, if you present the other person with a choice, he can decide for himself. If he genuinely has no interest in discussing his feelings, he may indicate this. However, it is often helpful to facilitate a release of feelings. What is so awful about feelings? Perhaps these worries or distress were so bottled up that it is a great relief to be able to talk about them or have a good cry. The misunderstanding is often that the person who has heard all this thinks he then has to *do* something. This is usually unnecessary. The most important thing is to be there for a moment. Do not condemn what the other person says at that moment. Show understanding and try to accept that the other person finds something difficult. If someone is distressed, a glass of water, a handkerchief and a comforting hand are usually of more help than an objective response.

Exercise 11. Reproducing: reflecting feelings

Aim:	to show awareness of reflections of feelings.
Number of persons:	individually; and discuss afterwards in the group.
Materials:	fragment of conversation below.
Time required:	reflection of feelings, 5 minutes; subsequent discussion, 15 minutes.
Procedure:	part of a conversation between a nurse and a patient is given below. The patient is talking.
	Reflect the emotions which emerge in this fragment of conversation, as if you are the nurse. Write down the reflection of feelings.

'Oh, you know the way it is, nurse. They have their own lives. My daughters all have young children, and that doesn't leave you with much time. I know that all too well from when they were little themselves. You're running round after them all day long. No, that doesn't always leave you with time to go and see your mother in hospital.
All the same it's hard, you know...'

Swap the reflections of feelings which have been written down. Discuss them afterwards. What are the features of a good reflection of feelings?

4. Reacting and contributing

Reacting goes further than acknowledging what you have heard. Reacting means that, having perceived what the other person wants to say and having indicated this in your initial responses to him, you now proceed to respond to those 'messages' you have received with your own 'messages'. However in good communication, particulary in a therapeutic or caring situation, it is not enough to be reactive all the time. You must be *proactive* as well. That is, you must *contribute* something yourself – explaining something or conveying information in such a way that the other person understands it. A number of rules have to be observed. We will deal with these rules one by one.

a. Speaking on your own behalf

When you want to make something clear to the other person, it is best to speak on behalf of yourself. Do not conceal yourself behind some authority or other. Only if you speak on your own behalf can you really motivate the other person to acknowledge and accept what you want to make clear to him. You are in a better position then to find out what the other person's views are, having given your own ideas. You can help him to assess the pros and cons of his situation and you can exchange ideas with him.

Figure 5.2.6
Explaining

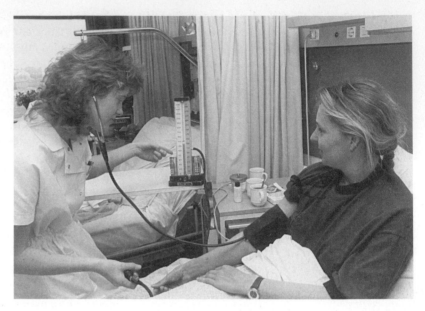

If you speak on behalf of someone else or on behalf of an authority ('the doctor says that it's better'), you are no more than a postman delivering the letter.

b. Do not ask questions if you want to convey something

If you want to tell the other person something, tell him straight. This is better than circling round the problem, asking questions. There are two reasons for this. Firstly it is very annoying for the other person to be aware that you have news for him but that you cannot get to the point. This is not to the benefit of the other person and you make it more and more difficult to break the news afterwards. (See also Chapter 3, Section 7, the bad news conversation.)

Secondly you suggest by asking questions that the other person has a choice. You make it seem as though he has an input to make, which he does not have if you want to inform him of something. He can obviously react later, but you must first convey the message as clearly as possible.

c. Do not read thoughts

If you have to tell someone something, take account in your mind of how this person will react. You almost automatically have a picture of this. It is very tempting to let this picture affect your presentation of the message. To a certain extent sympathizing is good, because

you obviously take some account of how the other person will react. However, you must not go too far with this and put a reaction into the other person's mouth. Do not formulate your message as follows: 'You will obviously find this bad news, but you will have to stay for a few more days. You will probably think: how am I to tell my wife? But it really is necessary!' The likelihood of your hitting the target with this predicted reaction is not very great, and you run the risk of doing more harm than good.

d. No veiled use of language

If news is bad, it is commonly 'packaged', as it were. Thus you talk in such cases not about, 'a bad result from the test' but of 'a little patch on the X-ray'. Or the message is generalized: 'after all's said and done, smoking is not good for people'.

Call things by their name, since that benefits clarity and ultimately serves the interests of the other person best.

e. Formulate your criticism positively

People accept criticism more readily if it is formulated positively. There are a number of rules which the formulation of criticism must meet for it to be taken to heart. The most important of these are:
– formulate your criticism in sentences containing the word 'I';

- state what you are critical about in terms of behaviour;
- along with your criticism say also what you would rather see.

f. Make your wishes concrete

If you say, 'Be a bit more relaxed', it is difficult to imagine what precisely you have to do to meet this wish. If the wish is formulated as behaviour, for example 'Breathe very calmly, stay sitting and pay attention to your body posture...' the other person will know better what you mean. The other person can obviously always decide not to comply with this wish; that is his own choice. The fact that he does not conform to your wish has nothing to do with the way in which you have made your wish clear.

g. Use metacommunication when communication does not run according to your wishes

If you stick to the guidelines described in the preceding sections, there is a good chance that communication will proceed smoothly. However, this is not always the case and a conversation may not run smoothly, despite all the good rules. One way of getting out of this is to use metacommunication. Metacommunication means communication on communication; it is thus the comments that you make on the way in which the other person says something. These sentences illustrate this: 'We can't get out of it that way. Whenever I suggest something, you reject it. Why is that?' This is sometimes precisely what you must do if communication does not run smoothly, despite your applying all the rules correctly. If you notice that the conversation constantly becomes stuck or if you notice that certain subjects are systematically avoided by the other person, you must bring that into the open. Say that you have noticed this and ask the other person whether he also is aware of it. Ask whether he wishes to talk about it, or tell him that it is (for this or that reason) important to talk about it, even if it is very difficult for him. Finally it may also be useful to apply metacommunication in the case of positive experiences. It is very pleasant to note together that a conversation has been good. Even if you just remark that the conversation always runs smoothly

when you are talking to the patient about his work, this can provide considerable insight into the things that are important to the patient.

h. Attuning use of language to the reference framework of the other person

We have defined reference framework earlier as the whole of the thoughts, emotions and attitudes with which each individual perceives the world. It is the spectacles through which you perceive the world. Your reference framework determines how you view words such as 'operation' and 'examination'. It is helpful if you adapt your use of words to what words the other person uses. This certainly applies to the use of technical jargon: for someone to whom the medical world is completely alien, it is best to avoid the word 'ECG', whilst you would not talk to a fellow nurse about 'a kind of recording of the heart'. This applies just as much when you are talking to other people about more sensitive subjects, such as making love. It improves effective communication particularly in this connection, if you find out what words the other person uses, so that you yourself can use these words as well.

Study activity
2. Think of four examples of use of language which are not suited to a particular person you know, such as a relative or a patient

i. Use consistent, non-paradoxical communication

We have indicated that paradoxical communication does not always take place consciously. As you may recall, even when we say something clearly, the way we say it and our non-verbal cues may be telling the other person something entirely different! It is important to ensure that your words can only be interpreted in one way. Avoid hidden meanings in your words and your use of language. We have already given examples of this in Chapter 1, Section 5, where we discussed communication problems. It may be tempting to voice your disapproval by a small remark to make a dig or to try via a question to make something clear. Be fully aware that these are diversions which probably do more harm than good. Be clear and unambiguous. Ensure that your verbal and non-verbal transmissions are consistent. Only then have you done everything to make your information understandable to the other person.

Study activity
3. Think of four examples of inconsistent communication you have recently witnessed. Consider each case and decide the ways in which they were inconsistent or inadequate.

j. Avoid use of disqualifications

We have already discussed disqualifications in Chapter 1 Section 5. As you will recall, these are comments which denigrate what the other person says and by so doing have the effect of sanctioning or punishing him. For example, if the patient says he is in pain, the nurse may respond by saying, 'Oh come on now, it's not that bad is it? You're being childish now!' You should always respond to the patient with genuine concern. The problem may seem trivial to you but it is very real to him.

Assertive behaviour
In your dealings with other people, you soon recognize the presence or absence of a particular characteristic which we call 'self-assurance'. It is a characteristic which is fundamental to all social skills which are described in this book. With some justification you could call it a character trait, although in different situations the same person can display very different degrees of self-assurance. The technical term for self-assurance is 'assertiveness'.

Assertiveness refers to your decision about whether you will react or not. Are you prepared to stand up for yourself, or would you rather let this chance pass by? Does it matter towards whom you have to stand up for yourself? These are questions which are concerned with assertiveness. Ultimately, if you dig deep into the reasons for your behaviour, what it will come down to is that this choice, whether or not to react, has a great deal to do with your belief in yourself. You constantly draw up the balance between your own interests and those of the other person. You perhaps assume that if you choose the interests of the other person, you will not be bothered by this person. Generally this may often be the case. Very often you may well feel a little frustration at this but in many cases it is very understandable to choose the interests of the other person rather than your own interests. We are thinking here of situations of people in need.

You must obviously choose the interests of the other person in this type of case, even if they do not entirely coincide with yours. This is a sacrifice which is inherent in your work and which you therefore have to accept. However, situations can also be imagined in which your first reaction is to give way, although you later regret it. You have then done something which was entirely unnecessary, which the other person could easily have done himself. When you think back on it later, you perhaps feel like a servant who has been used because she was unwilling to say no.

At moments like this it is right to examine your motives. What were the reasons why you did what you were asked (or told), without really wanting to? Was it because you were brought up to do what you were asked to do without grumbling? Or was it the

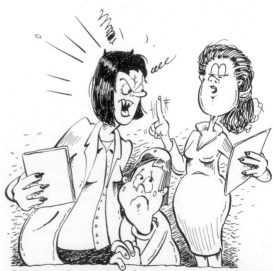

AGGRESSIVE — SUBORDINATE — ASSERTIVE

memory of the one time when this person you are interacting with lost his temper - something you do not want to experience again? Or is it perhaps the prospect of the fuss which a refusal would entail and which is probably out of proportion to the small trouble of just doing it?

Examine your motives and try to determine the boundary between the things which you do ('Oh, come here, I'll do it. No, it's no trouble') and the things which you no longer do for someone else. After you have found out why you do these things, it is perhaps sensible to ask yourself if it is sensible to continue doing them. There will, of course, be situations in which you cannot do otherwise. But look at the situations about which you were dissatisfied later, when you looked back. Are there not rather too many of these? If you swallow a little frustration from other people every day, is that not rather too much in the long run?

If questions of this kind apply to you or if you answer them all in the affirmative, it may be useful to read a few tips on assertive behaviour. These tips follow below:

- Assertiveness is not simply making a scene. It is simply standing up for your rights. You have rights to things like anyone else. We are talking here about very basic rights, some of which are even laid down in a job description. They are rights which you can demand and you are unwise if you do not do so.

- We have talked about more cautious or less self-assured behaviour than was necessary. The technical term for this is sub-assertive behaviour. You can also exaggerate it and act in too self-assured a fashion. We call this super-assertive or aggressive behaviour and this means that you attack the other person. That is not necessary either. By attacking you invite a counter-attack. You ask the other person as it were to react to your attack. Most people react to aggression with aggression. Such conversations will eventually finish up with angry or hurt people who are no longer listening to each other.

- The best way of standing up for yourself is therefore what is known as assertive behaviour. By this we mean telling the other person calmly and with self-assurance that he is asking you something or instructing you to do something which you do not need to do and which you therefore do not intend to do. In a subsequent chapter a number of rules are described which you must think about when you comment on someone else's behaviour. We call these the feedback rules. You must make sure during assertive behaviour that you observe these feedback rules closely. Other important rules for your assertive behaviour are:
  • summarize what the other person wants from you in the most concrete possible terms;
  • say that you are not doing that;
  • stay calm and substantiate your point of view;
  • avoid making a judgment of the other person and avoid condemning the other person; this does not concern the other person - it concerns you; what you know for certain is that you must make your position clear;
  • feel satisfied afterwards; do not fall into the trap of feeling guilty yourself; obviously it is unfamiliar and obviously the other person was surprised by you; at least he now knows your point of view.

k. React to resistance appropriately

Study activity

4. What does the word 'resistance' say about the person who is resisted?

In Module 1 you learnt what resistance was and what functions it can have. If people display resistance, how must you react to it?

Resistance tends not to be clearly expressed. People do not always say straight out that they do not want something. Resistance more often takes the form of sneaking opposition, unwillingness, setting about a task laboriously. When you observe this, it is no good trying to convince the other person that he had better do what you tell him. That does not work. You do not try to

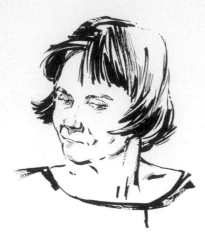

Figure 5.2.7
Nevertheless,
I no longer agree...

force the other person, because he may have good reasons for his unwillingness, for displaying resistance. This is nevertheless done a great deal. There are innumerable fruitless discussions conducted with people who are well aware that what is proposed is perhaps better, but who for other reasons are unwilling to co-operate.

We have seen in Chapter 1 of this module (see for example sickness gain, compliance and non-compliance) what the reasons for this might be.

If you observe resisting behaviour in a patient, it may be possible for you to help to limit this behaviour Mention the behaviour and ask why the patient is doing it, and ask about the background to this attitude. You may perhaps get an answer which gives more of an insight into his motives. If you know his motives, you are also able to give him the correct care. The patient may persevere in his opposition. But the likelihood of a patient giving up his opposition is small if you do not give him the opportunity to discuss the motives for his behaviour. Only then are you likely to help him overcome his resistance.

5. Summary

Every person perceives constantly: passively and actively. Passive perception takes place casually, without great effort. Active perception takes far more trouble. It is a conscious activity in which it is important to perceive accurately. This is not particularly easy. Just think of the football referee who has to correct his perception afterwards with the aid of the action replay.

In this chapter we have addressed the importance of perception in interpersonal communication. Important elements which assist us in perceiving accurately were discussed. Means of reproducing and thus confirming what is perceived were considered; in particular, paraphrasing, summarizing and reflecting feelings. The chapter concludes with a section on reacting and contributing during interpersonal communication.

The professional application of communication skills

3

1. Introduction

Nurses conduct innumerable conversations with patients, colleagues and other professionals. The importance of a chapter on professional communication therefore does not require further explanation. For the conducting of a conversation it is important for a nurse to master the sub-skills of structuring a conversation well:
– agreeing an agenda;
– summarizing;
– announcing procedure;
– distributing time;

During the actual interaction, the nurse must be able to commence, conduct and conclude an interaction appropriately. In this chapter we identify the various skills involved and discuss how the nurse might address these. The chapter includes a discussion of the various kinds of conversations:
– history-taking conversation;
– problem conversation;
– advisory conversation;
– bad news conversation;
– supporting conversation.

In the final section before the summary, the nature of the nurse-patient relationship is addressed.

Learning outcomes

After studying this chapter the student should be able to:
– recognize the following skills with regard to structuring:
  • agreeing an agenda;
  • summarizing;
  • announcing procedure;
  • distributing time;
– describe the social skills involved in beginning, conducting and concluding social interactions;
– describe two phases of the history-taking conversation;
– describe the following conversations:

- history taking conversation;
- problem conversation;
- advisory conversation;
- bad news conversation;
- supporting conversation;
- conduct conversations of all five types in simulated situations;
- discuss the nature and major components of the therapeutic nurse-patient relationship.

2.   Structuring

In this section the various aspects of structuring are discussed. Structuring is giving form to a conversation or social encounter in such a way that the nurse maintains sufficient control over progress and the topics discussed.

a. Phases in a conversation

Conversations which you conduct as a nurse are conducted with a particular aim. In order to achieve this aim you need a particular route by which the aim is achieved in the most efficient way. Depending on the purpose of the conversation, particular conversation structures are available to you. We shall only touch on a few here, the various types of conversations being discussed at greater length later.

Structuring

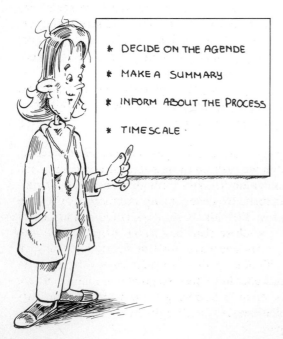

You can always discover various phases in a conversation. The phases are generally to be distinguished from each other by different social skills shown in each phase.

The various types of conversations which you conduct to achieve different aims can be distinguished by different phasing. For example, in a history-taking conversation the desired sequence of the different social skills is as follows:

- In the first phase you must find out properly what the patient wants to ask you. You must make it possible for the patient to tell you what is on his mind. The important thing in this phase is putting the patient at ease and conveying your respect for and acceptance of him. The relationship between you and the patient is established in this phase. You can ensure a good start by making use of the skills mentioned under 'Perception', Section 2 of the previous chapter.

- Then, in the second phase, it is important to obtain answers to the questions on the history-taking form. You must ask specific, closed questions for this purpose. The patient then only needs to answer briefly, so that there is less strain on him.

  Here you are using the questioning skills described in Chapter 2, Section 2 *and* establishing the accuracy of the answers (i.e. what you perceive) as explained in Section 3 of the same chapter.

- Finally, in the third phase, you discuss together with the patient how appropriate help can be given. In doing so the nurse gives more information (see 'Reacting and contributing', Chapter 2, Section 4).

You thus note that in a history-taking conversation there are three phases which can be distinguished, in which the nurse in each phase does something differently, making use of different skills. This also applies to other types of conversations such as the bad-news conversation, the problem conversation and the advisory conversation. These will be discussed in later sections.

b. Skills

All conversations have their own desired structure and this must be monitored during the course of the conversation. The nurse is the appointed person to do that, the patient having other things on his mind. You must keep to this desired sequence so that you do not cause any harm in conversation, or spend too much time on it. The skill with which you do this is called structuring. By structuring you prevent a conversation becoming literally endless. You indicate by means of structuring where the beginning and end of the conversation are. You indicate what belongs to the topic of the conversation and what does not. You thus as it were make clear the limitations within which the conversation will take place. This means that you must have a picture beforehand of what it will be possible to achieve with the conversation. You do not need to know precisely what will be presented as the content of the conversation. But you must know beforehand in what phases the conversation could run. Structuring means in other words that you yourself make a kind of agenda in which you distribute the available time and to which you adhere as closely as possible. Structuring is a combination of the following skills.

Agreeing an agenda
You can tell the other person beforehand what is going to happen. By agreeing such an agenda beforehand and keeping to it you make it easy for the patient to realize what is happening.

Summarizing
By summarizing you give the other person an insight into the structure of the conversation. In Section 3 of the previous chapter we indicated how a good summary must be given.

Announcing procedure
If for example you change over to different types of questions, inform the patient of this. In so doing you mark the transition from one phase to another, from one procedure to another. You ensure in this way that the patient does not have difficulty in adjusting to the changed nature of the conversation.

Distributing time
Try to distribute time as evenly as possible between the different phases. We intentionally say 'evenly' and not 'equally', because you obviously cannot predict precisely how long the discussion of a particular topic will last. However, if you have made it clear beforehand what will come and – approximately – how long it will last, it is easier to keep to it.

3. Use of communication skills

In Chapters 1 and 2 of Module 5 various aspects of communication skills were considered. If you scan these chapters again you will recall the importance of two-way communication. In fact there is a *communication loop,* as illustrated in Diagram 5.3.1.

When Person A initiates a communication, Person B responds. For the conversation to continue, when Person A receives feedback he in turn responds, and so on, until the social encounter ends. During this encounter the participants look, listen, receive and perceive messages, and transmit their own messages in responses.
Messages involve not only verbal messages, but also non-verbal, paralinguistic and meta-communication messages.

It is widely assumed, as is indeed often the case, that we pick up these social or communication skills incidentally through processes of socialization. However, many ordinary people have great difficulty with social skills, in some cases so much so that they never integrate well into society and have great difficulty in getting on with other people. In some cases difficulties in this area have been so great that individuals are labelled as suffering from mental illness, particularly personality disorders or even schizophrenia.

Diagram 5.3.1
The communication loop

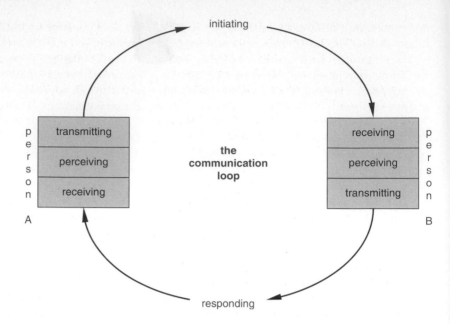

It is only fairly recently that some have argued that much maladaptive social behaviour is a result of social skills deficits and that the most appropriate approach may be educational rather than medical. For example, Authier et al. (1975) state that: 'the educational model means psychological practitioners seeing their function not in terms of abnormality (or illness) → diagnosis → prescription → therapy → cure; but rather in terms of dissatisfaction (or ambition) → goal setting → skill teaching → satisfaction (or goal achievement)'.

The recognition that the elements of good communication are social skills which can be learned rather than some intrinsic and almost innate property of the individual has been well argued in recent times. Good examples can be found in the work of Trower et al. (1978), Ellis and Whittington (1981) and Hargie (1986).

It you have not already become conscious of the fact that nursing is essentially an interpersonal activity you will very soon appreciate this. In effect, nursing is an occupation which involves communicating with patients or clients, fellow professionals, patients' families and others. Indeed, in some instances the communication itself is the actual therapeutic tool the nurse is using, rather than a wound dressing or a medicine. These communication skills can, as argued above and in Chapter 1, be learned. In the case of nursing we must learn to apply these skills in a very special and professional way which will benefit patients.

This is of course true for most of the caring professions. For medical students, Irwin and Bamber (1984) emphasize the importance of learning social skills in the medical interview or consultation situation. They emphasize the importance of beginning, conducting and concluding an interaction with a patient appropriately and effectively. The elements of such a communication encounter are worthy of a brief review here. As we proceed to consider the broad structure of particular types of encounter, we must keep in mind the important elements which make up such encounters.

The main elements can be summarized, as follows:
1. *Beginning the interaction.* This relates to how a nurse might commence an interaction. Factors such as the physical approach, the nurse's countenance, how she introduces herself and the topic, use of nonverbal 'welcoming' activity, e.g. appropriate touching or shaking hands, are pointers to effectiveness.

2. *Body posture*. This is how the nurse uses bodily position throughout the interaction. Features such as proximity, state of relaxation, sitting at eye level as opposed to standing above, looking down, may be pointers to effectiveness.

3. *Eye contact*. The presence or absence of eye contact, the frequency of contact, the 'naturalness', warmth and expressiveness of gaze are all important factors in effectiveness.

4. *Attentive listening*. It is important not only to actually listen to the patient but to demonstrate this by non-verbal cues, e.g. nodding, visibly concentrating on what the patient is saying.

5. *Use of facilitation*. This relates to the extent to which the nurse stimulates and encourages the patient to contribute. Such factors as allowing the patient time to respond, actively encouraging a response through verbal requests and non-verbal gestures may be pointers to effectiveness.

6. *Confrontation*. This is in essence facing the patient with issues in an appropriate manner. Thus, the nurse may demand an answer or acknowledgement of some fact, or present the patient with a proposition and ask for a response. The extent to which the nurse can enable the patient to confront an issue while avoiding undue distress is an important pointer to effectiveness.

7. *Use of silence*. This relates to the nurse's capacity to tolerate silence, and even to bring about and maintain silence if this is the appropriate thing to do in a particular situation. Effective use of silence may be demonstrated by the nurse's capacity to sit in a quiet and relaxed manner while allowing the patient time to collect his thoughts and decide on how to respond, without forcing the pace; or perhaps the capacity to sit quietly, holding a patient's hand when he is distressed.

8. *Style of questions*. This involves the nurse's capacity to pose questions in a clear and concise manner, using language and explanation appropriate to the patient and the circumstances. Questions may be closed and aimed at obtaining concrete information or open and aimed at encouraging a patient to be more expressive about a particular issue. Factors such as how questions are sequenced, e.g. starting off with open questions and zeroing in on specific issues with increasingly more closed questions; avoidance of leading or suggestive questions, i.e. questions which encourage the patient toward a particular answer (e.g. 'You don't really want to go home this weekend, do you?'); and avoidance of a threatening demeanour (e.g. 'What exactly do you think you are doing?') are pointers to effectiveness.

9. *Absence of jargon*. The nurse should avoid jargon which may be meaningless to the patient. This is particularly the case with complex technical terminology (e.g. 'We will be needing an ESR, a CAT-scan and an MSSU'). Some jargon is of course acceptable and indeed the patient may expect you to use it. For example a term such as 'loo' may be more acceptable to an adolescent than the term 'water closet', which he/she may not even understand. Conversely, saying to an adult male, 'Just pop your tiddly in this bottle', may be viewed as disparaging and offensive.

10. *Appropriateness of interrupting the patient*. Such appropriateness is often dependent on the actual social situation. In some circumstances it may be appropriate and necessary to intrude when a patient is doing something (e.g. at the toilet) or talking to someone else (e.g. his wife or girlfriend); at other times this might be most inappropriate. Appropriateness is also a factor in the course of interaction with a patient. It may for example be necessary to cut in when a patient is saying something important which you wish him to elaborate upon. Important factors in effectiveness are how the nurse quickly identifies the need and how smoothly and inoffensively she interrupts the patient.

11. *Keeping the patient to relevant matters*. This relates to the nurse's capacity to keep a patient's attention directed toward an issue. The nurse may use such devices as interrupting, asking questions which bring the patient back to the topic, or diplomatically

referring back to the original issue herself. The nurse must of course have the capacity to interpret reasons behind the patient straying off the topic. Sometimes, this is just a situation where the patient has difficulty in attending. However, it may also be the case that digressing is a meta-communication message, i.e. the patient is conveying the message that he does not want to remain with a very painful topic, such as his incurable cancer. In such circumstances careful judgement must come to bear in deciding whether or not it is the right time and right place to insist on the patient returning to a topic he is not ready to cope with yet.

12. *Picking up verbal cues*. The nurse achieves this by active listening and then perceiving and interpreting what the patient is saying. Confirming that verbal utterances have been received by nodding, repeating what the patient has said in different words or asking questions about what the patient said are all effective means of letting the patient know that he has been listened to.

13. *Picking up non-verbal cues*. The nurse achieves this by being actively observant. This includes the capacity to interpret general countenance, facial expression or – more easily – hand waving and gestures. It is very important that the nurse is sensitive to such 'messages' as tearfulness, pallor, pinched expression, the way in which the patient grasps her hand.

14. *Ability to clarify*. This is an important communication skill, the capacity to explain clearly to a patient. Effectiveness can be demonstrated by: the use of clear, simple language; taking time to explain carefully and in a relaxed manner; giving the patient time to respond and to ask questions; checking that the patient has understood by asking him questions on the information conveyed; repeating aspects of the message in more simple or different language where necessary (i.e. paraphrasing) until it is clear that mutual understanding has been achieved.

15. *Covering of psychological aspects*. This relates to the nurse's capacity to address and respond appropriately to observed psychological needs in the patient. That is, to re-

spond to the patient's expression of distress, fear, anxiety, boredom, inactivity, happiness. For example, does the nurse accurately identify particular verbal and non-verbal cues as expressions of great fear about a surgical operation and respond appropriately by taking time to sit with the patient, perhaps hold his hand, discuss and explain, get the surgeon or theatre Sister to come out and have a chat with him?

16. *Covering of physical aspects*. The nurse must address and respond appropriately to observed physical needs in the patient. That is, she must respond to the patient's state of need for food, fluids, excretion, elimination, rest, freedom from physical pain, warmth, cleanliness, etc. Most patients will ask for a drink when they are thirsty. However, the nurse may not always pick up non-verbal cues such as a dry mouth, furred tongue or cracked lips from the patient who is afraid or unable to ask for a drink. Even in cases when patients can and do ask for assistance, the nurse's response is an essential element in effectiveness. For example, returning with a bed-pan 30 minutes after a request would be a serious breach of good nursing standards of care.

17. *Covering of social issues*. This relates to the nurse's capacity to address and respond appropriately to observed social needs in the patient. That is, she must respond to the patient's need for social intercourse, self-esteem and social relationships. This may involve the nurse in activities which sometimes in the past were not only considered unimportant but actively frowned upon. Such activities may include chatting with patients, amusing them, stimulating conversation, playing board games, discussing current affairs, dealing with social problems at work, school or home.

18. *Presence of empathy*. This is the extent to which the nurse has insight into, or understanding of, the patient's situation from the patient's point of view. Authier (1986) defines 'being this as attuned to the way another person is feeling and conveying that understanding in a language he/she can understand.' Empathy is a vital component

of the nurse-patient relationship – for only by understanding the patient in his social world, from his point of view, can the nurse truely proceed to relate to him and help him. Many of the skills identified above are necessary for empathy: careful, active listening; constructive questioning; close observation and accurate interpretation of verbal and non-verbal cues; analysing what the patient says. All these are important skills for developing true understanding of the patient. But empathy must also be confirmed by sharing. The nurse must reiterate what the patient has conveyed; she must reflect back to him verbally and non-verbally that she appreciates what he is thinking and feeling; and most important of all, she must convey to the patient that she is truly and genuinely concerned about his feelings and concerns. It is only when this occurs that a therapeutic nurse-patient relationship begins to develop.

19. *Quality of exposition*. This relates to the nurse's overall contribution to the verbal element in communication. This concerns the capacity to: speak clearly and at a desirable speed; use short, simple sentences; avoid of large or complex words and convoluted grammar; speak in a relaxed and non-threatening manner; mesh her speech with that of the patient, i.e. leaving openings for the patient to contribute at appropriate points, ensuring that comments and responses flow smoothly throughout the conversation and avoiding embarrassing silences while not forcing the pace when silence is the right and most comfortable state at a particular point. In short, nurses must be good talkers as well as good listeners.

20. *Terminating the interaction*. Final 'completion' or 'closure' of a social encounter is one of the most difficult social skills to master. There is firstly the need to sense that a conversation should naturally come to an end at a certain point. There is next the need to choose the most appropriate closure behaviour. This should usually involve ensuring that the patient is also ready to end the exchange; indeed, it may be important to allow the patient to take the initiative in commencing the closure behaviour. It is highly important that the nurse makes appropriate departure or farewell statements. In a brief encounter with a patient who is an old friend, a squeeze of the hand may suffice. In a more detailed and lengthy encounter with a new patient just commencing treatment, there may need to be clear, verbal farewell statements preceded by a closing summary. This summary may involve confirming what was agreed between nurse and patient and agreeing to reopen communication at a later time.

A social encounter may be split up into elements differently to the 20-item breakdown presented above. And of course not all 20 items may be involved in each encounter. However, where elements are excluded, it must be because they have no part to play. Exclusion of psychological aspects when telling a patient the choice of dishes for lunch may be in most cases quite acceptable. But exclusion of attention to psychological needs when explaining to a patient about an impending major operation would almost always be totally indefensible. As you proceed to consider the major types of social interactions in the sections which follow, keep in mind the components of social encounters. Remember that all encounters must be opened and closed appropriately. Remember also that they will involve listening and exposition on your part. Remember, too, that there are elements of verbal and non-verbal communication which must be recognized, responded to, and utilized by you as well. Remember the importance of pacing and meshing in the smooth unfolding of an encounter. And remember most of all the need to respond appropriately to the patient's psychological, physical and social needs as and when they unfold during the encounter.

Exercise 1. Assessing your own social skills

Aims: to gain some insight into how well you interact with others; to start to develop skills in such situations.

Numbers of persons: the student alone, or two students with one assessing the other and vice versa.

Materials: copies of the checklist illustrated below.

Time required: 30-60 minutes.

Procedure: the following is a checklist of some of the 20 items identified in social encounters above.Make some copies of the checklist. As you will see, it presents a scale of scores for each item, ranging from 0 (*Negative*, or poorest performance) up to 3 (*Positive*, or the best performance). Interact with another person, a patient if possible. If there are two of you, one interacts and the other stands apart and scores. You then change places.Try to get in at least two interactions each. (If you are working alone, score yourself immediately after each interaction. But the activity works best if there are two of you.) You can then spend some time discussing your scores, how you performed, how you might improve your skill in a particular area. It is better discussing this with a colleague who observed you rather than having to address these issues alone. The checklist is used as follows. If in doubt, refer to the explanation of items above. Score each item by circling the appropriate score; 3 is maximum score for each item. Remember each target behaviour may not be needed. For example, item 1 will always come up, but 5 may not. If only 6 items are involved, for example, you would score out of a maximum score of 18 rather than 24.

After you have completed each interaction your partner (or yourself, if working alone) should arrive at a total score. Consider or discuss overall performance and performance in particular items. But remember the scoring here is a very crude device. The main benefit is in discussing details of the use of the skills involved and how you might improve on these.

Interaction checklist

Target behaviour	Evaluation of target behaviour (Circle a score as appropriate)		
	NEGATIVE		POSITIVE
1. Beginning the interaction	0	1	2	3
2. Body posture	0	1	2	3
3. Eye contact	0	1	2	3
4. Style of questions	0	1	2	3
5. Absence of jargon	0	1	2	3
6. Presence of empathy	0	1	2	3
7. Quality of exposition	0	1	2	3
8. Terminating the interaction	0	1	2	3

Total score:

Total =

4. The history-taking conversation

The patient is in a difficult situation when the list of questions in connection with the case-history is being put. Someone who has just been admitted to hospital has questions of his own and is very uncertain. He has often come to hospital on his own initiative and one hour after leaving home is in bed in pyjamas, in broad daylight; the dependence is already beginning. He must remain constantly alert at first because people keep wanting information from him. One of these people is the nurse, who wants to conduct a history-taking conversation. You must make allowance for this background when you come to the patient for such a conversation. You must be aware that the patient is full of questions, but that he does not know whether he can ask these questions at this moment. Everyone around him appears to know exactly how things go in hospital, apart from him. If you start asking the questions from the history-taking form in these circumstances, you will get an answer but you will probably not learn anything beyond that answer. If people feel alone and dependent, they hold back. A nurse who restricts himself or herself to running through a questionnaire does not really *invite* the patient to ask questions or mention worries. You will note that we have deliberately used the term conversation rather than interview here

Figure 5.3.1
The history-taking conversation

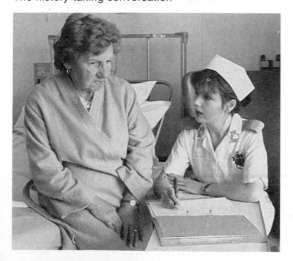

You may ask yourself whether it is so important to find out about these questions and worries. They are important for the following reasons. Firstly there may be a great many questions which you can answer directly, thus helping the patient to feel at ease sooner in his new situation. Secondly there is a positive relationship between how patients feel during an admission and the healing process. The less the patient has on his mind during admission, the quicker the cure. It is thus of major importance even for the healing process that everything is done to make the patient feel at his ease right from the start.

a. First phase

You help the patient to feel at ease by first giving him the opportunity to talk about what concerns him. This is an essential aspect of the history-taking conversation: start by inviting the patient to tell you something or to ask you questions. Try to imagine what is going through this patient's mind. Ask him specific, everyday things, ask for details. Mention the feelings you see or sense in him. Demonstrate your interest. Show that you are willing to listen to him and accept what he has to say. In doing so, you can make use of the basic skills described in the section on 'perception' in the previous chapter.

It may not always be the case that the patient will then actually open up and ask his questions and confide his worries at once; it may well be that he still holds back. But you have given him an opportunity, and started to build up empathy with him, as described at Section 3 above. This is the beginning of a mutual understanding with your patient. This is sometimes referred to as establishing a *rapport*.

When you have heard everything he had so say, you can summarize this. With this summary you give him the opportunity to add what is still missing from his story, or to correct what is not right. You also mark with this summary the transition to the next phase.

b. Second phase

In the second phase you have the opportunity to ask questions from your history-taking form. This is a completely different procedure from that applied so far in the conversation. Until now you have listened, summarized, conducted general open questioning and reflected feelings. But now you must firmly and efficiently find out about a number of practical matters. You suddenly have to start asking closed questions which are aimed at certain specific issues or phenomena.

Preparing

It is best to prepare the patient for the closed questions. If you say, 'I just want to ask you a few other questions. It may seem to you that they have nothing to do with what you have come for, but we have to know these things so that we can care for you as well as possible,' you let the patient know what is coming. He will then answer the questions with greater motivation, because you will have prepared him for them.

Variation in types of questions

There is another point which you must not forget during this phase of the history-taking conversation. People often have a tendency to fall into a kind of 'answering routine'. If they are given a series of questions to answer, it takes some concentration to fully take in each question and then to give the correct answer to it. Quite often they end up in a kind of rhythm in which the answer 'no' is automatically given, without having taken in the individual questions properly. This is called a 'response set', a readiness to engage in a certain type of response unthinkingly. Obviously, you must prevent people ending up in such a response set during your history-taking conversation. You can do this by varying your questions, and by alternating the type of questions. For example if you alternate a series of closed questions with a single open question, this interruption can prevent the onset of a 'yes', 'no' or 'don't know' response set. You can also break up the routine and help the other person to concentrate again by making a different kind of comment such as 'It won't take much longer now.'

In the history-taking conversation you must be aware that you are constantly demanding something from the patient, not only literally but also figuratively. By 'figuratively' we mean that the patient is entirely dependent on you. He must answer the questions which you ask him, and other than that there is little he can do. Bear this in mind during the conversation, perhaps commenting on it occasionally. Show understanding and if necessary divide the history-taking into smaller instalments. You can interrupt the whole thing with a different activity. In this way you refresh the patient's attention, as it were, so that he is again able to concentrate properly on your questions.

c. Third phase

It is important to end the procedure by allowing the patient the opportunity to both wind down and take stock. Here, any final question the patient may have can be addressed. You can also discuss with the patient what he will be faced with during his period in hospital and how he will be able to cope.

Answer any queries he may have, or if you cannot, undertake to find out and come back to him about this. But remember – do not use this as an avoidance strategy. Do find out; and do come back to him about it. Your developing therapeutic relationship with the patient depends on him seeing that you are dependable and have a genuine concern for him, *right from the start!* Finally, do not forget to thank the patient for his cooperation.

d. Hetero-history-taking

A special circumstance can arise in the history-taking conversation. It may happen that you do not take all or part of the history from the patient himself but that you have to obtain the information from others, such as members of the patient's family. This is called hetero-history-taking. In principle this does not differ greatly from history-taking with a patient; you simply have to be aware that another person obviously cannot feel precisely what the patient feels. The answers will probably be slightly less reliable, simply because they are not 'first hand'. It is different again when you are confronted with a group of members of the family or acquaintances. You then have to decide whom to talk to.

Make sure that you divide your attention between those who wish to give answers, and if

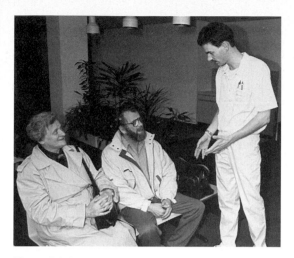

Figure 5.3.2
Hetero-history-taking

can hold a free conversation with the patient in which everything can be discussed, provided it gives information on possible nursing problems. These different forms are known as *structured conversation* and the *free-narrative conversation*. A mixed form, in which the topics of conversation are fixed but the precise questions are not, is called the *semi-structured conversation*.

The advantages and drawbacks of these forms can be guessed:
- *Structured conversation*
  Advantage: you obtain precisely the information you consider necessary, without needing to spend time on other things which are not of interest for the hospital admission. Drawback: you do not know after this conversation what the patient still has on his mind. You do not know whether other pressing matters (such as anxieties or concerns of the patient) will play an important part during the patient's stay in hospital.
- *Free-narrative conversation*
  Advantage: you can find out precisely what is preying on the patient's mind in this conversation.
  Drawback: you do not know precisely whether you have been given all the relevant information. The free-narrative conversation often takes longer than a structured conversation.
- *Semi-structured conversation*
  Advantage: it may contain the advantages of both the above forms. You might regard it as a number of small free-narrative conversations on fixed subjects.
  Drawback: it could also contain the drawbacks of both the above forms. This happens if you do not listen well or if the basic skills described under 'Perception' in Chapter 2 are not used well.

necessary make arrangements for separate interviews if you want to hear everyone. This will of course often depend on ward policy. It is often the case that history-taking – because of limited time and resources – has to be limited to the patient and his/her spouse, parent or friend.

Finally the mixed form can also occur: you want to take a history for a patient and the family is present. See first whether you can speak to the patient alone. If this is not possible, you must make it clear that you find everyone's input important, but that you can only talk to one at a time. Agree an order beforehand, and keep to it.

e. Different degrees of structure

Various degrees of freedom can occur in the history-taking conversation. The following extreme situations and mixed forms all occur. At one extreme you must regard the history-taking as a kind of survey: you have a list of questions and you must see that the patient gives answers to these questions. The other extreme is that you

Exercise 2. Types of conversations. The history-taking conversation

Aim: to be able to conduct a history-taking conversation.
Number of persons: 3.
Materials: the observation list presented below.
Time required: preparation, 10 minutes; role play, 15 minutes; subsequent discussion (depending on the possibility of using sound or video recordings), 30–60 minutes.

Procedure: one person plays the part of the patient. How he will fulfil this role is not told to the others. The role must in any case contain information on the complaint, the direct reason for admission, the emotions and the patient's questions.

The second person must take a history from this patient. He may use a list of questions from the nurse's history-taking form for this purpose. The third person is the observer, filling in the observation list. Start right in; assume that normal introductions have taken place.

After the conversation, the observer leads the discussion.

Use the features of the history-taking conversation described above for the subsequent discussion. These also appear in brief on the observation list. Discuss also to what extent this conversation pleased both participants.

The observer puts the questions below first to the 'nurse' and then to the 'patient'. Finally he gives his own observations. Did they have the impression that justice was done to all the aspects of the conversation? If aspects were left out, how bad was that?

Is this as bad for the nurse as for the patient? Why, or why not? How could things have been done differently? Try it out!

Observation list for history-taking conversation

(Circle 'yes' or 'no', as appropriate, for each item)

Phase 1

The nurse:

1. invites the patient to say what is on his mind .... yes   no
2. particularly uses open questions for this .... yes   no
3. continues asking questions within the reference
   framework of the patient .... yes   no
4. paraphrases the patient's information .... yes   no
5. summarizes the patient's information .... yes   no
6. reflects the patient's feelings .... yes   no

Phase 2

The nurse:

7. announces the procedure during the second phase .... yes   no
8. asks questions in the second phase in an alternating
   way .... yes   no
9. summarizes the information from the second phase .... yes   no

Phase 3

The nurse:

10. asks the patient if he has any final questions .... yes   no
11. discusses with him his period in hospital .... yes   no
12. thanks the patient .... yes   no

5. The problem conversation

We use the term *problem conversation* to refer to one concerned with difficult issues where the patient cannot cope on his own. These issues need not necessarily be exceptionally problematic or negative, they may be normal day-to-day problems on which you wish to exchange ideas. As you have read, patients can ask you many different questions. If you wish to differentiate these by content, you can group them firstly as questions on information and secondly as questions on a solution. The questions on a solution where the patient cannot manage himself often arise from problems. The conversation which you conduct with a patient on such a problem must comply with a number of guidelines. Let us first describe such a problem for clarity. Imagine the following occurs to you.

Patient A is in the ward after an operation to remedy a phimosis. You have got to know him during the admission as a 21-year-old cheerful, good-looking man. The operation has gone well. You notice that he has had few visitors in the two days he has been here: only his family has come to see him. You come up to his bed and suddenly he asks if you could see to it that his friends do not come to visit him. You think: perhaps he feels visitors would be too tiresome and you say; 'Well, how would it be if you allowed them to visit only for a short time?'

a. Clarifying the problem

Firstly we cannot emphasize it enough: make sure that you have understood the problem properly. Do not make the mistake of mentioning a solution before you know exactly what is preying on the patient's mind. Do not think that you can see through the patient. Do not think that you have no time to go into the problem in depth, and that you can quickly suggest something. Remember that this is the most common mistake in hospital, and not just there! It is better not to listen to a problem at all than to half-listen to it and then propose a solution.
The likelihood of a solution of this kind being the right one is minimal. Make sure when conducting a problem conversation that you start by asking the patient exactly what is preying on his mind. Use the basic skills described in Section 2 of the previous chapter on 'Perception'. This will require you to:

- look at the patient and listen actively and carefully;
- paraphrase his statements when appropriate;
- summarize what he tells you;
- continue asking questions within his reference framework;
- mention what you perceive of feelings in his story and be curious. Do not think too early on that you have grasped the problem, even if it appears quite obvious to you.

Back to Mr A.
After his initial request to exclude his friends from visiting, you go and sit with him and ask what he means by it. He says that he simply does not want his friends to come and visit him. You ask why he does not want to see them, but he does not answer. He merely says that his parents have told one of his friends that he is in hospital. Having heard this, you have a brainwave and ask; 'What would happen if they came?' He hesitates and finally says; 'Then they would see me like this.' You ask whether he would find that unpleasant, and he says yes.

You can only assume that you have analysed the patient's problem properly if you have summarized it properly. This summary has the function for yourself of checking whether you have actually heard and understood everything. It is also important for the patient for two reasons:

- he notices in this way that you have listened to him properly;
- you give him the chance to correct you if you have perhaps misunderstood something.

Make sure that you end your summary with a question (see also the description of summarizing in Chapter 2 of this module).

You may say to Mr A.; 'So you don't want your friends to know what you are here for?' He answers yes, but by now knows that you are going to carry on asking questions. He tries to prevent this by asking once again whether you

Figure 5.3.3
'I do not want my friends
to come and visit me'

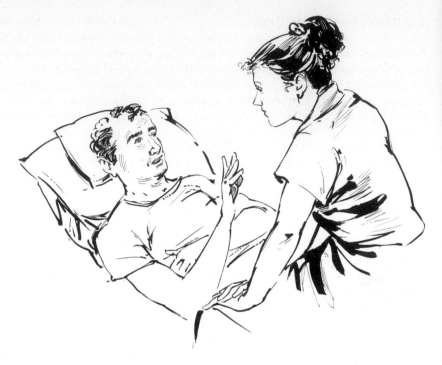

could see to this. You say that you do not really understand the reasons; 'After all we all have problems and can't you be calm and open about yours?' He evidently finds this a disappointing reaction, because he shrugs his shoulders and turns his face away.

You decide to break off at this moment, and later the same morning go back to him. He appreciates this. You ask him calmly how he is and what exactly was the matter. He decides to take you into his confidence and tells you that he has always boasted to his friends about his girl-friends, how he has been to bed with many women and so on. If his friends discovered why he was in hospital, they would realize that he had been making up some of these stories. You say; 'If your friends came, it would turn out that your stories were pure bravado, is that it?'

You have spent a good deal of time on obtaining information. By good continued questioning when the patient puts his problem to you, you help him to see it in sharper focus. The problem not only becomes clearer to you yourself, but also to the patient. If people only think about their own problems, their thoughts often go round in circles. You therefore often hear some-

one say, 'I can't get out of this.' The continued questioning on which you have to spend so much time has the function of breaking through this circle. Someone with problems can no longer cope with them because he does not dare to ask questions. This 'daring' must not be taken too literally. Think back to what you have read in Module 1 about defence mechanisms. All these defence mechanisms can be used if you come close to a 'difficult' question.

It is far easier for you, as an outsider in a problem of this kind, to ask the 'difficult' questions. They are generally far more apparent to an outsider ('Why don't you just say that?'). The patient may react to such a question in an unexpected way; it is quite possible that he will let this question sink in and later, in his thoughts, try to find an honest answer to it. Continued questioning in itself does not always have the benefit that the patient is helped to easily break out of his vicious circle. It is thus quite possible that the patient afterwards will himself continue to try to solve his problem himself, and may even solve it. However, this will not always be the case. There are problems which, although they can be defined very clearly, persist beyond this stage of definition.

b. Looking for a solution together

When certain problems arise, it is of the greatest importance that you and the patient look for a solution together. Good communication always involves reciprocity, so it is doubtful whether you alone, as an outsider, will find a good solution for the patient's problem. Everyone who has thought a little about his own problems has considered some solutions for himself. The likelihood that he will receive your first solution with jubilation is not great.

This is a different type of pitfall to those we have mentioned above. There we were concerned with giving a solution too early, but here we are concerned with a one-sided answer. What would be a solution in your situation need not be a solution for the patient.

If you are confronted with such a problem – very clear but not immediately solvable – it is sensible to ask yourself whether the patient wants to solve it. See the section on 'Sickness Gain' in the previous chapter. Try to find out what possible benefit the patient may have from keeping his problem unsolved. People are in principle able to adapt to changed circumstances. If your patient does not do so, it may be because he benefits in some way from not adapting. In the case of Mr A. above, you might ask him, even if it is difficult to do so, whether there are not also pleasant aspects to a visit from his friends. What would happen, or how would it be if his problem was solved? Continue asking questions. There is a good chance that your patient will give you an odd look if you ask such questions but he will generally be able to answer you.

Mr A. can then, in a period of reflection, become aware that he would prefer his friends not to shatter his public image, because they might then drop him. When you have obtained this information you can, together with the patient, look at how the advantage of seeing his friends can be achieved without having to take any drawbacks into the equation.

We have already used the words 'together with the patient' a number of times. This is an ongoing process we sometimes call *negotiating*. True negotiating is a process of give and take, of haggling, so that you arrive at the most suitable solution together.

With Mr A. you will look for ways of coping with his friends, short of keeping them away from his bedside. You suggest for example that he need not say anything about why he is here. But according to him this is not possible. Then you say that it is his turn to think up a solution. He thinks that perhaps he can mention something different than what is actually the matter. You comment that that too is risky and involves being dishonest to his friends. Finally the two of you decide that he should keep the reasons for his admission rather vague for his friends.

This example illustrates how thoughts can run. All kinds of problems are obviously possible. There are problems in which people become aware that they make things very difficult for themselves; problems in which people have no appreciation at all of their own contribution; there are also problems about which people find it very difficult to talk. These are often subjects which people are ashamed about. One way of identifying such a subject is to try to find a lead. This may for example be provided by the contradiction between what the patient says and what he does. If you notice someone saying something which he should be happy about and he looks distressed or dissatisfied about it, you comment on this. Or if someone tells you something unpleasant and he looks pleased or satisfied, this too raises a question. Pay close attention to feelings of this kind. Do you find what the other person tells you understandable or not? If not, ask for an explanation.

Exercise 3. Types of conversations. The problem conversation

Aim:	to be able to conduct a problem conversation.
Number of persons:	3.
Materials:	the observation list presented below.
Time required:	preparation, 10 minutes; role play, 30 minutes; subsequent discussion (depending on the possibility of using sound or video recordings), 30–60 minutes.
Procedure:	one person plays the part of the patient. He must not give details of this role to the other players. The role is concerned with a particular problem experienced by the patient. The role contains information on the complaint (for example, severe haemorrhoids), the direct reason for admission, the emotion (for example, shame and embarrassment) and the patient's questions.

Another player, playing the part of the nurse, conducts a problem conversation with this patient. She must be guided by the description of the problem conversation given in this section.

The third person is the observer, filling in the observation list in the same way as described for Exercise 2. Start right in; assume that normal introductions have taken place.

After the conversation, the observer leads the discussion.

Use the features of the problem conversation described in this section for the subsequent discussion. These also appear in brief on the observation list.

Discuss also to what extent this conversation pleased both players.

The observer puts the questions below first to the 'nurse' and then to the 'patient'. Finally he gives his own observations. Did they have the impression that justice was done to all the aspects of the role in this way? If aspects were omitted, how bad was that?

Is this as bad for the nurse as for the patient? Why, or why not? How could things have been done differently? Try it out!

Observation list for problem conversation/advisory conversation

(Circle 'yes' or 'no', as appropriate, for each item)

The nurse:

1. invites the patient to say what is on his mind	yes	no
2. particularly uses open questions for this	yes	no
3. continues asking questions within the reference framework of the patient	yes	no
4. paraphrases the patient's information	yes	no
5. summarizes the patient's information	yes	no
6. reflects the patient's feelings	yes	no
7. together with the patient defines the problem	yes	no
8. searches for solutions together with the patient	yes	no
9. negotiates with the patient a choice from the alternatives	yes	no

6. The advisory conversation

Obviously we cannot offer advice in a dogmatic way, 'You must do it, then everything will be fine!' Advice only works if it is tailored. We can, however, distinguish a number of points which you must take account of when you have to advise.

a. Acceptance

Firstly, and this is something which always applies, a piece of advice is seldom followed because it is intrinsically such good advice in qualitative terms. Following advice is always dependent on whether the patient accepts it or not. However good your advice is, if the patient does not accept it, or does not realize why it is good advice, or even does not believe it, nothing comes of the advice. It is apparent from this that a very important activity precedes advice. A first condition to be met for advice to be followed is that the patient must realize that it is necessary that something changes. If that is not accepted by the patient, it is probably useless to advise at all, because there will be no possibility of the advice being followed.

b. Guidance and advice

Ultimately it is always the patient himself who decides whether advice is followed or not. For example in this connection it has been found that 50 to 70% of the advice of GPs is not followed or is incorrectly followed! Patients often choose for themselves in the end.

This issue of co-operation in treatment is a controversial one. It is addressed – perhaps unfortunately – in medical sociology as the issue of *compliance* or *non-compliance* in treatment (an issue we addressed briefly in Chapter 1 of this module). In the past, and particularly in regard to those who were less educated or were members of the lower social classes, there was a tendency to recognize what Parsons (1970) described as the *competence gap*. That is, the doctor's greater expertise in the matter of health care was recognized and his perscriptions and instructions were implicitly followed. However, this situation would appear to be changing. As people become better educated and more

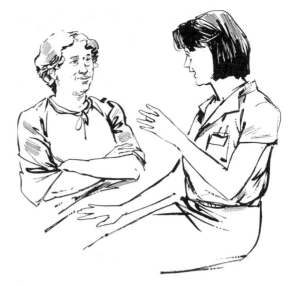

Figure 5.3.4
Advice is only followed
if it is accepted

consumer-orientated in their attitudes to health care, they become more critical of doctors. The competence gap has narrowed sufficiently for many people to start judging (perhaps quite erroneously) that they know as much as the doctor. They are also more conscious of their rights as clients or consumers and less in awe of the physician. This may lead to non-compliance with medical instructions, a situation described by Wilensky (1969) and Stimson (1974). Bearing this in mind, as in the case of doctors, nurses cannot expect that patients will always comply with their advice or instructions.

It is therefore important in an advisory conversation to make the patient aware of the purpose of the advice, so that he understands why it is being given. Here again it is important that you look out for reactions and signals from the patient which can tell you his attitude. This gives you information which you can draw on in later conversation with the patient. In this connection it is useful to read the section on 'negotiating' in the problem conversation (page 448). In the advisory conversation too it is a question of bargaining, of give and take. The procedure by which you have the greatest chance of success in the advisory conversation is the following:

– make sure that you offer the patient a number of alternative options for achieving a desired aim;
– more importantly, encourage the patient to suggest options himself;
– make sure that you discuss the advantages and drawbacks of the options with the patient;
– then let the patient choose from the various options.

Here again, this is similar to negotiating in the problem conversation: identify solutions with the patient, help the patient to realize what this or that option means in practice, and help the patient to make a choice. Only by doing this do you make it possible for the patient to choose the piece of advice which is most suitable for him, and the likelihood of the patient keeping to it is then greatest. You notice that in this case not so much advice is actually given, it is actually the patient giving himself advice. It is thus more correct in this case to speak of guidance.

The extent to which guidance or advice is given is in fact a fundamental issue in this type of caring relationship. The term *guidance* suggests that one person analyzes a situation and then tells the other what they should do. This would by definition be a predominantly directive activity. However, you will have noted that the suggestion above is that the nurse offers a number of options, and encourages the patient or client to choose. This is a much less directive activity than guidance in its narrowest sense. Indeed, it has become accepted that for such non-directive approaches the term *counselling* rather than guidance is preferable.

Perhaps the most significant counselling approach is that devised by Carl Rogers (1967, 1983). This is usually referred to as a *client- or person-centred* therapy or counselling. You will find that this approach is particularly popular in psychiatric nursing. Here the relationship between nurse and patient is an intimate person-to-person situation; the patient is seen as an individual in his own right and the relationship is a vehicle for patient and nurse exploring and developing understanding of problems. The nurse's role is to assist the patient in identifying and analyzing problems and a range of alternative solutions. The patient or client, however, has total autonomy of self-direction in deciding on the solution which he or she finds most acceptable. The nurse's role is essentially facilitative but never directive.

In reality it is often difficult to decide exactly how directive you need to be, or how non directive it is possible to be. This depends on the difficulty of the problems, the difficulty of operating solutions, the capacity of the patient and various environmental factors. It is desirable that where possible the patient decides. As suggested above, the patient is more likely to operate a solution he can accept ownership of. However, you may come across situations where the patient requires more guidance in terms of deciding on courses of action.

c. Motivation

There are obviously situations in which you must give advice which does not arise from wishes to change on the part of the patient. After the explanation on guidance and advice, you will understand that this is a difficult task. The first step here again is to try to help the patient realize that what is proposed is necessary, that a situation is undesirable and requires improvement. Try to make clear what improvement or benefits would ensue. In this way you can help the patient realize that help is necessary. This process is also known as 'motivation'.

As you can see, up to now we have taken as our basis a view which could be called a 'cooperation model'. This view does not include what you must do if a patient definitely does not wish to comply. Help-providers and care-providers then generally become a little touchy; they mean so well and yet the patient does not do what they consider good for him. The patient sometimes even does the opposite: this is going too far!

If you think along these lines, it is time to look at your own view of nursing. Who is the boss, do you think, nurse or patient? Who is responsible for what? Are you responsible if someone, despite being on a strict diet, secretly eats some sweets which a visitor has brought in? Would you ban him from doing so? Under what circumstances do you change your point of view on this? What do you do if it is very pleasant patient, or if he puts himself in mortal danger of complications by doing this?

We do not claim to have the right answers here; there are no correct answers. However, it is important that you examine for yourself what your own view is, in other words what your answers are to the above questions. Do not be satisfied with answers such as: 'It all depends.' Practise by asking further questions. What does it depend on? Under what circumstances do you answer yes, and under what circumstances no?

Exercise 4. Types of conversations. The advisory conversation

Aim: to be able to conduct an advisory conversation.

Number of persons: 3.

Materials: the observation check-list presented below.

Time required: preparation, 10 minutes; role play, 20 minutes; subsequent discussion (depending on the possibility of using sound or video recordings), 30–60 minutes.

Procedure: one person plays the part of the patient. She must not disclose details of this role to the other participants. The role must include information on the complaint (e.g. breast cancer), the direct reason for admission (mastectomy), the emotion (fear of surgery and anxiety about skin mutilation and how her husband will react to this) and the patient's questions.

Another player must advise this patient. She must be guided by what is said about the advisory conversation in this module.

The third person is the observer, filling in the observation list as described at Exercise 2. Start right in; assume that normal introductions have taken place.

After the conversation, the observer leads the discussion.
Use the features of the advisory conversation described in this section for the subsequent discussion. These also appear in brief in the observation list.
Discuss also to what extent this conversation pleased both players.
The observer puts the questions below first to the 'nurse' and then to the 'patient'. Finally she gives her own observations.
Is the patient going to follow the advice?
Did the players have the impression that justice was done to all the aspects of the advisory process?
If aspects were omitted, how bad was that?
Is this as bad for the nurse as for the patient? Why, or why not? How could things have been done differently? Try it out!

Observation list for problem conversation/advisory conversation
(Circle 'yes' or 'no' as appropriate, for each item.

The nurse:
1. invites the patient to say what is on her mind .... yes   no
2. particularly uses open questions for this .... yes   no
3. continues asking questions within the reference
   framework of the patient... yes   no
4. paraphrases the patient's information........................... yes   no

5.   summarizes the patient's information .... yes   no
6.   reflects the patient's feelings .... yes   no
7.   together with the patient defines the problem .... yes   no
8.   searches for solutions together with the patient .... yes   no
9.   negotiates with the patient a choice from the
     alternatives .... yes   no

7.   The bad-news conversation

By bad-news conversations we mean all conversations conducted in connection with an unpleasant piece of news. This appears simpler than it is. If you want to say it more precisely, a bad-news conversation is concerned with news which you think the other person may consider distressing. Generally what it comes down to is news which you find difficult to give.

We have now reached the core of the bad-news conversation. It is not the structure of such a conversation which makes it difficult, but the reaction which we may get to it. You can appreciate from this that bad news need not all be restricted to news on serious illnesses, loss, or an unfavourable result from a test. These are probably the worst things you will ever have to report to another person. However, items of news which have less of an impact on the life of someone may be very bad news for him. Think for example about trying to buy a new house or flat. The conversation which is conducted with you when you are informed that you have been unsuccessful is obviously a bad-news conversation.

a.   Guidelines

In conversations of this type it is best to keep to the guidelines which we shall discuss in the following sections. Then you know that you limit the suffering for the other person to what is necessary. At least you do not make it any worse because of your method of giving the news.

Do not beat about the bush
Deal the 'blow' early in the conversation. The longer you beat about the bush, the more difficult it becomes to get the message out.
Use no more than one or two introductory sentences, depending on how bad the news is, and then tell the news at once.

Figure 5.3.5
'I have some bad
news for you'

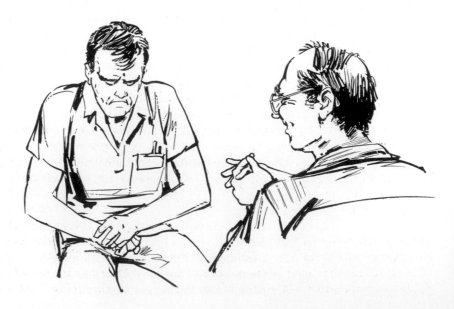

Look after the other person

When you have dealt the 'blow', stay with the other person. Since this person has just received a blow which has to be processed, he may now wish to let off steam and should be given the opportunity to do so. Give him this opportunity by staying with him. Your presence is in fact even more important than what you do or say. Make it clear that you too find it unpleasant – bad or terrible – for the other person. Ask whether he wants to talk about it, but above all react calmly to what you see or hear.

In particular there are a number of things you must not do:
– explain why...;
– say that it could have been worse...;
– say that you too have experienced...

Comments of this type are often made with the best of intentions, but really the other person has other things on his mind. In many cases these comments have the purpose of easing the burden for the bringer of the bad news rather than the victim. In his situation it serves little purpose to utter platitudes or saddle the latter with your problems. Try to be of service to the other person, that is better for him. The most commonly made mistake in the bad-news conversation, it should be noted, is that this phase of attending to the patient, is missed out! This may be done with the best of intentions. Generally the reasoning is, 'I cannot help him to come to terms with it, he has to do that himself.' However true this is in the long term, coming to terms begins immediately after the bad news has been heard. The person bringing the news can make a major contribution towards a start being made straightaway on coming to terms. The best way to make this start is at least to allow the patient to express everything that comes up in him prompted by this news. It is best for him to be invited to do so by the person bringing the bad news. The patient can always choose whether or not he wishes to make use of this offer.

Discuss 'where we go from here'

The last step in a bad-news conversation may only be taken when the patient indicates he is ready. Discuss where we go from here if the

patient asks something like, 'What do I do now?' You can introduce this with a comment such as 'A lot of things will change..., do you want to talk about that?' Let it depend on what the patient needs. If necessary offer him the chance to talk about it later and make sure that he knows that he can approach you when he is ready.

b. Possible reactions to bad news

Anything is possible. The whole scale of behaviour which has been described under defence mechanisms in Module 1 can be used. Violent emotions are often dreaded most, but in practice it is found that this is not the form of reaction with which people have the most trouble. If a patient remains in complete silence after receiving bad news, it is far more difficult to offer help. It is best to stay quiet for a while in such cases. At most you can ask him questions about it, without imposing on him. Just stay near to the other person. A general guiding principle for looking after someone who has just received bad news is to respect his emotions and tolerate them. If someone reacts very angrily, and perhaps even against you, try to understand that he is doing this to let off steam. Do not start defending yourself in a contrived way. Bear in mind above all that it is a defence reaction by the other person. If the patient repudiates the news or even pretends not to have heard it, do not go so far as to forcefully repeat it. It is also difficult to know exactly what others have told the patient, but in these cases it is of the greatest importance, for the welfare of the patient, that all those involved work as a team in bringing and confirming the bad news.

c. Evasion

A final comment on all the possible ways we have and use for beating about the bush when giving bad news. Although it may sound incredible, various forms of evasion, sometimes utilized very creatively, are thought up to avoid letting the dreaded words pass your lips. This may appear to help us for a short time, but not the patient, and in the long term we let ourselves down too. The patient then does not receive the information to which he is entitled. He will find out about it later. He will probably then think back to the time he asked you how he was or what was the matter. It is very likely that he will blame you for not being open with him.

The most common forms of evasion are:

Postponing
We tend to make use of all possible excuses for not giving the unpleasant news; the over-long introduction which was warned against above is an example of this. We also make use of very fine motives, such as: 'If I give him the news tomorrow, I can prepare for it better first...', but this actually serves mostly our own (short term) purposes.

Packaging
We sometimes use words which conceal from the patient what we actually mean. Just think how the following words are used: 'an inflammation, a patch on the X-ray, a spot...' It is a way of packaging the bad news. We use a word which does not sound too brutal and forget that the message may therefore not be understood by the patient. Or we present the best possible scenario: 'As many as 60 percent of people recover from this type of cancer with treatment.'

Avoidance
This is a method by which you ask questions in such a way that the patient eventually himself comes to the conclusion which you do not dare to say. 'You know what I told you last week? And what did you say then? Do I have to tell you again?'

Justification
You may try to justify yourself by saying that above all it is not your fault, perhaps even saying that it is the patient's own fault. For example: 'After all, you have been smoking all your life....'

'It's your own fault'

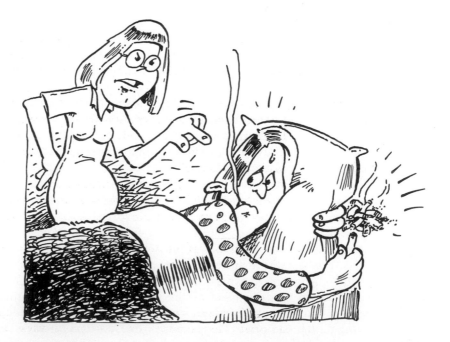

Exercise 5. Types of conversations. The bad-news conversation

Aim:	to be able to conduct a bad-news conversation.
Number of persons:	3.
Materials:	the observation checklist presented below.
Time required:	preparation, 10 minutes; role play, 20 minutes; subsequent discussion (depending on the possibility of using sound or video recordings), 30–60 minutes.
Procedure:	one player takes the patient role. The role must in each case contain information on the complaint, the direct reason for admission, the emotion and the patient's questions. In addition there must be bad news to give. Make sure that you do not make it too difficult, or it will be wearisome to play.

Examples are given below:

–   patient A would like to go home but cannot because the X-ray has not been successful and must be redone;
–   patient B's husband phoned to say that he cannot visit;
–   patient C is due to have her long-awaited operation this morning. However because of an emergency admission it is now being postponed indefinitely.

One player (the nurse) must bring the bad news to the 'patient.'

The third person is the observer, filling in the observation list, as described at Exercise 2. Start right in; assume that normal introductions have taken place.

After the conversation, the observer leads the discussion.

Use the features of the bad-news conversation described in this section for the subsequent discussion. These also appear in brief in the observation list.

The observer puts the questions below first to the 'nurse' and then to the 'patient'. Finally she gives her own observations. Were the pitfalls described successfully avoided?

Did the players have the impression that justice was done to all the aspects of the nurse's role?

If aspects were omitted, how serious were they?

Were they as serious for the nurse as for the patient? Why, or why not? How could things have been done differently? Try it out!

Observation list for problem conversation/advisory conversation
(Circle 'yes' or 'no', as appropriate, for each item)

The nurse:

1. gives a brief introductory statement ....   yes   no
2. gives the bad news immediately afterwards ....   yes   no
3. states the bad news briefly and clearly ....   yes   no
4. stays with the recipient of the bad news after giving it   yes   no
5. reflects the feelings of the recipient ....   yes   no
6. avoids forcing discussion too early ....   yes   no
7. asks whether the recipient wants to carry on talking
    about it ....   yes   no
8. discusses the future only if the patient initiates this ....   yes   no

8. The short, supporting conversation

A short, supporting conversation need not last long at all. The form of conversation we are describing here is not known as a separate form of conversation, yet a little conversation of this type is generally experienced as being very consoling and helpful. This is a brief conversation, usually lasting no more than five minutes, in which the nurse shows the patient that he is not alone. The chief purpose is to show that you take the patient seriously and are sympathetic towards him. He sees this in a number of small but very important things. These are things such as: knowing the name of the patient; being curious about more things than are only important for the illness, such as family circumstances and so on; maybe also being willing to speak honestly about yourself. However, one of the most important things is that you know how to bring out the important points from a patient's comments briefly and 'to the point'.

What makes a short, supporting conversation good is that you dare to look the patient's worries or anxieties in the eye and talk about them. If you think the patient is preoccupied with something, ask about it. Show that you appreciate it if he asks or tells you things. Show that you do not reject it or find it odd. One of the most important properties of the good nurse is her capacity to accept the patient irrespective of his personal failings or how unpleasant he appears. The nurse must not judge or condemn, but accept the patient as a person in need. The patient must be able to sense that he can depend on his nurse, that she at least will not reject him or let him down.

Most of the pointers identified above relate to things which are *said* while you are being supportive to the patient. However, often the most powerful supportive interventions are in fact non-verbal. This is particularly so when patients or their relatives are very distressed. For example an elderly lady whose husband has just died may need more than anything someone to just sit with her, holding her hand. Even the mere presence of the nurse, without touch being involved at all, can be an immensely

supporting experience for the distressed patient. Yet we often feel that if we just sit beside the patient doing nothing we are not properly occupied. Indeed, providing emotional support is one of the most vital functions of the nurse. You will find that how you relate to the patient, and the nurse-patient relationship in general, is a central aspect of nursing care.

9. The nurse-patient relationship

Earlier in this chapter and in Chapter 2 we discussed particular communication skills and how these can be utilized in helping patients. If you pause here for a minute, you will begin to realize that nursing is about helping people in some real or potential difficulty and that you do this through interacting with them. In essence when two people communicate, particularly on a relatively sustained basis, a relationship starts to build up between them. You will increasingly come across the phrase 'nurse-patient relationship' in the nursing literature. Indeed, as suggested at the end of Section 8 above, a therapeutic relationship is the very essence of good quality nursing care.

The problem here is in defining what is meant by a therapeutic relationship. Unfortunately this has not been accomplished with a great degree of success. It is interesting to note that in attempting to explain the therapeutic relationship, Rogers (1951) chose to concentrate on the 'therapeutic' aspect, taking the 'relationship' element as given. However, he was able to suggest that central to any therapeutic relationship was an expectation by the client that help would be given and a commitment on the part of the therapist to provide help and support. There was also a realization that therapy is not a one-way process with the therapist administering some miracle cure; the client has to contribute in partnership with the therapist. In addition the most successful relationships, i.e. those in which therapy goals were partially or wholly achieved, were those in which clients perceived in the therapist a real and genuine interest in them. It can be seen already that some of the activities described earlier in this chapter are important elements in that particular therapeutic partnership which is the nurse-patient caring relationship. Concepts such as helping, advising, supporting, agreeing solutions together, genuine interest on the part of the nurse can be seen in the examples of nurse-patient encounters described earlier in this chapter.

Altman and Taylor (1973) adopt a broader approach by defining relationships in terms of disclosure of information, which in essence involves cognitive or knowledge as well as affective or emotional elements. The argument here is that a relationship develops through a process of communication involving *self-disclosure* between the participants. As more information becomes available the participants view each other in discriminatory or differentiating ways as individuals rather than as anonymous others or sterotypes. In close relationships this can reach the stage where individuals can make predictions about each other. We say they know what each other is thinking. Such willingness to share your own ideas and feelings with the patient (i.e. self-disclosure) is addressed briefly at Section 8 above.

Another important element in relationships is the extent of sharing of views and outlooks which goes on. Morton et al. (1976) refer to this as '*the mutuality of relationship definition*'. This refers to the consensual rules and modes of communication which develop between individuals. This 'mutuality' is a multimodal process involving different forms of communication (e.g. verbal, non-verbal – speech, touch, gaze, etc.) and different domains of interaction (e.g. cognitive, affective, moral, ethical, etc.). As the forms of communication and domains become shared and are extended, the social bond between two people strengthens to the stage that they come to intimately know one another. This is common with husbands and wives, brothers, sisters, close friends, and sometimes in work-based relationships such as between nurse and patient.

Drawing from these important contributions in the literature on relationships, it is possible to identify elements which are major components of the therapeutic or caring relationship. These are:

(i) mutuality or consensus about the nature of the relationship and the rules which apply within it;

(ii) multimodality in terms of communication process (verbal, non-verbal, etc.) and domains of interaction (cognitive, affective, physical, ethical, moral, etc.);

(iii) discriminatory recognition, i.e. participants seeing each other as unique individuals rather than as anonymous others or sterotypes;

(iv) self-disclosure and intimacy between the participants;

(v) mutuality in relation to giving (by the nurse or therapist) and receiving (by the patient) help, and a genuine and perceived understanding and concern of one person for another.

To the extent that the above five elements or conditions are met, the relationship is close, personal and helping-orientated. When the nurse knows and understands her patient and when he accepts, understands and trusts her, there is a basis for helping. Nurses may learn verbal and non-verbal communication skills. They may even become familiar with the desired structure of particular social encounters – such as the problem, guidance, and 'bad news' encounters outlined earlier in this chapter. But these skills must be brought to bear in such activities as counselling, guiding and supporting the patient. It is very difficult to do these with total strangers. The 'relationship' is thus the vehicle by which social skills are brought to bear on meeting the patient's needs.

Study activity 1
Elements in a close relationship

Get together with a person you consider to be a personal friend. Choose a fellow student if possible. Each of you take a blank sheet of paper. Work separately. For each of the five elements of the caring relationship identified above, write down the extent to which your relationship meets the conditions of these elements. State whether or not it meets the conditions and list information which supports this, e.g. under (i) define the nature of the relationship (friend, colleague, lover, etc) and list rules which apply in the relationship. Take about 15 minutes. Then come together and compare notes. Discuss the extent to which you have both agreed or disagreed about your relationship.

Study activity 2
Advantages and disadvantages of close relationships with patients

Get together with 4-5 of your fellow students and a teacher if possible. All sit in a circle with a chalkboard or chart-stand and paperboard in the circle. First go around the group quickly, so that each person quickly shouts out an *advantage* in having a close personal relationship with a patient. List advantages on the board. Take about 3 minutes and try to get a list of at least 12 items. Next do the same, but try for at least 12 *disadvantages* and list these on the board beside the advantages. (This activity is know as brainstorming; you will meet it again in Chapter 5.) When you have got the two lists, discuss (over about 30 minutes) the various advantages and disadvantages identified. As you discuss you may as a group make deletions or additions to the lists. You may find it helpful if each of you note the final agreed lists so that you can think more about them in private study.

10. Summary

The following types of conversations have been discussed at length in this chapter:
– history-taking conversation;
– problem conversation;
– advisory conversation;
– bad news conversation;
– supporting conversation.

Before describing the various types of conversations, attention was focused on the skills which must be mastered in order to able to structure a conversation.

In the final section before the summary, the caring relationship was considered. This was addressed as a vehicle for using interpersonal skills to undertake caring activities such as problem-solving, counselling, supporting. Important elements of a caring or therapeutic relationship were identified and you were asked to consider advantages and disadvantages of having close relationships with patients.

It should be clear from this chapter that there is a great difference between knowing something and doing something. In other words: knowing how you should conduct a bad-news conversation does not mean that you have actually mastered the skill.

The consultative conversation

4

1. Introduction

If you seek the views or opinions of a colleague regarding a problem, we call this consultation. It is in principle slightly different from seeking advice from an expert. You consult among colleagues. You ask one or other of them how he or she would tackle a particular situation with which you have problems. The chief message in a consultative conversation is that you must first make clear to the other person precisely what you require from her. You are in essence asking for her (expert) opinion. The consultative conversation is discussed in this chapter.

Learning outcomes

After studying this chapter the student should be able to:
- identify the aim of consultation;
- recognize a consultative conversation;
- put into words the pitfalls that can arise in a consultative conversation;
- state four skills which are necessary to conduct a consultative conversation;
- conduct a consultative conversation under simulated conditions.

2. Aim of the contact

The aim of a consultative conversation is to obtain information or insight with which the person consulting can resolve a particular problem or dilemma. It thus remains the responsibility of the person consulting whether she will actually make use of this information.

The aim of the consultative conversation is thus not to solve the other person's problem. In the vast majority of consultative conversations the person consulting will at most gain an insight or obtain suggestions with which she can solve or reduce the problem. Another person generally cannot solve the problem of the person consulting.

We do not wish to claim here that giving advice is prohibited in all cases. It is obviously best to give a concrete answer to practical questions. If your colleague asks you how she can make it clear to Mr E. that it is better for him to put those flowers in water himself, then you need to offer a suggestion. However, there are many problems for which the solutions are not obvious. The person asking you something has probably tried everything and is only now coming as a last resort to you. The likelihood of your being able to suggest a good solution straightaway is not great. It is obviously the wish of the other person to see a problem solved. But if the person consulting indicates that she wants the other person to solve the problem for her, the first thing that must be made clear by the person being consulted is: what you require from me is not realistic; your problems may be best solved by you and no-one else.

3. Pitfalls in the consultative conversation

The most significant pitfall in a consultative discussion is giving advice too early. As we saw earlier, our inclination is to give an answer as soon as the question has been asked. But we are all too willing to give advice. Research into conversations between doctors and their patients has shown that doctors devote 70% of their time in such situations to giving advice. However, between 50 and 70% of this advice is not followed by patients. This is in fact the issue of *compliance*, a concept we addressed briefly in Chapter 3.

Let us for the sake of convenience assume that these doctors have given advice clearly; the fact that the patients did not follow the advice was not due to inadequate explanation. One of the reasons why advice is not followed is that the person receiving the advice does not know whether it represents the best advice which the other person can give. Is it the best possible solution? Has it been chosen out of a number of possibilities? People are more likely to follow advice if they have had a 'say' in it. If one has been able to join in deciding what is to be done, there is a far greater chance that the person receiving the advice will also keep to what has been agreed.

In this connection it is also relevant to note that the effect of a piece of advice depends not only on its quality but also on its acceptance by the person being advised. If the advice is totally unacceptable to the person being advised, the effect of the advice will be zero: it will not be followed. Although this appears very obvious, a great deal of advice is given which is unacceptable to the person receiving it: 'Try to do more about your fitness'; 'Just carry on working this evening'; 'You don't need to worry about that'; etc. We shall not examine here the reasons people may have for not accepting advice, some of which have been made clear in previous parts of this book.

Our concern here is with the fact that things quite often go wrong in the consultative conversation. The chief pitfall consists of giving the answer without precisely knowing the problem or issue contained in the question. The easiest way of avoiding this pitfall is therefore to obtain enough detailed information so that you know exactly what the other person is asking you. You do not know that until the other person has told you, or until she has confirmed it when you ask. Thus when your colleague asks how she should react when Mr Vincent gets awkward again, first ask more questions. What does she mean by getting awkward? What exactly does Mr Vincent do? How did she react? What has she already tried? What was the effect? Does she dislike Mr Vincent? Perhaps you will discover that she cannot get along with Mr Vincent because fundamentally she has no sympathy for this patient. Perhaps the two of you will then come to quite a different solution from the one you would have given to her first question, if you had not carried on asking questions.

4. Skills in the consultative conversation

The most important thing in a consultative conversation, and it will come as no surprise after reading the previous section, is that the person consulted should not start giving advice or an opinion at once. When being consulted, you must first carefully examine what exactly the issue is, and only then can advice be given. You use the skills of continued questioning (within the reference framework), concretizing, summarizing and explaining.

a. Continued questioning within the reference framework of the other person

By *reference framework* (see page 425) we mean the whole of the thoughts, feelings and attitudes with which the other person perceives the world. This reference framework is determined by a large quantity of experiences and impressions throughout a whole life. All these experiences and impressions which you have been through in your life determine your reference framework. They determine how you give meaning to the world. Someone who has grown up in a shopkeeper's family chooses different reports from the newspaper to read compared with someone whose parents were in teaching. It is very likely that these two people have learned to focus their attention on different things in their upbringing. They look at the world from a different perspective. We call this a different reference framework.

It is of course not an easy task to identify the other person's reference framework, especially if you both come from very different social backgrounds. To some extent, the other person will help us in this regard. If you refer back to Role Theory in Module 3, you may recall the important concept of 'taking the role of the the other' as advocated by Mead (1934). This means that how we play out our role is to a large extent determined by our interpretation of the other person's expectations of us. In effect, we behave as others expect us to behave. Or, using the terminology presented in this chapter we fall in with their frame of reference.

A particular problem arises where the patient comes from a different cultural background to that of the nurse. Under these circumstances the patient may have different beliefs about health, illness, treatment and care etc. This may require the nurse to have particular skills in adopting the patient's reference framework or – putting it another way – providing care within the patient's cultural context. This is especially important in modern multiracial societies and it has resulted in a particular perspective referred to as *transcultural nursing* (see for example: Leininger, 1978; Leininger, 1984).

As indicated above, it is dangerous to make assumptions on the basis of incomplete information. It is necessary to converse with the other person, to ask her questions about her position, to paraphrase her statements and ask her to confirm them, seek clarification as necessary, etc. And then it is necessary to reflect her statements and opinions back to her so that you can both confirm that you understand her position, that you can actually experience the person's 'universe' with her. This idea will be familiar to you. It is the concept of empathy discussed in the previous chapter, and as described by authors such as Rogers (1975) and Authier (1989). It is only by being able to pick up from the other

person's role expectations, by entering into a relationship which facilitates empathic understanding, that you can accurately identify her reference frame. You are then in a position to address with her the problems from her point of view.

The intention behind continued questioning within the reference framework is that you link your questions to what the other person is concerned with. You therefore do not directly ask the things which seem important to you but the things which follow on from what has already been said earlier. An example can perhaps make this clear.

If you hear from a colleague that she has trouble with Mr B. in room 5, because he moans so much, it is tempting to ask – from your own reference framework – whether she has tried being 'curt' with Mr B. That is something that has always worked well for you. However, your colleague has a different reference framework. She finds that she cannot be curt with a patient and she tried to make it clear to Mr B. in a different way that he must not moan so much, but this unfortunately did not have the desired effect; that was the background to her question. If you had continued asking questions you would have heard that from her. She could then have articulated her question to you more specifically as follows: 'How can I make it clear to Mr B. that he must not moan so much, without being curt towards him?' Only then could you both have thought up a solution to her question together. Questions within the reference framework of the other person work more effectively than questions which come from your own reference framework.

It is also important that these questions are formulated in an open way. To remind ourselves of a previous comment (see page 423): the other person can give any answer to open questions, so long as no suggestion is made within the question itself as to the answer the questioner would prefer to hear. Only 'yes' or 'no' or similar specific and limited responses are possible as answers to closed questions. An example of a closed question is: 'Do you like reading?' An open question, on the other hand, is: 'What kind of hobbies do you have?'

The subject of questions within and outside the reference framework was discussed in Chapter 2, of this module (see pages 425, 426). The exercise contained in that section can also be used for *continued* questions within and outside the reference framework.

b. Concretizing

By *concretizing* we mean a special type of continued questioning. You concretize when you want to make vague statements *precise,* impersonal statements *personal* and general things *specific.*
Whenever the person who asks you for advice makes a statement which is vague, impersonal or general, you must concretize it. You can recognize such vague statements because they

are packaged in such words as, 'They say..., people..., one..., in general...' and so on.

Concretizing takes the form of continued questioning. If the other person says, 'You cannot be curt towards a patient', a concretized follow-up question is, 'What exactly do you call "being curt"?'
When the other person says, 'I do not smoke that much', the concretizing response is, 'How much is that?' Bear in mind that you can also make concretizing sound silly. Concretizing is an intervention which is not automatically appreciated by the other person. She may be irritated by excessive use of this device. You should therefore make sure that you do not carry on concretizing to an excessive degree; restrict your concretization to those subjects where it is genuinely of great importance to obtain the precise, specific or personal information.

Exercise 1. Concretizing

Aim:	to be able to use concretization.
Number of persons:	individually and to be discussed afterwards in the group.
Materials:	the statements below.
Time required:	10 minutes; subsequent discussion, 15 minutes.
Procedure:	a number of statements appear below which must be made more concrete. Imagine that you as a nurse are in conversation with someone who makes such statements. Formulate questions with the intention of specifying these statements, making them more concrete. When you have finished, exchange these concretizations with your fellow group members. Discuss the different versions.

- In some way or other it's not quite right.
- I would simply like it to be more fun.
- Things are getting worse and worse.
- People no longer pay any attention to it these days.
- I mustn't complain.
- I can't really say how much I eat.
- Sometimes more, sometimes less.
- I have had trouble with it.

c. Summarizing

- By regularly *summarizing* you achieve order in what the other person has said. You run a comb through it, as it were, and give yourself an insight into or overview of what has been presented.
- Secondly you show by a summary that you

are following what the other person is saying. You show that you are doing your best to understand the other person, that you are still there.
- Finally: a good summary is not a summing-up of the total information which the other person has given, but a shortened statement of

the *core* of what has been said, in your own words.

For example: if a person has said in a lot of words that his wife has run off with another man, that he no longer sees his children, that he has to leave his old house and that things are not going too smoothly at work either, a good, succinct summary is: 'So you're having a hard time just now. Is that not so?' In so doing, you give a collective name to what he has just told you. This makes it clear to him that you understand him.

It is thus important when summarizing that you do not start repeating what the other says parrot-fashion, but that you restate the core of what has been said succinctly and in your own words. A good summary finally ends with a question, for example, 'Is that right?' In this way you offer the other person the opportunity to make additions or corrections to your summary.

Exercise 2. Summarizing

Aim: to be able to use summaries.
Number of persons: individually and to be discussed afterwards in the group.
Materials: fragment of conversation below.
Time required: summarizing, 5 minutes; subsequent discussion, 15 minutes.
Procedure: part of a conversation between a nurse and a patient appears below. The patient is speaking.
Write a summary of what is said below.

'Yes, you know, I haven't felt at my best recently, with this dizziness. And my wife has always said take that walking stick with you, then at least you have a bit of support. But whenever I take it with me I am bothered by it. I don't like walking with it, because that makes you an invalid, I reckon. People look at you when you walk with a stick. No, I'd rather stay at home.'
Swap summaries. Discuss them afterwards. Pay attention to the features of a good conversation. These are described on pages 427-9.

Do the same with the following piece of text:
'But now he's out of work, and that takes some getting used to, you know. At first I thought: fine, now he can do a few jobs around the house and collect the children from school. But that's not the way it's gone at all. He just sits around. I don't like the person he's turning into...'

d. Explaining

Often in a consultative conversation so much definition is already given to the problem by the summary, or so much insight into the problem has arisen as a result of concretization, that the person consulting can then carry on herself, without the person consulted having given any advice. However, this is not always the case. The next skill which you, as the person consulted, require is *explaining*. In the context of consultation, this relates to explaining the problem (as you see it), and the options for solution (again as you see them).

Good explanation depends on many factors. The clarity with which you say something, the level of comprehension of the other person and the gravity of what you say are all things which influence whether the other person grasps what you mean. You will understand that we cannot give guidelines for all the different circumstances for a good explanation. What we can do is give guidelines or advice which apply to every explanation. These are as follows:
– Give your explanation in short pieces. Break up the information you wish to convey into smaller amounts and mention these one by

one. Nothing is worse in an explanation than a 20 minute 'lecture'; the other person cannot listen to you with concentration for that long.

– Regularly ask whether the other person has understood. Not after every sentence, but at every chunk of information which you give, it is important that you check whether it reaches the other person.

– Mention the most important thing first. People remember best what is said to them first. Make sure that you mention the most important thing early in your explanation and that you reserve the remainder of your explanation for support or background.

– Keep a close watch on how the other person reacts to what you are saying. Is she still looking interested or is she gazing out of the window? In this way you receive direct information on the effectiveness of your account and you can adjust your explanation to these reactions.

– Use an illustration or drawing for things which lend themselves to this. Something which is difficult to explain can often very quickly be made clear with a comparison, a metaphor, an analogy or an illustration. Examples also have this function: they make difficult, abstract or vague things understandable.

– Finally an 'exercise tip': the best way of

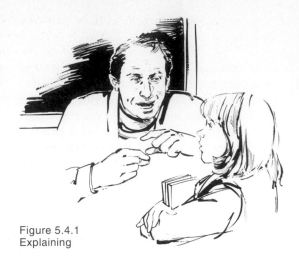

Figure 5.4.1
Explaining

practising explaining is to try to make something clear to a six year-old child. You must not become infantile, but make a clear distinction between principal (the most important) and secondary (supporting or background) matters.

When you have explained how you see the problem, your analysis of it, and also explained the options for solution which may be available, it is decision time! This is a matter for the other person, with or without your support or advice.

Exercise 3. Explaining

Aim   to be able to use the skill of explaining.
Number of persons: 3.
Materials: list of subjects below and observation checklist below.
Time required: explanation per round, 5 minutes; subsequent discussion, 5 to 10 minutes.
Procedure: the first person does the explaining. The second listens to the explanation and decides whether she finds the explanation clear. The third person is the observer and follows the explanation with the observation checklist.

Not all the guidelines necessarily have to be followed, they are aids in explanation.

Change roles after an explanation. Do this at least often enough to give each player one turn. Afterwards, discuss each explanation, making use of the completed observation checklist.

Each explanation can be concerned with one of the following topics (obviously you can also think up your own subjects):

– What are clouds?
– Why is it said that the National Health Service is based on what is known as the solidarity principle?

- Why does a higher gear ratio on the back wheel of a racing bike have less teeth than a lower gear ratio?
- What is an 'optic chiasma'?
- What do the two measurements you obtain when you measure blood pressure mean?
- Explain to a patient why only two people can visit him at the same time.

Observation checklist for explanation
(Circle 'yes' or 'no', as appropriate for each item)

When the person gives an explanation:

1. Is the information given in small amounts? .... yes   no
2. Does the person giving the explanation ask
    if it is understood? .... yes   no
3. Is the most important thing mentioned first? .... yes   no
4. Does the person giving the explanation pay attention to
    the other person's reaction? .... yes   no
5. Does the person giving the explanation make a distinction
    between principal and secondary matters? .... yes   no
6. Does the person giving the explanation make use of
    illustrations, comparisons, metaphors or analogies? .... yes   no

5. Summary

In a nursing department or team you encounter different knowledge, skills and interests among the various nurses. It is essential, in solving complex health care problems, that this expertise can be shared and fully utilized. Hence the consulting of professional colleagues is an important skill, which has been described in this chapter. The aim of consultation, some common pitfalls and useful skills in the consultative process are all discussed. The chapter emphasizes that, although when consulted you are helping the other person to clarify the 'problem', analyze it, and identify possible solutions, it is best that he or she makes the final decision. You may advise the other person, but you should not yourself make the decision for him/her.

5

Co-operating in groups

1. Introduction

In this chapter we discuss co-operation in groups, seen through the eyes of the participants in this co-operation. How a person leading the conversation must keep this co-operation with the group along the right lines is discussed in Chapter 6.

The organization of this chapter is as follows:
– firstly important conditions for co-operation are mentioned: decision-making and involvement;
– the pitfalls in co-operation are then discussed;
– then co-operation is divided into two parts: ways of decision-making and evaluation;
– finally the skills which belong to the two parts of co-operation are described.

Learning outcomes

After studying this chapter the student should be able to:
– name two functions and two aims of a group;
– state three pitfalls which can arise in co-operation in groups;
– recognize and apply the skills with regard to decision-making and evaluation.

2. Functions and aims of co-operation in groups

As we have already described at length in Module 3, people belong to innumerable groups in their everyday lives. School classes, football clubs, music societies, conservationists, these are all examples of groups of which you may be a member at a certain moment in your life. Obviously all these groups have particular aims, and exist for a particular reason. You can say that the reason for the existence of a group is its function. The function of a student group may be to co-operate in order to achieve learning outcomes. The 'official' function of a football club may be to receive coaching on how to play football and to take part in competitions. However, for individual members of a football club this group may have quite different functions: for one person an opportunity to get physical exercise in a relaxed way, for another a good way of getting rid of the frustrations which he has built up at work, for a third person a way of not having to do any shopping on Saturdays and for a fourth a pleasant way of having a chat with other people after the match and having a few beers.

Thus one group can have many different functions. Two well-known functions of groups are:

- the task function (which is to do with the group's main purpose or aims);
- the binding function (which is to do with social intercourse and the need for relationships with others – an affinity for the group and its members).

As a nurse you will often work in groups which above all have particular tasks to perform. In this chapter, we shall therefore examine the skills which you need as a participant in groups with a task function. A task of this kind may be: ensuring together that a department in the hospital runs well, or attending to the hand-over from the night shift to the day shift. The quality of this kind of co-operation can easily be established. If it goes well, the department runs smoothly or the day shift knows exactly what has happened to the various patients during the previous night.

Why do people work so much in groups? Why is it not just individuals who take decisions? In answering these obvious questions we must go into the aims which are attained by working in groups. Two aims are achieved by working in groups:
- (the best) decision-making;
- (the greatest) involvement.

a. Decision-making

Decision-making, which is the way in which people come to a decision, benefits from a large amount of information. For the best decision it is necessary to know about all the aspects of the matter. It is self-evident that the likelihood of more information is greater if more people join in the decision-making. This obviously does not go on for ever, and at a given moment there are enough people and more participants would simply get in the way. A meeting at which a decision is going to be taken has an optimum number of participants. This optimum situation is achieved when all the information necessary to make the best decision is available within and distributed among all the participants.

One brief word of warning here. It is not always the case that group-work is the best type of decision-making. Group responsibility for a

cognitive task can sometimes lead to diminished effort. This is sometimes related to the phenomenon of '*social loafing*'. That is the tendency – particularly in larger groups – for individuals to make less of an effort than they might in an individual or small group situation in which their responsibility is highlighted and visible to a greater extent. There are also some situations where a group has been together as a separate entity for such a long time that they are inward thinking, entrenched in their attitudes and tend to come to a consensus opinion because of relational influences rather than logical argument. Such groups are by definition usually closed groups which do not benefit from new members with new ideas coming in. Janis (1972) describes this phenomenon as '*group-think*'. Obviously while such groups may be very co-operative, the soundness of their decision-making may be questionable.

b. Involvement

Involvement means the degree to which you feel partly responsible for the success of the decision. It is concerned with the will of the participants to implement the decision, to back it. The will to implement a decision is found to be closely bound up with the degree to which you have assisted in the taking of that decision. You can broadly say that decisions which have been taken by third parties meet with far greater resistance than decisions which have been taken by those involved themselves. It is logical therefore that the implementation of a decision goes better if the implementers have taken part in the decision-making. This is another reason why people do not always take decisions alone, but often in groups composed of, or recognized as being representative of those who must implement the decisions.

3. Pitfalls in co-operation in groups

A number of clear pitfalls can also be distinguished in group co-operation. Here again it is a case of learning early on to recognize a number of common mistakes and thus learning not to fall into the traps. With an eye to co-operation in groups we shall discuss the following common problems:

- the hidden agenda;
- failing to recognize group dynamics;
- fighting out at content level what exists at the relational level.

a. The hidden agenda

By a hidden agenda we mean that someone has his own aim at a meeting, something which he wants to achieve, without the others being informed of this. You can think of many different things here: underhandedly aiming to get the night shift swapped because you cannot cope with it properly; underhandedly trying to make an impression on a new colleague who is attending the meeting for the first time today; underhandedly agreeing to all the proposals, making sure that the meeting is over quickly today, so that you have time to do some shopping. As you can see, there are plenty of examples.

It is characteristic of a hidden agenda that the others are not informed of it. You can see that in the examples the word 'underhandedly' recurs; a hidden agenda is thus a pitfall at a meeting. If the others are not informed of your intentions, they may think for example that you really are in agreement with all the proposals. They thus think that a decision has been taken which everyone supported, whilst you (assuming you had a hidden agenda) might well want to come back on that later. Perhaps you will later find that it is difficult to carry out the decision, or that you are not completely behind it. You will understand that if you take decisions at a meeting at which a hidden agenda (possibly of various participants) plays a role, you are actually building in a large number of problems.

b. Failing to recognize group dynamics

Dynamics is the science of movement. The term *group dynamics* means that processes are always taking place within groups which influence: the way in which people deal with each other; the relationships between group members; the way in which group members deal with each other; the way in which the group members behave when a new group member joins them. Because you have participated in a large number of groups all your life, you probably recognize some of these group dynamics processes, as they

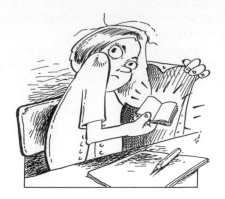

Hidden agenda

are called. Just think of your first week in a new class at school. It was all rather unfamiliar; you all adopted a wait-and-see attitude. Existing group members were sounding each other out: what can you do here, and what can you not do? Who dares most, and where do I stand in the class pecking order? A few weeks later this situation has settled down much more. Relationships have stabilized, the hierarchy is fixed. This is a well-known group dynamics phenomenon: it is known as *the incipient group process*.

If you want to know more about group dynamics, we refer you to Chapter 2 in Module 3. If you have time for a more detailed consideration of the research into group dynamics you will find the work of Blumberg et al (1983) an invaluable source of information. For this chapter, however, it is important that you realize that co-operation in a group is largely dependent on the development of this group. The influence of group dynamics on co-operation in a group is very great. Failing to recognize this influence can thus represent a pitfall. If you are not aware that in an incipient group other things are taking place between the lines apart from the task for which the group has been set up, faulty decisions may be taken.

c. Fighting out at content level what takes place at relational level

In Chapter 1 of this module (page 401) we touched on the fact that two levels can be distinguished in how people deal with each other: what is (literally) said and what is said between the lines. We define that here as the content level and the relational level.

The *content* relates to what was said and how it was understood, the *relation* to how people feel about it.

It is not usual in our culture to say much out loud about the relational level. We evidently prefer to do that between the lines. It is very unusual to express your feelings at a meeting. It seems as though this is forbidden. Yet everyone has feelings with regard to his colleagues. We usually deal with this in a very particular way in work situations: we translate these feelings. We tend not to say that the other person has played a nasty trick on us. We try to thwart the other person in a very polite and decent way by making objections to his proposal. What has in fact happened is that we are fighting out at content level (with pragmatic arguments) what exists at relational level.

An example of this is Doctor A, who said repeatedly that a wound dressing with natural cotton wool had to be put on patient B. When he was told that this was not the best course for this patient, he expounded detailed reasoning to justify his instructions – on one occasion explaining about practices in another hospital, on another quoting research into wound dressings. If we had seen into Dr. A's mind, we would have seen that he was actually unsure about his reputation in the hospital. When he made this blunder on the dressing as well, for the sake of his need for self-esteem he had to resort to all sorts of contortions to put himself in the right. He did this by attempting to 'prove' that he knew a lot about wound dressings. At content level it was a case of the choice of type of bandage, but at relational level Dr A wanted to be seen as an expert and accepted within the professional team of doctors and nurses.

This too is a situation which can spoil co-operation in groups. What is actually happening is that while arguments may be taking place at the level of content, in terms of disputing decisions etc, these are being greatly influenced by relational or interpersonal factors. For example, a person may be agreeing or disagreeing with a decision just because he has a liking for or commitment to someone else in the group. It is this relational factor which is influencing the person's decision rather than his independent and objective consideration of the content-matter or data being presented. The difficult thing about this state of affairs is that the motive behind his decision is often something primary and intuitive which the person will rarely admit to. He is often not even aware of it himself. The best thing you can do is therefore to try to prevent it. This may involve trying to keep discussion at the level of content, ensuring that when individuals express opinions they back these up with rational arguments and avoiding the group rushing to a final decision on a vote until all members have had opportunity to consider the rational arguments and counter arguments.

4. Important components of co-operation in groups

There are many components to be distinguished in co-operation in groups. You only need to bring to mind all the different types of groups, with all the different aims and all the different functions for the members. We shall not consider all of these. We shall present the two most important components, because you will encounter them a great deal in group co-operation. The two most significant components of co-operation in groups are:
– decision-making;
– evaluation.

a. Decision-making

By decision making we mean the way in which a decision comes about. Decision-making can take place in many ways. The various ways of decision-making can be distinguished for example by the extent to which those attending the meeting are brought in. Is everyone allowed to join in the decision or is it ultimately the chairman who has the final say? An argument can be made for every kind of decision-making. It is not that one form is always better than another.

The choice between the different ways of decision-making is in theory determined by the following three factors:

– The *time available* to spend on decision-making. Obviously the quality of the outcome is considered in all decisions, but there are situations where it is highly important that something is decided quickly. In nursing you will be faced with life or death situations where sound descision have to be made within seconds.

– The *quality or soundness* of the final decision reached. Where the time criterion is not one of urgency, the quality or soundness criterion should prevail. This means that the group should take sufficient time for discussion and analysis of a problem, consider different possible solutions or decisions, try to make sound judgements about the probable effectiveness of each, and carefully select the decision which has the best fit under the circumstances.

– Finally the *involvement* of the participants is of great significance for the outcome of a decision. Involvement, as we have already said earlier, influences the extent to which the participants are committed to a decision which has been taken. A decision may be good qualitatively, and also be taken quickly, but if the participants are not willing to carry it out, all the trouble taken may have been to no avail.

It is necessary for a good choice to be made in regard to the above three factors or criteria. Does the decision have to be taken quickly or can a long time be taken over it? Does the decision have to be of the very highest quality or is it more important that the participants are all behind it? Only if this kind of assessment is made can a determination be made on the best method of decision-making in a particular situation.

Skills in decision-making

Remember that in this chapter we are concerned with the skills of the participants in a meeting. The next chapter is concerned with the skills of the person leading the discussion at a meeting. The group participant skills identified here are as follows:

– *Collecting information.*
One condition to be met in order to reach a good decision is that it is based on a sufficient amount of relevant information. If you read on the agenda of a meeting what will be discussed at the meeting, and you consider it important, make sure that you are informed about the subject. Go and search in the library, read the newspaper on this topic, talk to this or that person, run through all the arguments you can think of; in this way you can join in the decision-making.

– *Reporting.*
You can only do something with this information if you succeed in conveying it to others. Two aspects to reporting can also be distinguished: content and form.
The following skills are important features regarding *content*:
• Give a brief introduction. Do not go straight to the point, but say what you want to make a comment on and only then say what your comment is.
• Make sure that you structure your reporting. Mention the most important thing first, do not tell too much at the same time and use examples of what you want the other participants to respond to.
• Finish with a statement in which you refer again to what you wanted to say. Indicate to what extent you feel that your contribution answers the problem stated.
With regard to *form*, the following skills are important:
• Speak clearly and intelligibly. Avoid your voice becoming quieter during what you have to say.
• Do not speak too quickly. Grant the others the opportunity to listen to your argument.
• Use short sentences. In this way you 'catch' the other group members' attention. You are more likely to lose the thread of the argument if you use long sentences with many qualifications. Decide what your important points are and make them briefly and appositely.
• Use concrete language. Talk about things, people and specific instances, avoiding phrases as 'generally' or 'most people'.

- Look at the others. This is probably the best aid you have for capturing the attention of the others. At the same time you can observe in this way whether the others are still following what you are saying.

– *Brainstorming.*
Brainstorming is a skill which many of us find difficult to get used to. This is a technique which is intended to allow all sensible and non-sensible ideas with regard to the topic of the meeting to emerge. In a brainstorming session all the participants are invited to mention all the ideas they can think of for solving a particular problem. The most important rule is that no discussion is allowed in this phase. The quality or inaptness of the ideas must not be discussed at this time: that comes later. Brainstorming thus demands that we lower our usual thresholds. At this stage we do not ask the obvious questions like for instance 'would this idea really work?' In effect, members of the group quickly, without premeditation, present single word or brief phrase statements related to the problem to be solved. We must also try to keep the first rejecting reactions to ourselves, as immediate analytic reaction is banned in this phase of brainstorming. In this situation we must stimulate and invite. Be curious in brainstorming about the train of thought of the other person. You can do this by asking for further explanation in an open manner. It is best to note down the participants' comments so that you can make use of these later. If noted down, these can be organized, combined, and discussed afterwards when problem-solving proceeds.

– *Combining solutions.*
After the brainstorming phase a slightly more structured approach must be taken. The ideas which have come up during the brainstorming must now be turned into workable and realistic solutions. For this to be done it is necessary for all the participants to see what kind of ideas have been put forward. Let everyone think about it, and ask the participants in turn to state their solutions for the situation on which a decision has to be taken. Note down the solutions. They will often consist of combinations of the ideas which have been stated in the previous phase. Make sure that the original purpose is mentioned regularly during this itemization; it should not be lost sight of in the heat of the meeting!

– *Choosing solutions.*
Having reached this phase, a choice must be made as to which of the proposed solutions we prefer. At this point problem-solving reaches the stage of decision-making. Here in particular the original problem and the possible limitations must be recalled. In this way an assessment can be made of which solution appears best. If there are two or more people who are emphatically not in

Brainstorming

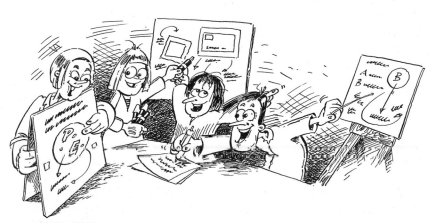

agreement, try to dissociate the points of view from the persons. Quite often the individuals are entrenched against each other and the points at issue become less significant when they are talked about in an objective and rational manner.

– *Planning*.

By planning we mean clearly identifying the problem, indicating the aims or objectives to be achieved and making agreements on how the solution is to be tried out. In regard to such agreements the following things are necessary.

• Make agreements which can be checked. An agreement such as: 'And then we'll have a look in a couple of months at how things are going' gives nothing to grasp onto. This kind of agreement is not a good basis on which to judge whether a solution

has been successful or not. The following agreement is therefore better: 'We will consider it to have been successful if in three months the average period of stay of patients in our department has fallen by one day.'

• Make actions specific. Agree when and what steps must be taken, and take account of what is feasible. Agree also who alerts whom if a step is not reached and what must then happen.

• Make sure that the contributions of the participants are well distributed. Appoint people who are responsible for the whole task and/or for parts of the task. Take account again of what is feasible. Offer those who are responsible support by regularly giving them the opportunity to report how the task is progressing.

Exercise 1. Decision-making

Aim: to be able to recognize decision-making processes in a group.

Number of persons: 8 to 16, of whom 2 are observers.

Materials: the observation checklist below..

Time required: exercise, 45 minutes; break, 15 minutes; subsequent discussion, 30 minutes.

Procedure: the group chooses two observers. These are equipped with the attached observation checklist. If necessary they read through the section on decision-making once more.

The other group members choose a discussion leader.

The group looks at the following situation:

The group is asked to assume that they have been given £20,000 on condition that they agree on how it is to be used. They must not use the money for themselves, the purpose must be to benefit the patients in their own hospital.

Each group member first decides for himself how he would prefer to spend the money. The group members spend five minutes individually on this. Note that no talking is allowed during this period. The decision-making then starts. The observers each fill in the observation list separately.

When the lists are completed the observations are then discussed. Make sure that you do not go back to re-examining the content of the arguments again. The emphasis must now be on the process of decision-making.

If the observations of the two observers differ, let them each explain how they arrived at these judgements.

Observation checklist for decision-making groups
(Circle 'yes' or 'no', as appropriate, for each item)
The following skills were correctly put to use in the meeting:

Information:

1. Sufficient information was collected to take the decision	yes	no

Brainstorming:

2. The participants were invited to state their ideas and/or views	yes	no
3. Discussions were interrupted	yes	no

Combining solutions:

4. Possible solutions were assessed in the light of the original aim	yes	no
5. A structure was applied to the solution strategies	yes	no

Choice:

6. Opinions were dissociated from individuals	yes	no
7. A decision was taken	yes	no

Planning:

8. A time path was made	yes	no
9. The contributions of the participants were distributed to the satisfaction of each	yes	no

Outcome:

10. The decision taken was the best in terms of		
Time (available)	yes	no
Quality (of decision)	yes	no
Involvement (of group members)	yes	no

A final comment is worth noting. People often use the terms problem-solving and decision-making interchangeably, as indeed we have tended to do above. However, there is a subtle difference. An individual or group can often solve a problem and identify action needed, but lack the conviction, assertiveness and courage to actually make the decision to 'carry it through'. Having the courage to take risks, acknowledge responsibility and accept accountability for decisions will be an important aspect of your nursing work. You should give this matter some attention in your follow-up work reviewing literature on risk-taking and professional accountablity.

The issues of problem-solving and decision-making are also discussed further in Chapter 6.

b. Evaluation

We normally make an evaluation when we have the idea that co-operation is not running as we would have wished or foreseen. However, it is not advisable to wait until a conflict erupts or problem arises. Some groups regularly organize a meeting to get feedback from participants or evaluate how things are going. An evaluation often only deals with whether the tasks involved in co-operating have been the most efficient way of achieving a particular aim, and whether all the tasks were or can be carried out. Less self-evident but just as necessary is to consider how those involved related to each other. In other words, alongside the evaluation of the task-oriented process an evaluation of the group-oriented process is also desirable.

The function of an evaluation – both of the task-oriented and the group-oriented process – is firstly to obtain information via the judgements of the participants. There is also an important second stage: an evaluation is only meaningful if it is followed by a plan and particular activities to remedy any situation with which there is dissatisfaction.

The content of the evaluation

It is useful to run through the following content-related steps in an evaluation:
– Have we achieved the task or the aim? To what

extent have we succeeded in keeping to the agreements we have made? If this has not been successful or not completely successful, why was this? Were the agreements not realistic; were there unforeseen circumstances as a result of which it proved impossible to achieve our aim? How must these circumstances be adapted, or what alternative aims are feasible?

– What is the evaluation of the means of achieving the aims? Are the participants satisfied that the resources and facilities for carrying forward the work were adequate? It is necessary to think here about time, money, material and other resources.

– What was the distribution of contributions in the group? Were the tasks in general evenly distributed? Were the unpleasant jobs evenly distributed?

– What comments can be made in regard to personal feelings?

In the above items we have spoken about satisfaction or dissatisfaction with regard to a number of more or less practical matters. However, dissatisfaction can also exist at the interpersonal level. Although you can assume that most people succeed in limiting this to manageable proportions, you will understand after reading the section about group dynamics that these feelings can lead to problems. It is thus of great importance to the progress of co-operation

to help shed light on these personal feelings. Be tactful when you bring up the subject of interpersonal relationships within the group; some of the skills in the section 'Skills in group evaluation' (pages 477, 478) will be useful in this respect. A certain amount of care is needed but it is nevertheless often illuminating to talk about these matters in the group. In so doing you may avoid personal distress and may also avoid failure to achieve the planned outcome of the problem-solving project.

The time of evaluation

Within the group you may have agreed on a specific time for evaluating, but do not restrict evaluation to such times; it should be an ongoing process. You must constantly keep your eyes open for information from the group members from which an assessment of the co-operation may become apparent. If you notice something which bothers the group members and it appears that they do not bring it out into the open, it is good to raise this. The best times for evaluation often arise spontaneously. On the principle, 'Strike while the iron's hot', it is best to talk about an incident as soon as it occurs. There are sound reasons for doing this. Firstly, there is the damage-containment argument. That is, if difficulties arise, they can be resolved before they place the planned outcomes of a project in jeopardy. Secondly, when difficulties arise people at

Figure 5.5.1
Evaluation

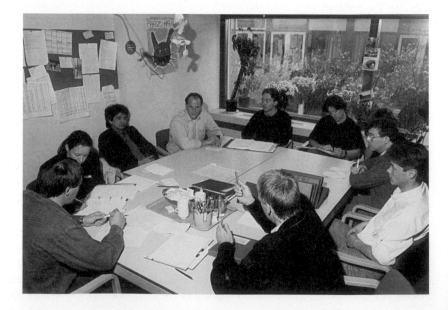

that point of time are often at their most vocal and are more likely to be open about the problems. If the matter is left until later, there is the possibility that individuals will consciously or unconsciously disguise their initial feelings.

You may want to refer back to the discussion of mental defence mechanisms in the psychology modules here. This will help you to recall how, given sufficient time, individuals may repress their true feelings or come up with rationalizations for how they behaved during a crisis. You will find when you study psychiatric nursing practices that it is often necessary to address major personal or interpersonal difficulties at or soon after they arise before the underlying problem is covered up. The same principle applies in group decision making. We used the phrase 'Strike while the iron is hot' above. The technical term psychiatric nurses use is *crisis intervention*. If you are interested in following up this term, Aguilera and Messick (1978) is a useful reference. However, one word of warning. Crisis intervention is a highly-charged situation and problems may be heightened and get out of control. There is sometimes a need to let the situation settle deliberately and address problems later when group members are more in control.

Another issue of timing is essentially all about the type of evaluation. There are in fact two types of evaluation:

Formative evaluation
This is evaluation which is ongoing and which takes place all the time or at regular intervals throughout the planned programme for achieving aims or resolving problems. This is essentially a diagnostic activity. The rationale is that it is too late waiting to the end, when the programme has to a greater or lesser extent failed, to do an evaluation. Formative evaluation allows for problems to be identified as (or even before) they arise, so that remedial action can be taken.

Summative evaluation
This is a major evaluation which takes place at the end of a planned programme for achieving aims. The purpose in this end-evaluation is to ascertain how successful the programme was in achieving its aims. However, it is not just about judging success. As in the case of formative evaluation, summative evaluation will almost always lead to further decision-making and subsequent action. If aims have not been achieved, a modified plan to resolve the problems remaining must be instituted; if the activities for problem resolution were not highly effective, different approaches may have to be adopted.

Skills in group evaluation
In evaluation, whether it happens in a planned or spontaneous way, you always need the following social skills:
- Introducing. Evaluation involves a specific judgemental way of talking about an issue. It is thus important to indicate to the other group members that you now want to talk about the effectiveness of the co-operation.
- Keep your comment descriptive. Talk about behaviour, make sure that the others can recognize what you talking about. Keep your description separate from your judgement, for example: 'I saw such and such happen, and I think it means as follows...'.
- Express your observations in 'I' terms. 'I consider...', 'it seems to me that...' sounds more open than 'You are always...'. The other person will probably feel attacked by the latter, and will thus show a tendency to start defending himself. This does not benefit open communication.
- Mention first the positive part of what you have to say. Make it clear that you do not want to demolish everything. Then mention the negative part, i.e. problems which have arisen, and failures in terms of achieving set aims.
- Ask the others for reactions. Be aware that your views could be wrong, so let others contribute as well. Remember, this is a group activity.
- Consider the following points, according to the meeting techniques described at Section 4a above. Remember that in *evaluating* how successful our problem identification – problem analysis – decision making – problem resolution programme has been, we are using the exact same techniques. That is – we are

identifying and analyzing problems, arriving at decisions and agreeing programmes for resolving problems or achieving aims. Thus, the same group activities are involved in group evaluation activities as were involved in the original group activities when the programme we are evaluating was formulated. This sounds all very formal. However, whether you have agreed a formal meeting for a major summative evaluation or are having an informal discussion in the staff rest room as part of ongoing formative evaluation, the same basic rules apply.

The techniques involved are:

- *Collecting Information*. A shared group activity; all members should bring their contribution to the meeting.
- *Reporting*. Each person contributes:
  - do group members share views about how well or badly things have progressed?
  - do group members share the conclusion that something must be done in relation to failures or problems which have arisen?

These two processes in fact reflect the essence of evaluation which is first to judge or assess success, and second to take action in resolving problems or improving success.

- *Brainstorming*. This technique, as described earlier, can be used in the group evaluation for two reasons. Firstly, it can be used as a means of collecting information quickly on group-members' judgements and feelings about the success or otherwise of the programme. Secondly it can be used to start off the problem-resolution process, as described at Section 4a above.
- *Combining solutions*. As you will recall, this is the amalgamating of ideas gained in brainstorming into possible or viable solutions.
- *Choosing solutions*. Here possible solutions are prioritized, and a 'first choice' is made.
- *Planning*. Even in evaluation there is a need for a plan which includes making an agreement (i.e. on aims to be achieved and actions to be taken), time schedules, distribution of contributions among group members. The important thing to remember is that in evaluation the agreement being made, i.e. the aims to be achieved and action to be taken, is concerned with prob-

lems which were identified at the judgement stage of the evaluation process.

Study activity

1. Problem solving in nursing practice. One of the areas in which nurses cooperate is concerned with patient-care problems. In your nursing studies you will be introduced to the *Nursing Process Method*. This is in fact a problem solving approach. It is usually divided into stages of *Assessment, Planning, Implementation* and *Evaluation*. Read descriptions of the nursing process method in your nursing textbooks. Write a brief rationale (about 500 words) for using the group co-operation principle in this chapter when applying the nursing process approach.

5. Summary

Co-operation in groups has been addressed chiefly by discussing the conditions necessary in order to make co-operation possible. We considered group functions in terms of task function and binding function. A rationale for group co-operation in terms of decision-making and involvement was explicated.

We have also dwelt on the pitfalls which can arise during co-operation.

Finally the following subjects were discussed:

- ways of decision-making and evaluation;
- the skills which are necessary with regard to decision-making and evaluation.

Directing meetings

6

1. Introduction

Directing meetings is a complicated business. If you expect one person to master all the skills necessary for keeping a meeting going along the right lines, you are expecting a lot from that person. This view nevertheless often prevails among those attending a meeting. If it does not run smoothly, the person directing the meeting is soon blamed and no blame is attached to the participants.

It is commonly believed that there are people who can lead a discussion and others who will never learn how to do it. There is an element of truth in this, but it is certainly not entirely true. There are obviously people who lead a discussion better than others, but this is only partly due to their character or personality. Generally these people have also simply learnt this skill. There are also groups which are easier to lead or guide. All the members of the group jointly determine how co-operation in this group will proceed. If the group members make smooth progress of the meeting dependent on the discussion leader, this means that he has to simultaneously take care of the agenda, the procedural rules, the process of interaction between the group members and possibly his own view of the problem or item on the agenda which is being discussed. This is too big a job for most people.

You may well wonder why a chapter on leadership, especially one which addresses leading or chairing group discussions, is included in a module on communication skills for nurses. However, nurses do not always work in an isolated one-to-one relationship with their patients. Each hospital ward has a team of nurses, which is part of a wider multidisciplinary team including doctors, nurses, occupational therapists, physiotherapists, social workers and others. In community settings nurses also work with each other and with others such as General Practitioners, social workers and voluntary care workers. We have already seen in the previous chapter that a number of issues which arise are dealt with on a group discussion basis. It often also falls on a nurse to adopt the role of discussion leader or chairman of such groups. This is therefore a skill you will have to develop for proceeding in your nursing career. Even in the narrower situation of patient-care some nursing situations involve working with groups rather than individual patients. Those of you who are proceeding to qualify as psychiatric nurses will find that group therapy techniques will be an important aspect of your education. Here too, the issue of leading group activities is an important skill area.

Learning outcomes

After studying this chapter the student should be able to:
– understand the aim of discussion leadership;
– recognize and describe the following styles of leadership:
  • autocratic;
  • democratic;
  • laissez-faire;
  • functional;
– recognize and describe seven task-oriented skills in the directing of meetings;
– recognize and describe five group-oriented skills;
– begin to develop skills of group leadership.

2. Aim of discussion leadership

Study activity
  1. a. Itemize what experience you have of leading discussions and put the experience into words.
  b. Try to sketch a profile of personal characteristics and skills which according to you a good leader should have.

It is evident from the previous chapter that group co-operation decisions are taken on the basis of all the relevant information, and the commitment of the participants is greater the more they are allowed to join in deciding. The aim of leadership in discussion is actually to ensure that the group's goals and aims are achieved. Ultimately the leader is the person who is responsible. We say 'ultimately' here because we wish to emphasize once again that all group members must contribute. Only if this does not happen, does not happen sufficiently or does not happen on time must the discussion leader intervene. The following sections must also be read in this light.

A discussion leader can behave in a number of different ways. You have already read in Module 3 about the different types of leadership. We shall briefly repeat this here:
– *Autocratic leadership*. A discussion leader who behaves autocratically (literally: ruling with his/her own power) assumes the right to make the final decision for himself. He will at most listen to the group members and generally not even that. They have to do what they

are told, and that is the end of it. Do not make the mistake of confusing this form with task-oriented leadership. A discussion leader who acts autocratically can take decisions both in the field of the task and in the field of interaction. The characteristic feature is merely that he is the only one who makes the decision.
– *Democratic leadership*. The leader here uses interventions which are directed towards giving the group members the maximum input. The leader occupies himself particularly with signals which he gets from the group on the satisfaction and involvement of the various participants. A discussion leader who in a particular situation chooses a democratic style of leadership stimulates the group members and invites them to take part actively in the solution of the problem which exists at that moment. The final decision is shared by the members.
– *Laissez-faire leadership*. To translate this term freely, it means something like, 'Let things go'. This is actually the absence of leadership. The group leader does not intervene and allows the meeting to take its course. The decision is often taken by the one who is most assertive. In effect a final decision can be taken by anyone or (not infrequently) by nobody! That is, no final decision is taken at all.

We also wish to draw another term to your attention: *functional leadership*. We indicated in Module 3 that the three styles of leadership mentioned are not fixed personality features, but that you must be able to choose a particular style at particular moments.

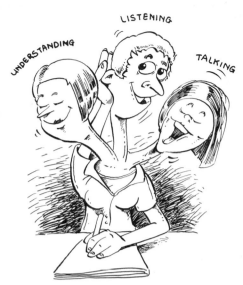

LISTENING
UNDERSTANDING
TALKING

The discussion leader has to do
a lot at the same time

There can be said to be functional leadership if:
- the group members are jointly responsible for the progress of the meeting, and
- the chairman or group leader from time to time can make a choice among the various styles of leadership.

The question naturally arises on what basis this choice for one or other style is to be made. You can take the following factors into consideration.
- *Situation.*
  One situation demands a different style of leadership to another. In the case of something which has to be decided quickly, the discussion leader must behave more autocratically than in the case of a decision which can take longer. In an adult group which runs well and whose members of are well accustomed to each other, it is best for the chairman to adopt a 'laissez faire' attitude for a while, so long as he is ready if necessary to intervene.
- *Requirements.*
  The group members may also have differing and sometimes even changing requirements. An item on the agenda which they have already dealt with earlier will probably proceed more easily with a chairman who employs a democratic style of leadership, whilst a new

subject, with many unfamiliar aspects, makes a more autocratic style desirable.
- *Habits.*
  Finally you must not lose sight of the fact that solution habits soon arise in a department which form part of the 'department culture'. You should also review the phenomenon of groupthink at this point (see page 469). We are not arguing here that habits should be prevented, but it can be quite salutary to discuss them. Bear in mind, however, that habits are often very stubborn. Someone who weighs in strongly against particular ingrained patterns of behaviour may pay heavily for it in a co-operation situation. So make sure that you tackle habits with tact and caution.

3. Skills in directing or chairing meetings

These are discussed in two parts. Firstly there are the skills necessary to bring the task to a successful conclusion, the *task-oriented skills*. These are skills with which you work efficiently and with which a correct solution is striven for. They are not the skills which serve the co-operation itself. The social skills which are necessary for co-operation for its own ends are called *group-oriented skills*. These are the interventions by which the participants in a meeting can be allowed to flourish as much as possible.

a. Task-oriented skills

Preparation

The discussion leader can only chair the meeting well if he has prepared himself as well as possible. Good preparation consists of:
- gathering information;
- identifying and formulating the problem;
- thinking of issues which must be addressed and strategies for doing this;
- ensuring that the goals or aims and terms of reference (i.e. what the group has to do) are clarified in advance or identified as issues for discussion.

It is also useful in the meantime to sound out a few opinions, and to think of possible solutions to the problem which is to be dealt with.

Setting an agenda

A second condition for a meeting to run well is to distribute an agenda well in advance (for example one week before the meeting). This of course requires that the group membership (i.e. those who will receive the agenda) has been determined in advance. Such an agenda might contain the following items:
- the subject or subjects which will be brought up at the meeting;
- the order in which items will be discussed;
- what the purpose of the discussion is (for example: sounding out initial opinion, or decision-taking);
- where any further information on these subjects can be found.

It may also be necessary to circulate other documentation with the agenda, e.g. discussion papers.

It is not always the case, of course, that formal, detailed typewritten agendas are used. In some cases, for example daily meetings of a ward nursing team, only a single handwritten agenda is drawn up – perhaps in the ward diary or a notebook in which brief notes of the meeting are also kept. In some cases, where for example a group meets frequently to discuss a single subject, a formal agenda may be unnecessary.

Organizing the meeting

To ensure that the meeting runs smoothly you will need to address general organizational issues. These will include:
- ensuring that the meeting room is suitable and adequately equipped with table, chairs, etc;
- making sure that reference books which may be required, a set of standing orders or rules of meeting (if such has been agreed in advance), pencils and paper, are provided;
- arranging refreshments if a long meeting is anticipated;
- particularly in a more formal setting, ensuring that someone has been identified to take the minutes or at least an informal record of the meeting.

You are now ready to proceed with the meeting. As chairman or group leader you will be:
- welcoming members
- noting apologies
- doing a brief chairman's or group leader's opening address, which briefly identifies the business to be conducted, the terms of reference (i.e. goals or aims) and standing orders.

The meeting can then proceed with each agenda item in sequence or agreed order. The remainder of this section addresses the task-orientated skills for dealing with each individual item.

Introduction

An agenda item should be introduced.
The following issues are brought up in an introduction:
- Why is the subject on the agenda? What has led to this situation and what is the purpose of the discussion?
- What can and cannot be changed at this meeting? These circumstances must be clear before it is known how the subject can be handled.
- Propose a procedure. Make agreements on the time which it is proposed should be spent on the discussion. Where appropriate agree how a decision can be taken: must everyone be agreed or does a majority of votes apply?
- Finally, ask a neutral initial question. Make sure that no opinion is indicated by this; you have already said a great deal as chairman. It is now time for those attending to be invited to express their opinions on the subject. You know from the previous module that it is best to invite people by asking an open question.

Problem-solving

As already discussed in Chapter 5, this process runs along fairly fixed lines. We called the component parts:
- collecting information;
- reporting;
- brainstorming;
- combining solutions;
- choosing solutions.

In Chapter 5 we describe the skills which you use in these phases as a participant in such a meeting. Here we consider the skills which you need as a discussion leader at such a meeting. Problem-solving starts with *reporting,* whilst the *collecting of information* happens outside the meeting.

– *Reporting.*

The reporting generally begins after the discussion leader has asked who would like to speak. If the participants have prepared themselves (and this is highly likely if there is a good agenda), there will certainly be participants who want to say something. The discussion leader must restrict himself to clarifying – if necessary – what is said. He must make sure that only questions for further information are asked, and no others. After everyone who wanted to has reported his findings, it is possible to move on to the next phase, brainstorming.

– *Brainstorming.*

The discussion leader must introduce this phase by briefly defining the procedure: in brainstorming the participants do not ask each other for further information on solutions. Individuals provide brief short phrase or even one-word suggestions for dealing with the issue. There is no discussion. The goal is to get as many of these as possible.

The chairman or group leader first asks an introductory question: how could we solve this problem? After this he monitors the rules that have just been described.

In brainstorming it is important that the suggestions are recorded. The way in which it is done does not matter, but it is necessary to agree who does it. This person is not able to take part in the content of the brainstorming session. Consequently it is not advisable for the discussion leader himself to do this reporting. He already has his hands full leading the brainstorming session. In this phase too it is important to monitor the time and to draw attention to the fact if time threatens to run out.

When the brainstorming session has burnt itself out – you notice that when less ideas come – the discussion leader asks whether there are any last suggestions. It is then possible to move on to the next phase.

– *Combining solutions.*

It is useful for this phase if the discussion leader has some overview of the requirements to be met by a solution. He must in particular first refer back to the original statement of the problem. This is in effect the follow-up stage of brainstorming. Discussion and analysis may now take place. Here the listed solutions are analyzed, added to, deleted, joined together, etc.

The leader must help to identify solutions which really appear to reduce or solve the problem. If there are strong personal conflicts in the group, it is particularly important in this phase that the discussion leader tries to dissociate the opinions from the persons who proclaim these opinions. Make sure you do not talk about 'Peter, who said this', but about what has been said.

Finally it is possible to discover in this phase of the decision-making process that the original statement of the problem was incorrect. In this case it is necessary to re-formulate the problem. The proposed solutions can perhaps be of good service, but it may even be necessary to think up alternatives. If problems were indeed so clear that you were able to see the way to the solution at once, less meetings would be needed.

– *Choosing a solution or solutions.*

Now the group must choose what it agrees is the best solution or solutions. Where different solutions are available, the group must prioritize these and select the best one. This is in fact the stage at which problem-solving becomes decision-taking or decision-making. This important activity is elaborated upon below.

It is worth noting that not everyone uses an orthodox brainstorming approach in which ideas for solving a problem are first generated without discussion and there is then discussion in a combining solutions stage. Indeed these two stages are often combined and discussion is allowed to flow in a much less structured way. However, it is important to ensure that the stage which we are now going on to consider, the decision-making stage is kept separate and distinct from the earlier problem-solving activities.

It is important that a definite decision can be identified when all discussion has ended.

Decision-making

The various forms of decision-making have to some extent already been presented in the previous chapter, from the point of view of the person attending a meeting. We discussed choice and planning. In addition we looked at how far the participants could be involved in the taking of decisions. It came down to the decision being made in the meeting only in the case of joint decision by the group members; in all other cases the discussion leader decides. We therefore restrict the discussion here to the phase of decision-making in group situations.

In group decision there are a number of other options for decision-making open to you. Depending on what sort of procedural agreements you have made with the group at the introduction, a choice has been made for: decision by ordinary majority (half plus one); general agreement or consensus; unanimous, i.e. the decision is only taken if everyone is in agreement. In the latter case each group member has what is known as the right of veto: the right to prevent a decision if he or she is not in agreement with it. If voting is to take place, an agreement must also be reached on how votes are to be cast. It is usual that if the matter you are voting on concerns people, it is done in writing. In most other cases voting takes place by raising a hand. The discussion leader must formally state all the alternatives, so that the participants are also given the opportunity to abstain from voting.

Decision-making ends with the planning of its implementation. Someone may perhaps be released, or partially released, from other activities in the group in order to fulfil the tasks; otherwise tasks have to be divided up among the participants. A schedule must be drawn up so that each person knows when results are to be expected. All must be clear about when a solution is accepted. The criteria which a solution must meet are set by a number of questions. What must be achieved within what time before one is satisfied? What are the steps which must be taken? Who should be informed if these steps are not taken? What happens then? Does the item return to the agenda or does a contingency plan come into effect? All these questions form part of the conclusion of the decision-making phase of a meeting. The task of the discussion leader in this is to see to it that all these items are dealt with.

Decision-making in the absence of reaction

In the decision-making described above it is assumed that all the participants join in properly where they have something to say on the subject. In fact the reality may be somewhat more complicated. It is often found that participants in a meeting do not react or hardly react despite many invitations.

You may observe the following in such a meeting. The discussion leader works extremely hard to get the group moving but members do not respond. They may sit watching, some with amusement, and let the meeting roll by, while enjoying a cup of coffee. The attitude of the group members is certainly willing, provided nothing needs to be done. On the pretext that 'very sensible things are being said' they do not feel obliged to join in. This is in fact an example of the 'social loafing' phenomenon described on page 469. The discussion leader, at his wits' end, as a last resort addresses one of the group members personally with: 'What do you think about it?' The reaction can be predicted: 'I agree with it.' This can go on for a long time. The discussion leader often does not see what is happening. He is aware that the group cannot be got moving, and he tries harder to encourage and draw out responses. The group notices this and the members think (consciously or unconsciously), 'There he goes, let him carry on.' Instead of feeling encouraged, they consider this an invitation to make even less of an effort. After all, someone else is hard at work!

If this goes on, the discussion leader and the group members are in a vicious circle. The behaviour of one part provokes the behaviour of the other part. The meeting drags itself on, completely dominated by the discussion leader.

At a particular moment a decision will have to be taken. The type of decision-making which takes place here occurs so often that we designate it as decision-making in the absence of reaction. The discussion leader makes a proposal. There is no reaction. The discussion leader makes a proposal again. Again no real reaction, at most some murmuring. The discussion leader, not yet tiring, tries once more: 'Do I take from this that you are in agreement?' Once again murmured assent. The discussion leader has now had enough: the decision has been taken. You will understand that this decision may not have a great chance of being implemented by the participants.

In addition the mood in such a meeting is not quite right. It is therefore something that needs to be prevented, and this need not be too difficult. If you chair such a meeting, you need to be able to observe and recognize this kind of behaviour. What you must do about it is to bring the behaviour itself up for discussion. Require the participants to participate. Cut short the meeting if this does not happen and reserve the right to take a decision yourself in this case. It is very likely that the group members will then wake up and will start to join in.

Evaluation

The function, content, and time of the evaluation and the skills required for it were discussed in Chapter 5 from the point of view of the participants in a meeting. We also explained there why it is better to evaluate too often than too little. Even if the meeting has gone well, it is sometimes useful to look back. We shall be concerned here again with what the discussion leader must do to contribute to a successful evaluation, in the context of a meeting.

The leader must again briefly introduce this part of the discussion. This introduction should culminate in a question, for example: 'Looking back on this discussion, how did you find it went?' or something similar. You can in fact regard evaluation as a phase of decision-making in itself: the same things actually happen. Here again information is obtained, albeit far briefer;

solutions are found for any problems and agreements reached on how such things are to be tackled subsequently.

Checking and where necessary adjusting

If the preceding phases of the meeting have proceeded well, the checking and adjustment need not pose any problem. It has been agreed what must be done and by whom. It has also been agreed what must happen if an agreed course of action is not complied with. The discussion leader needs to ensure that any action agreed is or will be carried forward. Nevertheless, this may not be so simple. This is due usually to the fact that the previous phases in the meeting were not covered as conscientiously as described here.

Closing the meeting

When each item on the agenda has been discussed, it is time to call the meeting to a close. Of course, all the business may not have been completed, and in many cases it is not expected that all will have been achieved at a single meeting. It is important to:

– ensure that some time has been set aside for any other business e.g. urgent matters which members wish to draw attention to;
– agree a date, time and venue for a subsequent meeting, if required;
– thank members for their contributions;
– clearly declare the meeting closed.

b. Group-oriented skills

In the treatment of the skills of a discussion leader above we mentioned the skills which are concerned with efficiently achieving the aim. Whether people scratched each other's eyes out or sat flirting was not of importance, so long as it did not get in the way of achieving the aim. Reality is obviously once again more complicated. Read through Module 3, Chapter 2 once more: people in groups always react to each other and together make a group a whole, which is constantly in motion. Mutual attraction and repulsion occur commonly in groups. This obviously also affects (task-oriented) co-operation. It is sometimes necessary to say something which explicitly has the intention of influencing these group dynamics. We call these types of comments 'group-oriented skills'. We explain some of these skills below.

Following what the other person has to say

Do not make do with your own judgement but continue asking questions as to precisely what a group member means. In this way you do justice to the other person. In addition, by summarizing a point being made, you help to keep the matter clear for each participant.

Encouragement

By encouraging you stimulate co-operation. The participants feel less inhibited to say things on topics about which they know little. The mood becomes less judgemental and more constructive. In the most favourable case a common mood arises, one of 'all hands to the wheel'. Encouragement consists of the following components:
– Acknowledging that the other person has an opinion which must be listened to.
– Offering help. Invite the other person to put forward his opinion if you see that he is hesitating. Stand by the other person if there is a threat of his being attacked too early by other group members. Stimulate him to finish off his train of thought. Be aware that conflicts remain lurking under the surface if they are not openly expressed.
– Rewarding. Honour the usable elements in the other person's argument. Do not use this as a dodge: your credibility as group leader is at risk if it is obvious that you do not mean it. Do not be afraid of showing your enthusiasm if you like the idea someone puts forward. However, one problem with rewarding is that you may be more enthusiastic for one proposal than you are for another. We call this 'selective rewarding' and although it is quite natural to be better disposed towards one thing rather than another, your rewarding may be seen by some members of the group as favouritism or a bias towards someone in the group whose arguments (it may seem) you are always supporting.

Responding to group feelings

There are occasions when the meeting does not run smoothly. It is difficult to find out exactly what is wrong, but the participants react stiffly to each other. Things are not understood and attention is lost. You can see this from the non-verbal behaviour of the participants. Looks of disapproval, distracted people and even sleeping or dozing may also occur. These are all signs that it is not working. It is sensible to mention this as the discussion leader. Take your own feeling as a guide. This is generally a good 'thermometer' for moods. Make sure that you only do this when you feel familiar with your role as discussion leader. Some tension at the start of the discussion is natural, and you only make this worse if you speak about your uncertainty when this is not shared by the others!

Controlling interactions in the group

You will often find that some people threaten to monopolize the discussion, while others are easily subdued and are fearful of contributing. Some members of the group may be positive in their criticism while others may have a habitually negative and cynical attitude towards most proposals and arguments. It is difficult to be prescriptive about all strategies which may work in different situations to ensure that group interaction proceeds smoothly and effectively. You will have to use your own judgement and discretion. However, there are two simple devices you can use here:
(i)   Directional control. Deliberately and openly ask one member to comment, while asking the others to listen; if necessary cut in if attention drifts and reiterate a question to the particular member, perhaps using paraphrasing.
(ii) Bringing in and shutting out. Use the chairman's veto to 'give the floor' to under-contributors and cut out the over-contributors. It is of course important that in bringing in you do not place undue pressure on members, and that in shutting out you do not offend a highly motivated and constructive colleague whose only 'crime' is over-enthusiasm!

Promoting relaxation

If you can bring about a relaxed atmosphere in a natural way, this is by far the best way of positively influencing the mood. We cannot give any recipes such as 'Two jokes per meeting'. We can only advise you that, if it seems appropriate, you should not hold back a joke.

Mediating

If conflict arises in the group it is of the greatest importance that the conflict is resolved within a short time. Conflicts are not unusual, but they can negatively influence the meeting if nothing is done about them. When we say, 'Do something about conflict', we certainly do not mean that the conflict should be soothed without being tackled. Comments such as, 'Well, let's not talk about it any more' do not solve the conflict.

For conflict to be solved it must be talked out. This obviously need not necessarily take place in the group, but if an eruption occurs during a meeting, you need not always step aside from it either. The most important thing, however, is that someone, for example the discussion leader, prompts people to express their conflict. Offer to support them in this talking out.

The function of the discussion leader during such mediation is that of referee, with the remark that you must above all avoid taking sides, however much you are tempted to do so. Make sure that you allow both parties to formulate what according to them is wrong. Let them then both formulate what must be done according to them and ensure also that the rules of fair play are observed.

Study activity

1. The nurse as group leader. Although it may seem a long way off now, someday you may be a ward manager and have to use group leadership skills. However you may be faced with leadership responsibilities much sooner. In *Primary Nursing* a nurse is responsible for the care of one or more patients. In new approaches to community care, described as *Care Management*, a nurse may find herself to be the member of the multi-disciplinary team who is the *key worker* or *case manager* for a particular patient. In regard to this patient's care she will have to adopt the group leader role.
   a. Review the literature on primary nursing and care management. Write a brief (300 word) description of each of these concepts.
   b. Select one of these concepts and write a brief (400 word) explanation of how the group leadership skills described in this chapter are important in operating the particular concept you have chosen.

4. Summary

Participating in a meeting is not always a pleasant activity. Participation becomes a (co-)responsibility if the aim of the meeting has to be achieved quickly and efficiently.

Co-responsibility of this kind often creates (emotional) problems, and this is intensified if you have to chair a meeting as a discussion leader. The leadership styles involved in this role were discussed.

The skills needed in chairing a meeting can be learnt and these were described. The skills involved were considered from both task-oriented and group-oriented perspectives.

Various problems associated with chairing meetings were discussed, including the absence of reaction in the groups and the imbalance in the level of contributions from the individual group members. Obviously personal characteristics also have an important role to play.

7 Negotiating

1. Introduction

Negotiation is essentially about resolving conflicts or settling disputes. It is a process of joint decision-making characterized by bargaining, the success of which is a decision or agreement. This is usually marked by some degree of compromise for the parties concerned. According to interactionist sociology (see Module 3) all social phenomena – rules, norms, role behaviour, etc – are the outcome of negotiation. Negotiation is thus a very important sociological concept and is, according to interactionists, the process by which social norms and social order is established; in fact their technical term for this is 'the negotiated order'. Negotiation may relate to the swapping of a shift, the purchase of a car or the motivating of a patient. It is a skill which everyone needs and uses in many aspects of everyday life.

In this chapter we describe negotiation in the work context of the nurse in a health care setting.

Learning outcomes

After studying this chapter the student should be able to:
– describe what is understood by integrative and distributive negotiation;
– describe three pitfalls during negotiation;
– recognize and describe the skills of negotiation and negotiation strat–
  egies.
– explain negotiation as an influential process in nursing;
– operate negotiation strategies in dyadic (two-person) and group situations.

2. Aim of negotiation

By negotiating you try to achieve particular aims with someone who has different interests from yourself, so that you can continue co-operating with this person. The trust between the two people is not damaged. To make this clear we make a distinction between the two extreme forms of negotiation:

– *integrative negotiation;*
– *distributive negotiation.*

We shall first give an example of both an integrative and a distributive way of negotiating. Imagine that you are going to put together the duty roster for the coming period with a colleague. It will make a difference if you are talking to someone who will only continue working in the department for two months or someone who will be staying for years. In the first case you will do your best to get the most out of your colleague. You will probably negotiate harder and concede less than with someone with whom you will be working in the department for a long time to come. In the latter case something else is involved. You will later regularly encounter this person, and you are dependent on each other. To put it differently, you will have to be a little friendly towards this other person. You do not do that by trying to get the most you can out of her.

The type of negotiation on the duty roster with someone you will not see for much longer falls into the category of *distributive negotiation.* The relationship between the two negotiating partners is one of 'my gain is your loss'. What one person gets is at the cost of what the other person loses. Something is *distributed* between two people. Hence the term 'distribution'. The negotiations can best be described as 'fighting' or 'bargaining'.

The second type of negotiation, with someone you will see for a long time, falls into the category of *integrative negotiation.* In this type of negotiation the aim is for both to get a good deal. A gain for one is also a gain for the other. Nothing is distributed, both benefit from it. The wishes of both are merged or integrated. Co-operation between colleagues in this way remains on-going. These negotiations can be best described as 'co-operation'.

3. Pitfalls in negotiation

Negotiation itself is actually a hornet's nest. It is a subtle skill which has a great many possible ways of going wrong. We shall mention a few of these:

– It is quite possible that you go so astray in a negotiation that you limit your strategy to thwarting the other person. Instead of ensuring that you achieve your own aims, you direct all your attention to preventing the other person achieving his. You may well prevent the other person attaining what he had planned. But do you emerge from the conflict satisfied? If you direct your activities towards thwarting the other person, so that this person in any case does not achieve his aim, you can easily fail in your own aim. If you look at what comes out of such an action, compared with what should come out of it, it generally comes as an enormous shock. Not only have you thwarted the other person, so that he did not attain the best possible result, you yourself have achieved far less than was possible for yourself.

– A second important pitfall is negotiating too

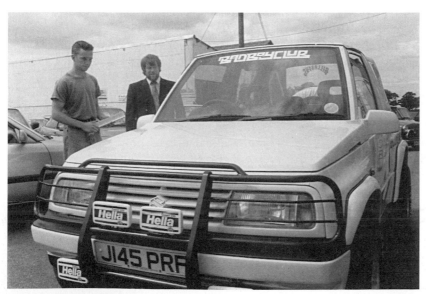

Figure 5.7.1
Negotiating

hard, too distributively. In the long run this will be to your detriment. You do not make any friends by doing this. Particularly in a co-operative situation it is not advisable to antagonize colleagues. You will pay for it later.

However, you must understand that we are not advocating indiscriminately staying friends with everyone, if that were possible. As we have already said, negotiation is a subtle game of give and take. You are constantly balancing costs and benefits. What does this move do for me and what does it cost me? How do the scales balance between what I owe the other person and what he owes me? It should be noted that the balance is not only maintained by factual matters but also by emotional matters.

4.   Negotiation as a nursing skill

We have illustrated in earlier chapters that nursing is in fact an interpersonal activity. All nursing work involves interacting with others, directly or indirectly. Much of this interaction is in fact negotiating. Nurses negotiate with nursing colleagues to provide staff cover on the wards and to agree patient care plans. They negotiate with doctors and other professionals in agreeing treatment and care regimes. And they negotiate with patients – sometimes to achieve compliance and co-operation in care programmes.

It may be helpful to consider two of these examples in a little more detail. Firstly, the example of negotiating with doctors. Doctors have in most instances the final say in patient management. The balance of power is in their favour. There is also sometimes a male (doctor) and a female (nurse) potential conflict here. Many nurses see themselves as autonomous professionals in their own right. Yet many doctors, and indeed some more traditional nurses, aspire to the situation in the past in which the nurse was 'the doctor's handmaiden'. The problem here is that, because of her greater degree of contact and intimacy with the patient, the nurse often knows much more about the patient than the doctor. The doctor needs the nurse's advice. But asking for it can be difficult as there is a 'balance of power' status quo to be

maintained. As a result a complex form of negotiation has to be undergone.

This situation was excellently illustrated by Stein (1978) in his paper entitled 'The doctor-nurse game'. In this game the nurse makes recommendations on patient treatment which have to appear to come from the doctor. They both achieve this by a complex game of subtle and indirect questions and answers, veiled recommendations and almost tongue-in-cheek confirmation of recommendations. Note the following conversation:

Nurse: She is becoming increasingly agitated – very disruptive for the other patients.
          We had this problem with her before.
Doctor: What was prescribed for her previously?
Nurse: Chlorpromazine worked quite well when she was in before.
Doctor: Perhaps we should try her on 50 mg Chlorpromazine three times daily.
Nurse: 50 mg did not really hold her last time. We had to increase it in the end.
Doctor: I'll try her on Chlorpromazine 100 mg three times daily.

This was of course what the nurse wanted all along. It was her intention to get this patient on a relatively high dosage of Chlorpromazine (a tranquillizing drug). Indeed she actually wanted 100 mg administered three times a day. But she could not come out and directly suggest this. That would have got the doctor's 'back up'; it would not have been playing the doctor-nurse game. The recommendation in its final form had to be seen to be initiated by the doctor.

In the second example of nurse-patient interaction, the balance of power is in the nurse's favour. However, here again, by subtle negotiation activities the patient can manage to exert some control over his circumstances. This is well illustrated in the paper by Roth (1971) to which you were first introduced in Chapter 3 of Module 3. This was one of the earliest and still often quoted pieces of research on negotiation in the health care situation. You are again strongly encouraged to read this important work in your follow-up studies. Roth found that patients quickly learn bargaining strategies which work. They find out which nurses will give them medication they want and negotiate with them rather than others. The nurses may attempt to avoid complying by stalling tactics, pretending to forget or giving the patient a placebo (e.g. an aspirin rather than a sedative). However, the patient has his counter-strategies: he keeps on nagging until the nurse gives in, or he makes the threat of going 'over the nurse's head' to the doctor if she does not give in. Sometimes it all just does not work. But often the patient's bargaining is successful and he gets exactly what he wants, or waits and tries another nurse!

You may have formed the opinion from this that much nursing work is about negotiating with doctors, patients and others; and that much of it comes down to striking bargains and agreeing deals.
In a nutshell, you are quite correct! It is therefore very important that you learn negotiating skills.

5. Skills in negotiation

In this chapter we discuss a number of skills which have a large part to play in negotiation.

a. Preparation

As might have been predicted, the more expert you are with regard to a subject, the less hold the other person has on you and the firmer your footing. A good negotiating position thus comes closer if you prepare yourself well. Preparation for negotiation must cover the following items:
– Seek information on the subject and your partner (or adversary) in negotiation. What is his interest? What does he wish to achieve? What is he sensitive to? What does he know? What does he not know? What does he know about you?
– Formulate different solutions for yourself, including less desirable ones. Make sure you do not have only one card to play. Imagine beforehand how the negotiation might go, and what might come out of it. Do not be

obsessed by what is the best solution for you: think about solutions which may be less good as well. Then you can react more flexibly in negotiation. You have already considered this and that option, which may perhaps signify new and unexpected turns in the conversation for the other person.
– Establish for yourself what outcome would satisfy you and what outcome would not be acceptable. This dividing line is the most important thing for you to hold onto during the negotiation itself. The most important thing of all in the whole negotiation is that you keep this dividing line strictly secret from the opposing party. Make sure that it is impossible for him to get to know anything about it. He must not know what your are prepared to accept, i.e. what is the limit to which you are prepared to go in accommodating him. If the opposing party knows the *limits of your acceptance* he will not be prepared to accept any less and you will not be able to negotiate a better deal or bargain from your point of view.

b. Who bids?

Start the negotiation with an opening bid.
State a possible outcome about which you wish to talk with the other person. This *stake* must satisfy a number of conditions:
– Bid as far as you have arguments for doing so. Be aware that after making your bid you can only go down, so start as high as possible. The likelihood of finishing in a position with which you are satisfied is then all the greater. Bear in mind that you must have arguments for your opening bid. It makes your position weak if you have to backtrack, because your opening bid then looks implausible. In other words, make sure that you yourself believe in what you are saying. This has much to do with your preparation, such as the amount of information and the secrecy of your dividing line, i.e. how far you are prepared to drop.
– Build *'small change'* into your bid. Be prepared to drop a little, do not stick at all costs to your opening bid. We cannot stipulate when you have to climb down. You have to learn this from experience, but if you have the idea that the other person is on the point of

stopping the negotiation, you can decide to concede something. We call this *'making a concession'*.

c. Keeping negotiation integrative

This is the most difficult and also the most important skill. You must for example never talk about negotiation, but always about co-operation. Make sure that you do not create the impression of being against the interests of the other person. The way you do this is as follows. Identify a common interest. Make sure that the common interest is as close as possible to your own position. If the task is to divide up a budget for your department together with your competitor, do not talk about everything you disagree on, but emphasize that it is a department which is running well, and that you are both agreed on that. Refer constantly to what you have in common. This is the basis on which you will have to give form to the co-operation. This is the only way in which you can keep the negotiation integrative.

d. First choice of position

After both parties have made their bids, it is time to make a first choice of position. Is there anything in the other person's proposal? What do you and he agree on? You must pass through the following steps here:

– Itemizing joint criteria. By this we mean stating the underlying principles which the other person is evidently adopting.
State your own underlying principles too. Express what you initially disagree on and what you agree on. Make sure that the other person also sees and acknowledges the agreements. In this way you already start unravelling the other person's bid, and this can later come in useful for you. The intention is to make the other person give up bits of his bid. If you succeed in dividing the bid up into bits, this is to your advantage. Formulate clearly what underlying principles you agree on. After you have stated the common aim, this is thus the second component on which you are agreed.
– Try to define the problems on which you are negotiating in an objective way. Facts and arguments, that is what negotiation is about

and these facts and arguments can be compared with each other to some extent; you can more or less weigh them up against each other. Negotiation only works if choices can be made. In the extreme situation, when there is really no more choice for you, it is best to let the other person know that you cannot negotiate any further. This may apply for example in cases in which difficult ethical decisions have to be taken, and where there is a stage beyond which you cannot agree on further compromise. Make sure the other person clearly understands this.

– Formulate requirements. When it is found that you are agreed on what must be achieved and on the criteria which a solution must fulfil, requirements can be formulated. These are the conditions which you feel (or wish) that a solution must fulfil.

e. Intensifying points of view

After the points of view have become a little clearer in the previous phases of the negotiation, the opposing points of view are now intensified. You must be aware of the following aspects:

– Make a distinction between the requirements which are compatible with each other and the requirements which are in conflict with each other. State again that there are points of agreement. State also what points you do not appear to agree on. Something will have to be done about the latter.

– Make clear what requirements are important to you. The benefit of good preparation is apparent here too. A little bit becomes known here of what is your 'small change' and what is not. In this way you reveal something about your dividing line between what is and what is not acceptable. Be very careful with this and only drop those requirements or conditions which you feel you can give in on, and only drop them one by one. Watch very closely each time what the reaction is.

– Once again, do not reveal with what minimum outcome you would still be satisfied, i.e. do not expose your bottom limits of acceptance.

– Emphasize that you must get on with each other. You are dependent on each other and must thus try to reach a solution together.

That is, promote an integrative and co-operative rather than distributive and adversarial climate in the negotiation.

f. Phase of crisis and rounding-off

Inevitably a 'bend or break' phase arrives in every negotiation. Ideally, this phase comes when everything on which you are agreed has been stated. Now it is necessary to work on what remains of the difference of opinion. This is the phase of actual negotiation. The previous phases can best be regarded as clearing away irrelevant ballast. That is what you were agreed on. In this phase of actual negotiation, a rounding-off will be worked towards via a 'crisis'. It may be that this rounding-off means the participants moving apart, although that is not aimed for. It is more pleasant if the negotiators reach an agreement at this stage. The skills needed in this phase are as follows:

Alternative thinking

In order to face up to conflicting requirements, alternative solutions must be thought up. In the previous stage the negotiators stated which requirements conflicted with each other. Before the negotiators start to climb down, possible solutions must first be searched for in which both (conflicting) requirements can be satisfied. In other words, are the requirements really in conflict or can a creative solution be imagined in which both parties will get what they want?

At a particular time the negotiators must start to bargain. They take turns in running through the previous positions of the original stakes or bids and the areas of agreement. It is important here that they take turns in making a move. Each person may consider what other concession he can make. Often this is dependent on whether or not the other person shows willingness to reciprocate.

You can avoid a stalemate situation here by having ready a particular concession you are prepared to make which you view as no great loss. This pressures the other person to respond perhaps by conceding on a much more significant issue. When no further areas of difference can be removed, the protagonists must then proceed to identify alternative solutions or compromises they may be able to accept.

Choosing solutions

If the thinking up of alternatives is done well, this results in one or more desirable or best possible solutions. There is nothing wrong if there is only one; this simply becomes the agreement reached. If there are more, a choice must be made among them. This too must be done carefully. This means that a fresh phase of negotiation starts, but now at micro-level; the best has to be sought from the possible solutions. The awkward thing about it is, of course, that what is the very best of the possible solutions for one person may perhaps be the least good of all the possible solutions for the other negotiator. As you can see, it then starts all over again. For the phases which you must then go through, we therefore obviously refer you back to what has been described above.

Co-operation

When you start to work towards a compromise in the negotiation, it is important that you emphasize the atmosphere of co-operation. Recall your agreement on a large number of matters and the fact that you are working together towards a solution with which you can both make progress. You can draw attention to the following points:

– Focus attention on the future. Point out that you will regularly need each other.
– Point out that you recognize the interests of the other person. Ask for example whether the other person will have trouble discussing a particular proposal with his colleagues, or show understanding if the other person points out that he does not expect a particular proposal to be accepted.
– React more personally. Do not leave all your feelings out during this phase of the negotiation. React in a relaxed way. Avoid being aggressive or antagonistic and treat the other person with sincerity and respect.

Recording results

We have already touched on this: when the negotiations have been completed and an agreement has been reached, this result must be recorded in a way which is acceptable to both parties. Make sure that the agreement is recorded in such a way that no more difference of opinion is possible in the future on the interpretation of this document. Both parties sign the document, and only then has the negotiation been completed.

Recording is of course a gesture of formal negotiation situations – for example, between staff and management. You must bear in mind that on a more informal level negotiations and bargaining are going on all the time. Recall the example of the doctor–nurse game and nurse–patient bargaining given earlier in this chapter. In such situations there are no written agreements. Indeed, often the protagonists will not concede that they are bargaining at all.

Negotiation is a difficult skill which you will nevertheless often need to have. Not all negotiations take such strict and formal forms as we have described in this chapter. All these stages nonetheless occur in each negotiation. Often, however, they are blocked or are passed through very quickly. You generally suffer as a result later on. Passing through a phase too quickly or passing over it generally leads to a less desirable result in a later phase than would have been possible.

Finally, one last point. Negotiation is to some extent about people trying to overcome each other under the pretext of co-operation; in addition, they know this about each other. To make the whole thing even less clear, you can add that they also have to continue working with each other, for example in a department or hospital ward. You can imagine that in this way there are a lot of hidden meanings in the skill of 'negotiation'. You can only learn to negotiate by doing it. You can give yourself the greatest chance of succeeding from the outset by making use of all the procedures we have mentioned.

Negotiating strategies

Negotiation is a delicate set of skills. It is rather like playing chess. There are sides, in which each takes turns to make a move. Sometimes a move is made in order to gain a direct advantage, sometimes the reason for it is to keep the other person from making a gain. A move may also be made in order to put the other person on the

wrong track. This could be called a *diversionary move*. These are statements which one of the negotiating partners makes to put the other person out of his stride. The intention is to influence the other person imperceptibly, so that he will be more ready to do what you want rather than what he himself wants. Skilled negotiators demonstrate a good understanding of some applications of psychology in this way.

Although the term would be appropriate, 'manipulation' is rarely mentioned in this context. We prefer to talk about 'negotiating strategies'. We shall mention some of these strategies below. We do not wish to suggest that you can apply them entirely to your own benefit. The reason why we are considering negotiating strategies here is that there is no doubt that you will encounter them in such a many-sided community as the hospital. In our view, the better you recognize them, the less likely you are to fall victim to them.

– *Delaying*. This strategy is particularly effective if the other person is in a hurry. Say that you cannot decide on this proposal alone, but that you have to speak to your colleagues about it. A drawback of this procedure is that the opposing party has an opportunity to think up an effective counter-strategy.
– *Creating division*. A divided opponent is always weaker. If you discover a trace of conflict within the camp of your negotiating partner, say that you can well understand it. Point out subtly that you have heard (and mention the name of the person in the opposing camp who is not in agreement with the negotiator) that someone thinks completely differently, thus showing that you are familiar with the position in their ranks too.
– *Thinking with your opponent*. You can try to make it clear to the opposite side that their proposals or points of view could have disastrous consequences, with a comment such as, 'Think for example about the effect on your colleagues if it turns out that no agreement could be reached because of your stubborn refusal to make any concession.'
– *Attacking individual arguments*. Points of

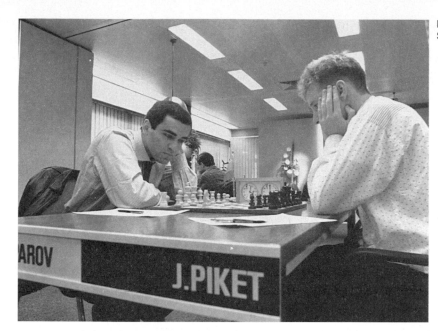

Figure 5.7.2
Strategies

view are generally backed up with a number of arguments. There are good arguments and not so good ones among them. Concentrate on the weaker arguments; make the other side explain them at length. Use strategies for overcoming or weakening arguments, for example:

• 'soft-soaping': nodding benevolently until you have encouraged the opposite side so much that he traps himself. It is then not very difficult to attack and bring all the arguments into doubt.

• right from the beginning giving sceptical looks, shaking your head often during your opponent's argument, raising your eyebrows and occasionally laughing sympathetically. Here too the time comes when the weak argument is no longer felt to be tenable and is abandoned.

However, it is important that you do all this in a genuine and courteous way. If you smirk, mock and deride colleagues, and resort to rudeness and discourtesy you will not win arguments. You will simply demean yourself and make enemies into the bargain.

Exercise 1. Negotiation between two people

Aim: to be able to recognize and practise negotiating processes between two people.

Number of persons: 3

Materials: the observation checklist below.

Time required: preparation, 10 minutes; negotiation, 15 minutes; subsequent discussion, 20 minutes.

Procedure: one of the three is an observer. The other two agree what is to be negotiated. This may be anything, provided it is of sufficient value to both.

Examples are:
- Duty during the Easter weekend, which one of them would like to swap;
- Shopping which one of them would like to do, but her duty lasts until after the shops have closed.
- Help in a busy period due to illness of a colleague.

The two negotiators think up arguments for their negotiating bids during the preparation. Remember the principles of good negotiating: do not expose your bids and fall-back positions to your opponent in advance.

The observer observes the negotiations and fills in an observation checklist for each 'negotiation'. When completed, the observations are discussed. The observer leads this discussion. He asks the negotiators to show their hands and say what their bid was, and the minimum with which they would have been satisfied. He also asks what would need to have been done to make the partner agree to this minimum.

Observation checklist for negotiation between two persons
(Circle 'yes' or 'no', as appropriate, for each item)

The following skills were correctly used in the negotiation.

1. The bid can be argued
   (that is, a viable argument is presented)........................ yes   no
2. A joint aim is formulated................................. yes   no
3. It is stated what is agreed on .... yes   no
4. Concessions are made .... yes   no
5. What outcome would have been ajudged
   satisfactory remains concealed...................................... yes   no
6. Arguments favourable to the other person
   are also stated .... yes   no
7. Agreement is established .... yes   no

Exercise 2. Negotiation in a group

Aim:	to be able to recognize the processes of negotiations in a group.
Number of persons:	8, 7 for role-play and 1 acting as observer.
Materials:	agenda: description below.
Time required:	negotiation, 45 minutes; break, 15 minutes; subsequent discussion, 45 minutes.
Procedure:	in this exercise one person acts as independent observer while the others act as members of a ward team. One takes the role of ward sister, three the roles of staff nurses, two the roles of enrolled nurses and one the role of nursing auxiliary.

It has been proposed that primary nursing will be introduced on the ward. This involves a named nurse accepting primary responsibility for a patient or patients on a 24 hour day, 7 day week basis. He/she is the person directly responsible for planning and managing care, assisted by 'associate' nurses who also continue with her prescribed care when she is off duty.

The ward sister fears her authority may be usurped under this new system. The staff nurses feel primary nursing should be introduced – it will give them more responsibility and autonomy. But they feel enrolled nurses would not be capable of taking on the primary nurse role. The enrolled nurses feel this may be another attempt to undermine their professional status. The auxiliary feels that once again she will be left to do all the basic care work.

Proceed, in a simulated ward team meeting, to discuss if and how primary nursing will be implemented. Take 45 minutes. The observer makes notes of how negotiations proceed. Afterwards the observer leads a 45 minute discussion. This should address how the negotiation skills identified at Section 5 above were utilized.

6. Summary

In this chapter negotiation was defined and the characteristics of distributive and integrative negotiation were explained.

The skills relating to negotiation were described. After the purpose of negotiation had been presented, the various pitfalls in negotiation were considered. Negotiation was identified as a process for establishing social norms and maintaining social order. The importance of negotiation in the practice of nursing was emphasized, particularly from the important points of view of the nurse–doctor and nurse–patient relationships.

The chapter then proceeded to consider negotiation skills and concluded with a consideration of particular negotiating strategies.

8

Dealing with group conflicts

1. Introduction

This chapter addresses situations in which interpersonal tensions, antagonism and disharmony arise in groups. It suggests that such conflicts can have functional and dysfunctional aspects and proceeds to examine common pitfalls when dealing with such conflicts. The chapter describes how you can manage group conflicts and lists the skills needed to identify and resolve them.

With these skills you do not need to wait until conflict has arisen. They may also be used to prevent conflict.

Learning outcomes

After studying this chapter the student should be able to:
– describe the function of group conflicts;
– describe four pitfalls in group conflicts;
– recognize and describe the skills in resolving conflicts in the group.

2. Function of group conflicts

It is tempting to view conflict within the group in terms of antagonism between individual group members. However, conflict is, within normal limits, a natural property of all human groups. People do not agree on everything and by working through differences the group members become more accepting of each other and start to function as a cohesive entity. In this sense conflict has a positive function in the group. However, it is often a sign of group discord and dissatisfaction. This is the chief message which we wish to put across in this chapter: make sure that you do not ignore conflicts in the group. You must take them seriously, because they are sometimes symptoms of how discord and problems of failures in co-operation arise in the group. That is, they can be dysfunctional as well as functional processes. They are processes the group must face up to and work through if it is to develop cohesion and achieve its aims.

Conflicts can be productive!

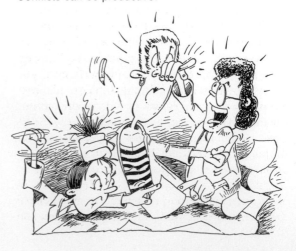

The major pitfalls applicable to co-operation in groups were described in Chapter 5, Section 3.

We were concerned there with the following features:
- the hidden agenda;
- failing to recognize group dynamics;
- fighting out at content level what exists at relational level.

In Chapter 5 we identified these three topics and discussed their function and how they can be dealt with.

You may find it helpful to review the relevant sections now.

3. Pitfalls in group conflicts

The following are some of the most significant pitfalls which can occur.

a. The conflict is not recognized

It is not necessary for the discussion leader to be asleep for a conflict to escape his notice.

Some conflicts take place so subtly and some people are so good at wrapping up their malice that a conflict is not noticed at all. You may ask whether it is then necessary to try to solve the conflict. It appears to have no effect on co-operation in the group.

We would warn against being too cautious about discussing conflicts in the group. The fact that you do not recognize a conflict firstly need not mean that others do not recognize it and secondly a conflict which is not recognized as such can nevertheless have an effect on the group process. If, for example, a critical atmosphere prevails in the group along the lines of, 'If you can't express yourself well here you are punished mercilessly', this may not be recognized as a dormant group conflict which keeps the participants on their guard and perhaps makes some so anxious that they are incapable of participating at all. The participants will obviously not feel completely free to express their opinion in this group. They will keep quiet. In such situations group co-operation may benefit from the issue being brought into the open and discussed.

b. The conflict is not understood

The conflict may also be recognized but not correctly interpreted. An example of this was given in Chapter 5, Section 3c: disputes may appear to be at content level while the real source of conflict is at relational level, i.e. it is all to do with relationships and how people get on with each other. In such cases this is often not diagnosed: a different conflict is found to exist apart from the one that needs to be solved. The diagnosis was: these people do not agree on the *content* problem. The solution which ensued from this was therefore: they must talk it out, i.e. solve the content problem. However, since the diagnosis was incorrect or at least incomplete (i.e. it took no account of the underlying *relational* conflict), the solution did not work either. The question in this diagnosis should have been: why are these two adult people disagreeing so much over a trifling subject?

Why are they making such an issue of it? Do not think you alone can find an answer to this; this must come from the participants themselves although an apt observation from the discussion leader may help the participants to recognize that the real issue here is a relational one.

c. The conflict is suppressed

In certain situations people try by smoothing over the conflict to disguise the underlying cause as well. There are many reasons to explain why people do that. You may have acquired in your upbringing and development a certain fear of entering into conflicts. Inequality of power between the participants in a conflict may also have a part to play. For example, think of a group of trainees who completely disagree with the approach of the head of department. They do not enter into conflict because they are afraid of adverse consequences in their practical assessments.

d. The conflict is solved wrongly; a scapegoat is selected

It also sometimes happens that one person or a subgroup is held responsible for the tensions in the group. This is known as *the scapegoat phenomenon*. Scapegoats are generally people who in one way or another are both conspicuous and weak in the group.

By selecting a scapegoat, it is denied that the problem is shared by the whole group. It is assumed that if the scapegoat is out of the way, the tensions and therefore the problems will be gone. This is obviously not normally the case.

4. Skills in resolving conflicts in the group

Dealing with group conflicts and giving feedback have a great deal to do with each other. The connection between them is that feedback (which is another word for exchanging comments on each other) is necessary for solving conflicts in co-operation. You can regard group conflict as the 'behaviour' of a group as a whole. The way of discussing this is therefore commenting on 'group behaviour', in other words by giving feedback. Hence we are largely concerned here with feedback skills. We shall consider the principal *feedback skills* below.

a. Not trivializing

Trivializing means 'presenting as a trifling matter'. Making a conflict appear smaller than it is in reality is generally completely wrong. In so doing you deny that someone is considerably bothered by it. What you are in fact saying, when you trivialize is, 'What nonsense, why are you getting upset over something so silly?' Between the lines you are saying: 'Aren't you childish.' As we argued earlier, this is not the attitude by which you put people at their ease. All you achieve by this is to make people defend themselves. And that is precisely what you do not need when you want to help resolve a conflict, because you explicitly need the trust of the participants. Take the conflict seriously and recognize, for example by continued questioning, that the participants may be bothered by it.

b. Conflicts can be productive

Help the participants to realize that conflicts can be beneficial. It is frequently assumed that conflicts must be removed. We tend to be afraid of conflicts; it seems like having a row, and that is something we are not used to. It can therefore be

an enlightening insight that a conflict may be a useful step towards better co-operation. If you lead the discussion during such a meeting, start by declaring that the conflict proves that people are involved in the matter in hand, which is good. Differences of opinion at least mean people have an opinion and that is a sign of commitment.

The next stage which must be made clear is that the conflict can become even more annoying if it causes one's own life to suffer. If the participants do not resolve it, the conflict can continue to lurk beneath the surface, and that has the consequence that the participants easily become entrenched in their disagreement. A characteristic feature of this kind of situation is that people no longer listen to each other; their only contacts consist of denigrating others. If a conflict has reached this stage, it is very difficult to overcome it without the active co-operation of both parties to the dispute.

It should also be stressed that conflict will have to be talked out among the participants. Sometimes the members are reluctant to accept that conflict exists and are unwilling to agree to talk about it. The resistance generally appears in the form of wanting to tone down the conflict slightly, with reactions such as, 'That was to be expected', 'You are making it bigger than it was' and so on. Do not allow yourself to be distracted from dealing with the conflict. If you keep to the rules, you do not make the conflict greater than it was, you just make it more open.

c. Make the conflict common

We now come to the stage of the real conflict handling conversation. The purpose of this is to help to discover the source and function of the conflict. Only if you uncover this can you start to solve the conflict. You can help the participants to clarify the source and function of the conflict by discussing with them precisely what is wrong, what must be done and why this does not succeed. Source and function are discussed one by one below.

– *What precisely is wrong?*
    This appears to be a question with an obvious answer. But this is not entirely true. Just think

back to the pages we have given over to explaining why the phase of 'problem clarification' was necessary. If you give each participant the opportunity to say when he first noticed that something was not quite right and how he noticed this, you will get lots of different stories. For many people it is quite a discovery when they hear that there are so many differences. But all too often we think that it must be very clear to everyone what is going on.

With these different versions of what is wrong, you make it clear that there are differences of interpretation in the stories. We must assume that the facts in the stories are easy enough to check. We would in any case advise you against arguing over that for long. You can either ascertain the facts or state that two opinions exist on what precisely happened. State that the interpretations vary. Try, and this is the most important point, not to say that one of the interpretations appears more likely than the other. An interpretation is the private explanation which someone gives to an event. You can only ascertain whether this interpretation is correct by asking the person whose behaviour is being interpreted. So, if John says of Marie that she finished off her shift carelessly yesterday and left him to sort out the mess, then (when it has become clear what 'carelessly' means) Marie must be asked whether this really was the case. Only Marie can confirm or deny this assuming of course that she is prepared to give an honest account.

– *What must be done about it?*
Ask the participants what they consider to be a favourable outcome of the conflict. What do they want to achieve? Here you must fervently hope that John does not say that the most desirable thing would be for Marie to be dismissed immediately. That is not particularly constructive. Try to convince the participants of the fact that they have to try to get on with each other and just hope that they have the decency to keep secret wishes of this kind to themselves. If something like that is nevertheless mentioned, the best thing to do is to treat it as real malice: that's how far the conflict has gone! You must certainly

treat this seriously and not trivialize it. A second condition at this stage of the handling of the conflict is to give the most concrete possible description of what is desirable. Agreements can be improved if everyone knows precisely what these agreements are. Try to aim towards desirable behaviour being described.

– *Why does it not succeed?*
In order to completely survey the conflict, it is right to discuss also why the solution which is seen as desirable has not yet got off the ground. What has stopped them from already taking steps themselves to solve this conflict? Were the parties already somewhat entrenched or is there perhaps something wrong with the solution? Is this capable of being solved quickly or is it necessary to look for a more acceptable solution?

d. Negotiation

Now that the source and function of the conflict have become clear, thanks to the above skills, the time has come to do something about it. Even now it is not out of the question that the sides involved have gained enough insight into their conflict in the previous phase that this now appears much less severe. Perhaps they can now resolve it themselves. However, we would advise against leaving them to it. There could be a form of resistance to the changes made or against too much interference from outside, but there could also be an attempt to put off the solution (often the changing of behaviour). These need not all be attempts which are made consciously; it can sometimes also be an unconscious manoeuvre.

If the parties decide to talk out the conflict, this talk has precisely the same structure as negotiation, to which we have devoted the whole of Chapter 7. Read this chapter once more since these are precisely the steps which are necessary in this stage of conflict resolution. However, you must be aware of one thing: the chapter on negotiation discusses the situation from the point of view of the participant in the negotiation. In this chapter you are addressed as the person who leads a conflict handling discussion.

e. Monitoring the rules

When running through each of the stages referred to above, the discussion leader must make sure that the sides listen carefully to each other. There are some guidelines for this. These guidelines apply during the whole conflict handling discussion. In a conflict situation listening is generally obstructed by emotions. People do not want to listen, they want to convince. In a conflict the tendency is to want to argue. Try not to oppose this: it is a hopeless task. However, the discussion leader in a conflict handling discussion of this kind can make sure in particular that the sides keep to the rules of 'etiquette'. The discussion leader explicitly has an adjudicator's role. The rules which he must monitor are as follows:

– Listen to the discussion leader.
    A conflict handling discussion only succeeds if the sides are prepared to recognize the discussion leader as such. Without recog-

Figure 5.8.1
Monitoring the rules

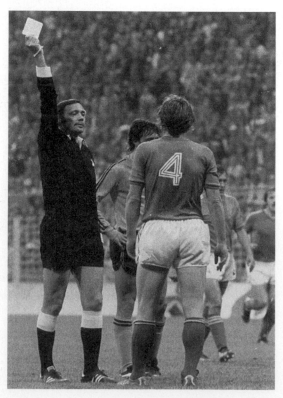

nition you have already fallen into a trap. This is an unenviable position for any discussion leader; all his work is to no avail if his role is not recognized.

– Make a distinction between facts and interpretations. Make sure that you also make this distinction clear to both parties; this is the whole basis of conflict handling. It is very likely that this distinction is not known, since the whole conflict would probably otherwise not have gone so far. Draw attention to the fact when a statement from one of the parties contains an interpretation.

– If there are interpretations, these must be checked with the person whose behaviour was interpreted.
    The example we gave above concerning Marie and John makes this clear. Behaviour is often interpreted very differently from the way it was intended. The person explains the interpretation he has placed on the behaviour of the other person. This other person in turn interprets this reaction. Perhaps she also makes it an incorrect interpretation. From this point of view there are so many possible ways of misunderstanding one another that you wonder how a message ever gets across properly!
    The discussion leader must be very alert. He must intervene immediately if there is a direct reaction to an interpretation. This is very hard work. You have to be on top and nothing must escape you. You must also be daring, because as soon as you let something go because you do not dare to intervene, the incident escalates. It is incredible how quickly people who are already in a conflict can drive each other into a frenzy. If you allow this to happen once as the discussion leader, you actually lose your credibility as a discussion leader. You may perhaps be able to save yourself by saying, 'That's precisely why you need an adjudicator', but this is your last chance.

Finally a few remarks. Managing conflict in the way described above can go very well. You can help the parties who are in conflict to realize with relatively little difficulty that they themselves also view the behaviour of others from their own particular point of view. The likelihood of a change in the way of looking at the other person is better if you succeed in working in this way.

The difficulty with this kind of discussion is that it demands a firm position from you. It is perhaps a complete change-over from the way you pay attention to the wishes patients have. In handling conflict you have to react far more directively than you do towards most patients. It requires some flexibility to be able to make this change-over. However, it is possible that group conflicts will also involve patients. This is commonly found in group therapy situations or in situations where mental health problems arise from family conflicts.

Study activity
  1. Group conflict involving the patient. Sometimes group conflict revolves around the patient. You may particularly meet this in mental health settings where a patient's emotional problems seem to be caused by conflict within the family.
    a. Consider how conflict has arisen within your own family in the past. Did family members collude against or 'scapegoat' an individual family member? Was the situation discussed openly and resolved positively, or was it never resolved satisfactorily?
    b. Search the literature for the Family Centred Therapy approach to resolving family conflict. Write a brief (500 word) description of this approach.

5. Summary

In this chapter the functions of and pitfalls in group conflicts were briefly discussed. The idea of group conflicts or disharmony was viewed from the perspective of group dynamic processes. It was shown how conflicts can have a functional influence, helping members towards group cohesion; or dysfunctional influences, leading to disruption and lack of co-operation. Pitfalls in managing group conflicts were identified.

The chapter concluded by addressing some of the skills necessary to help solve these group conflicts.

Final test Module 5

Instructions
- This section comprises 90 yes/no questions.
- Each proposition, claim, statement, etc. may be *true* or *false,* either *yes* or *no.* There is no middle way: you must make a choice.
- Your assessment of whether one of the 90 items is true or false should be based on your reading of the book.
- The questions are arranged in order relating to subjects or chapters.
- Check that all questions have been answered.
- Finally, mark the test yourself. You will find the answers at the end of the book.

1. Reciprocity in communication means that people always react to each other.
2. Communication takes place between transmitter and receiver.
3. The word message also means verbal information
4. One of the underlying principles of communication theory is: you cannot communicate by verbal means alone.
5. Non-verbal messages are also conveyed in a letter.
6. Non-verbal messages are also conveyed in a telephone conversation.
7. In communication theory 'content level' refers to what is said.
8. In communication theory 'relational level' refers to what is not said.
9. People only react to each other on the content level.
10. Communication on communication is called 'paralinguistics'.
11. There is said to be horizontal communica-

tion when both partners in a conversation are sitting.
12. Vertical communication is characterized by one-way traffic.
13. The door-knob phenomenon refers to the fact that people mention the most important thing first.
14. In hospital the hopes and expectations of the patient are the same.
15. 'Sickness gain' refers to the fact that a patient can also become financially better off from his sickness.
16. 'Not understanding dialect' is an example of a communication problem in the phase between the expression of words and the hearing of these words.
17. By making a good punctuation, you find out who has started a conflict.
18. 'Be spontaneous' is an example of a paradoxical task.
19. Inadequate communication with a patient has an adverse effect on the co-operation of this patient.
20. The halo effect is the phenomenon that conclusions are drawn about the whole person on the basis of one or two characteristics.

Attentive behaviour involves:
21. looking at the other person.
22. sitting quietly.
23. relaxed body posture.
24. following verbally.

When two people carry on a conversation with each other, they generally do not talk at the same time, but speak in turns.
25. This speaking in turns is brought about more

by breaks in speech than by eye contact between the partners in the conversation.

26. Widening of the pupils indicates that the other person is calm.
27. You get to hear the most information in a conversation if you sit forward with your elbows on your knees.
28. By interpreting the behaviour of another person, you attribute feelings and attitudes to this other person which are more applicable to yourself than to this other person.
29. Keeping perception and interpretation apart becomes easier if the speaker transmits a very emotional message.
30. A question is open if you can answer it with yes or no.
31. 'Do you find that annoying?' is an example of a closed question.
32. Continued questioning within the reference framework of the other person means asking for information which this other person does not mention himself.
33. A continued question is asked to obtain more detailed information on a subject which the speaker has already touched on.
34. Paraphrases are most effective if they are expressed in a questioning tone.
35. A summary only has a stimulating effect on the flow of information of the other person if the content is correct.
36. In a good reflection of feeling both the content and intensity of the emotion are correctly reproduced.
37. In a free-narrative interview the questioner must not interpret.
38. The way of conducting a conversation is partly dependent on the purpose of the conversation.
39. Closed questions lead to more relevant information than open questions.
40. If a patient repeats himself, this generally means that he is uncertain whether the other person has taken in this information.
41. The effectiveness of communication is promoted if the meaning of a sent message is explained and tested back and forth.
42. In a reflection of feeling the speaker shows his own feelings about the other person's problem.

43. It is best to give criticism impersonally.
44. Assertive behaviour is creating a scene.
45. In a history-taking conversation which runs well, various phases can be discovered.
46. By regularly summarizing, you give your partner in conversation an insight into the structure of the conversation.
47. Closed questions are most effective in the first phase of the history-taking conversation.
48. In a problem conversation an attempt is made to find a solution together.
49. Concretization must be avoided as far as possible during a problem conversation.
50. A piece of advice is only followed if it is of high quality.
51. The likelihood of a piece of advice being followed is greatest if alternatives are offered.
52. In a correct bad-news conversation the bad news is given early in the conversation.
53. In a correct bad-news conversation the future is talked about immediately after the bad news has been received.
54. If a patient is unwilling to accept bad news, it is best for the bringer of the bad news to argue why the news is bad.
55. If the recipient of bad news reacts angrily to the bringer, the bringer must mention his own emotions.
56. The aim of the consultative conversation is for the person consulted to solve the problem of the person consulting.
57. All of the advice given by the doctors is correctly followed.

Concretization is the skill required if you receive information which is:
58. vague;
59. impersonal;
60. specific.

A good concretization of a statement from a patient: 'It all deteriorates when you get older' is:
61. 'Do you feel you are getting older?'
62. 'Do you notice that you are deteriorating?'
63. 'What exactly deteriorates with age?'
64. 'Who says that?'

65. A good explanation ends with the most important information.
66. The sole aim of co-operation in groups is to achieve the best decision.
67. A hidden agenda is unknown to all the participants at a meeting.
68. An incipient group can co-operate best.
69. A group decision is always best if its quality is optimum.
70. If you explain something to group members, it is best to use short sentences.
71. In brainstorming one important requirement is that you do not discuss the brainstorming responses initially.
72. If two participants in a meeting disagree, the likelihood of a solution is greater if the opinions are dissociated from the persons.
73. In an evaluation of a meeting the description of behaviour and the assessment of it must be separate.
74. In an evaluation of a meeting it is best to mention the negative aspect first and then the positive.
75. The agenda for a meeting must include for each item an explanation of the purpose of placing this the item on the agenda.
76. A procedural proposal belongs to the introduction of an item on the agenda.
77. In decision-making by consensus each participant in the meeting has the right of veto.
78. An important group-oriented skill is encouragement.
79. In integrative negotiation the strategy of both participants is to thwart the other.
80. The harder you act in a negotiation, the greater the gain you obtain.
81. It is best when preparing for a negotiation to formulate more than one desired solution.
82. When preparing for a negotiation you must know precisely what is and what is not acceptable for you.
83. In a negotiation you can seldom make a greater gain than is represented in your opening bid.
84. In order to solve stagnation in a negotiation, reference must be made to a common interest.
85. Group conflicts are sometimes productive.
86. The guilty person in group conflicts is the scapegoat.
87. It is best to soothe group conflicts quickly.
88. A good way of taking a conflict seriously is continued questioning.
89. When handling group conflicts it is important to make a distinction between facts and interpretations.
90. Empathy refers to one person's capacity to influence another person's decision making.

References

Aguilera, D. and Messick, J. (1978). *Crisis Intervention: Theory and Methodology* (3rd Ed.). St. Louis, C.V. Mosby Company.

Altman, I. and Tayler, D.A. (1973). *Social Penetration: The Development of Interpersonal Relationships*. New York, Holt.

Argyle, M. (1972). *The Psychology of Interpersonal Behaviour*. London, Penguin.

Authier, J., Gustavson, K., Guerney, B. and Kasdorf, J.A. (1975). The psychological practitioner as a teacher: a theoretical-historical and practical review. *The Counseling Psychologist*, 5, 31-49.

Authier, J. (1989). Showing warmth and empathy. In O'Hargie (Ed.), *A Handbook of Communication Skills*. London, Routledge.

Bateson, G. and Jackson, D.D. (1964). Some variations of pathogenic organisation. In McRioch, D. (Ed.), *Disorders of Communication*. Baltimore, Association for Research in Nervous and Mental Disease.

Bernal, G. and Baker, J. (1979). Towards a metacommunication framework of couple interactions. *Family Processes*, 18, 293-302.

Blumberg, H.H., Hare, A.P., Kent, V. et al. (Eds.) (1983). *Small Groups and Social Interation* (Volumes One and Two). Chichester, John Wiley and Sons.

Egan, G. (1975). *The Skilled Helper*. Monteroy, Brooks Cole.

Ellis, R. and Whittington, D. (1981). *A Guide to Social Skill Training*. Beckenham, Croom Helm.

Hargie, O. (1986). *A Handbook of Communication Skills*. London, Routledge.

Irwin, W.G. and Bamber, J.H. (1984). An evaluation of medical student behaviours in communication. *Medical Education*, 18, 90-95.

Janis, I. (1972). *Victims of Groupthink*. Boston, Houghton Mifflin.

Leininger, M. (1978). *Transcultural Nursing Concepts, Theories and Practices*. New York, Wiley.

Leininger, M. (1984). Transcultural nursing: an essential knowledge and practice field for today. *Canadian Nurse*, 80 (11), 41-45.

McClintock, E. (1983). Interaction. In Kelley, H.H., Bercheid, E., Cristensen, A. et al. (Eds.), *Close Relationships*. New York, W.H. Freeman and Co.

Morton, T.L., Alexander, J.F. and Altman, I. (1976). Communication and relationship definition. In Millar, G.R. (Ed.), *Explorations in Interpersonal Communication*. London, Sage Publications.

Parsons, T. (1970). On becoming a patient. In Parsons, T., *The Social System*. New York, Macmillan.

Pfeiffer, J.W. and Jones, J.E. (1977). *A Handbook of Structured Experiences for Human Relations Training*. San Diego, University Associates.

Rogers, C.R. (1951). *Client-centred Therapy*. Boston, Houghton Mifflin.

Rogers, C.R. (1967), *On Becoming a Person*. London, Constable.

Rogers, C.R. (1975). Empathic: an unappreciated way of being. *Counselling Psychologist*, 5, 2-10.

Rogers, C.R. (1983), *Freedom to Learn for the 80's*. London, Charles E. Merrill.

Roth, J. (1971). The treatment of tuberculosis as a bargaining process. In Rose, A.M. (Ed.), *Human Behaviour and Social Processes*. London, Routledge and Kegan Paul.

Stein, L. (1978). The doctor-nurse game. In Dingwall, R. and McIntosh, J. (Eds), *Readings in the Sociology of Nursing*. Edinburgh, Churchill Livingstone.

Trower, P., Bryant, B., Argyle, M. and Marzillien, J. (1978). *Social Skills and Mental Health*. London, Methuen & Co Ltd.

Key to final test Module 1

1 No	9 Yes	17 Yes	25 Yes	33 Yes	41 No
2 Yes	10 Yes	18 No	26 Yes	34 No	42 Yes
3 No	11 No	19 No	27 Yes	35 Yes	43 Yes
4 Yes	12 No	20 Yes	28 Yes	36 Yes	44 No
5 Yes	13 Yes	21 Yes	29 Yes	37 Yes	
6 Yes	14 No	22 Yes	30 Yes	38 No	
7 No	15 Yes	23 Yes	31 Yes	39 No	
8 Yes	16 No	24 No	32 No	40 Yes	

Key to final test Module 2

1 No	15 Yes	29 Yes	43 No	57 No	71 Yes
2 No	16 Yes	30 No	44 No	58 Yes	72 Yes
3 Yes	17 No	31 No	45 Yes	59 Yes	73 No
4 No	18 Yes	32 No	46 No	60 No	74 No
5 No	19 Yes	33 No	47 Yes	61 No	75 Yes
6 Yes	20 Yes	34 Yes	48 No	62 No	76 No
7 No	21 No	35 Yes	49 Yes	63 Yes	77 Yes
8 Yes	22 Yes	36 No	50 No	64 No	
9 No	23 Yes	37 No	51 Yes	65 Yes	
10 Yes	24 Yes	38 Yes	52 Yes	66 Yes	
11 Yes	25 No	39 Yes	53 No	67 Yes	
12 No	26 Yes	40 No	54 No	68 No	
13 Yes	27 Yes	41 No	55 Yes	69 No	
14 No	28 No	42 Yes	56 No	70 Yes	

Key to final test Module 3

1 No	13 Yes	25 No	37 No	49 Yes	61 Yes
2 Yes	14 Yes	26 No	38 No	50 Yes	62 Yes
3 No	15 No	27 No	39 Yes	51 No	63 No
4 Yes	16 Yes	28 Yes	40 Yes	52 No	64 Yes
5 Yes	17 No	29 No	41 Yes	53 Yes	65 Yes
6 Yes	18 No	30 No	42 No	54 Yes	66 Yes
7 Yes	19 No	31 No	43 No	55 No	67 No
8 No	20 No	32 Yes	44 Yes	56 Yes	68 No
9 No	21 Yes	33 Yes	45 No	57 Yes	69 Yes
10 No	22 Yes	34 No	46 No	58 No	70 Yes
11 No	23 No	35 No	47 No	59 Yes	
12 No	24 Yes	36 Yes	48 No	60 Yes	

Key to final test Module 4

1 No	18 No	35 No	52 No	69 Yes	86 No
2 No	19 No	36 No	53 Yes	70 No	87 Yes
3 Yes	20 Yes	37 Yes	54 No	71 Yes	88 Yes
4 Yes	21 Yes	38 No	55 Yes	72 Yes	89 No
5 Yes	22 No	39 Yes	56 No	73 No	90 Yes
6 Yes	23 No	40 Yes	57 Yes	74 Yes	91 Yes
7 No	24 Yes	41 Yes	58 Yes	75 No	92 Yes
8 Yes	25 Yes	42 Yes	59 Yes	76 No	93 No
9 Yes	26 Yes	43 No	60 Yes	77 No	94 Yes
10 No	27 Yes	44 Yes	61 Yes	78 No	95 Yes
11 Yes	28 Yes	45 Yes	62 Yes	79 Yes	96 No
12 Yes	29 No	46 Yes	63 Yes	80 No	97 Yes
13 No	30 Yes	47 Yes	64 No	81 Yes	98 No
14 Yes	31 No	48 No	65 Yes	82 Yes	99 Yes
15 No	32 Yes	49 No	66 Yes	83 Yes	100 Yes
16 Yes	33 Yes	50 Yes	67 No	84 Yes	
17 Yes	34 No	51 Yes	68 Yes	85 No	

Key to final test Module 5

1 Yes	16 Yes	31 Yes	46 Yes	61 No	76 Yes
2 Yes	17 No	32 No	47 No	62 No	77 Yes
3 No	18 Yes	33 Yes	48 Yes	63 Yes	78 Yes
4 Yes	19 Yes	34 Yes	49 No	64 No	79 No
5 No	20 Yes	35 No	50 No	65 No	80 No
6 Yes	21 Yes	36 Yes	51 Yes	66 No	81 Yes
7 Yes	22 No	37 No	52 Yes	67 No	82 Yes
8 No	23 Yes	38 Yes	53 No	68 No	83 Yes
9 No	24 Yes	39 No	54 No	69 No	84 Yes
10 No	25 No	40 Yes	55 No	70 Yes	85 Yes
11 No	26 No	41 Yes	56 No	71 Yes	86 No
12 Yes	27 No	42 No	57 No	72 Yes	87 No
13 No	28 Yes	43 No	58 Yes	73 Yes	88 Yes
14 No	29 No	44 No	59 Yes	74 No	89 Yes
15 No	30 No	45 Yes	60 No	75 Yes	90 No

Index

Page numbers in bold type indicate definitions and core references.